THIRD EDITION

ESSENTIALS OF ATHLETIC TRAINING

DANIEL D. ARNHEIM, D.P.E., A.T., C.

Professor Emeritus, Physical Eduction
California State University
Long Beach, California

THIRD EDITION

With 416 illustrations and 268 photographs

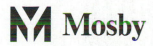

St. Louis Baltimore Berlin Boston Carlsbad Chicago London Madrid
Naples New York Philadelphia Sydney Tokyo Toronto

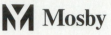

Mosby

Dedicated to Publishing Excellence

Publisher: James M. Smith
Acquisitions Editor: Vicki Malinee
Developmental Editor: Christy Wells
Project Manager: Mark Spann
Production Editors: Jerry Schwartz and Jennifer Doll
Designer: David Zielinski
Manufacturing Supervisor: Theresa Fuchs

This text was based on the most up-to-date research and suggestions made by individuals knowledgeable in the field of athletic training. The author and publisher disclaim any responsibility for any adverse effects or consequences from the misapplication or injudicious use of information contained within this text. It is also accepted as judicious that the coach and/or athletic trainer performing his or her duties is, at all times, working under the guidance of a licensed physician.

Printed in the United States of America
Composition by Clarinda Company
Printing/binding by William C. Brown Publishers

Mosby–Year Book, Inc.
11830 Westline Industrial Drive
St. Louis, Missouri 63146

Library of Congress Cataloging-in-Publication Data

Arnheim, Daniel D.
    Essentials of athletic training / Daniel D. Arnheim.—3rd ed.
        p.   cm.
    Includes bibliographical references and index.
    ISBN 0-8151-0301-8.—ISBN 0-8151-0300-X (pbk.)
    1. Sports injuries.   2. Sports injuries—Prevention.   I. Title.
RD97.A76   1994   94-35662
617.1'027—dc20   CIP

95 96 97 98 99 / 9 8 7 6 5 4 3 2

Preface

The third edition of *Essentials of Athletic Training* provides the reader with the most current information possible on the subject of prevention and basic care of sports injuries. *Essentials* is designed as a primary text for the student going into the field of coaching and/or physical eduction. Its major thrust is toward injury prevention and the immediate care of the most common sports injuries. Basic foundations are also provided for the student interested in more substantive areas of rehabilitation.

Organization and Coverage

Essentials of Athletic Training was created from the foundations established by *Principles of Athletic Training*. Whereas *Principles of Athletic Training* serves as a major text for athletic trainers and those individuals interested in sports medicine, *Essentials of Athletic Training* is written for the coach and physical educator.

The general approach of the text is that adverse physical problems arising from sports participation should be prevented whenever possible. When adverse problems do arise, quick and proper care can reduce their seriousness.

Essentials of Athletic Training is divided into three parts: Foundations; Sports Injury Causation, Response, and Management; and Sports Conditions. Overall, this text is designed to take the beginning student from general to more specific concepts. All chapters promote an understanding of the prevention and care of athletic injuries.

In the third edition, the order of chapters has been reorganized and two new chapters have been added. Part One, Foundations, gives the reader an overall look at athletic training as it relates to sports medicine and the major aspects of injury prevention. Chapter 1 introduces the student to the origins and basic principles of athletic training and the status of athletic training and sports medicine today. Chapter 2 focuses on physical conditioning. Psychological considerations now makes up retitled Chapter 3, Psychological Stress and Sports Injuries. Chapter 4 covers basic principles of sound nutrition, nutrition problems, and concerns unique to the athlete.

Part Two, Sports Injury Causation, Response, and Management, includes six chapters. These chapters provide an understanding of how the body is susceptible to traumatic musculoskeletal injuries and how these injuries are classified, recognized, and evaluated. Chapter 5 presents basic injury prevention with sport-specific recommendations for protective devices. Chapter 6 reviews anatomy so that the reader will have the information necessary to recognize injury and injury potential. Chapter 7 supplies an organized guide to emergency procedures, and Chapter 8 presents additional information specific to healing and follow-up care. Chapter 9 is allocated to wound dressing and bandaging. All of the taping information has been gathered into Chapter 10, making taping instruction easier and more comprehensive.

Part Three, Sports Conditions, includes ten chapters covering major sports injuries that occur to the different body regions. Each of these chapters presents related anatomy, methods of prevention, and immediate and follow-up care.

New Features

As mentioned previously, there are two new chapters in this edition:
- A new chapter on the psychology of sports injuries (Chapter 3) discusses overtraining, staleness, and the conditions under which sports participation becomes a psychological stressor. The roles of the coach and athletic trainer are also discussed.
- Discussion of the spine has been expanded and separated into its own chapter (Chapter 16).

In addition to updates throughout, other new features in the third edition include the following:
- A discussion of AMA's recognition of Athletic Training as an Allied Health Profession.
- Common names of muslces (with Latin names in parenthesis), so students no longer have to rely solely on Latin names.
- Thoroughly revised illustrations that are clear, easy to use, and better represent cultural diversity.
- Updated photographs that show only the latest in sports equipment.
- Revised exercises that include only currently accepted exercises that are safe and beneficial.
- An updated First Aid section that details only the currently recommended procedures.

Pedagogical Features

A number of teaching devices are included in this text:
1. *Chapter objectives.* Objectives are presented at the beginning of each chapter to reinforce learning goals.
2. *Boxed material within chapters.* Important information is emphasized by placing it in a box.
3. *Marginal information.* For greater emphasis, key concepts, selected definitions, helpful training tips, salient points, and some illustrations have been placed in margins throughout the text.
4. *Illustrations, numerous photographs and line drawings.* These crucial tools are presented to facilitate the student's comprehension of athletic training.
5. *Color throughout the text.* A second color appears throughout the text to enhance the overall appearance and accentuate illustrations.
6. *Review questions and class activities.* A list of questions and suggested class activities follows each chapter for review and application of the concepts learned.

7. *References.* All chapters have a bibliography of pertinent references that includes the most complete and up-to-date resources available.
8. *Annotated bibliography.* To further aid in learning, relevant and timely articles, books, and topics from the current literature have been annotated to provide additional resources.
9. *Glossary.* A comprehensive list of key terms and their definitions are presented at the end of the text.
10. *Appendix.* The appendix provides the students with helpful vitamin tables and conversion tables for units of measure.

Ancillaries for the Instructor

Instructor's Manual: An Instructor's Manual designed specifically for the *Essentials* text has been added to the ancillary package. Practical features include the following:

- Brief chapter overviews
- Learning objectives
- Key terminology
- Discussion questions
- Class activities
- Appendixes (answer keys, additional resources, and transparency masters)
- Perforated format, ready for immediate use

Computerized Test Bank: In addition, a computerized Test Bank, with over 900 questions is available to qualified adopters. This software enables the the instructor to select, edit, add, or delete questions and to develop test and answer keys. Each chapter contains multiple-choice, true-false, and short essay questions, keyed according to level of difficulty.

ACKNOWLEDGEMENTS

Special thanks are extended to Christy Wells, Developmental Editor. She provided invaluable assistance in the preparation of the third edition of *Essentials of Athletic Training*. Also deserving of special acknowledgement is Renee Reavis Shingles of Central Michigan University, who generously donated her time in preparing many new photographs for the third edition. I wish to extend my deepest thanks to Denise Fandel of the University of Nebraska at Omaha, who is preparing the Instructor's Manual. Acknowledgement is also extended to the following reviewers of the second edition whose suggestions have been carefully incorporated into the third edition.

Denise Fandel, University of Nebraska
Julie D. Felix, Virginia Tech
Jennie Gilbert, California State University
Michael Hanley, East Carolina University
Anne Hutchins, University of Mary

Daniel D. Arnheim

Contents in Brief

Contents

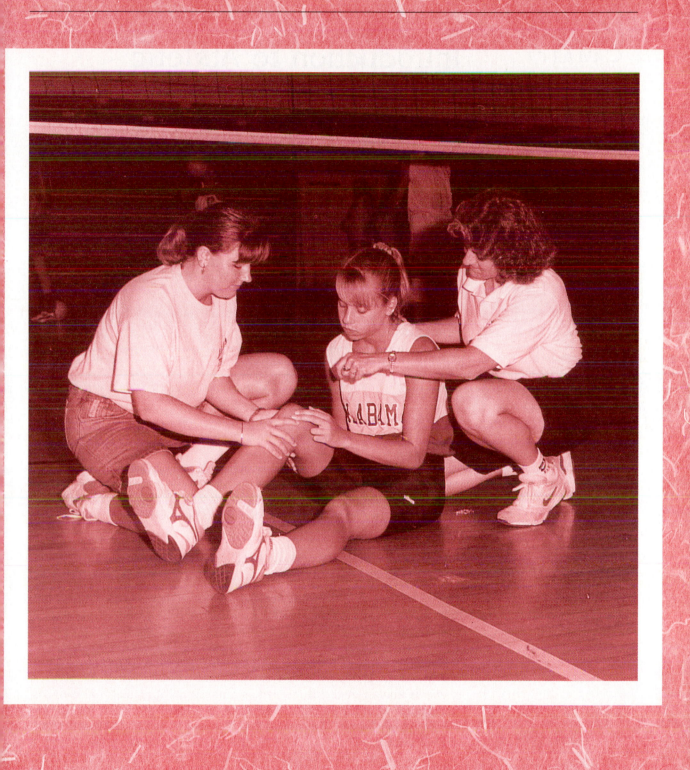

Introduction to Athletic Training

When you finish this chapter, you will be able to:

- Describe the historical foundations of athletic training
- Describe the role of a coach, athletic trainer, and team physician and their functions within an athletic training program
- Describe the major legal concerns of the coach and the athletic trainer in terms of sports injuries and how negligence can be avoided
- Identify major administrative tasks, including preparticipation examinations, facility management, insurance requirements, and budget concerns
- Define collision, contact, and noncontact sports and the types of injuries they commonly induce
- Define epidemiological data gathering of sports injuries

Chapter 1 is concerned with introducing the field of sports medicine/athletic training primarily to the coach and physical educator.

Sports medicine, of which athletic training is a major part, can be traced back in history to the earliest period of human existence. These early humans spent their daily lives in the pursuit of basic survival. A healthy, able body was absolutely necessary to forage for food effectively.

HISTORY OF ATHLETIC TRAINING

Sports medicine and athletic training in early civilizations are best reflected in the civilizations of ancient Greece and the early Roman empire. With the rise of the Greek civilization and its emphasis on achieving physical perfection through athletics came the professional specialties of coaching and the development of athletic training specialists. Professional coaches and athletic trainers also played an important role in the life of the gladiators of the early Roman period. Galen, the greatest name in Roman medicine, served as a physician at gladiatorial contests, in addition to other pursuits. Herodicus, a Roman physician for the ancient Olympic Games, was considered by many to be the first sports medicine physician.

After the fall of the Roman empire there was a complete lack of interest in sports competition. It was not until the beginning of the Renaissance that sports activities slowly regained popularity. Athletic training as we know it came into existence during the late nineteenth century with the firm establishment of intercollegiate athletics in the United States.

Modern Sports Medicine and Athletic Training

Modern athletic training, although having roots in ancient Greece and the Roman empire, is for the most part unique to North America. The first athletic trainers of the era were hangers-on who rubbed down the athlete. Since they possessed no technical knowledge, their athletic training techniques were mainly composed of massage and home remedies.

The growth of athletic training in the United States generally has followed the growth of American football.

The Field of Sports Medicine

Sports medicine has become a term that has many connotations depending on which group is using it. It is a generic term that encompasses many different areas of sports related to both performance and injury. Among the areas of specialization within sports medicine are athletic training, biomechanics, exercise physiology, the practice of medicine relative to the athlete, physical therapy, sports nutrition, and sports psychology. The American College of Sports Medicine (ACSM) has defined sports medicine as multidisciplinary, including the physiological, biomechanical, psychological, and pathological phenomena associated with exercise and sports. The clinical application of the work of these disciplines is performed to improve and maintain an individual's functional capacities for physical labor, exercise, and sports. It also includes the prevention and treatment of diseases and injuries related to exercise and sports (Figure 1-1.

> American College of Sports Medicine (ACSM) has defined sports medicine as multidisciplinary, including the physiological, biomechanical, psychological, and pathological phenomena associated with exercise and sports.

The Field of Athletic Training

Athletic training is a subspecialization of sports medicine providing a major link between a sports program and the medical community for the implementation of injury prevention, emergency care, and rehabilitation procedures.[11] It had evolved as a major paramedical profession when the National Athletic Trainers' Association (NATA) was formed in 1950.[13] Currently the athletic trainer is recognized by the American Medical Association.

> The American Medical Association has recognized the athletic trainer.

THE ATHLETE'S HEALTH AND SAFETY

Athletes, while participating in an organized sport, have every right to expect that their health and safety are of the highest priority at all times. A major rule to be considered by sports professionals is that the prevention of a health problem is much preferred over caring for the problem once it has occurred.

The three persons having the closest relationship to the athlete are the coach, the athletic trainer, and the team physician. Ideally, they should work together as an *injury prevention team*.

The Coach

The coach is directly responsible for preventing injuries by seeing to it that the athlete has undergone a preventive injury conditioning program. He or she must ensure that sports equipment, especially protective equipment, is of the highest quality and is properly fitted. The coach must also make sure that protective equipment is properly maintained. A coach must be keenly aware of what produces injuries in his or her particular sport and what measures must be taken to avoid them. A coach should

Figure 1-1

One aspect of the field of sports medicine is the care and prevention of injuries.

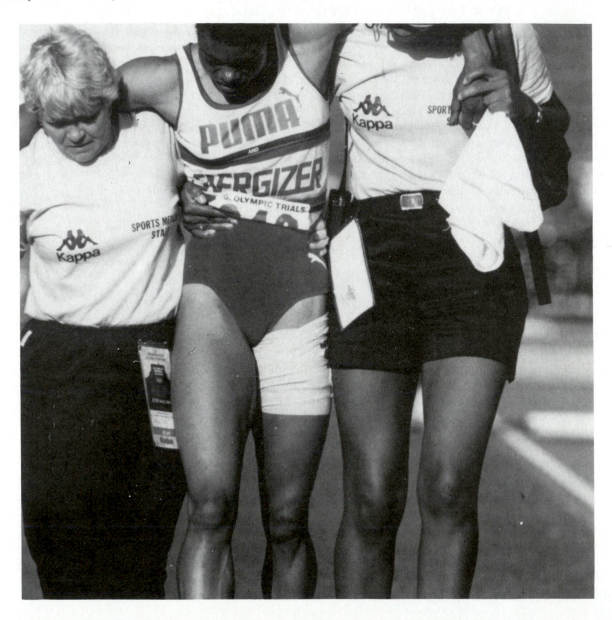

be able, when called upon, to apply proper first aid. This is especially true in cases of serious head and spinal injuries (Figure 1-2).

It is essential that a coach have a good understanding of skill techniques and environmental factors that may adversely affect the athlete. Poor techniques in such skill areas as throwing and running can lead to overuse injuries of the arms and legs, whereas overexposure to heat and humidity may cause death. The fact that a coach is experienced in coaching does not mean that he or she knows proper skill techniques. It is essential that coaches engage in a continual process of education to further their knowledge in a particular sport. When a sports program or specific sport is without an athletic trainer, the coach often takes over this role.

In the absence of an athletic trainer the coach must be able to carry out preventive measures such as taping; recognize signs of major injuries, especially those that may be life threatening or catastrophic; perform first aid; and properly get the injured athlete to medical care. To do so the coach must have a first aid certification and must have taken an introductory course in athletic training.

Coaches work closely with athletic trainers; therefore each must develop awareness of and insight into the other's problems so that there is optimum care of the athlete. Athletic trainers must also avoid questioning the abilities of the coaches and must restrict their opinions to athletic training matters. To avoid hard feelings, the coach must coach and the athletic trainer must deal with athletic training matters. To ensure the health and well-being of the athlete, the athletic trainer and the physician, when available, have the "last word." This position must be backed at all times by the athletic director.

> When a sports program is without an athletic trainer, the coach very often takes over this role.

> Coaches and athletic trainers must work together so that there is optimum care of the athlete.

> To ensure the health and well-being of the athlete, the athletic trainer and the physician, when available, have the "last word."

Figure 1-2

The coach is directly responsible for preventing injuries in his or her sport.

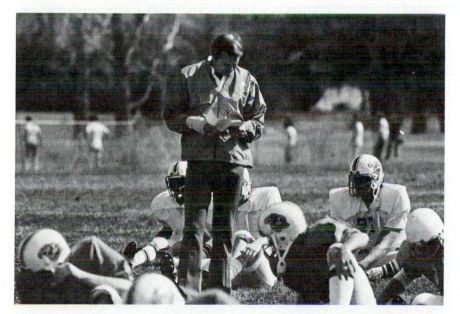

The Certified Athletic Trainer

Athletic training, more specifically the athletic trainer, is a major link between the athletic program and the medical community for the implementation of preventive measures, emergency care, and injury management. Ideally, every organized sports program should have a certified athletic trainer on its staff. Too often, however, a coach or student trainer assumes these responsibilities.

As mentioned earlier, the athletic trainer is a highly educated and well-trained professional. The titles *athletic trainer* and *athletic training* remain because of tradition. In reality, *trainer* is synonymous with *coach*, and *training* with *coaching* or *teaching*. A better title to describe the role of an athletic trainer is *sports therapist* or perhaps *sports medicine therapist* (Figure 1-3).

Qualifications of the NATA-Certified Athletic Trainer

The NATA-certified athletic trainer is a highly qualified paramedical professional educated and experienced in dealing with the injuries that occur with participation in sports. Certification requires an extensive background of formal academic preparation and supervised practical experience in a clinical setting, according to NATA-approved guidelines. Many certified athletic trainers choose also to become certified as emergency medical technicians (EMT) and to be educated as teachers and/or physical therapists. (For the most current information on certification, contact the NATA board of certifications.*)

The Athletic Trainer's Functions

The prevention of injury is a major goal of athletic training.

Today's professional athletic trainer performs numerous and diverse functions. In general, he or she is concerned with seven major task areas: *prevention* of athletic injuries and illness; *evaluation* and *recognition* of athletic injuries and illnesses and medical referral; *first aid* and *emergency care;* rehabilitation and *reconditioning; organization, counseling,* and *guidance;* and *education.*

The athletic trainer is considered a paramedical specialist in sports medicine.

Athletic trainers are employed by individual high schools, school districts, colleges and universities, professional teams, and in industrial settings. Many sports medicine clinics work closely with school sports programs, providing routine and event coverage.

Many states now license athletic trainers and officially establish their relationship with the physician, their scope of function of athletic training, and the use of therapeutic methods. Ideally, every organized sports program should have a certified athletic trainer on its staff. This is especially true at the secondary school level.

The Team Physician

The physician has full authority over the coach and athletic trainer.

The team physician must have a full understanding of sports injuries. Ideally the team physician has a background in sports medicine. Currently

---

*NATA Board of Certification, NATA Headquarters, 2952 Stemmons Freeway, Suite 200, Dallas, TX 75247-6103.

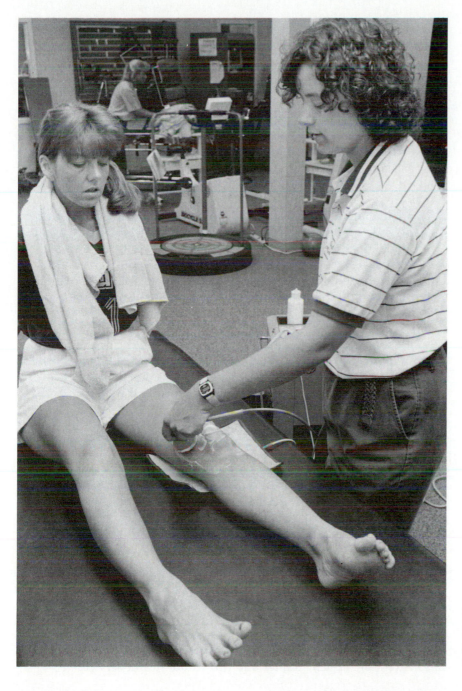

Figure 1-3

The athletic trainer is a major
link between the athletic
program and the medical
community.

physicians with varied specializations act as team physicians. These may
be family physicians, pediatricians (specialists with children), internal
medicine specialists, or orthopedic surgeons (specialists in the **musculoskeletal** system). These physicians may be medical doctors (M.D.) or
doctors of osteopathy (D.O.) The physician working with teams has full

musculoskeletal
Pertaining to muscles and
the skeleton

authority over the coach and athletic trainer in health matters in the athletic setting. Their primary duties entail the following:

1. Seeing that a complete medical history of each athlete is compiled and is readily available
2. Determining through a physical examination the athletes' health status
3. Diagnosing and treating injuries and illnesses
4. Directing and advising the athletic trainer on health matters
5. Acting, when necessary, as an instructor to the athletic trainer, assistant athletic trainer, and student athletic trainers on special therapeutic methods, therapeutic problems, and related procedures
6. Attending all games, athletic contests, scrimmages, and practices; if this is not feasible, arranging for attendance by other qualified medical personnel; when personal attendance is not possible, being available for emergency call
7. Deciding when, on medical grounds, athletes should be disqualified from participation and when they may be permitted to reenter competition
8. Serving as an advisor to the athletic trainer and the coach and, when necessary, as a counselor to the athlete
9. Working closely with the school administrator, school dentist, trainer, coach, and health services personnel to promote and maintain consistently high standards for the care of the athlete

Other Specialists Concerned with Athletic Health and Safety

A number of support health services may be used by a sports program. They may include a nurse, school health services, orthopedist, dentist, podiatrist, nutritionist, equipment personnel, and officials.

The Nurse

Support personnel concerned with the athlete's health and safety:
Nurse
School health services
Team orthopedist
Team dentist
Team podiatrist
Team nutritionist
Equipment personnel
Biomechanist
Strength and conditioning coach
Sport psychologist
Physical therapist
Exercise physiologist
Referees

In the absence of a physician or athletic trainer the school nurse may be the first person to see the injured athlete. Under these circumstances the nurse must be competent in giving first aid, recognizing serious injuries, and expediting the appropriate medical care. The nurse usually works in liaison with the athletic trainer and under the direction of a physician.

As a rule, the nurse is not usually responsible for the recognition of sports injuries. Education and background, however, render the nurse quite capable in the recognition of skin disease, infections, and minor irritations. The nurse works under the direction of the physician and in liaison with the athletic trainer and the school health services.

School Health Services

Colleges and universities maintain school health services that range from a department operating with one or two nurses and a physician available on a part-time basis to an elaborate setup comprised of a full complement of nursing services with a staff of full-time medical specialists and complete laboratory and hospital facilities. At the high school level health services are usually organized so that one or two nurses conduct the program under the direction of the school physician, who may serve a number of schools in a given area or district. This organization poses a problem, since it is often difficult to have qualified medical help at hand when it is needed. Local policy determines the procedure of referral for medical care. If such policies are lacking, the athletic trainer should see to it that an effective method is established for handling all athletes requiring medical care or opinion. The ultimate source of health care is the physician. The effectiveness of athletic health care service can be evaluated only to the extent to which it meets the following criteria:

1. Availability at every scheduled practice or contest of a person qualified and delegated to render emergency care to an injured or ill participant
2. Planned access to a physician by phone or nearby presence for prompt medical evaluation of the health care problems that warrant this attention
3. Planned access to a medical facility—including plans for communication and transportation

Team Orthopedist

Often the team physician has a specialty in family medicine or is an internist. In such cases serious musculoskeletal injuries are referred to an orthopedic surgeon. Many colleges and universities employ a team orthopedist.

Team Dentist

The role of team dentist is somewhat analogous to that of team physician. He or she serves as a dental consultant for the team and should be available for first aid and emergency care. Good communication between the dentist and the coach or athletic trainer should ensure a good dental program. There are three areas of responsibility for the team dentist:

1. Organizing and performing the preseason dental examination
2. Being available to provide emergency care when needed
3. Conducting the fitting of mouth protectors

Team Podiatrist

Podiatry, the specialized field dealing with the study and care of the foot, has become an integral part of sports health care. Many podiatrists are trained in surgical procedures, foot biomechanics, and the prescribing and construction of orthotic devices for the shoe. Like the team dentist, a podiatrist should be available on a consulting basis.

Team Nutritionist

Increasingly, nutritionists are becoming a part of the professional teams of large universities. They serve as consultants on eating programs and advise athletes who need special diets.

Equipment Personnel

Sports equipment personnel should be specialists in the purchase and proper fitting of protective equipment. They must work closely with the coach and the athletic trainer.

Biomechanist

An individual who possesses some expertise in the analysis of human motion can also be a great aid to the athletic trainer. The biomechanist uses sophisticated video and computer-enhanced digital analysis equipment to study movement. By advising the athlete, the coach, and the athletic trainer on matters such as faulty gait patterns or improper throwing mechanics, the biomechanist could reduce the likelihood of injury to the athlete.

Strength and Conditioning Coach

Many colleges and universities and some high schools employ full-time strength coaches to advise athletes on training and conditioning programs. Athletic trainers should routinely consult with these individuals to advise them about injuries to a particular athlete and exercises that should be avoided or modified relative to a specific injury.

Sports Psychologists

The sports psychologist can advise the athlete trainer on matters related to the psychological aspects of the rehabilitation process. The way the athlete feels about his or her injury and how it affects his or her social, emotional, intellectual, and physical dimensions can have a substantial effect on the course of a treatment program and how quickly the athlete may return to competition. The sports psychologist uses different intervention strategies to help the athlete cope with injury.

Physical Therapists

Some athletic trainers use physical therapists to supervise the rehabilitation programs for injured athletes while the athletic trainer concentrates primarily on getting a player ready to practice or compete. A number of athletic trainers are also physical therapists.

Exercise Physiologists

The exercise physiologist can significantly influence the athletic training program by giving input to the trainer regarding training and conditioning techniques, body composition analysis, and nutritional considerations.

Referees

Referees must be highly knowledgeable regarding rules and regulations, especially those that relate to the health and welfare of the athlete. They work cooperatively with the coach and the athletic trainer. They must be capable of checking the playing facility for dangerous situations and equipment that may predispose the athlete to injury. They must routinely check athletes to ensure that they are wearing adequate protective pads.[11]

In recent years negligence suits against teachers, coaches, athletic trainers, school officials, and physicians because of sports injuries have increased in frequency and in the amount of damages awarded. An increasing awareness of the many risk factors present in physical activities has had a major effect on the coach and the athletic trainer in particular. A great deal of care must be taken in following coaching and athletic training procedures that conform to the legal guidelines governing liability.

Liability

Liability is the state of being legally responsible for the harm one causes another person. It assumes that the coach and athletic trainer acts according to the standards of a reasonably prudent person. These standards require the coach or the athletic trainer to function as any reasonable person of ordinary prudence (with comparable education, skills, and training) would act in a comparable situation. In most cases in which someone has been charged with **negligence,** the actions of a hypothetical, reasonably prudent person have been compared with the actions of the defendant to ascertain whether the course of action followed by the defendant was in conformity with the judgment exercised by such a reasonably prudent person. The key phrase has been "reasonable care." Individuals who are charged with the well-being of the athlete and who have special education and experience in their profession must act in accordance with this background. The courts generally acknowledge that hazards are present in sports through the concept of **assumption of risk**. In other words, the individual, either by expressed or implied agreement, assumes the danger and hence relieves the other individual of legal responsibility to protect him or her; by so doing he or she agrees to take his or her own chances. This concept, however, is subject to many and varied interpretations in the courts, especially when a minor is involved, since he or she is not considered able to render a mature judgment about the risks inherent in the situation. Although athletes participating in a sports program are considered to assume a normal risk, this in no way exempts those in charge from exercising reasonable care and prudence in the conduct of such activities or from foreseeing and taking precautionary measures against accident-provoking circumstances. In general, the courts have been fairly consistent in upholding waivers and releases of liability for adults unless there is evidence of fraud, misrepresentation, or duress.

Negligence

Negligence is the failure to use ordinary or reasonable care—care that persons of ordinary prudence would exercise to avoid injury to them-

liability
State of being legally responsible for the harm one causes another person

negligence
Failure to use ordinary or reasonable care.

assumption of risk
The individual, through expressed or implied agreement, assumes some risk or danger will be involved in the particular undertaking. The individual thus relieves the other individual of legal responsibility to protect the first individual. In other words, a person takes his or her own chances

selves or to others under similar circumstances. This standard assumes that the individual is neither an exceptionally skillful individual nor an extraordinarily cautious one but is a person of *reasonable* and *ordinary* prudence. Put another way, it is expected that the individual will bring a commonsense approach to the situation at hand and will exercise due care in its handling.

Torts

tort
Legal wrongs committed against the person or property of another

Torts are legal wrongs committed against the person or property of another.[29] Such wrongs may emanate from an act of *omission,* wherein the individual fails to perform a legal duty, or from an act of *commission,* wherein he or she commits an act that is not legally his or hers to perform. In either instance, if injury results, the person can be held liable. In the case of omission, a coach or athletic trainer may fail to refer a seriously injured athlete for the proper medical attention. In the case of commission, the coach or athletic trainer may perform a medical treatment not within his or her legal province and from which serious medical complications develop.

The tort concept of negligence is held by the courts when it is shown that an individual (1) does something that a reasonably prudent person would not do or (2) fails to do something that a reasonably prudent person would do under circumstances similar to those shown by the evidence.

It is expected that a person possessing more training in a given field or area will possess a correspondingly higher level of competence than, for example, a student. An individual will, therefore, be judged in terms of his or her expected level of competence in any situation in which legal liability may be assessed.[16]

Warning of Risks

Athletes must know the risks, understand the risks, and appreciate the risks involved in their sport.

At the beginning of each season the coach must sufficiently warn players of the possible risks inherent with that sport. This is not limited to playing within the rules of the game but should also include the dangers they may face when using improper and dangerous techniques. Three levels of comprehension exist for the players: knowing the risks, understanding the risks, and appreciating the consequences of the risks. In other words, the players must have a clear understanding of the injuries that may occur as a result of participating in the sport, the nature—including the extent and severity—of those injuries, and the long-term disability that may arise from those injuries.[8]

Coaches can avoid injury risks involved in sport participation in a variety of ways. Some examples are shown in the box on page 14. Many schools state the risks of participation in written form and require that the parents or guardians of the athletes, and the athletes themselves, read and sign the form. Warning athletes of the risks does not stop here. Continual reinforcement throughout the season is necessary to remind the players frequently and regularly of the risks of the activity. The language

SAFEGUARDING AGAINST LIABILITY

The School Should Follow These Guidelines:

1. Hire a certified athletic trainer for injury care. If one is not available, designate one person who is adequately trained in emergency care to assume this role.
2. Have an established participation plan, including the following:
   a. Yearly preparticipation health examination
   b. Insurance verification form
   c. Medical history form
   d. Standard injury referral form
   e. Documentation of medical clearance from a physician after an injury has been sustained
3. Provide a safe environment for practice and play, including proper field maintenance.
4. Hire adequate and qualified supervisors for all practices and games, including supervision of weight training rooms and gymnasiums during and after school hours.
5. Post warning signs in plain view around equipment. These should describe both risks and proper use of the equipment.

The Coach Should Follow These Guidelines:

1. Warn the athletes of the dangers inherent in the sport.
2. Get informed consent from the athlete's parents or guardians before participation in sports.
3. Properly prepare and condition each athlete.
4. Progress through skill instruction as the players improve. Teach acceptable skills and proper techniques with frequent mention of risks involved.
5. Ensure that proper and safe equipment and facilities are used by the athlete at all times.

The Athletic Trainer Should Follow These Guidelines:

1. Develop and carefully follow an emergency plan, including the following:
   a. Make sure there is access to phones and emergency telephone numbers at each sport area.
   b. Designate staff responsibilities in an emergency.
   c. Document all injuries and subsequent actions.
2. Make it a point to become familiar with the health status and medical history of the athletes; be aware of any particular problems an athlete may have that could present a need for additional care or caution.
3. Establish and maintain qualified and adequate supervision of the training room, its environs, facilities, and equipment at all times.
4. If the distribution of nonprescription medications is allowed by law, exercise extreme caution and do not dispense prescription drugs.
5. Use only those therapeutic methods that you are qualified to use and that the law states you can use.
6. Do not use or permit the presence of faulty or hazardous equipment.
7. Work cooperatively with the coach and the team physician in the selection and use of sports protective equipment and insist that the best be obtained and properly fitted.
8. Do not permit injured players to participate unless cleared by the team physician. Players suffering a head injury should not be permitted to reenter the game. In some states a player who has suffered a concussion may not continue in the sport for the balance of the season.
9. Do not under any circumstances give a local anesthetic to enable an injured player to continue participation. It is dangerous, as well as unethical.
10. Develop an understanding with the coaches that an injured athlete will not be allowed to reenter competition until in the opinion of the team physician he or she is mentally and physically able. Do not permit yourself to be pressured to clear an athlete until he or she is fully cleared by the physician.
11. Follow the express orders of the team physician at all times.
12. Use common sense in making decisions about the athlete's health and safety.

In the case of an injury the coach or athletic trainer must use reasonable care to prevent further injury until medical care is obtained.[7]

and manner of informing players of the risks will vary with the age, maturity, and skill level of the players.

Foreseeability of Risk

Regular checks must be made to ensure that athletes have a safe environment in which to function. Coaches and/or designated health and safety personnel should do regular checks of the gymnasium and field areas to note hazardous conditions that may lead to injury for participants and spectators. Examples of these hazards may include lack of adequate padding on the gymnasium walls under the baskets, glass in doors leading into the gymnasium, potholes or glass on the playing fields, deteriorating steps or walkways, unsecured goal cages, and unsafe bleachers. Hazards should be documented in writing and appropriate individuals should be notified so that the hazards can be repaired or removed. Coaches should keep accurate records on all actions taken on an injured athlete.

At all times the athletes' health and welfare should be the number one priority.

Coaches should keep accurate records of all actions taken on an injured athlete.

Insurance Requirements

Since 1971, there has been a significant increase in the number of lawsuits filed, caused in part by the steady increase in individuals who have become active in sports.[5] The costs of insurance have also significantly increased during this period. With more lawsuits and much higher medical costs there is a crisis in the insurance industry.[6] The major types of insurance about which individuals concerned with athletic training and sports medicine should have some understanding are general health insurance, catastrophic insurance, accident insurance, and liability insurance, as well as insurance for errors and omissions. There is a need to protect adequately all who are concerned with sports health and safety.

General Health Insurance

It is essential that the athlete be fully insured.

Every athlete should have a general health insurance policy that covers illness, hospitalization, and emergency care (Figure 1-4). Some so-called comprehensive plans do not cover every health need. For example, they

---

A REASONABLE, PRUDENT COACH SHOULD:

1. Warn the athlete of the potential dangers inherent in the sport. A videotape demonstration on the hazards of the sport should be shown to both athlete and parent.
2. Supervise constantly and attentively.
3. Properly prepare and condition the athlete.
4. Properly instruct the athlete in the skills of the sports.
5. Ensure that proper and safe equipment and facilities are used by the athlete at all times.

may cover physicians' care but not hospital charges. Many of these plans require large prepayments before the insurance takes effect.[5]

Accident Insurance

Besides general health insurance, low-cost accident insurance is available to the student. It often covers accidents on school grounds while the student is in attendance. The purpose of this insurance is to protect against financial loss from medical and hospital bills, to encourage an injured student to receive prompt medical care, to encourage prompt reporting of injuries, and to relieve a school of financial responsibility.[5]

The school's general insurance may be limited; thus accident insurance for a specific activity such as sports may be needed to provide additional protection.[5] This type of coverage is limited and does not require knowledge of fault, and the amount it pays is very limited. For very serious sport injuries requiring surgery and lengthy rehabilitation, accident insurance is usually not adequate. This inadequacy can put families with limited budgets into a real financial bind. Of particular concern is insurance that does not adequately cover catastrophic injuries.

> For very serious sport injuries requiring surgery and lengthy rehabilitation, accident insurance is usually not adequate.

Catastrophic Insurance

Although catastrophic injuries in sports participation are relatively uncommon, when they do occur, the consequences to the athlete, family, and institution, as well as society, can be staggering. In the past when available funds have been completely diminished, the family was forced to seek funding elsewhere, usually through a lawsuit. Organizations such as the NCAA and NAIA provide plans that deal with the problem of lifetime medical and rehabilitative care because of a permanent disability.[6]

Figure 1-4

Sample insurance form.

Insurance Information on Student Athletes
Student's Name_____Date of birth_____
Address_____
Social Security Number_____Sex: M_____ F_____
Names of Insurance Companies_____
Address of Insurance Company_____
Certificate Number_____Group_____Type_____
Policy Holder_____Relationship to Student_____
Employer or Policyholder_____
Should my son/daughter require services beyond those covered by the Sports Medicine Program, I give permission to the Division of Sports Medicine to file a claim for such services with the above health care insurer.
According to NCAA regulations, I understand that any insurance payments I receive must be returned to be placed on my child's account.
Date_____   _____
                                                    Parent's Signature

Benefits begin when expenses have reached $25,000 and are then extended through the individual's lifetime. At the secondary school level a program is offered to districts by the National Federation of State High School Associations (NFSHSA). This plan provides medical, rehabilitation, and transportation costs that are in excess of $10,000 and that are not covered by other insurance benefits.[1]

Personal Liability Insurance

Because of the amount of litigation for alleged negligence, all professionals involved with the sports program must be fully protected by personal liability insurance.

Most individual schools and school districts have general liability insurance to protect against damages that may arise from injuries occurring on school property. It covers claims of negligence on the part of the individuals. Its major concern is whether supervision was reasonable and whether unreasonable risk of harm was perceived by the sports participant.

Because of the amount of litigation based on alleged negligence, premiums have become almost prohibitive for some schools. Typically when a victim sues, the lawsuit has been a shotgun approach, with the coach, athletic trainer, physician, school administrator, and school district all named. If a protective piece of equipment is involved, the product manufacturer is also sued.

To offset this shotgun mentality and to cover what is not covered by a general liability policy, *errors and omissions* liability insurance has evolved. It is designed to cover school employees, officers, and the district against suits claiming malpractice, wrongful actions, errors and omissions, and acts of negligence. Even when working in a program having good liability coverage, each person within that program who works directly with students must have his or her own personal liability insurance.

Even when working in a program having good liability coverage, each person within that program who works directly with students must have his or her own personal liability insurance.

The Preparticipation Health Examination

An important component of athletic training is the preparticipation health examination.

The primary purpose of the preseason health examination is to determine whether an athlete is at risk for injury, reinjury, illness, or even death when participating in a specific sport. Preseason health examinations must be given not only at the entry level but must be conducted during each season in which an athlete competes. Three types of examinations are commonly given—the locker room examination, an examination by a personal physician, and a station examination.

Locker Room Examination

Locker room examination refers to mass examination. Groups of athletes are examined by a team or volunteer physician in a cursory manner to satisfy the requirements of a particular sport. This method lacks a standardized history form and involves an examination that is less than thorough (Figures 1-5 and 1-6). However, this is a screening examination that is highly specific and sports related. It should never be viewed as a complete physical examination.[16]

```
Name _____        Date _____

1.  BP (sitting) _____/_____
2.  Vision:  L 20/_____  R 20/_____              CHECK IF
3.  Skin _____              NEGATIVE
                                                                  ☐
    Mouth _____                 ☐
    Eyes:  Pupils  L _____  R _____
4.  Chest: PMI _____                ☐
          Pulses _____
          Rhythm _____
          Murmurs _____
          Lungs _____
5.  Lymphatics:  Cervical _____               ☐
                 Axillary _____
    Abdomen:  Organs _____                 ☐
              _____
    Genitalia: _____                 ☐
    Maturation Index _____
6.  Orthopedic (conduct according to Figure 2-10):                 ☐
    Cervical spine/back _____
    Shoulders _____
    Arm/elbow/wrist/hold _____
    Knees _____
          _____
    Ankles _____
          _____
7.  Other _____                  ☐
```

Figure 1-5

Preparticipation health
examination—physical
evaluation.

Personal Physician Examination

Examination by a personal physician has the advantage of providing an
in-depth history and an ideal physician-patient relationship. A disadvantage of this type of examination is that it may not be directed to detection of factors that predispose the athlete for a sports injury.[8]

Station Examination

The most thorough and sport-specific type of preparticipation examination is the station examination (Figure 1-7). This method can provide a
detailed examination of an athlete in a short period of time. A team of
nine people is needed to examine 30 or more athletes. The team should
include two physicians, two medically trained nonphysicians (nurse,
athletic trainer, physical therapist, or physician assistant), and five
managers, student athletic trainers, or assistant coaches (Table 1-1).

Orthopedic Screening

Orthopedic screening is an essential part of the preparticipation health examination (Figure 1-8). Its purpose is to reveal past injuries that are inadequately rehabilitated or that have not been previously detected. The examination requires 90 seconds per individual athlete.

Maturity Assessment

Maturity assessment should be part of the preparticipation health examination as a means of protecting the young athlete.[4] Most commonly used

Name _____ _____ Date _____

Completed by *athlete* or *parent*   YES   NO
1. Have any members of your family under age 50 had a "heart attack"   ☐   ☐
   or "heart problems"?
2. Have you ever been told you have a heart murmur, high blood   ☐   ☐
   pressure, extra heartbeats, or a heart abnormality?
3. Do you have to stop while running around a (¼ mile) track twice?   ☐   ☐
4. Are you taking any medications?   ☐   ☐
5. Have you ever "passed out" or been "knocked out" (concussion)?   ☐   ☐
6. Have you ever had any illness, condition, or injury that:
   a. Required you to go to the hospital either as a patient overnight ☐   ☐
      or in the emergency room or for x-rays?
   b. Required an operation?   ☐   ☐
   c. Lasted longer than a week?   ☐   ☐
   d. Caused you to miss a game or practice?   ☐   ☐
   e. Is related to allergies (hayfever, hives, asthma, or medicine)? ☐   ☐

Completed by *physician*

Physician's name _____

Item #

_____   _____

_____   _____

_____   _____

_____   _____

Disposition

1. No participation in _____

2. Limited participation in _____

   _____

3. Requires: _____

   _____

4. Full participation _____

   _____

                              _____
                              Physician's signature

                              _____
                              Date

Name _____ S.S. # _____

Height _____ Weight _____

	CHECK IF NEGATIVE
1. Blood pressure _____ / _____	☐
2. Vision	
Without glasses: R 20/_____ L 20/_____	☐
With glasses: R 20/_____ L 20/_____	☐
3. Skin _____	☐
Mouth _____	☐
Pupil size: R _____ L _____	☐
4. Chest: Pulses _____	☐
Heart rhythm _____	☐
Lungs _____	☐
Breast _____	☐
5. Lymphatics: Cervical _____	☐
Axillary _____	☐
Abdominal organs _____	☐
Genitalia _____	☐
6. Orthopedic: Postural alignment _____	☐
Cervical spine/back _____	☐
Leg _____	☐
Joint deformity/swelling _____	☐
Joint laxity _____	☐
Decreased range of motion _____	☐
7. Urinalysis (Lab-Stix) _____	☐
8. Other points noted _____	

Disposition

1. No participation in _____

2. Clearance withheld until _____

3. Limited participation _____

4. Full, unlimited participation _____

Additional comments _____

_____

Physician's signature

_____

Date

Figure 1-7

Preparticipation health
examination—station report.

methods are the circumpubertal (sexual maturity), skeletal, and dental assessments. Of the three, Tanner's five stages of assessment, indicating maturity of secondary sexual characteristics, is the most expedient for use in the station method of examination. The Tanner approach evaluates pubic hair and genitalia development in boys and pubic hair and breast development in girls. Other indicators that may be noted are facial and axillary hair. Stage one indicates that puberty is not evident, whereas stage five indicates full development. The crucial stage in terms of collision and high-intensity noncontact sports is stage three, in which there is the fastest bone growth. In this stage, the growth plates are two to five times weaker than the joint capsule and tendon attachments.[4] Young athletes in grades 7 to 12 must be matched by maturity, not age.[4]

Tanner's stage three is crucial in terms of collision and high-intensity noncontact sports. Bone growth is fastest in this stage and athletes in grades 7-12 must be matched by maturity, not age.

TABLE 1-1 Station preparticipation examination

Station	Points Noted	Personnel
1. Individual history; height, weight	Yes answers are probed in depth; height and weight relationships	Physician, nurse, or athletic trainer
2. Blood pressure, pulse	Upper limits: ages 6 to 11—130/80; 12 and older—140/90; right arm is measured while athlete is seated	Student athletic trainer or manager
3. Snellen test	Upper limits of visual acuity—20/40	Student athletic trainer or manager
4. Skin, mouth, eyes	Suspicious-looking skin infections and/or rashes, dental prosthesis or caries, unequal pupils	Physician, nurse, or athletic trainer
5. Chest	Heart abnormalities (e.g., murmurs, latent bronchospasm)	Physician
6. Lymphatics, abdomen, male genitalia	Adenopathy (cervical and axillary), abnormalities of genitalia, hernia	Physician or physician's assistant
7. Orthopedics	Postural asymmetry, decreased range of motion or strength, abnormal joint laxity	Physician, athletic trainer, physical therapist, or nurse practitioner
8. Urinalysis	After its collection in a paper cup, urine is tested for positive with a Lab-Stix	Student athletic trainer or manager
9. Review	History and physical examination reports are evaluated and the following decisions are made: (a) No sports participation (b) Limited participation (no participation in specific sports such as football or ice hockey) (c) Clearance withheld until certain conditions are met (e.g., additional tests are taken, rehabilitation is complete) (d) Full, unlimited participation is allowed	Physician

Sport Disqualification

As discussed previously, sports participation involves risks. Most disqualification conditions that are ascertained by a preparticipation health evaluation are noted in the medical history (Table 1-2).

In general, the athlete who has lost one of two paired organs such as eyes or kidneys is cautioned against playing a collision or contact sport.[7] Such an athlete should be counseled into participating in a noncontact sport. The athlete with one testicle or one or both that are undescended must be apprised that the small risk of serious injury can be substantially minimized by the use of an athletic supporter and a protective device.[16]

Budgetary Concerns

One of the major problems faced by athletic trainers is to obtain a budget of sufficient size to permit them to perform a creditable job of athletic training. Most high schools fail to make any budgetary provision for athletic training except for the purchase of tape, ankle wraps, and a training bag that contains a minimum amount of equipment. Many fail to provide a room or any of the special facilities that are needed to establish an effective athletic training program. Some school boards and administrators fail to recognize that the functions performed in the athletic training quarters are an essential component of the athletic program and that even if no specialist is used, the facilities are nonetheless necessary. Colleges and universities are not usually faced with this problem to the same extent as high schools. By and large, athletic training is recognized as an important aspect of the collegiate athletic program.

Budgetary needs vary considerably within programs; some require only a few thousand dollars, whereas others entail spending of hundreds of thousands of dollars. The amount spent on building and equipping a

A major problem often facing athletic trainers is obtaining a budget of sufficient size.

Figure 1-8

The orthopedic screening examination. Equipment that may be needed includes reflex hammer, tape measure, pin, and examining table.

ORTHOPEDIC SCREENING EXAMINATION	
Activity and Instruction	**To Determine**
Stand facing examiner	Acromioclavicular joints; general habitus
Look at ceiling, floor, over both shoulders; touch ears to shoulders	Cervical spine motion
Shrug shoulders (examiner resists)	Trapezius strength
Abduct shoulders 90° (examiner resists at 90°)	Deltoid strength
Full external rotation of arms	Shoulder motion
Flex and extend elbows	Elbow motion
Arms at sides, elbows 90° flexed; pronate and supinate wrists	Elbow and wrist motion
Spread fingers; make fist	Hand or finger motion and deformities
Tighten (contract) quadriceps; relax quadriceps	Symmetry and knee effusion; ankle effusion
"Duck walk" four steps (away from examiner with buttocks on heels)	Hip, knee, and ankle motion
Stand with back to examiner	Shoulder symmetry; scoliosis
Knees straight, touch toes	Scoliosis, hip motion, hamstring tightness
Raise up on toes, raise heels	Calf symmetry, leg strength

TABLE 1-2 Disqualifying conditions for sports participation

Conditions	Collision*	Contact†	Noncontact‡
General Health			
Acute infections (respiratory, genitourinary, infectious mononucleosis, hepatitis, active rheumatic fever, active tuberculosis)	X	X	X
Obvious physical immaturity in comparison with other competitors	X	X	
Hemorrhagic disease (hemophilia, purpura, and other serious bleeding tendencies)	X	X	X
Diabetes, inadequately controlled	X	X	X
Diabetes, controlled	§	§	§
Jaundice	X	X	X
Eyes			
Absence or loss of function of one eye	X	X	
Respiratory			
Tuberculosis (active or symptomatic)	X	X	X
Severe pulmonary insufficiency	X	X	X
Cardiovascular			
Mitral stenosis, aortic stenosis, aortic insufficiency, coarctation of aorta, cyanotic heart disease, recent carditis of any etiology	X	X	X
Hypertension on organic basis	X	X	X

*Football, rugby, hockey, lacrosse, and so forth.
†Baseball, soccer, basketball, wrestling, and so forth.
‡Cross country, track, tennis, crew, swimming, and so forth.
§No exclusions.

TABLE 1-2 Disqualifying conditions for sports participation—cont'd

Conditions	Collision	Contact	Noncontact
Previous heart surgery for congenital or acquired heart disease	‖	‖	‖
Liver, enlarged	X	X	
Skin			
Boils, impetigo, and herpes simplex gladiatorum	X	X	
Spleen, enlarged	X	X	
Hernia			
Inguinal or femoral hernia	X	X	X
Musculoskeletal			
Symptomatic abnormalities or inflammations	X	X	X
Functional inadequacy of the musculoskeletal system, congenital or acquired, incompatible with the contact or skill demands of the sport	X	X	X
Neurological			
History of symptoms of previous serious head trauma or repeated concussions	X		
Controlled convulsive disorder	**	**	**
Convulsive disorder not controlled moderately well by medication	X		

‖Each individual should be judged on an individual basis in conjunction with his or her cardiologist and surgeon.

**Each patient should be judged on an individual basis. All things being equal, it is probably better to encourage a young boy or girl to participate in a noncontact sport rather than a contact sport. However, if a patient has a desire to play a contact sport and this is deemed a major ameliorating factor in his or her adjustment to school, associates, and the seizure disorder, serious consideration should be given to letting him or her participate if the seizures are moderately well controlled or the patient is under good medical management. *Continued*.

TABLE 1-2 Disqualifying conditions for sports participation—cont'd

Conditions	Collision	Contact	Noncontact
Neurological—cont'd			
Previous surgery on head	X	X	
Renal			
Absence of one kidney	X	X	
Renal disease	X	X	X
Genitalia			
Absence of one testicle	††	††	††
Undescended testicle	††	††	††

††The committee approves the concept of contact sports participation for youths with only one testicle or with undescended testicle(s), except in specific instances such as an inguinal canal undescended testicle(s), following appropriate medical evaluation to rule out unusual injury risk. However, the athlete, parents, and school authorities should be fully informed that participation in contact sports for youths with only one testicle carries a slight injury risk to the remaining healthy testicle. Fertility may be adversely affected following an injury. But the chances of an injury to a descended testicle are low, and the injury risk can be further substantially minimized with an athletic supporter and protective device.

training facility, of course, is entirely a matter of local option. In purchasing equipment, immediate needs and availability of personnel to operate specialized equipment should be kept in mind.

Budget records should be kept on file so that they are available for use in projecting the following year's budgetary needs. They present a picture of the distribution of current funds and serve to substantiate future budgetary requests.

Expenditures for individual items vary in accordance with different training philosophies. An annual inventory must be conducted at the end of the year or before the ordering of supplies and equipment takes place. Accurate records must be kept to justify future requests.

Supplies

Supplies are expendable and usually are for injury prevention, first aid, and management. Examples of supplies are athletic training tape, germicides, and massage lubricants.

Equipment

The term *equipment* refers to those items that are not expendable. Equipment may be fixed or nonfixed. The word *fixed* does not necessarily mean that it cannot be moved but that it is not usually removed from the athletic training facility. Examples of fixed equipment are icemakers, exercise devices such as the Universal machine, and various therapeutic modalities. *Nonfixed* equipment refers to nonexpendable items that are moved as needed. Examples are blankets, scissors, and training kits.

Supplies are expendable and usually are for injury prevention, first aid, and management.

Purchasing Systems

Purchasing supplies and equipment must be done through either *competitive bid* or *direct buy*. For expensive purchases an institutional purchasing agent is sent out to competing vendors who quote a price on specified supplies or equipment. Orders are usually placed with the lowest bidder. Smaller purchases or emergency purchases may be made directly from one single vendor.[9]

Purchasing supplies and equipment must be done through either competitive bid or direct buy.

THE ATHLETIC TRAINING PROGRAM

Most high schools and colleges have some type of athletic training program. They may range from basic offerings to highly complex ones. The degree to which the athletic training program provides services to the athlete depends on the philosophy of the administration, the availability of a professional trainer, available facilities, and the budget. Athletic training and sports medicine form a health care unit that requires careful organization and administration.

Athletic training and sports medicine form a health care unit that requires careful organization and administration.

Record Keeping

Record keeping is a major responsibility of the athletic training program. When the athletic training program has an athletic trainer, record keeping generally is his or her responsibility. Records kept include injury reports and how the athlete is disposed, treatment logs, supply and equipment inventories, and annual reports on program functioning. A major concern to the coach without an athletic trainer is keeping accurate records of emergency procedures that were carried out.

The Athletic Training Facility

The major use for the athletic training facility is the prevention and care of sports injuries and related health functions. The athletic training room is a special facility, often with many rooms designed to meet the many requirements of a sports training program. Larger, more complex facilities found in some universities and those for professional teams have areas for first aid, physical examinations, pregame and prepractice bandaging and taping, and one where a variety of therapeutic techniques can be carried out (Figure 1-9). In these complexes there also may be separate offices for athletic trainers and physicians. In contrast, some high schools may have only one small room to carry out a multitude of health and safety functions. Above all, an athletic training facility should never become a club room for athletes, a meeting room for coaches and athletes, or a storage room for athletic equipment. Unless strict rules on the function of the athletic training room are made and kept, the training room soon loses its major purpose. A major goal is that the training room be kept in a hygienic and sanitary condition at all times. The following are some general rules to which athletes should adhere:

The only use for the training room is the prevention and care of sports injuries and related health functions.

1. No cleated shoes are allowed.
2. Game equipment is kept outside.

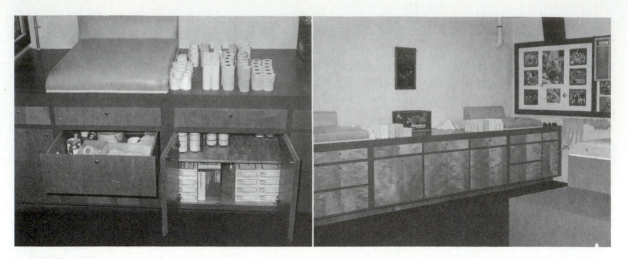

Figure 1-9

An effective athletic training program must have appropriate, highly organized storage facilities.

3. Shoes are kept off treatment tables.
4. Athletes must shower following activity and before receiving treatment except in an emergency situation.
5. Roughhousing and profanity are never allowed.
6. Food, drink, and tobacco products are not allowed.

Example of Service Areas

Modern athletic training rooms are usually organized into service areas. Some examples of special service areas follow:

1. Taping, bandaging, and orthotics section
2. Superficial thermal and mechanical therapy section—moist heat pads, paraffin bath
3. Electrotherapy section—ultrasound and electrostimulation machines
4. Hydrotherapy section—whirlpool baths, ice machine, sinks, and in some cases a steam room
5. Exercise rehabilitation section—resistance apparatus, stationary bicycle
6. Computer and record-keeping area

In addition to these service sections, there must be a trainer's office and plentiful storage facilities.

SUSTAINING SPORTS INJURIES

Understanding sports injuries requires knowledge of the types of sports involved and how injuries are sustained.

An **accident** is defined as an unplanned event capable of resulting in loss of time, property damage, injury, disablement, or even death.[3] On the other hand, an **injury** may be defined as damage to the body that restricts activity or causes disability to such an extent that the athlete is confined to his or her bed.[2]

accident
Occurring by chance or without intention

injury
An act that causes damage or hurt

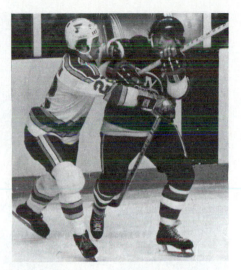

Figure 1-10

In collision sports, athletes use their bodies to deter or punish opponents.

An athlete runs a 50% chance of sustaining some injury. Of the 50 million estimated sports injuries sustained each year, approximately 50% require only minor care with no activity restriction.[3] Ninety percent of sports injuries are considered minor, while 10% are of the more serious type. It should be noted, however, that repeated **acute** minor injuries can eventually lead to more serious **chronic** conditions in later life.

Sports Classification

Sports injuries cannot be studied without an examination of the different types of sports classifications. Sports can be classified in many different ways. The classifications that best describe the extent to which a sport produces situations for accidents and subsequent injuries are collision, contact, and noncontact sports. In **collision sports** athletes use their bodies to deter or punish opponents (Figure 1-10). American football, ice hockey, boxing, and rugby are common American collision sports. In **contact sports** athletes make physical contact, but not with the intent to produce bodily injury (Figure 1-11). Examples of contact sports are soccer, basketball, baseball, and touch and flag football. As the name implies, **noncontact sports** have no physical contact. Archery, crew rowing, and cross-country running are examples of noncontact sports (Figure 1-12).

Sports Injury Information

By their very nature many sports activities invite injury. The all-out exertion required, the numerous situations requiring body contact, and play that involves the striking and throwing of missiles create hazards that are either directly or indirectly responsible for the many different injuries suffered by athletes.

In general, accurate assessment of why sports injuries occur is very

acute injury
An injury with sudden onset and short duration

chronic injury
An injury with long onset and long duration

collision sport
Athletes use their bodies to deter or punish opponents

contact sport
Athletes make physical contact, but not with the intent to produce bodily injury

noncontact sport
Athletes are not involved in any physical contact

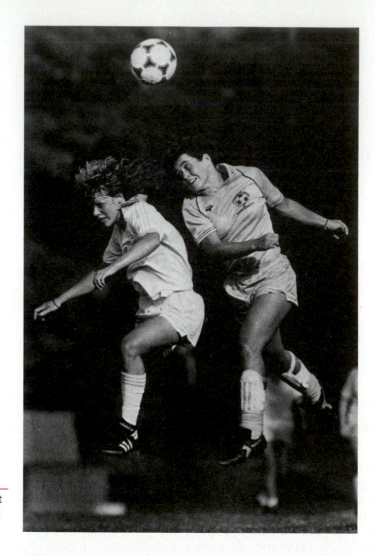

Figure 1-11

There is some bodily contact in contact sports but without intent to produce injury.

epidemiological approach
The study of sports injuries involving the relationship of as many injury factors as possible

difficult. As many factors as possible must be known about why the injury occurred. Knowledge of the skill level of the athlete, how much exposure to an injury was sustained by the athlete, and environmental conditions represents just a few of the bits of information needed before a complete understanding can be accomplished.

Vast numbers of people involved with organized and recreational sports become injured. However, the collection of accurate data that stem from these injuries is weak for the most part. Most data collection systems report that an injury occurred, but they do not collect details of the occurrence. A good data collection system is one that takes an **epidemiological approach,** such as the NATA's High School Athletic Injury Registry conducted by John Powell, Ph.D. This system documents sports-related injuries in six scholastic sports: football, wrestling, girls and boys basketball, and girls and boys soccer. It not only documents an injury's

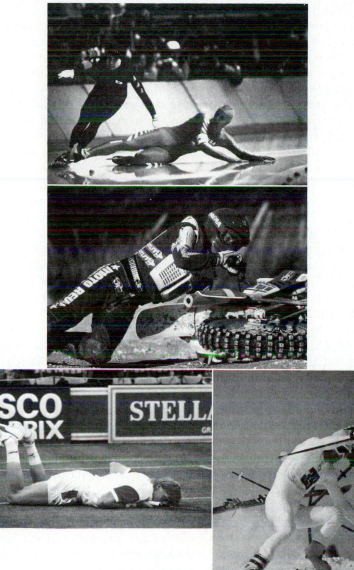

Figure 1-12

Noncontact sports do not involve physical contact with an opposing player.

occurrence but also collects as many factors related to the injury as possible.

Collision sports, primarily American football, are associated directly with causing catastrophic injuries and even death. However, fatalities in organized football have dropped significantly since rules were adopted that prevent the head from being used as a primary and initial contact area.[15] Deaths in sports are attributed primarily to head injuries, most of which occurred in high school football.[13] Since 1977 there has been a

time-loss injuries
Injuries that require the player to suspend activity the day of an injury or the day after the onset

catastrophic injury
A permanent injury to the spinal cord that leaves the athlete quadriplegic or paraplegic

gradual decline in minor injuries due to stricter adherence to the rules of play, better conditioning, medical supervision, and continued research in the improvement of protective equipment (e.g., the helmet).

Time-loss injuries are defined by NATA as those that require the player to suspend activity for at least the remainder of the day the injury occurred or the day after onset of injury.[14] Of the injuries 60% occurred during practice, and 40% occurred at games. The incidence of surgical cases remained fairly constant, averaging one per school, 64% being knee related, and 45% occurring during practice.

The highest incidence of indirect sports death stems from heat stroke. Other less common indirect causes include cardiovascular and respiratory problems and congenital conditions not previously known. Since 1976 there has been a steady decline in permanent spinal injuries leading to quadriplegia. The expression **catastrophic injury** refers to permanent spinal injuries.

It should be noted that although millions of individuals participate in organized and recreational sports, there is a relatively low incidence of serious injuries. Ninety-eight percent of individuals with injuries requiring hospital emergency room medical attention are treated and released immediately. Deaths from sports have been attributed to chest or trunk impact by thrown objects, other players, or nonyielding objects. Deaths have occurred when players were struck in the head by sports implements (bats, golf clubs, hockey sticks) or by missiles (baseballs, soccer balls, golf balls, hockey pucks). Deaths have also resulted when an individual received a direct blow to the head from another player or as a result of falling to the ground. On record are a number of recreational sports deaths in which a playing structure, such as a goalpost or backstop, fell on a participant.

In general, in most popular organized and recreational sports activities, the legs and arms are most at risk, with the head and face next. Of the game-related injuries, 65% suffered by boys and 67% suffered by girls occurred in the second half. Most injuries were to the lower extremity with ankle and foot injuries being the most prevalent.[20] Of all reported injuries, 15% were classified as major, precluding participation for 3 weeks or more; 17% were moderate; and 68% were minor (players being out 7 days or less). Most of the injuries (68%) occurred during practice, and half of all injuries involved the upper extremities. Muscle strains, joint sprains, contusions, and skin abrasions are the most frequent injuries sustained by the active sports participant.

SUMMARY

Modern sports medicine and athletic training have their roots in the civilizations of ancient Greece and early Rome. Today athletic training is a specialization within sports medicine, its major concern being the health and safety of athletes. The primary athletic training team consists of the coach, the athletic trainer, and the team physician.

The coach is directly responsible for preventing injuries to the athlete by obviating hazardous situations, providing well-made and properly fitting protective equipment, and making sure the athlete is in top physical condition and capable of withstanding the rigors of the sport. The athletic trainer provides the major link between the athletic program and the medical community. It is important that the athletic trainer be well educated in the prevention and care of sports injuries and be nationally certified by the National Athletic Trainers' Association.

At all times, the coach and the athletic trainer must act in a reasonable and prudent manner. A person who fails to act with reasonable care is considered negligent. The coach and the athletic trainer must always consider as paramount the health and well-being of the athlete. Legal liability or responsibility varies in its interpretation from state to state and from area to area.

The team physician can be in varied specializations. Team physicians, depending on the time they are committed to a specific sports program, can perform a variety of duties. Some key responsibilities are performing the preparticipation health examination, diagnosing and treating illnesses and injuries, advising and teaching the athletic training staff, attending games, scrimmages, and practices, and counseling the athlete about health matters.

The athletic training program forms a health care unit requiring careful organization and administration. Of major concern are the maintenance of facilities, provision of proper supervision of special service sections, and performance of an effective preparticipation health examination. Insurance, budget, accident reporting, treatment logging, and annual reports are some of the record-keeping responsibilities required of the athletic training program.

Athletic training facilities vary in size from a small room to a complex of many rooms. The athletic training program has as its major concern the health and safety of the athlete. It provides services such as first aid, physical examinations, preventive taping, and the carrying out of therapeutic procedures.

REVIEW QUESTIONS AND CLASS ACTIVITIES

1. The role of the athletic trainer has changed a great deal since earlier days. How do you perceive athletic trainers and their contribution to the total development of athletic programs?
2. Why is it so important that the athletic trainer be NATA certified?
3. What qualifications of education, certification, and personality should the athletic trainer have?
4. Why is it so important that the coach, athletic trainer, and team physician all work together to care for the athletes?
5. Chart the line of responsibility for health care of an athlete at your school and what chain of command must be followed in referring the athlete to the team physician or to another specialist.
6. What are the major legal concerns of the coach, athletic trainer, and other school personnel in giving health care?
7. Invite an attorney familiar with sport litigation to your class to discuss how

you can protect yourself from lawsuits. You may want to make this guest speaker available to other students in the department who can also benefit from discussing this topic.

8. What tests and activities should the team physician employ in a preseason physical examination?
9. Design a station preparticipation exam that will be given at your school during the summer for your football squad (approximately 90 athletes). Allow for privacy at some of the stations, provide any special equipment and supplies that will be needed, and place supervisors at each station.
10. What conditions may preclude an athlete's participation in an athletic program? Who determines this at your school? Do the athletes have a right to appeal that decision?
11. What factors constitute a collision sport, contact sport, and a noncontact sport? Can you identify the sports in each of the categories?
12. Why does the epidemiological approach to the collection of data about injuries help us understand the risks involved?
13. American football is the nation's, if not the world's, most injurious sport. What rule changes have made it safer for young athletes? What other things might we do to make it even safer?

REFERENCES

1. Berg R: Catastrophic injury insurance, an end to costly litigation, *Ath J* 8:10, 1987.
2. Borkowski RP: Coaches and the courts, *First Order* 54:1, 1985.
3. Borkowski RP: Lawsuit less likely if safety comes first, *First Aider* 55:11, 1985.
4. Caine DJ, Broekhoff J: Maturity assessment: a viable preventive measure against physical and psychological insult to the young athlete? *Phys Sportsmed* 15:67, 1987.
5. Chambers RL et al: Insurance types and coverages: knowledge to plan for the future (with a focus on motor skill activities and athletics), *Phys Educator* 44:233, 1986.
6. Clement A: Patterns of litigation in physical education instruction. Paper presented at the American Association of Health, Physical Education, and Dance, National Convention and Exposition, Cincinnati, April 1986.
7. Dorsen PJ: Should athletes with one eye, kidney, or testicle play contact sports? *Phys Sportmed* 14:130, 1986.
8. Drowatzky JN: Legal duties and liability in athletic training, *Ath Train* 20:11, 1985.
9. Frost R et al: *Administration of physical education and athletic programs,* Dubuque, Iowa, 1988, Wm C Brown.
10. Hawkins J, Appenzeller H: Legal aspects of sports medicine. In Mueller F, Ryan A, eds: *Prevention of athletic injuries: the role of the sports medicine team,* Philadelphia, 1991, FA Davis.
11. Kegerreis S: Sports medicine: a functional definition, *J Phys Educ Rec Dance* 52:22, 1981.
12. McKeog DB: Preseason physical examination for the prevention of sports injuries, *Sports Med* 2:413, 1985.
13. O'Shea ME: *A history of the National Athletic Trainers' Association,* Greenville, N.C., 1980, National Athletic Trainer's Association.
14. Public Relations Committee: NATA 3 year study of high school sports injuries, *Ath Train* 24:61, 1993
15. Torg JS: Epidemiology, pathomechanics, and prevention of athletic injuries to the cervical spine, *Med Sci Sports Exerc* 17:295, 1985.
16. Yasser R: Calculating risk, *Sports Med Dig* 9:5, 1987.

ANNOTATED BIBLIOGRAPHY

Arnheim DD, Prentice WA: *Principles of athletic training,* ed 8, St Louis, 1989, Times Mirror/Mosby College Publishing. Discusses the history of athletic training and surveillance of sports injuries as well as personnel and their administrative tasks.

Bilik SE: *The trainers bible,* ed 9, New York, 1956, TJ Reed. A classic book by a major pioneer in athletic training and sports medicine. It was first published in 1917.

Bloomfield J et al, eds: *Text book of science and medicine in sports,* Champaign, Ill: Human Kinetics, 1992. A sports medicine text divided in five sections including basic sciences, athletic training, nutrition, and environmental stresses.

Contu RC, Micheli LJ, eds: *ACSM's guidelines for the team physician,* Lea & Febiger, Malvern, Pa, 1991. Covers most aspects of the information needed for the team physician, including precompetition, postcompetition, and medicolegal aspects, as well as other health-related topics.

Herbert DL: *Legal aspects of sports medicine,* Canton, Ohio, 1992, Professional Reports. A discussion of sports medicine, policies, procedures, responsibilities of the sports medicine team, informed consent, negligence, insurance and risk management, medications, drug testing, and other topics.

Myers GC, Garrick JG: The preseason physical examination of school and college athletes. In Strauss RH, ed: *Sports medicine,* Philadelphia, 1984, WB Saunders. An excellent discussion of what a preseason physical examination should contain. The American Medical Association's "disqualifying conditions for sports participation" are also included.

Nygaard G, Boone TH: *Coaches guide to sport law,* Champaign, Ill, 1985, Human Kinetics. Provides general information on the legal responsibilities of coaches and physical educators.

O'Shea ME: *A history of the National Athletic Trainers' Association,* Greenville, NC, 1980, National Athletic Trainers' Association. An interesting text on the history of the NATA. Any student interested in athletic training as a career should know something about the pioneers in this field.

Shahody EJ, Petrizzi MJ: *Sports medicine for coaches and trainers,* Chapel Hill, 1991, University of North Carolina Press. A general guide to the management of sports medicine.

Shephard RJ: *The 1992 year book of sports medicine,* Chicago, 1992, Mosby-Year Book. Covers the year's most important publishers literature in the area of sports medicine.

Stopka C, Kaiser D: Certified athletic trainers in our secondary schools: the need and the solution, *Ath Train* 23:322, 1988. Presents information on frequency of injuries and the medical, legal, and educational benefits of employing a certified athletic trainer and describes how to hire a certified trainer.

Injury Prevention: Physical Conditioning

When you finish this chapter you will be able to:

- Identify the major conditioning seasons
- Identify and explain the major components of a conditioning program
- Explain the major procedures in warm-up and cool-down
- Describe the major aspects of developing flexibility, strength, and endurance for performance and injury prevention
- Identify overexertional muscle problems

Chapter 2 is concerned with physical conditioning as a means to preventing athletic injuries.

CONDITIONING AND ATHLETIC TRAINING

Physical conditioning for sports participation, besides preparing athletes for high-level performance, also prevents injuries (Figure 2-1). Coaches now recognize that improper conditioning is one of the major causes of sports injuries. Muscular imbalance, improper timing due to faulty neuromuscular coordination, inadequate ligamentous or tendinous strength, inadequate muscle or cardiovascular endurance, inadequate muscle bulk, problems of flexibility, and problems related to body composition are some of the primary causes of sport injury directly attributable to insufficient or improper physical conditioning and training.

Physical training is usually defined as a systematic process of repetitive, progressive exercise or work, involving the learning process and acclimatization. The great sports medicine pioneer Dr. S.E. Bilik[2] correctly stated that the primary objective of intense sports conditioning and training must be as follows: *"To put the body with extreme and exceptional care under the influence of all agents which promote its health and strength in order to enable it to meet extreme and exceptional demands upon it."*

Through the use of systematic work increments, improved voluntary responses by the organs are attained; through constant repetition, the

Lack of physical fitness is one of the primary causes of sports injuries.

Training is a systematic process of repetitive, progressive exercise or work, involving the learning process and acclimatization.

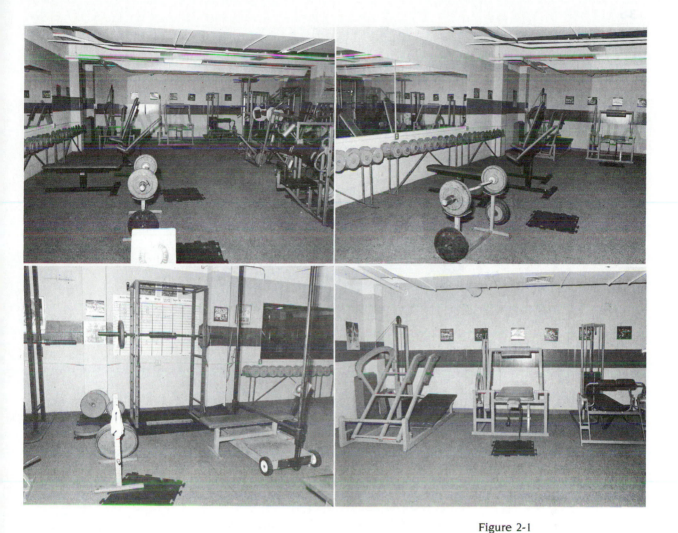

Figure 2-1

Modern sports programs often require elaborate conditioning facilities and equipment to provide sound injury prevention methods.

conscious movements become more automatic and more reflexive, requiring less concentration by the higher nerve centers and thus reducing the amount of energy expended through the elimination of movements unnecessary for performance of the desired task. Increasing the strenuousness of exercise in the ways suggested is an application of the overload principle, which holds that an activity must always be upgraded to a consistently higher level through maximum or near-maximum stimulation. In this way the metabolic level and the organic responses can be increased.

Properly graded conditioning can positively affect both the soft and bony tissues of the body (Figure 2-2). Connective tissue, comprising tendons, ligaments, and joint capsules, becomes increasingly more dense and, as a result, stronger. Stretched muscle fibers increase in their cross-sectioned width and in blood and nerve supply. Bones that are positively stressed will also increase their density and become stronger over a pe-

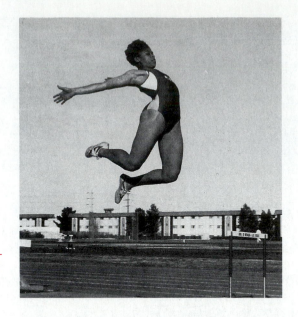

Figure 2-2

Properly graded conditioning positively affects soft and bony tissues.

riod of time. Conversely, *soft tissue and bony tissue that are adversely stressed will become weakened over time.*

It takes time and careful preparation to bring an athlete into competition at a level of fitness that will preclude early-season injury (see box on p. 39). The most dangerous period in any sport is the first 3 or 4 weeks of the season, primarily because athletes frequently are lacking in flexibility, are often overweight, and many times are out of good physical condition when they report for initial practice. Another factor is lack of familiarity with most of the fundamentals of a sport, resulting in awkwardness and a consequent proneness to potential injury-provoking situations.

Athletes are lacking in flexibility, strength, and cardiovascular conditioning during the first 3 to 4 weeks of the season. This is the most dangerous time.

Conditioning Seasons (Periodization)

No longer do serious athletes engage only in preseason conditioning and in-season competition. Sports conditioning is now a year-round endeavor. The concept of periodization is an approach to conditioning that attempts to bring about peak performance while reducing injuries and overtraining in the athlete by developing a training and conditioning program to be followed throughout the various seasons. The idea of periodization takes into account that athletes have different needs relative to training and conditioning during different seasons and modifies the program according to individual needs. For the athlete, the conditioning program often encompasses four training seasons: postseason, off-season, preseason, and in-season. This plan is especially appropriate for collision-type sports such as football. For American football, the postseason generally is from February to May; off-season, May to July; preseason, July to September; and in season, September to January.

Periodization allows athletes to train year-round with less risk of injury and staleness.

Postseason

The postseason period is immediately after a sport season. It is often dedicated to physical restoration, especially for athletes who have been injured during the season. This is a time for postsurgical rehabilitation and detailed medical evaluation.

Off-Season

It is not essential that athletes continue an intensive conditioning program during the off-season. It is, however, a good idea for the athlete to engage in another sport during this period. Such sport activity should be physiologically demanding so that strength, endurance, and flexibility are maintained. If it is not feasible for athletes to participate in an off-season sport, a *detraining program* should be planned. A moderate to strong weekly workout is usually all that is required. Keep in mind, however, that caloric intake must be decreased accordingly with the amount of exercise load that is decreased, because not as much energy is being expended. In this way extreme overweight and poor fitness can be avoided.

Preseason

If the athlete has maintained a reasonably high level of physical fitness during the off season, the preseason work will not be especially difficult. During this period the athlete should achieve the highest possible level of conditioning and training specific to the position played. At the high school level, 6 to 8 weeks of preseason conditioning afford the best insurance against susceptibility to injury and permit the athlete to enter competition in a good state of physical fitness; however, 2 to 3 weeks is most common. This is a period when the majority of muscle strength and bulk are achieved. During this preliminary period, flexibility, endurance, and strength should be emphasized in a carefully graded developmental program.

In Season

It should be noted that the intensive preseason conditioning program that brought the athlete to the competitive season may not be maintained by the sport itself. Unless there is conditioning throughout the season, a problem of deconditioning may occur. In other words, athletes who do not undergo a maintenance conditioning program may lose the ideal entry level of physiological fitness.

Cross-Training

The concept of cross-training is an approach to training and conditioning for a specific sport that involves substitution of alternative activities that have some carryover value to that sport. For example, a swimmer could engage in jogging, running, or aerobic exercise to maintain levels of cardiorespiratory conditioning. Cross-training is particularly useful in both

Sports conditioning often involves four seasons:
Postseason
Off-season
Preseason
In-season

The majority of muscle bulk and strength is achieved in preseason.

the postseason and the off-season for maintaining fitness levels and avoiding boredom that would typically occur by following the same training regimen and using the same techniques for conditioning as in the preseason and competitive season.

Foundations of Conditioning

Injury prevention can be accomplished by increasing flexibility, strength, power, and endurance. *Flexibility* involves the range of motion of a specific joint or group of joints influenced by the associated bones, muscles, and other joint structures. *Strength* is the ability of a muscular contraction to exert force to move an object (dynamic) or the ability to perform work against a fixed object (static). *Power* denotes the ability to accelerate a load and is dependent on the strength and velocity of a muscle contraction. *Endurance* is the ability of the body to undergo prolonged activity.

The *SAID principle* relates to sports conditioning and training. SAID is an acronym for *s*pecific *a*daptation to *i*mposed *d*emands. The SAID principle directs conditioning and training toward the specific demands of a given sport.

Fat and the Lean Body

The human body is generally composed of fat and a lean body mass. *Essential fat* is the survival fat that is stored around vital organs and in the bone marrow and nervous system. This usually constitutes about 3% to 5% of the total body fat in adult males and 8% to 12% in adult females. Fat other than essential fat is primarily found subcutaneously. A normal total body fat of 13% to 15% has been shown for young adult males and 22% to 25% for young women. Obesity in males is considered 20% to 25% and in females, 30%.

In terms of sports injuries prevention, excess body fat should be avoided. Excess body fat is weight that is considered "dead" and not viable. This extra weight places an added stress on the body, especially the joints, and therefore increases susceptibility to overuse problems.

Warming Up and Cooling Down

The processes of properly warming up and cooling down are believed by many authorities to have major implications in the prevention of sports injuries.[13]

Warming Up   Although warm-up is still a subject of study and results are somewhat conflicting, most evidence favors its use. The use of warm-up procedures has been traditional in sports and is still advocated as the means of preparing the body physiologically and psychologically for physical performance, in the belief that it will not only improve performance but will lessen the possibilities of injury. The term *warming up* in this discussion refers to the use of preliminary exercise procedures rather than the use of hot showers, massage, counterirritants, diathermy, or other forms of passive warm-up.

PRINCIPLES OF CONDITIONING

The following principles should be applied in all programs of training and conditioning to minimize the likelihood of injury:

1. *Warm-up/cool-down.* Take time to do an appropriate warm up before engaging in any activity. Do not neglect the cool-down period following a training session.

2. *Motivation.* Athletes are generally highly motivated to work hard because they want to be successful in their sport. By varying the training program and incorporating different aspects of conditioning, the program can remain enjoyable rather than becoming routine and boring.

3. *Overload.* To see improvement in any physiological component, the system must work harder than it is accustomed to working. Gradually, that system will adapt to the imposed demands.

4. *Consistency.* The athlete must engage in a training and conditioning program on a consistent, regularly scheduled basis if it is to be effective.

5. *Progression.* Increase the intensity of the conditioning program gradually and within the individual athlete's ability to adapt to increasing workloads.

6. *Intensity.* Stress the intensity of the work rather than the quantity. Coaches and athletic trainers too often confuse working hard with working for long periods of time. They make the mistake of prolonging the workout rather than increasing tempo or the workload. The tired athlete is prone to injury.

7. *Specificity.* Specific goals for the training program must be identified. The program must be designed to address specific components of fitness (i.e., strength, flexibility, cardiorespiratory endurance) relative to the sport in which the athlete is competing.

8. *Individuality.* The needs of individual athletes vary considerably. The successful coach is one who recognizes these individual differences and adjusts or alters the training and conditioning program accordingly to best accommodate the athlete.

9. *Minimize stress.* Expect that athletes will train as close to their physiological limits as possible. Push the athletes as far as possible but consider other stressful aspects of their lives, allowing time for the team to be away from the conditioning demands of their sport.

10. *Safety.* Make the training environment as safe as possible. Take time to educate athletes regarding proper techniques, how they should feel during the workout, and when they should push harder or back off.

Warm-up is used as a preventive measure. Studies have shown that in preconditioned muscles greater force and increase in length of stretch were necessary to tear the muscle fibers than in unconditioned muscles. This supports the practice of warming up before exercise because the process stretches the entire muscle, which results in increased length at a given load and less tension on the muscle. It is believed that a proper warm-up will prevent or reduce strains and the tearing of muscle fibers from their tendinous attachments. Most frequently the antagonist muscles are torn. Their inability to relax rapidly, plus the great contrac-

A proper warm-up before exercise will reduce the tearing of muscle fibers and prevent muscle soreness.

tile force of the agonist muscles added to the momentum of the moving part, subject the antagonists to a sudden severe strain that can result in tearing of the fibers themselves as well as their tendinous attachments. Proper warm-up can also help to reduce or prevent muscle soreness.

Physiological purposes of warming up The main purposes of warming up are to raise both the general body and the deep muscle temperatures and to stretch connective tissues to permit greater flexibility. This reduces the possibility of muscle tears and ligamentous sprains and helps to prevent muscle soreness. As cellular temperature increases, it is accompanied by a corresponding increase in the speed of the metabolic processes within the cells, because such processes are temperature dependent. For each degree of internal temperature rise there is a corresponding rise of about 13% in the rate of metabolism. At higher temperatures there is a faster and more complete dissociation of oxygen from the hemoglobin and myoglobins, which improves the oxygen supply during work. The transmission of nerve impulses speeds up as well. Overloading the muscle groups before power activities results in improved performance. It is thought that there is an increased level of excitation of the motor units that are called into play to handle the increased load and that these motor units are then carried over into the actual performance. The result is an increase in the athlete's physical working capacity.

It takes at least 15 to 30 minutes of gradual warm-up to bring the body to a state of readiness with its attendant rise in body temperature and to adequately mobilize the body physiology in terms of making a greater number of muscle capillaries available for extreme effort and of readying blood sugar and adrenaline. The time needed for satisfactory warm-up varies with the individual and tends to increase with age.

Warm-up differs in relation to the type of competition. It is advisable for athletes to warm up in activities similar to the event in which they will compete. Accordingly, a sprinter might start by jogging a bit, practice a few starts, and use some stretching techniques and general body exercises. A baseball player might first use general body exercises, swing a bat through a number of practice swings, and do preliminary throwing, alternating these activities with stretching exercises. Both overload and the use of mimetic activities appear to be important for those events in which neurovascular coordination is paramount.

The process of warming up Generally, warm-up is considered as falling into two categories: (1) the *general,* or *unrelated,* warm-up, which consists of activities that bring about a general warming of the body without having any relationship to the skills to be performed; and (2) *specific,* or *related,* warm-up, which is mimetic, that is, similar to or the same as skills to be performed in competition (such as running, throwing, and swinging).

General warm-up General warm-up procedures should consist of jogging or easy running, gradual stretching, and general exercises. These procedures should mobilize the body for action and make it supple and free. They must be of sufficient duration and intensity to raise deep tis-

Warming up involves general body warming plus specific warming to the demands of the sport.

sue temperatures without causing marked fatigue. When athletes attain a state of sweating, they have raised their internal temperatures to a desirable level. The nature of the warm-up varies to some degree in relation to the activity. Some procedures lend themselves well to athletic activities of all types and should be performed along with others that are specifically designed for the sport in which the athlete is to participate.

The exercises described in this discussion provide balance and depth in procedures, so that total body warm-up may be achieved. The athlete's daily workout, either for practice or for competition, should begin with running and the static stretches and then proceed to the calisthenic exercises.

Specific event warm-up   After completing the general exercises in the warm-up, the athletes should progress to those that are specific for their events or activities. They should start at a moderate pace and then increase the tempo as they feel body temperature and cardiovascular increases taking place. The effects of warm-up may persist as long as 45 minutes. However, the closer the warm-up period is to the actual performance, the more beneficial it will be in terms of its effect on the performance. For the athlete to benefit optimally from warm-up, no more than 15 minutes should elapse between the completion of the warm-up and the performance of the activity itself.

Cooling Down   Cooling down applies to exercise of gradually diminishing intensity that follows strenuous work and permits the return of both the circulation and various body functions to preexercise levels. From 30 seconds to 1 minute of jogging, followed by 3 to 5 minutes of walking, permits the body to effect the necessary readjustments.

Physiologically, an important reason for cooling down is that blood and muscle lactic acid levels decrease more rapidly during active recovery than during passive recovery. Also, active recovery keeps the muscle pumps active, which prevents blood from pooling in the extremities (see Table 2-1). Empirical evidence seems to indicate that athletes who stretch

Proper cooling decreases blood and muscle lactic acid levels more rapidly.

TABLE 2-1 Suggested schedule for conditioning program for sports competition to reduce injuries		
Phase	**Estimated Time**	**Activities**
Warm-up	15-30 minutes	Jogging, gradual stretching, and general exercise followed by activities specific to the sport; gradually increasing intensity until the body begins to sweat
Activity	1-2 hours	No more than 15 minutes should elapse between warm-up and the activity
Cool-down	15-20 minutes	Jogging 1-3 minutes followed by 3-5 minutes of walking; end with gradual stretching of major muscle groups

during the cool-down period tend to have fewer problems with muscle soreness after strenuous activity, which can result from ischemia in the working tissues.

Flexibility

Flexibility is defined as the range of movement of a specific joint or group of joints influenced by the associated bones and bony structures and the physiological characteristics of the muscles, tendons, ligaments, and the various other collagenous tissues surrounding the joint. Studies have indicated that an increase in the flexibility of inflexible joints tends to decrease the injuries to those joints. In most instances it is also contended that an increase in flexibility contributes to better athletic performance. Both of these considerations are important to the coach and athletic trainer.

Good flexibility usually indicates that there are no adhesions or abnormalities present in or around the joints and that there are no serious muscular limitations. This allows the body to move freely and easily through the full range-of-joint flexion and extension without any unnecessary restrictions in the joints or the adjacent tissues. Examples of static flexibility exercises are shown on pp. 43-45.

Most authorities in sports consider flexibility one of the most important objectives in conditioning athletes.[13] Good flexibility increases the athlete's ability to avoid injury. Since it permits a greater range of movement within the joint, the ligaments and other connective tissues are not so easily strained or torn. It also permits greater freedom of movement in all directions. There appears to be a definite relationship between injury and joint flexibility. The "tight" or inflexible athlete performs under a considerable handicap in terms of movement, besides being much more injury prone. Tight-jointed athletes seem to be more susceptible to muscle strains and tears. Repetitive stretching of the collagenous or fascial ligamentous tissue over a long period of time permits the athlete to obtain an increased range of motion.

Conversely, **hyperflexibility**, defined as flexibility beyond a joint's normal range of motion, is of little performance value and can result in weakness of the joint at certain angles. Flexibility is usually specific to a given joint and varies among athletes.

IMPROVING FLEXIBILITY THROUGH STRETCHING TECHNIQUES

The maintenance of a full, nonrestricted range of motion has long been recognized as an essential component of physical fitness. Flexibility is important not only for successful physical performance but also in the prevention of injury.[1]

The goal of any effective flexibility program should be to improve the range of motion at a given articulation by altering the extensibility of the musculotendinous units that produce movements at that joint. It is well documented that exercises that stretch these musculotendinous units over a period of time will increase the range of movement possible about a given joint.[15]

Conditioning should be performed gradually, with work being added in small increments.

The "tight" or inflexible athlete performs under a considerable handicap in terms of movement.

hyperflexibility
Flexibility beyond a joint's normal range

Stretching techniques for improving flexibility have evolved over the years. The oldest technique for stretching is called *ballistic stretching*, which makes use of repetitive bouncing motions.

A second technique, known as *static stretching*, involves stretching a muscle to the point of discomfort and then holding it at that point for an extended period of time. This technique has been used for many years. Recently another group of stretching techniques, known collectively as *proprioceptive neuromuscular facilitation (PNF)* involving alternating contractions and stretches, has also been recommended.[10]

Ballistic Stretching

Ballistic stretching techniques have not been recommended during recent years because of danger in exceeding the extensibility limits of the muscle when performing these bouncing movements. Ballistic stretching should be avoided in sedentary individuals. However, in athletes who are highly conditioned there is little likelihood that a muscle can be injured by stretching ballistically.

ballistic stretching
Older stretching technique that uses repetitive bouncing motions

Static Stretching

The **static stretching** technique is extremely effective and popular. This technique involves passively stretching a given antagonist muscle by placing it in a maximal position of stretch and holding it there for an extended time. Recommendations for the optimum time for holding this stretched position vary from as short as 3 seconds to as long as 60 seconds.[10] Data are inconclusive at present; however, it appears that 20 seconds may be sufficient. The static stretch of each muscle should be repeated 3 or 4 times.

static stretching
Passively stretching an antagonist muscle by placing it in a maximal stretch and holding it there

STATIC FLEXIBILITY EXERCISES

Hamstring stretch Starting position—sitting with legs straight, feet 8 inches apart. Keeping the knees straight, the athlete reaches forward and grasps either ankles or toes, depending on the extensibility of the hamstring muscles. NOTE: The stretch must first be felt in back of the knees and then in the low back.

Upper hamstring stretch Starting position—sitting with legs extended and grasping the right ankle with the left hand and underneath the knee with the right hand. The athlete then brings the leg as a unit toward the chest, stretching the hamstring muscles. NOTE: No pressure should be placed on the knee and the knee should be kept close to the chest.

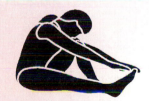

Hamstring stretch

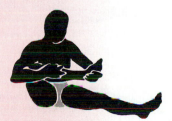

Upper hamstring stretch

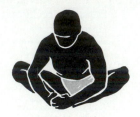

Groin stretch

Groin stretch   Starting position—sitting with knees bent and the soles of the feet together and grasping both forefeet with both hands. Both elbows should rest on the lower legs. The athlete then leans the trunk forward while pressing downward on the bent legs.

Achilles tendon (gastrocnemius) stretch   Starting position—while facing a wall or other similar support, one leg is positioned back while leaning toward the wall. With the left foot flat, heel down, and knee straight, the stretch is to the gastrocnemius with the right knee bent. Stretch is focused on the Achilles tendon. The stretch can be varied by first stretching with the foot straight ahead, then adducted and, finally, abducted.

Soleus stretch   Starting position—Using the same position as in the achilles tendon (gastrocnemius stretch), flex the left knee, keeping the left heel on the ground and leaning forward to stretch the soleus.

Hip flexor stretch   Starting position—with the right foot flat, the knee is bent, and the left leg is extended straight backward. The trunk is then lowered as far as possible and positioned as far forward as possible. The stretch should be felt in the groin region.

Quadriceps stretch   Starting position—first the body is positioned on the left side, and the right foot is grasped with the right hand while the right knee is bent. To add to the stretch the hip is moved forward. The stretch is then repeated on the left side. NOTE: Avoid putting stress on the knee joint.

Trunk and leg stretch   Starting position—with the arms extended overhead and legs straight, feet pointed, the athlete reaches overhead as far as possible and feet downward as much as possible. Stretching occurs to the posterior aspect of the arms, back, and legs.

Sitting low back stretch   Starting position—sitting in a cross-legged position, the athlete leans forward, stretching the low back.

Rocking low back stretch   Starting position—lying on the back, the knees are grasped with both hands, with the head curling forward far as possible toward the knees. In this position the athlete gently rocks back and forth.

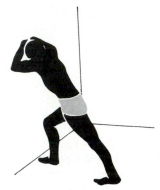

Achilles tendon (gastrocnemius) stretch

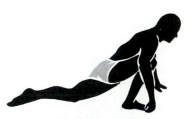

Hip flexor stretch

Quadriceps stretch

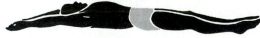

Trunk and leg stretch

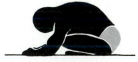

Sitting low back stretch

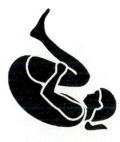

Rocking

Spinal twist   Starting position—sitting, legs fully extended; then the right leg is bent under the left leg. The heel of the left foot is then placed just in front of the bent right knee. Next, the trunk is twisted to the left, and the right elbow is positioned on the lateral aspect of the left knee. If possible, the foot or ankle of the right leg is grasped by the right hand. From this position the trunk and head are rotated toward the left while the right elbow pushes backward on the bent left knee. The back is kept straight. This sequence of movements is repeated on the opposite side.

Kneeling shoulder stretch   Starting position—taking a four-point position, the arm or arms are extended as far in front of the head as possible. At the same time the trunk and face are lowered as much as possible to accentuate the stretch.

Double anterior shoulder stretch   Starting position—both hands are grasped behind the back, with elbows fully extended. In this position both arms are slowly raised as far as possible while maintaining a fully upright posture.

Single anterior shoulder stretch   Starting position—standing fully upright, the left arm is placed behind the back, with the right arm raised to the side. In this position the right arm is pulled as far backward as possible, stretching the anterior shoulder.

Overhead shoulder stretch   Starting position—both arms are raised above the head. The left elbow is bent and is grasped with the right hand. The left upper arm is then gently pulled toward the midline of the body. Repeat with the other side.

Overhead/behind back shoulder stretch   Starting position—the left arm is raised overhead and the hand is positioned behind the head and as far down the back as possible. The right elbow is then placed behind the back, with the hand reaching upward as far as possible. Ideally, the fingers of both hands grasp. If grasping is not possible, connection can be made by holding onto a towel.

Neck rotation stretch   Starting position—standing or sitting with good posture, slowly rotate head to the right until a gentle stretch is felt. Repeat on the left side.

Lateral neck stretch   Starting position—standing or sitting with good posture, slowly bend the neck laterally and, if possible, touch the right ear to the tip of the right shoulder. Repeat on the opposite side.

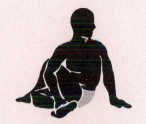

Spinal twist

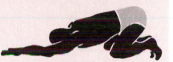

Kneeling shoulder stretch

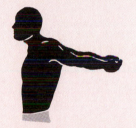

Double anterior shoulder stretch

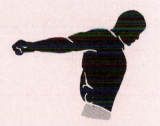

Single anterior shoulder stretch

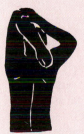

Overhead shoulder stretch

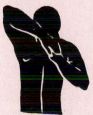

Overhead/behind back shoulder stretch

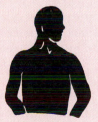

Neck rotation stretch

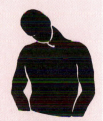

Lateral neck stretch

1. When to stretch
   a. After a general warm-up; before engaging in any vigorous conditioning activity or sports performance.
   b. After cooling down; following any vigorous activity.
2. How to stretch[1]
   a. Warm up musculoskeletal system through some repetitive activity, bringing skin to a light sweat (e.g., jogging, rope jumping).
   b. Begin with an *easy stretch*, holding for 20 to 30 seconds (this produces mild muscle tension and relaxation).
   c. When stretching, focus on muscle region that is pulling the body part into a stretch position (agonists).
   d. Following the easy stretch, proceed to the next phase—the *developmental stretch;* move to a moderate stretch position for 20 to 30 seconds.
   e. Avoid breath holding at all times. As the developmental stretch is performed, exhale the air from the lungs completely as the stretch is assumed; follow with breathing that is slow, relaxed, and rhythmic.
   f. Avoid severe, painful stretching. Overstretching an area will defeat the purpose of the activity.
   g. Each stretch may be executed one to three times per day. The minimum number of stretch sessions per week is three. Ideally, athletes who have severe restriction of range of motion should stretch daily until a more normal range has been attained.

proprioceptive neuromuscular facilitation (PNF)
Stretching techniques that involve combinations of alternating contractions and stretches

Isometric exercises are performed against a solid object.

Muscle stretching through PNF A number of **PNF** techniques are used for stretching—the slow-reversal–hold relax, the contract-relax, and the hold-relax techniques. All three involve various combinations of alternating the contraction and relaxation of both agonist and antagonist muscles. All techniques consist of a 5- or 10-second pushing phase, followed by a 5- to 10-second relaxation phase (Figure 2-3).

In using the slow-reversal–hold-relax technique on the hamstring muscle, the following steps are executed: the athlete lies on his or her back with the knee extended and ankle flexed at 90 degrees. The coach or teammate flexes the athlete's leg at the hip joint until mild discomfort is felt in the hamstring region. At this time, the athlete pushes against the operator's resistance by contracting the hamstring muscle. After pushing 5 to 10 seconds, the athlete relaxes his or her hamstring, and the agonist quadricep muscle is contracted while the athletic trainer applies a passive stretch to further stretch the hamstrings. This process is repeated three times.

In the contract-relax technique, the hamstrings are actively (isotonically) contracted, moving the leg toward a flat surface on the push phase. The hold-relax method consists of a hamstring contraction against an immovable (isometric) resistance during the push phase. With both the contract-relax and the hold-relax techniques, there is a relaxation of hamstring and quadricep muscles, followed by a passive stretch of the hamstring muscles.

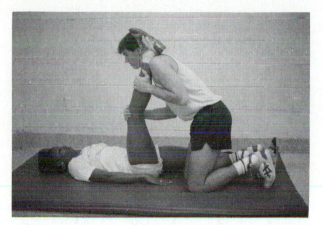

Figure 2-3

The slow-reversal–hold-relax
technique for stretching the
hamstring muscles.

Muscular Strength

The development of muscular strength is an essential component for the
competitive athlete. By definition, **muscular strength** is the maximum
force that can be applied by a muscle during a single maximal contraction.

Strength Differences Between Men and Women

A woman in weight training will probably see more remarkable gains in
strength initially, even though muscle bulk does not increase.

For a muscle to contract, an impulse must be transmitted from the
nervous system to the muscle. Each muscle fiber is innervated by a specific motor unit. By overloading a particular muscle, as in weight training, the muscle is forced to work efficiently. Efficiency is achieved by getting more motor units to fire, causing a stronger contraction of the
muscle. Consequently, it is not uncommon for a woman to see extremely
rapid gains in strength when a weight-training program is first begun.
These tremendous initial gains, which can be attributed to improved neuromuscular system efficiency, tend to plateau, and minimal improvement
in muscular strength will be realized during a continuing strength-
training program. These initial neuromuscular strength gains will also be
seen in men, although their strength will continue to increase with appropriate training.

Perhaps the most critical difference between men and women regarding physical performance is the ratio of strength to weight. The reduced
strength/body weight ratio in women is the result of their higher percentage of body fat. The strength/body weight ratio may be significantly
improved through weight training by decreasing the body fat percentage
while increasing lean weight. Strength training programs for women
should follow the same guidelines as those for men.

Techniques of Strength Training

The principle of overload is one of the basic premises of strength training. Frequent repetitions, if not coincidental with increases in work load,

muscular strength
Maximum force that can be
applied by a muscle during a
single maximal contraction

Perhaps the most critical
performance difference
between men and women is
the ratio of strength to
weight.

are of little value for this purpose, although the total work load may be equal.

Muscular strength can show an increase of three times or more without a proportional increase in muscle bulk necessarily being indicated. However, exercise must be performed against near-maximum and gradually increasing resistance. Such resistance can be obtained either by lifting, pulling, or pushing against some resistive force that requires near-maximum effort for the individual; by moving the body at an ever-increasing rate of speed that is approaching the maximum level of performance; or by a combination of the two. It is important for the coach to know that a number of factors are involved in strength training. The speed, duration, number of repetitions, and vigor or force with which exercises are performed will determine the outcome of the program. The variable of individual difference is another factor that will affect the final result. Two athletes of the same gender following identical programs will not develop strength at the same rate, in the same manner, or to the same degree, because of varying inherent characteristics.

Two athletes of the same gender following identical programs will not develop strength at the same rate, in the same manner, or to the same degree, because of varying inherent characteristics.

Muscle Contraction and Exercise

Exercise for the development of strength is related to the type of muscle contraction.

Isometric   An isometric muscle contraction is one in which there is no change in the length of the muscle or in the angle of the joint at which the contraction takes place. **Isometric exercise** (Figure 2-4) has been shown to be most effective when 6 to 10 maximal contractions are held for at least 6 seconds. After resting between each bout, the athlete repeats the exercise 5 to 10 times. Strength gained through an isometric exercise is specific to the joint angle at which the contraction takes place. It is commonly used in rehabilitation and not conditioning.

isometric exercise
Contracts the muscle statically without changing its length

Figure 2-4

In isometric exercise the muscle is contracted on a static position against resistance.

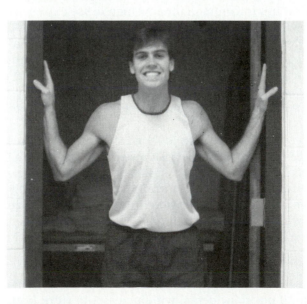

ISOMETRIC EXERCISES

Stationary press bar leg thrust   Starting position—angle-lying position under the press bar, balls of the feet in contact with the bar or bar platform, legs in a half-flexed position. Press bar is locked into place. Exert maximum force against the immovable bar, sustaining full pressure for 6 to 10 seconds. Following a short period of relaxation (5 to 10 seconds) repeat the procedure two or three times. NOTE: Hips may be elevated by a 2-inch pad.

Stationary press bar leg tensor   Starting position—a half-crouched position under the bar, which is locked into place, shoulders and neck in contact with the bar. Exert maximum pressure against the bar by using the leg extensors and sustain full pressure for 6 to 10 seconds. Following a momentary relaxation, repeat the exercise two or three times.

Wall press   Starting position—stand in a small side-stride stand in either the corner of a room or a doorway, placing the hands against the walls or the sides of the opening at about shoulder height. The elbows should be bent to about the halfway point in the normal range. Exert maximum force against the opposing surface, holding the position for at least 6 to 10 seconds. Relax pressure momentarily. Repeat two or three times.

Shoulder-arm tensor   Starting position—feet in a small side-stride stand. Hook the fingers of the hands together, elbows bent so that hands are above waist height. Push the hands together forcefully, at the same time tensing the arm, shoulder, neck, and abdominal muscles. Hold for 6 to 10 seconds. Relax momentarily and then repeat the tensing action but reverse the hand action by pulling against the fingers with as much force as possible. Repeat two or three times.

Isotonics   Shortening or lengthening the muscle, causing a skeletal part to be moved through a full range of motion, is an isotonic contraction. **Isotonic exercise** (Figure 2-5) involves moving a resistive force,

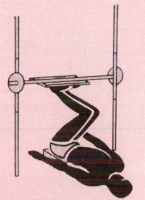

Stationary press
bar leg thrust

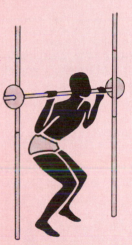

Stationary press
bar leg tensor

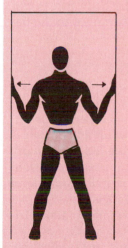

Wall press

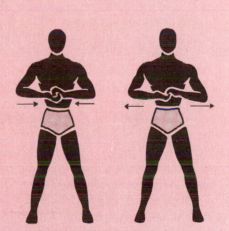

Shoulder-arm tensor

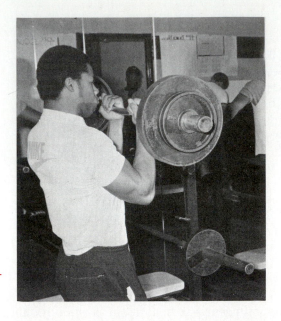

Figure 2-5

An example of an isotonic exercise.

isotonic exercise
Shortens and lengthens the muscle through a complete range of motion

either a body part or some object, and may also be referred to as *dynamic* contraction. An isotonic exercise does not involve the same muscle fibers throughout a particular movement because the load remains constant regardless of the angle of contraction and the degree of fatigue. Thus the greatest strength gain is in those fibers used in the initial part of the movement, when inertia is overcome. The least strength gain is at the midpoint of the contraction.

The major values of performing exercises involving isotonic contraction are that they promote joint range of motion and increase circulation and endurance. During an isotonic movement against resistance, the muscle should first be placed in a stretched position to ensure maximal innervation to the muscle fibers. After full stretch, the body part is *concentrically* moved as far as possible and then *eccentrically* moved to the beginning stretch position.

ISOTONIC EXERCISES

Military press   Starting position—feet in a side-stride stand, barbell raised to the bent-arm position in front of chest. Slowly extend arms overhead. Hold. Return to starting position; three sets of 10 repetitions.

Two-arm curl   Reverse or under grip and regular or upper grip. Starting position—feet in a side-stride stand, arms extended downward. Slowly flex elbows, bringing the barbell to a bent-arm position in front of chest. Return to starting position. NOTE: Keep elbows close to side of body. Alternate grasp on each series; three sets of 10 repetitions.

Half squat   Heels are elevated approximately 1½ inches, and a 20-inch bench is placed behind the buttocks to reduce the possibility of knee injury by serving as a "stop." Starting position—feet in a small side-stride

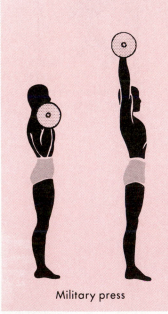

Military press

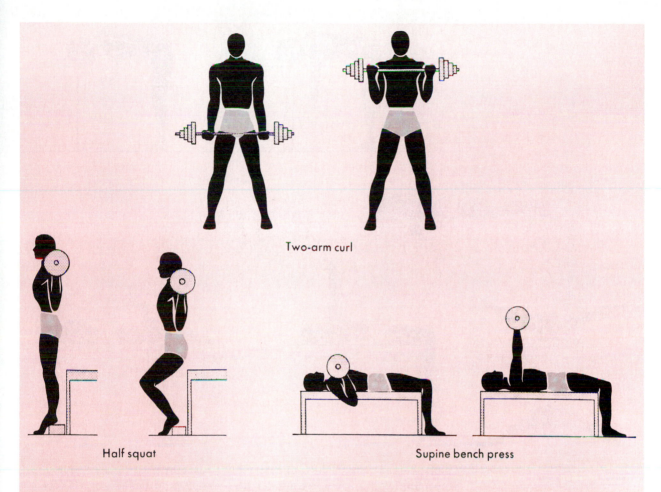

Two-arm curl

Half squat

Supine bench press

stand, barbell resting on back of neck and shoulders. Slowly bend knees to half-squat position. Hold. Return to starting position; three sets of 10 repetitions.

Supine bench press   Starting position—lying supine on a 20-inch bench, knees bent at right angles, feet flat on the floor, and barbell held at the chest. Slowly extend arms upward. Hold. Return to starting position; three sets of 10 repetitions.

Rowing exercise   Starting position—feet in a small side-stride stand, arms extended downward with hands centered and in proximity to the bar, head resting on a folded towel placed on a table. Slowly pull the bar up to a position in front of the chest. Hold. Return to starting position; three sets of 10 repetitions. NOTE: This may also be done with the lifter assuming and maintaining an angle stand—that is, trunk flexed forward at the hips at approximately a right angle.

Side-arm raises   Starting position—prone or supine position on a bench, arms downward, hands grasping 10-pound dumbbells. Slowly raise arms sideward to a horizontal position. Hold. Return to starting po-

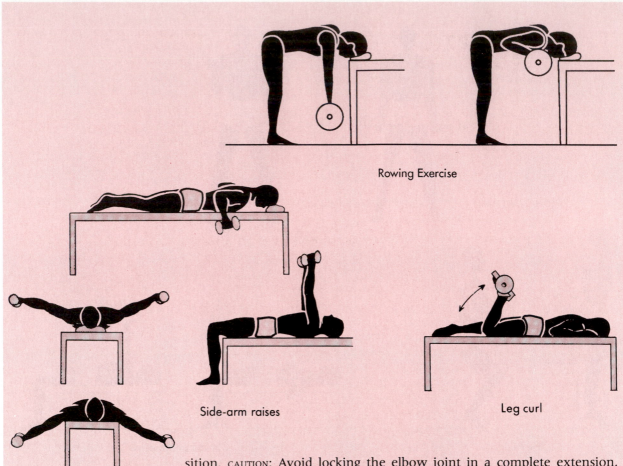

Rowing Exercise

Side-arm raises

Leg curl

sition. CAUTION: Avoid locking the elbow joint in a complete extension, since this exerts severe strain on the joint. Do three sets of 10 repetitions, alternating the prone and supine positions daily.

Leg Curl Starting position—face-lying position with boot weight fixed to one foot. The leg is curled upward as far as possible and then slowly returned to its original position; three sets of 10 repetitions and then repeat with other leg.

Heel raise Starting position—feet in a small side-stride stand, balls of the feet on a 2-inch riser, barbell resting on the back of the neck and shoulders. Slowly rise on toes. Hold. Return to starting position. Variations may be performed by having the feet either toes out or toes in; three sets of 10 repetitions.

Press bar leg thrust Starting position—angle-lying position under the press bar, balls of the feet in contact with the bar or bar platform, legs in a half-flexed position. Slowly extend the knees, keeping the buttocks in contact with the floor. Hold. Return to starting position; three sets of 10 repetitions. NOTE: To provide for better contact, fasten an 8-inch by 12-inch board to the bar. This prevents the feet from slipping off the bar.

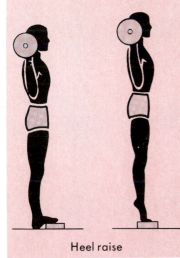

Heel raise

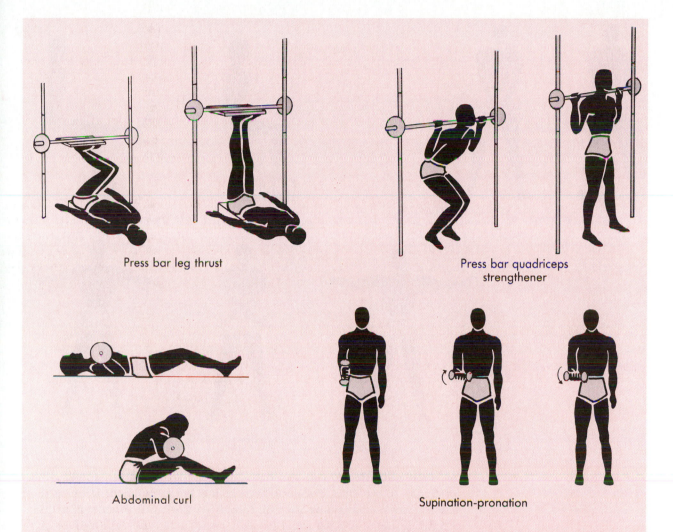

Press bar leg thrust

Press bar quadriceps
strengthener

Abdominal curl

Supination-pronation

Press bar quadriceps strengthener Starting position—a half-crouched position under the bar. Shoulders and neck in contact with the bar. (A folded towel may be used as a pad.) Slowly extend knees to an erect position. Hold. Return to starting position; three sets of 10 repetitions. CAUTION: Lift with the knee extensors, not the lower back muscles.

Abdominal curl Starting position—hook-lying, feet anchored, and dumbbell weighing 15 to 25 pounds held on the upper chest. Curl the upper trunk upward and as far forward as possible. Return slowly to the starting position. Maintain a moderate tempo and steady rhythm and avoid bouncing up from the floor; three sets of 10 repetitions. Number can be increased as capacity for more work increases.

Supination-pronation Start with feet in small side-stride stand, elbow bent at a right angle to upper arm, and hand grasping a 20-pound dumbbell. Rotate the dumbbell alternately left and right, using the muscles of the forearm and wrist only; three sets of 10 repetitions.

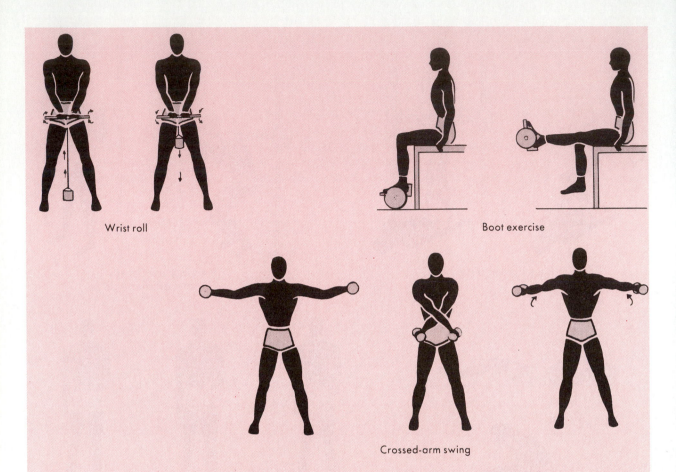

Wrist roll

Boot exercise

Crossed-arm swing

Wrist roll   Begin with feet in a small side-stride stand. Slowly wind up a cord to which a 25-pound weight has been attached. Reverse the action, slowly unwinding the full length of the cord; three sets of five repetitions. NOTE: A wrist roller is easily constructed by securing one end of a 30-inch length of sash cord to the center of a 12-inch length of broomstick or dowel of a somewhat thicker diameter and the other end to a 25-pound weight.

Boot exercise   Sit on plinth or table with lower legs hanging free over the edge and clear of the floor. A 20-pound boot is strapped to the foot. Do exercises involving knee flexion and extension and inversion, eversion, flexion, and extension of the ankle. The weight should be increased with the ability to handle it. Each exercise should be done for three sets of 10 repetitions.

Crossed-arm swings   Starting position—small side-stride stand, a 20-pound dumbbell in each hand, arms raised directly sideward to shoulder height. Slowly swing the arms forward in a horizontal plane, continuing until each arm has progressed across the other and is carried as far as possible. Arms are extended, but elbow joints should not be locked. Return slowly toward the starting position, carrying the arms horizontally as far backward as possible; three sets of 10 repetitions.

Concentric contraction, or **positive resistance,** refers to shortening of the muscle. Eccentric contraction, or **negative resistance,** refers to lengthening of the muscle. Eccentric muscle action enervates more muscle fibers, is capable of producing higher forces, and uses less oxygen than a concentric contraction. In pylometric exercise an eccentric contraction immediately precedes a concentric contraction. The forces generated by the subsequent concentric contraction significantly increase because of the apparent storage and recovery of elastic energy in the muscle fibers. Note that eccentric contraction tends to cause more muscle soreness.

Recovery from muscular fatigue is more rapid in isotonic than in isometric exercise. Isotonic exercises that involve increasingly greater resistance are known as progressive resistance exercises (PREs) and were introduced by DeLorme and Watkins.[4] Although there are many variations to the DeLorme method, it originally made use of a series of three exercise sets having 10 repetitions in each set. The first set is performed against a resistance equal to half of one's maximum effort, the second at three-fourths maximum effort, and the final set against a full maximum effort. When the athlete is easily able to perform the third set, the weight increment is increased by 2½ to 5 pounds. Workouts commonly take place every other day, or three to four times weekly. Although 10 repetitions will increase strength, four to eight repetitions will produce the greatest increase in strength.

The use of a lifting belt is strongly recommended for resistance training. During lifting, the belt increases intraabdominal pressure, which has been shown to reduce disc-compressive forces in the low back. This in turn reduces the risk of injury and increases safety while lifting.

Variable resistance is a common strength training method used with many commercial machines. It uses nearly total involvement of the muscle fibers because the resistance varies according to the angle of pull. The inertia of the resistance varies according to the angle of pull. The inertia of the resistance, a definite factor in other isotonic exercises, is not a factor in variable-resistance exercise, since the resistance is varied throughout the range of motion. Therefore the user can maintain a constant and consistent force throughout the various strength levels in the working muscles.[7] Both constant isotonic and variable-resistance machines allow lifting a weight in an eccentric manner that can result in significant gains in strength. However, one drawback of excessive eccentric loading is that it seems to create more muscle soreness than any other methods.

Nautilus, for example, uses a shell-shaped cam to alter the load throughout the range of motion. As the pulley chain moves around the cam, the distance of the resistance arm changes so that the resistance felt by the muscle at its strongest point is greater than at its weakest point (Figure 2-6). This allows for balanced resistance, both eccentric and concentric work, and a variable and rotary form of resistance.

Accommodating resistance is a form of **isokinetic exercise.** Like variable resistance, it uses total involvement of the muscle fibers. It

positive resistance
Slow concentric muscle contraction against resistance with muscle shortening

negative resistance
Slow eccentric muscle contraction against resistance with muscle lengthening

variable resistance
Resistance is varied throughout the range of motion

accommodating resistance
Form of isokinetic exercises where speed is an element

isokinetic exercise
Amount of resistance depends on the extent of force applied by the athlete, and speed is constant

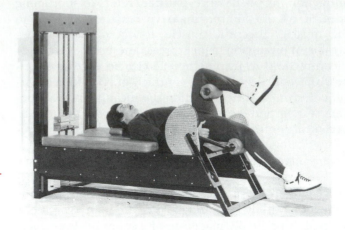

Figure 2-6

Nautilus training provides body stabilization and muscle group isolation.

produces resistance according to the exerted resistance of the working muscles and varies by range of motion and the degree of fatigue developed throughout the exercise. Speed is the key element distinguishing it from other forms of strength training. The rate of speed, not the amount of resistance, is selected on a dial. No matter how much force is exerted by the muscle tension, the machine will allow the movement to proceed only at the set speed. Using this method, a maximal contraction of the muscles at all joint angles will be matched by a maximal resistance at all joint angles. A major advantage of this method is the ability to train at different speeds, thus developing not only strength but also power and endurance. A major disadvantage is that results depend on the athlete's motivation to work at a maximal level throughout the training session.

Neither isotonic, variable resistance, nor accommodating resistance is superior to the others. The goal of training must be satisfied according to the SAID principle. Over the last few years accommodating resistance has found a valuable place in rehabilitation, just as free weights employing isotonic principles have become increasingly popular in sports conditioning. The hard-working athlete will derive benefits from either weights or machines; the athlete who is unwilling to extend a maximum effort will benefit from neither.

plyometric exercise
Maximizes the stretch reflex

Plyometric training Plyometric training is an exercise technique that includes specific exercises that encompass a rapid stretch of a muscle eccentrically, followed immediately by a rapid concentric contraction of that muscle for the purpose of facilitating and developing a forceful explosive movement over a short period of time. The greater the stretch put on the muscle from its resting length immediately before the concentric contraction, the greater the load the muscle can lift or overcome. Plyometrics emphasize the speed of the eccentric phase. The rate of the stretch is more critical than the magnitude of the strength.

Plyometric exercises   involve hops, bounds, and depth jumping for the lower extremity and the use of medicine balls and other weighted

TABLE 2-2 Comparison of strength exercises

	Isometric	Isotonic	Isokinetic	Variable Resistance (Nautilus)
Resistance	Accommodating at one angle	Constant	Accommodating through range of motion	Fixed ratio through range of motion
Velocity (speed)	Zero	Variable	Constant	Variable
Reciprocal contraction	None	None	Yes	None
Eccentric contraction	None	Yes	Yes	Yes
Safeness	Excellent	Poor	Excellent	Poor
Specificity to sport	Low	Medium	Very high	Medium
Motivation to exercise	Low	High	Medium	High

equipment for the upper extremity. Depth jumping is an example of a plyometric technique in which an athlete jumps to the ground from a specified height and then quickly jumps again as soon as ground contact is made.

Plyometric exercises tend to put a great deal of stress on the musculoskeletal system. To reduce the incidence of injury, the learning and perfection of specific jumping skills must be technically correct and specific to one's age, event, and physical and skill development.

Ways of Achieving Strength

Individuals can gain strength in numerous ways (see Table 2-2 for a comparison of strength exercises). This discussion briefly describes the more prevalent ways strength is developed; they are the nonequipment, equipment, and combined nonequipment and equipment approaches.

Nonequipment approaches Three nonequipment approaches are presently employed in sports conditioning: calisthenics, or free exercise; partner, or reciprocal, resistance; and self-resistance.

Calisthenics, or *free exercise,* is one of the more easily available means of developing strength. Isotonic movement exercises can be graded according to intensity by using gravity as an aid, ruling gravity out, moving against gravity, or using the body or body part as a resistance against gravity. Most calisthenics require the athlete to support the body or move the total body against the force of gravity. Push-ups are a good example of a vigorous antigravity free exercise. When isotonic movements are made, 10 or more repetitions are performed for each exercise and repeated in sets of two or three.

Some free exercises have a holding phase instead of employing a full range of motion. Examples of these are back extensions and sit-ups. When the exercise produces maximal muscle tension, it is held between 6 and 10 seconds and then repeated one to three times.

Partner, or *reciprocal, resistance exercise* requires no equipment other than a partner who is about equal in size and strength. It is often highly

Calisthenics, or free exercise, use the force of gravity as resistance.

Reciprocal exercise requires a partner who is about equal in size, weight, and strength.

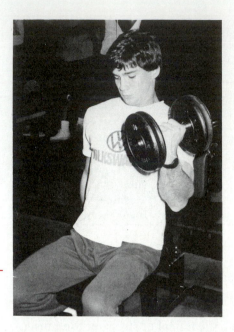

Figure 2-7

Dumbbells provide an excellent means for isotonic strength development.

motivating for both participants, and all types of exercise can be done using this method. When performing isokinetic resistance, the body part involved is taken into a stretched position by the partner. Resistance is accommodated through a complete range of motion. Three bouts of resistance usually are given for each exercise.

Equipment approaches Modern athletic training programs include numerous devices designed to overload the musculature and develop strength. These range from individual pieces to entire conditioning systems and generally are categorized as isotonic/isometric and isokinetic.

The different kinds of *isotonic/isometric equipment* are almost too numerous to mention. Some of the standard stationary apparatus—chinning bars, parallel bars, and stall bars—have numerous possibilities for increasing strength. Another standard piece of equipment is the wall-pulley weight, which progressively exercises the major joints and muscles.

Free weights are very popular and are used for developing strength through both isotonic and isometric contraction. Sports programs commonly use a variety of free weights, including dumbbells (Figure 2-7) and barbells (Figure 2-8). Dumbbells range from 2 to 2½ pounds to 50 to 75 pounds or more, and barbells range from 25 to 30 pounds to well over 200 pounds. Free weights help in the development of balance and coordination and exercise the stabilizing and accessory muscles, which machine systems often do not do.[11] Certain barbell exercises, such as squats, bench presses, and incline presses, should be performed with the assistance of a spotter, who can assist in taking the barbell from and return-

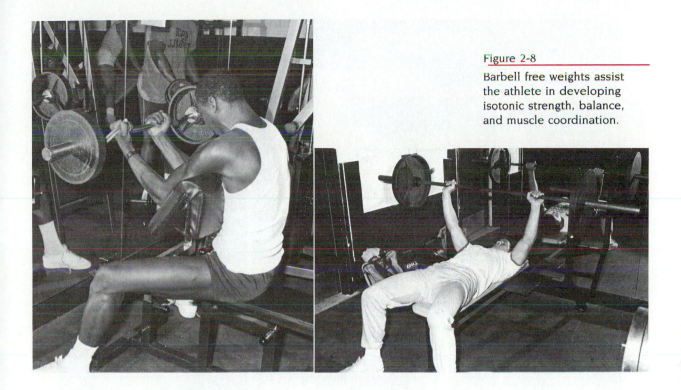

Figure 2-8

Barbell free weights assist the athlete in developing isotonic strength, balance, and muscle coordination.

ing it to the supports. The spotter is also a considerable safety factor in case the lifter gets trapped under a heavy weight.

Machine exercise systems such as the *Universal Gym* allow a variety of exercises such as sit-ups, parallel bar dips, bench presses, pull-downs, rowing exercises, knee extensions, knee curls, and biceps curls, as well as arm pressing (Figure 2-9). The Universal Gym employs graduated weights that are lifted by heavy cables as the athlete applies force against a bar. Newer Universal Gym machines provide variable resistance.

Fundamental Principles of Isotonic Weight Training

In a weight-training program certain fundamental principles must be followed by each athlete:

1. Precede all weight training with the general warm-up.
2. Begin all isotonic contractions from a position of stretch, immediately moving into the concentric contraction.
3. Perform isotonic movements slowly and deliberately, at approximately one-fifth maximal speed.
4. Apply the overload principle in all isotonic contractions. When you are able to complete the second or third series with some degree of ease, add more resistance.
5. Maintain good muscular balance by exercising both the agonist and antagonist muscles.

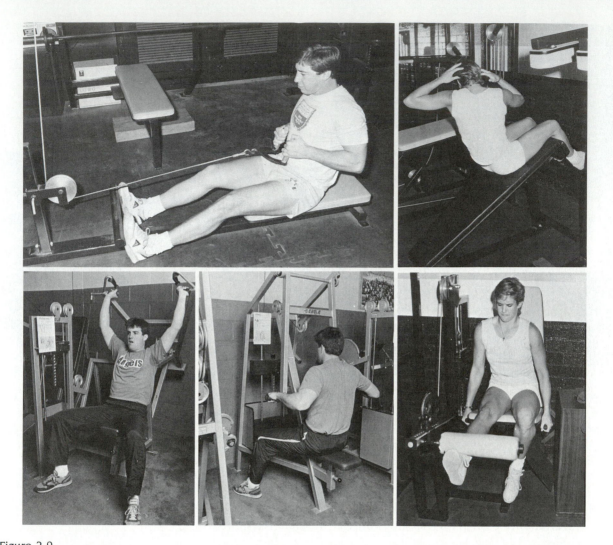

Figure 2-9

Many machine exercise systems provide a variety of exercise possibilities for the athlete.

6. Confine heavy work to the off-season and the preseason. A light to medium program can be maintained during the regular practice days of the competitive season, provided it is confined to use of the weight schedules after the regular practice.

7. Work with weights every other day, or no more than 4 days a week. This allows ample time for reduction of soreness and stiffness.

8. Initiate the training program first in terms of general body development and then progress to exercises tailored to the specific sport or event employing the SAID principle and geared to the type of muscle fiber involved in the activity.

9. After a general warm-up, begin a preliminary series of about 10 repetitions using approximately half of the weight normally used. This is usually a sound procedure.

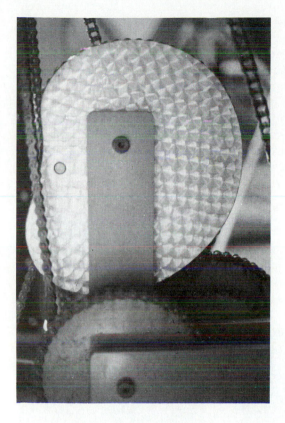

Figure 2-10

The cam system on the Nautilus equipment is designed to equalize the resistance throughout the full range of motion.

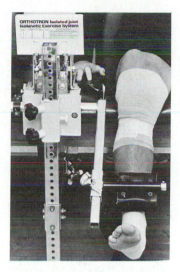

Figure 2-11

Nautilus variable resistance machine.

10. Observe proper breathing procedures during lifting to assist in fixing the stabilizing muscles of the trunk and therefore to give a firm base from which to work. Inhale deeply as the lift is being executed, and exhale forcefully and smoothly at the end of the lift.

11. Evaluate your progress at certain intervals of time by testing maximum lifts.

12. Develop a recording system using cards or a notebook.

Variable resistance machines, such as Nautilus, Soloflex, and some Universal machines, provide full range of movement and direct resistance to specific muscles or muscle groups. The Nautilus training machines provide both concentric and eccentric muscle contraction by special cams and counterweights (Figure 2-10).[17] In this system, negative, or eccentric, work is accentuated. Each machine provides body stabilization to afford isolation of a specific muscle or muscle group. Because the amount of resistance varies during a full range of motion, resistance is indicated by the number of plates lifted rather than the number of pounds (Figure 2-11).

Accommodating resistance machines provide an accommodating resistance through a full range of motion. A maximal load is produced as the athlete dynamically performs work. The amount of resistance depends on the extent of force applied by the athlete. Machines designed for isokinetic resistance develop flexibility and coordination as well as strength and power. The Mini-Gym, Orthotron, Cybex, and Kinkom machines make use of this exercise method (Figure 2-12).

Hydra-Fitness uses the term *omnikinetics* to describe its method of resistance training. Within these machines hydraulic fluid in cylinders provides positive resistance through the range of motion. The amount of resistance is regulated by the size of the aperture through which the fluid flows. It also provides reciprocal muscle work in the opposing muscle groups as they perform concentric contractions during the final stage of the repetition.

Resistance Training for Specific Activities

After the general program of weight training, exercises specifically designed to develop the muscle groups that are most important for successful performance in a given activity should be assigned. Sports demand rotational rather than linear elements of the body. Exercises must be se-

Figure 2-12

Cybex accommodating resistance machine.

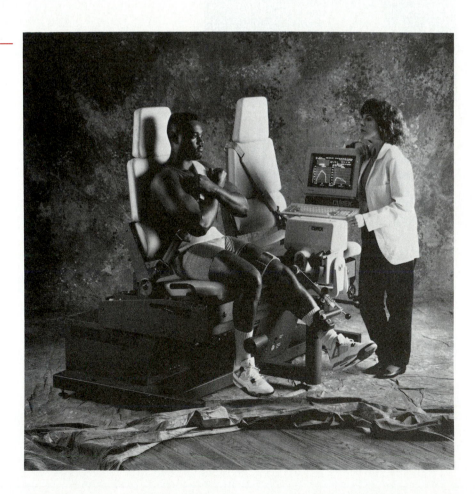

lected on the basis of their developmental construction, as well as memetic activity as specifically related to a given sport (Figure 2-13).

The Relationship of Strength and Flexibility

We often hear about the negative effects that strength training has on flexibility. For example, someone who develops large bulk through strength training is often referred to as "muscle-bound," an expression that has negative connotations in terms of the ability of that person to move. We tend to think of people who have highly developed muscles as having lost much of their ability to move freely through a full range of motion.

Occasionally a person develops so much bulk that the physical size of the muscle prevents a normal range of motion. It is certainly true that strength training, if done improperly, can impair movement; however, there is no reason to believe that weight training, if done properly and through a full range of motion, will impair flexibility. Proper strength training likely improves dynamic flexibility and, if combined with a rigorous stretching program, can greatly enhance powerful and coordinated movements that are essential for success in many sports activities. In all cases, a heavy strengthening program should be accompanied by a strong flexibility program.

Excessive muscle bulk can limit flexibility and range of motion.

Endurance and Stamina

Conditioning builds a given economy—an efficiency in body adaptability—which is important as the body adjusts to the continued and prolonged stresses put on it in performing an activity that requires all-out or near-maximal performance over a considerable period of time.

The degree of ability to withstand fatigue is inherited, and the basis of the fatigue pattern is in each individual's constitution. Endurance is comprised of two different components: muscular endurance and cardio-

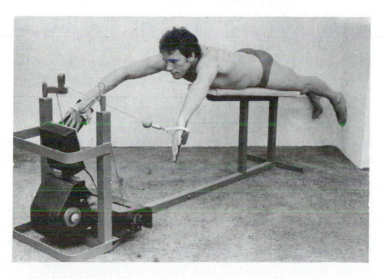

Figure 2-13

Exercise systems such as that provided by the Mini-Gym offer the athlete opportunities to concentrate on specific sports requirements.

Foundations

Cardiorespiratory endurance refers to the body's ability to transport and utilize oxygen efficiently.

Muscle endurance refers to the body's ability to perform repetitive muscular contraction against some resistance.

As a muscle tires, it loses some of its ability to relax.

stroke volume

The capacity of the heart to pump blood

respiratory endurance. Muscular endurance relates to a muscle's ability to engage in repeated muscle contraction. Cardiorespiratory endurance refers to the cardiorespiratory system's ability to transport and utilize oxygen throughout the body.

Muscle endurance   The ability to perform repetitive muscular contraction against some resistance is closely related to muscular strength and cardiorespiratory endurance. By definition, strength is the maximum force that can be applied by a muscle during a single contraction.

As with the physiological genetic components forming the foundation for cardiorespiratory endurance, muscle endurance has a genetic component of slow-twitch oxidative (SO) muscle fibers. SOs are aerobic, requiring oxygen for continued contraction. In comparison, there are fast-twitch oxidative-glycolytic (FOG) fibers and fast-twitch glycolytic (FG) fibers for activities requiring speed and power.

As a muscle tires, it loses some of its ability to relax and thus is more likely to tear. The character of a muscle is indicated not only by its ability to produce power over a period of time but also by its capacity to concurrently maintain its elasticity. As the muscle works, it restores its own oxygen and fuel supplies and disposes of metabolic products. As long as these two processes continue to operate at basically the same rate, the muscle can continue to work with efficiency. In fatigue the reaction time slows down and is accompanied by stiffening or inability of the muscle to reach a condition of relaxation, which is a contributing factor to some sports injuries.

Cardiorespiratory endurance   To perform whole-body activities for extended periods of time requires the ability to transport oxygen throughout the body. To do so effectively involves the coordinated function of the heart, lungs, blood vessels, and blood. Training increases vital capacity (the maximal volume of air the lungs exchange in one respiratory cycle) and aids materially in establishing economy in the oxygen requirement. The conditioned athlete operates primarily on a "pay-as-you-go" basis as a result of his or her increased **stroke volume** and reduced heartbeat. An increase in the contractile power of the respiratory muscles, particularly the diaphragm, results in deeper respiration per breath. This enables the athlete to use a greater lung capacity and consequently to effect increased economy in the use of oxygen. The untrained individual attempts to compensate by increasing the rate of res- piration and soon reaches a state of considerable respiratory indebtedness, which severely encumbers or even halts performance.

Endurance work improves circulation by calling into play more capillaries, thus providing the working muscles with more oxygen and fuel and facilitating removal of the metabolic by-products of the exercise.

Endurance training not only significantly improves maximal oxygen consumption and lowers blood pressure but is a key factor in injury prevention. The fatigued athlete not only as a diminished reaction capacity but because of muscular fatigue is less able to withstand extraneous forces, which means that such an athlete is more likely to sustain an injury under circumstances in which a better-conditioned performer will not.

Neuromuscular Coordination

Neuromuscular coordination is a complex interaction between muscles and nerves to carry out a purposeful action. Major aspects of this coordination are the proprioceptors that are located in muscles, tendons, joints, and labyrinth of the inner ear. Proprioceptors give the athlete a knowledge of where the body is in space.

Proprioceptive sense is the ability to discern where you are in space.

Athletes need to be able to recruit the appropriate muscles on demand. When recruitment of specific muscles is inappropriate, abnormal physical stresses can occur, leading to acute or chronic injuries. This is also very true for proprioception. When the athlete is unable to adequately perceive the body in space, serious injuries can occur.

Special Conditioning Approaches
Circuit Training

Circuit training is a method of physical conditioning that employs both apparatus resistance training and calisthenic conditioning exercises. It provides a means of achieving optimal fitness in a systematized, controlled fashion. The intensity and vigor of circuit training are indeed challenging and enjoyable to the performer. This system produces positive changes in motor performance, general fitness, muscular power, endurance, and speed.

Circuit training is based on the premise that the athlete must do the same amount of work in a shorter period of time or must do considerably more work within the limits of an assigned training period. Numerous variations of this system are in use, but all employ certain common factors: (1) the use of PREs; (2) the use of calisthenics and apparatus exercises, the former being performed either with or without weights; (3) a circular arrangement of the activities that permits progression from one station to another until all stations have been visited, the total constituting a circuit; and (4) a limiting time factor within which the circuit must be concluded.

The circuit is usually set up around the perimeter of the exercise area and consists of 8 to 12 exercise stations that encourage development of the body parts most commonly called into play in a particular sports activity as well as for total body fitness. Ten to 20 repetitions are usually performed at each station with a 20- to 40-second test interval (no exercise as the person moves to the next station). After a thorough orientation period, a target time, which is one third lower than the initial trial time, is assigned. A sample circuit program is shown in Figure 2-14.

Cardiorespiratory Improvement

A number of training methods are designed to specifically enhance cardiorespiratory performance according to the requirements of a particular sport. Those discussed here are continuous training and interval training.

Figure 2-14

Sample circuit program *Station* 1, Squat thrusts, 75% maximum number of repetitions performed in 1 minute; 2, general flexion exercise, performed for 1 minute; 3, jump rope for 1 minute; 4, abdominal curls with weights, 75% maximum number of repetitions; 5, two-arm curls, 75% maximum number of repetions; 6, vertical jump (sargent), 75% maximum number of repetitions performed in one minute; 7, wrist curls with weight for 1 minute; 8, half squat, heels raised, exercise with weight, 75% maximum number of repetitions; 9, general flexion exercises.

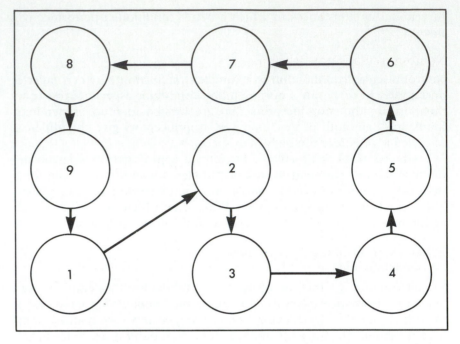

Continuous training   The continuous training approach is designed for long-endurance activities such as marathon running. Long, uninterrupted work is engaged in at a constant intensity. The steady pace in a situation of constant overload draws on the athlete's energy reserves over a long period of time. This method develops the athlete's aerobic capacity, functional stability, and energy reserves.

Interval Training   Unlike continuous training, interval training involves more intermittent activities. Interval training consists of alternating periods of relatively intense work and active recovery. It allows for performance of much work at a more intense work load over a longer period of time than if working continuously.

For best results, continuous training should be performed at 60% to 80% of maximal heart rate.

It is most desirable in continuous training to work at an intensity of about 60% to 80% of maximal heart rate. Obviously, sustaining activity at a relatively high intensity over a 20-minute period would be extremely difficult. The advantage of interval training is that it allows work at this 80% or higher level for a short period of time followed by an active period of recovery during which an individual may be working at only 30% to 45% of maximum heart rate. Thus the intensity of the workout and its duration can be greater than with continuous training.

Most sports are anaerobic, involving short bursts of intense activity followed by a sort of active recovery period (for example, football, basketball, soccer, or tennis). Training with the interval technique allows the athlete to be more sport specific during the workout. With interval training the overload principle is applied by making the training period much more intense.

There are several important considerations in interval training. The training period is the amount of time that continuous activity is actually being performed, and the recovery period is that time between training periods. A set is a group of combined training and recovery periods, and a repetition is the number of training/recovery periods per set. Training time or distance refers to the rate or distance of the training period. The training/recovery ratio indicates a time ratio for training vs. recovery.

An example of interval training would be a soccer player running sprints. An interval workout would involve running two sets of four 440-yard dashes in under 70 seconds, with a 2-minute 20-second walking recovery period between each dash. During this training session the soccer player's heart rate would probably increase to 85% to 90% of maximal level during the dash and should probably fall to the 30% to 45% level during the recovery period.

Overexertional Muscle Problems

One ever-present problem in physical conditioning and training is that which stems from overexertion. Even though the gradual pattern of overloading the body is the best way for ultimate success, many athletes and even coaches believe that if there is no pain, there is no gain.

Exercise overdosage is reflected in muscle soreness, decreased joint flexibility, and general fatigue 24 hours after activity. Any one of the above, or even all, can be present. Four specific indicators of possible overexertion are acute muscle soreness, muscle stiffness, delayed muscle soreness, and muscle cramping.

Muscle soreness has long been a problem for the person engaging in physical conditioning. Two major types of muscle soreness are associated with severe exercise. The first, occurring immediately after exercise, is acute soreness, which is resolved when exercise has ceased. The second and more serious problem is delayed soreness, which is related mainly to early-season or unaccustomed work. Severe muscular discomfort occurs 24 to 48 hours after exercise.[11]

The two major types of muscle soreness associated with severe exercise are acute and delayed.

Acute-Onset Muscle Soreness

Acute-onset muscle soreness is related to an impedance of circulation, causing muscular ischemia. Lactic acid and potassium collect in the muscle and stimulate pain receptors.

Delayed-Onset Muscle Soreness

Unlike acute-onset soreness, delayed-onset muscle soreness (DOMS) increases in intensity for 2 to 3 days until it has completely disappeared within 7 days.[5]

The cause of DOMS apparently is sublethal and lethal damage to a small group of recruited muscle fibers. The perception of soreness is caused by the activation of free nerve endings around selected muscle fibers.[6] The type of activity that causes the most soreness is eccentric exercise. Muscle fibers may take as long as 12 weeks to repair; therefore, athletes need abundant recovery time.[10]

There are many ways to reduce the possibility of delayed muscle soreness. One is a gradual and complete warm-up before engaging in vigorous activity, followed by a careful cooling down. In the early part of training, careful attention should be paid to static stretching before and after activity. If there is extreme soreness, the application of ice packs or ice massage to the point of numbness (for approximately 5 to 8 minutes) followed by a static stretch will often provide relief.

Muscle Stiffness

Muscle stiffness is different than muscle soreness in that it does not produce pain. It occurs when a group of muscles have been worked hard for a long period of time. The fluids that collect in the muscles during and after exercise are absorbed into the bloodstream at a very slow rate. As a result the muscle becomes swollen, shorter, and thicker and therefore resists stretching. Light exercise, massage, and passive mobilization assist in reducing stiffness.

Muscle Cramps

Like muscle soreness and stiffness, muscle cramps can be a problem related to hard conditioning. The most common cramp is **tonic,** in which there is continuous muscle contraction. It is caused by the body's depletion of essential electrolytes or an interruption of synergism between opposing muscles. **Clonic,** or intermittent, contraction stemming from nerve irritation rarely occurs.

tonic cramp
Muscle contraction marked by constant contraction that lasts a long time

clonic cramp
Involuntary muscle contraction marked by alternate contraction and relaxation in rapid succession

TRAINING AND COMPETITION IN CHILDHOOD

Parents and professionals in the areas of education, psychology, and medicine have long questioned whether vigorous physical training and competition are advisable for the immature child. Increasingly, children are engaging in intense programs of training that require many hours of daily commitment and may extend over many years. Swimmers may practice 2 hours, two times a day, covering 6,000 to 10,000 meters each season in the water; gymnasts may practice 3 to 5 hours per day; and runners may cover as many as 70 miles each week.

The American Academy of Pediatrics has indicated that the nearly universal participation of young children of both genders in competitive sports requires realistic guidelines. It is recognized that sports have an important effect on stamina and physiology and have lifelong value as recreational activities.[1] The American Academy of Pediatrics also indicates that there is no physical reason to separate preadolescent girls and boys by gender in sports activities or recreational activities; however, separation of the genders should occur in collision-type sports when boys have acquired greater muscle mass in proportion to body weight, making participation with girls hazardous. All participants should be properly grouped by physical maturation, weight, size, and skill (Figure 2-15).

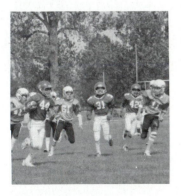

Figure 2-15

It is particularly important to properly group children according to maturity, size, and skill.

Of major importance is the physical examination that the child should be given before entering organized competitive sports. It is also important that coaches of children have some understanding of growth and development, injury causation, prevention of sports injuries, and the understanding and practice of correct coaching techniques.[11] Physical strength training and endurance training must be carefully coached and supervised to ensure proper execution and to avoid overdoing.

Physical Immaturity

Many professionals are concerned with the young athlete who has an immature skeletal structure and engages in highly competitive sports. The degree of maturation is commonly measured by skeletal ossification. The skeleton does not completely mature until early adulthood. An example of this is the femur, which reaches full ossification at approximately 19 years of age. The main concern of opponents of vigorous competitive youth sports programs, especially the contact or collision variety, is injuries that could cause a premature cessation of growth in a particular bone. *Epiphyseal injuries* affecting growth plates, which are primarily cartilaginous in their immature state, can result from a number of activities. The following activities should be performed with great caution.[11]

- Falling, jumping, and landing with straight legs
- Excessive stress to the shoulder and elbow from repeated throwing motions

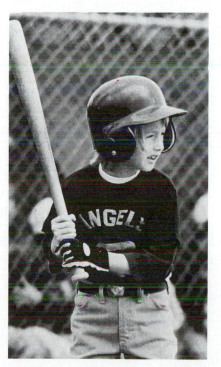

Figure 2-16

Unsupervised play is generally more dangerous than organized sports activities.

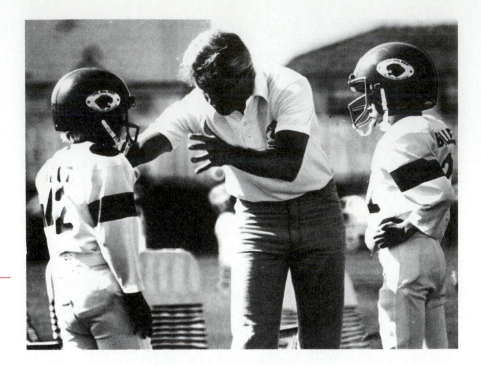

Figure 2-17

Constant high-level psychological pressure can lead to a child's becoming disinterested in sports and exercise.

- Long-duration exercise involving weight bearing, such as long-distance running
- Heavy weight lifting

Generally, according to the current data, youngsters adapt well to the same type of training routines used to train the mature athlete.

Many physicians also are concerned with repeated microtraumas that occur to the young athlete over a period of time. Such small traumas can compound and produce chronic and in some cases degenerative conditions within the immature musculoskeletal system.

Extreme training intensity can increase a child's chance of sustaining an overuse injury. Even though Wolff's law is at work when the growing child is experiencing intensive physical training, extreme care must be taken by coaches to avoid a considerable risk of injury. *Proper supervision* is the key term in these circumstances (Figure 2-16).

Of even more concern than the physical aspects of training in childhood are the psychological stresses that may be placed on children by overzealous parents and coaches. Enjoyment of the activity, rather than being winners at all cost, should be the focus of training and competition (Figure 2-17).

SUMMARY

Proper physical conditioning for sports participation should prepare the athlete for a high-level performance while helping to prevent injuries that are inherent to that sport. Injury-preventive physical conditioning must include concern for strength, flexibility, endurance, and neuromuscular coordination. Physical conditioning is a year-round task.

Physical conditioning must be concerned with the SAID principle—an acronym for *s*pecific *a*daptation to *i*mposed *d*emands. It must work toward making the body as lean as possible, commensurate with the athlete's sport.

A proper warm-up should precede conditioning, and a proper cool-down should follow. It takes at least 15 to 30 minutes of gradual warm-up to bring the body to a state of readiness for vigorous sports training and participation. Warming up consists of general unrelated activity followed by specific related activity.

Optimum flexibility is a necessary attribute for success in most sports. However, too much flexibility can allow joint trauma to occur, while too little flexibility can result in muscle tears or strains. Ballistic stretching exercises should be avoided. The safest means of increasing flexibility are the static and resistive (hold-relax) methods.

Strength is the capacity to exert a force or the ability to perform work against a resistance. There are numerous means to achieve strength development, including isometric, isotonic, and isokinetic muscle contraction. Isometric exercise generates heat energy by forcefully contracting the muscle in a stable position that produces no change in the length of the muscle. Isotonic exercise involves shortening and lengthening a muscle through a complete range of motion. Isokinetic exercise involves shortening or lengthening the muscle, causing a skeletal part to be moved through an accommodating resistance exercise (ARE). Plyometric exercise maximizes the stretch reflex by first lengthening a muscle and then immediately shortening the muscle against a resistance. To avoid athletic injury, the athlete must have a high level of neuromuscular coordination, which involves a complex interaction between muscles and nerves to perform a purposeful and safe action.

Too much exercising can lead to the problems of overexertional muscle soreness or injury. They include acute and chronic muscle soreness, muscle stiffness, and muscle cramps. Muscles that show signs of overexertion fail to function properly and are candidates for serious injuries.

Stamina, or endurance, is a necessary factor in most active sports, some more than others. It is the ability to undergo prolonged activity involving both the muscular and cardiorespiratory systems. Physical fatigue involves the loss of the ability to properly relax and coordinate muscles, making the athlete more prone to injury.

The child athlete/competitor who engages in intense physical activities is becoming more and more common. His or her physical immaturity must be taken into consideration when he or she undergoes conditioning and participates in a sport. Injuries to growth areas must be avoided.

REVIEW QUESTIONS AND CLASS ACTIVITIES

1. Why is year-round conditioning important for injury prevention?
2. Design a preseason conditioning program for a particular sport.
3. What types of activities should be included in your warm-up? How can extremes of temperatures affect your warm-up?
4. Take a single event or sport activity and design a warm-up and cool-down program for a practice session for it.
5. Why is cooling down just as important as warming up?
6. What are the different elements of a total fitness program?
7. What are the advantages and disadvantages of each strength training method? Develop a strength training program for one sport using the equipment at your school.
8. Have the students take one weight-training machine or single station and develop dos and don'ts for using this station properly so as to avoid injury. Combine them and post them in the weight room.
9. What is exercise overdosage? How can that produce muscle soreness? What can you do to reduce muscle soreness and muscle stiffness?
10. Discuss the advantages and disadvantages of training and competition for young children.

REFERENCES

1. Arnheim D, Prentice W: *Principles of athletic training,* ed 8, St Louis, 1993, Times Mirror/Mosby College Publishing.
2. Bilik SE: *The trainer's bible,* ed 9, New York, 1956, TJ Reed.
3. Chang DE et al: Limited joint mobility in power lifter, *Am J Sports Med* 16:280, 1988.
4. DeLorme TLK, Watkins ALK: *Progressive resistance exercise,* New York, 1951, Appleton-Century-Crofts.
5. Evans WJ: Exercise-induced skeletal muscle damage, *Phys Sportsmed* 15:89, 1987.
6. Fox E et al: *The physiological basis of physical education and athletics,* Philadelphia, 1988, WB Saunders.
7. Fleck SJ: Cardiovascular adaptations resistance training, *Med Sci Sports Exerc* 20:S146, 1988.
8. Hafen BQ: *First aid for health emergencies,* ed 4, St Paul, Minn, 1992, West Publishing.
9. Janda DH: Prevention has everything to do with sports medicine. *Clin J Sports Med* 2:159, 1992.
10. Knott M, Voss P: *Proprioceptive neuromuscular facilitation,* ed 3, New York, 1985, Harper & Row.
11. Kulund DN: *The injured athlete,* ed 2, Philadelphia, 1988, JB Lippincott.
12. Mc Ardle W et al: *Exercise physiology, energy, nutrition, and human performance,* Philadelphia, 1991, Lea & Febiger.
13. Mechelen VW et al: Prevention of running injuries by warm-up, cool-down, and stretching exercises, *Am J Sports Med* 21, 1993.
14. Prentice W: *Fitness for college and life,* St Louis, 1991, Mosby-Year Book.
15. Prentice W: A comparison of static and PNF stretching for improvement of hips joint flexibility, *Ath Train* 18:56, 1983.
16. Safran MR et al: The role of warmup in muscular injury prevention, *Am J Sports Med* 16:123, 1988.
17. Sale DG: Neural adaptation to resistance training, *Med Sci Sports Exerc* 20:S135, 1988.
18. Stone MH: Implication for connective tissue and bone alterations resulting from resistance exercise training, *Med Sci Sports Exerc* 20:S162, 1988.

19. Stone WJ, Steingard PM: Year-round conditioning for basketball. In Steingard PM, ed: *Basketball injuries clinic in sports medicine,* vol 12, Philadelphia, 1993, WB Saunders.

20. Wilmore JH, Seay MG: Strength training for the young athlete, *Sports Med Dig* 9:4, 1987.

ANNOTATED BIBLIOGRAPHY

Branner TT: *The safe exercise book.* Dubuque, Iowa, 1989, Kendall/Hunt.
  An easy-to-read book for the health professional. Covers the recommended and contraindicated exercises.
Di Nubile NA: *Clinics in sports medicine: the exercise prescription.*
  A series of publications published quarterly directed to the clinical practice of sports medicine.
Garhammer J: *Strength training,* New York, 1986, Harper & Row.
  Provides an excellent presentation on the basics of strength training and conditioning.
Mueller FO, Ryan AJ: *Prevention of athletic injuries: the role of the sports medicine team.*
  A text dedicated to preventing most aspects of athletic training/sports medicine.
Pearsall P: *Superimmunity,* New York, 1987, McGraw-Hill.
  An in-depth look at the relationship of emotions to health.
Walton CW, Martin D, eds: *Orthopaedic sports medicine 1993,* St Louis, 1993, Mosby-Year Book.
  A practical approach to athletic injuries of the musculoskeletal system, including acute care, rehabilitation, conditioning, and fitness.

Psychological Stress and Sports Injuries

When you finish this chapter, you should be able to:

- Describe why and under what circumstances sports participation is a psychological stressor
- Explain all the aspects of overtraining and staleness that stem from sports
- Define the conflict adjustments that may occur as a result of becoming overstressed in sports
- Identify physiological responses to stress
- Describe how an athlete may respond psychologically to injuries or illnesses
- Describe the role of coaches when dealing with an overly stressed athlete

Mens sana in corpore sano, or "a sound mind in a sound body," is the concept of mind-body relationship that we have accepted since the time of the early Greeks. In recent years we have become increasingly concerned with the effect of psychological stress and its relationship to injury prevention and causation.

SPORTS AS A STRESSOR

stress
The positive and negative forces that can disrupt the body's equilibrium

Recently, the word **stress** has had a negative connotation. Rather, stress refers to a change. Stress is not all bad, nor is it all good. According to Pearsall,[11] stress is not something that an individual can do to his or her body, but it is something that happens or that the brain tells the athlete is happening, which may be different from what has, in truth, been happening. When change occurs, the brain interprets that change and tells the body how to react to it. Selye[15] also considers stress as not necessarily implying a morbid change, but a change that could also be associated with intense pleasure. The concern here is the relationship between sports and abnormal stress (Figure 3-1).

Sports participation serves as both a physical and an emotional stressor. Stress can be a positive or negative influence. All living organisms are endowed with the ability to cope effectively with stressful situations. Pelletier[12] stated: "Without stress, there would be very little constructive activity or positive change." Negative stress can contribute to poor health, whereas positive stress produces growth and development. A healthy life

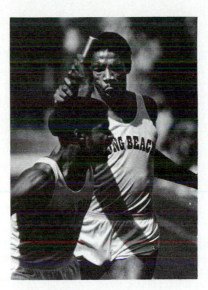

Figure 3-1

Stress in sports, as in other endeavors, can be either "bad" or "good," depending on the brain's interpretation of it.

must have a balance of stress; too little causes a "rusting out," and too much stress can cause "burnout."

Athletes place their bodies in countless daily stress situations. Their bodies undergo numerous "fight-or-flight" reactions to avoid injury or other threatening situations. Inappropriate adjustment to fight-or-flight responses can eventually lead to emotional or physical illness.

Sports participation is both a physical and an emotional stressor.

The Pregame Responses

Pregame stress is a response with which everyone connected with sports is familiar. Before any event that is of significance to the performer, the symptoms occur in varying degrees. Continued exposure to this stress somewhat lessens but does not stop the effects; veteran athletes, public performers, politicians, and others will attest to still feeling one or more of these effects of tension.

The pregame syndrome is one of nature's ways of preparing the individual for maximum effort. Key endocrine chemicals are released into the system producing dramatic results. These effects increase the physical performance of an individual in an emergency. This is accomplished through the following means:

Pregame syndrome is the body's way of preparing an athlete for intense performance.

1. Speed-up of circulation and respiration, which increases the delivery of fuel to the muscles and the removal of metabolites and other wastes
2. An increase in the blood sugar content and more fuel supplied to the muscles
3. An increase in mental alertness and in the speed of muscle responses, thus improving physical performance.

With the increase in blood pressure, heart rate, and endocrine stimulation, certain emotional symptoms appear, such as a feeling of anxiety, breathlessness, butterflies in the stomach, and trembling. An athlete in a

Before competition, athletes may experience anxiety, breathlessness, butterflies, or trembling.

state of readiness for competition will exhibit these signs in varying degrees.

Also associated with these physiological responses is an extremely dry mouth **(xerostomia).** Stress causes a lack of normal salivary secretion. This problem can be relieved by chewing gum or sucking on a lemon. When the stress has been relieved, normal moisture returns. Other typical responses to prevent stress are increased urine production and a nervous desire for bowel movements, which often accompany pregame tension and may be attributed to increased hormonal and nerve action. Once the sports event has begun, the vast majority of the pregame nervous responses subside.

xerostomia
Having a dry mouth

Overtraining and Staleness

Athletes who undergo prolonged stress because of overtraining can become stale. The term "stale" refers to a loss of vigor, initiative, and successful performance. Staleness is both a metabolical and physiological condition. This situation can be attributed to a wide variety of influences.

"Staleness" refers to a loss of vigor, initiative, and successful performance.

Causes of Staleness

The general cause of staleness in athletes is stress, usually occurring over a long period of time without adequate relief. Sometimes it is called athletic "burnout," much like psychological "burnout," which occurs in any field that has major responsibilities.

There are countless reasons why some athletes become stale. In fact, the athlete could be training too hard and long without proper rest or may not be eating properly.

Although poor eating habits are an important cause of staleness, and more often and most importantly, anxieties. **Anxiety** is one of the most common mental and emotional stress producers. It is reflected by a nondescript fear, a sense of apprehension, and restlessness. Typically the anxious athlete is unable to describe the problem. The athlete feels inadequate in a certain situation but is unable to say why. Increased heart rate with a strong, irregular beat, shortness of breath, sweaty palms, constriction in the throat, and headache may accompany anxiety. Children who are pushed too hard by parents may acquire a number of psychological problems. They may even fail purposely in their sport just to rid themselves of the painful stress of achieving. A coach who acts like a drill sergeant—who is continually negative—will more than likely cause the athlete to develop symptoms of overstress (Figure 3-2).

anxiety
A feeling of uncertainty or apprehension

A coach who is stingy with praise can develop overstressed athletes.

Athletes are much more prone to staleness if the rewards of their efforts are minimal (Figure 3-3). A losing season commonly causes many athletes to become stale.

Symptoms of Staleness

Staleness is evidenced by a wide variety of symptoms, among which are a deterioration in the usual standard of performance, chronic fatigue, apathy, loss of appetite, indigestion, weight loss, and inability to sleep or

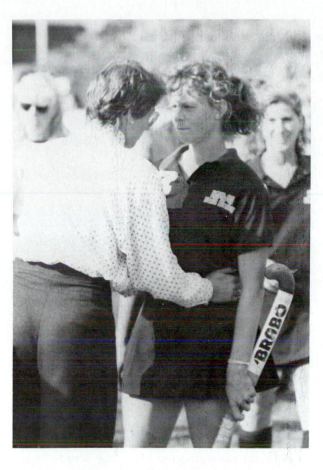

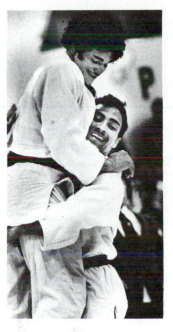

Figure 3-2
A coach with a negative attitude can add to overstressing the athlete.

Figure 3-3
Signs of staleness can be deterred if there are maximum rewards for the athlete.

rest properly. Often athletes will exhibit higher blood pressure or an increased pulse rate, both at rest and during activity. All these signs indicate adrenal exhaustion. The athlete becomes irritable and restless, has to force himself or herself to practice, and exhibits signs of boredom and lassitude in respect to everything connected with the activity[4] (see the box on p. 78).

Accident Proneness

Accident-prone athletes have more than an average share of injuries. Injuries seem to seek them out, and normally insignificant or innocuous situations assume significance when they occur. They are easily involved in situations wherein they receive some injury, although others emerge unscathed.

Accident-prone athletes are most likely to suffer an accident toward the end of a long or sustained period of work. Accident proneness apparently is caused by a lack of ability to coordinate properly, as the result of either fatigue or emotional imbalance. Often the discouraged or apathetic athlete is accident prone. Athletic trainers and coaches have long

Accident-prone individuals are most likely to suffer an accident toward the end of a long or sustained period of work.

RECOGNIZING SIGNS OF STALENESS IN ATHLETES

An athlete who is becoming stale will often display some or most of the following signs. He or she may

1. Show a decrease in performance level
2. Have difficulty falling asleep
3. Be awakened from sleep for no apparent reason
4. Experience a loss of appetite and a loss of weight; conversely, the athlete may overeat because of chronic worry
5. Have indigestion
6. Have difficulty concentrating
7. Have difficulty enjoying sex
8. Experience nausea for no apparent reason
9. Be prone to head colds and/or allergic reactions
10. Show behavioral signs of restlessness, irritability, anxiety, and/or depression
11. Have an elevated resting heart rate and elevated blood pressure
12. Display psychosomatic episodes of perceiving bodily pains such as sore muscles, especially before competing

observed that the competitor who is not emotionally stable stands an excellent chance of being injured. Accident proneness may also develop when the athlete becomes tense or depressed or is overly concerned about school, social, and home problems.[13]

Physiological Responses to Stress

psychophysiological
Involving the mind and the body

Stress is a **psychophysiological** phenomenon. In other words, it involves the mind and the body. As discussed earlier, sports, in every respect, are stressors. Physiologically, the body can experience three phases when stressed—alarm, resistance, and exhaustion. These reactions are commonly known as the General Adaptation Syndrome, or the GAS theory, as originally developed by Dr. Hans Selye.[15]

Alarm Stage

In the alarm phase, secretions from the adrenal gland sharply increase, creating the well-known "flight-or-fight" response. With adrenaline in the bloodstream, pupils dilate, hearing becomes more acute, muscles become more responsive, and blood pressure increases to facilitate the absorption of oxygen. In addition to these responses, respiration and heart rate increase to further prepare the body for action.

3 stages of stress:
alarm
resistance
exhaustion

Resistance Stage

Following the alarm stage, the body gradually changes to the resistance stage. During this stage, the body prepares itself for coping by diminishing the adrenocortical secretions and directing stress to a particular body site. This stage is the body's way of resisting the stressor. Physiological

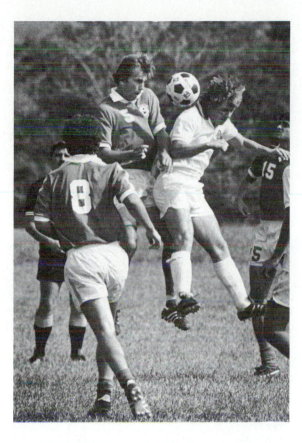

Figure 3-4

The highly competitive
athlete often has personality
qualities that have to be
carefully channeled to
improve performances.

response may remain high and could eventually lead to the final stage, exhaustion (Figure 3-4).

Exhaustion Stage

The exhaustion stage refers to an entire organ system, or a single organ, becoming dysfunctional and diseased as a result of chronic stress. It is generally accepted that chronic stress can adversely affect brain function, the autonomic nervous system, the endocrine system, and the immune system, eventually leading to a **psychosomatic** illness.

Thus it is concluded that there are two kinds of stress—acute and chronic. During acute stress, the threat is immediate, and response is instantaneous. Physiologically, the body remains in the alarm stage. The primary reaction of the alarm stage is produced by the epinephrine and norepinephrine of the adrenal medulla. Chronic stress primarily involves the stages of resistance and exhaustion. During chronic stress, there is an increase of blood corticoids from the adrenal cortex.

psychosomatic
Originating in the mind, although symptoms manifest in the body and are quite real

Stress can be acute or chronic.

STRESS RELATED TO INJURIES OR ILLNESS

An athlete who is taken out of a sport because of an injury or illness reacts in a personal way. The athlete who has trained diligently, has looked forward to a successful season, and is suddenly thwarted in that goal by an injury or illness can be emotionally devastated.

At the Time of Injury or Illness

At the time of serious injury or illness the athlete may normally fear the experience of pain or possible disability. There may be a sense of anxiety about suddenly becoming disabled and unable to continue sport participation.[9] An injury or illness is a stressor that results from an external or internal sensory stimulus. Coping with this stressor depends on the athlete's cognitive appraisal. Over time negative feelings can lead to chronic tension, loss of appetite, sleep, lack of motivation, and, overall, adversely affect the healing process.[17] There also may be a sense of guilt about being unable to help the team or "letting down" the coach. Becoming suddenly dependent and somewhat helpless can cause anxiety in the usually independent and aggressive person.[6] The athlete may regress to childlike behavior, crying or displacing anger toward the coach or athletic trainer who is administering first aid. Also, in the very early period of injury, and sometimes later, the athlete may deny the injury altogether. Reaction of the athlete to a sudden injury may require immediate emotional support as shown in Table 3-1.

TABLE 3-1 Emotional emergency care

Type of Emotional Reaction	Outward Signs	Care Giver Reactions	
		Yes	No
Normal	Weakness, trembling Nausea, vomiting Perspiration Diarrhea Fear, anxiety Heart pounding	Be calm and reassuring	Avoid pity
Overreaction	Excessive talking Argumentativeness Inappropriate joke telling Hyperactivity	Allow athlete to vent emotions	Avoid telling athlete he or she is acting abnormally
Underreaction	Depression; sitting or standing numbly Little talking if any Emotionless Confusion Failure to respond to questions	Be empathetic; encourage talking to express feelings	Avoid being abrupt; avoid pity

The Psychology of Loss

The athlete who has sustained an injury of such intensity that he or she is unable to perform for a long period will generally experience five reactions: denial or disbelief, anger, bargaining, depression, and acceptance of the situation (see box below). These reactions are typical for anyone who has experienced a sudden serious loss. The injured athlete initially may be in shock and unable to grasp the full consequences of the injury.[8] The athlete may not believe that he or she is vulnerable and not impervious to injury.[14] There may be a loss of self-esteem, a sense of worthlessness, and self-reproach.[14]

The coach must realize that reactions to a sense of loss are normal

Psychological reactions to serious injury may include denial or disbelief, anger, bargaining, depression, or acceptance.

PSYCHOLOGICAL REACTIONS TO LOSS

Denial or Disbelief

When suddenly becoming disabled and unable to perform, the athlete will commonly deny the seriousness of the condition. When indications are that the injury is serious and will not heal before the end of the season, the athlete might respond by saying, "Not so, I'll be back in 2 weeks." This irrational thinking indicates denial of the true seriousness of the injury.

Anger

Anger commonly follows disbelief. As the athlete slowly becomes aware of the seriousness of the injury, a sense of anger develops. The athlete begins to ask, "Why me?" "What did I do wrong?" "Why am I being punished?" "It's not fair." Commonly, this anger becomes displaced toward other people. The athletic trainer may be blamed for not providing a good enough tape job, or another player may be blamed for causing the situation that set up the injury.

Bargaining

As anger becomes less intense, the athlete gradually becomes aware of the real nature of the injury and, with this awareness, begins to have doubts and fears about the situation, which leads to a need to bargain. Bargaining may be reflected in prayer, "God, if you will heal this injury in 3 weeks instead of 6, I'll go to church every Sunday." Or it may be reflected by pressure being put on the athletic trainer or physician to do his or her very best for a fast healing.

Depression

As the athlete becomes increasingly aware of the nature of the injury and that healing will take a specific length of time, depression can set in. Crying episodes may occur; there may be periods of insomnia, and the athlete may lose the desire for food.

Acceptance

Gradually, the athlete begins to feel less dejected and isolated and becomes resigned to the situation.

and must allow the athlete to fully experience each reaction. A common error is to try to talk the person out of being angry or depressed. Athletic trainers must educate all of their injured charges to understand that rehabilitation and full recovery are a cooperative venture, with major responsibility resting on the athlete's shoulders.[17]

The athlete who finds himself or herself overstressed could experience mental depression. Along with the major signs of staleness, the athlete may have feelings of worthlessness, self-reproach, and/or excessive and inappropriate guilt. This depression could be a temporary situational reaction.[18]

It is generally accepted that sports are stressors to the athlete. There is often a fine line between the athlete's reaching and maintaining peak performance and overtraining. Besides performance concerns, many peripheral stressors can be imposed on the athlete, such as unreasonable expectations by the athlete, the coaches, and/or the parents. Worries that stem from school, work, and family can also be major causes of emotional stress.

The coach is often the first person to notice that an athlete is overstressed. The athlete whose performance is declining and whose personality is changing may need a training program that is less demanding. A good talk with the athlete by the coach might reveal emotional and physical problems that need to be dealt with by a counselor/psychologist or a physician.

Injury prevention is *psychological,* as well as *physiological.* The athlete who enters a contest while angry, frustrated, or discouraged or while undergoing some other disturbing emotional state is more prone to injury than is the individual who is better adjusted emotionally. The angry player, for example, wants to vent ire in some way and therefore often loses perspective of desirable and approved conduct. In the grip of emotion, skill and coordination are sacrificed, resulting in an injury that otherwise would have been avoided.

> The coach is often the first person to notice that an athlete is overstressed and must be continually alert for signs of serious depression that need to be dealt with by a counselor/psychologist or a physician.

Regaining Competitive Confidence

Psychological rehabilitation is often as important as the restoration of the physical body. This is a commonly neglected factor in the total rehabilitative process. Very often an athlete returns to participation physically ready but psychologically ill-prepared. Although few athletes will admit it, when returning to participation they often feel very anxious about getting hurt again (Figure 3-5). This very feeling may, in some ways, be a self-fulfilling prophecy. In other words, anxiety can lead to muscle tension, which, in turn, can lead to disruption of normal coordination, thus producing conditions that are favorable for reinjury or for injury to another body part.[13] One suggestion for helping an athlete regain competitive confidence is to allow the athlete to regain full performance by progressing in small increments. Return might include, first, performing all the necessary skills away from the team. This action may be followed by engaging in a highly controlled, small-group practice and then attempt-

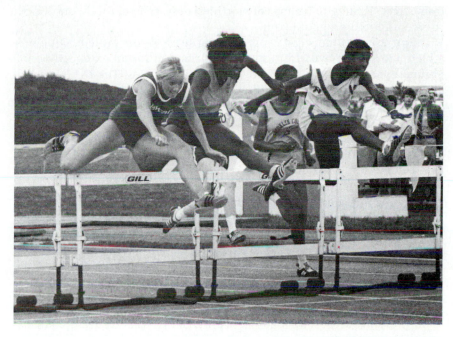

Figure 3-5

Anxiety can lead to adverse
muscle tension and
subsequent muscle injury.

ing participation in full-team noncontact practice. The athlete should be
encouraged to express freely any anxiety that may be felt and to engage
in full contact only when anxiety is at a minimum.

SUMMARY

Sports participation serves as both a physical and an emotional stressor.
As with other endeavors, sports can be both a negative and positive stressor. A normal response to stress is the pregame response. In this response
the body and mind speed up to meet the anticipated demands of competition.

An athlete who undergoes prolonged stress caused by overtraining
can become stale. Another term for staleness is "burnout." The symptoms of staleness can stem from a variety of reasons other than emotions, such as faulty diet or an unknown illness. A too-demanding coach
or an athlete who is too intense can also cause overtraining.

The athlete who is overstressed may respond in a number of physiological and psychological ways such as having a higher-than-usual blood
pressure, increased pulse rate, and increased catecholamine excretions.
The athlete who continues at the reactive phase of stress eventually will
become exhausted. Overstress can lead to adrenal exhaustion, causing a
variety of psychoemotional problems. Conflict adjustment is one type of
response to chronic stress.

The athlete may respond to chronic stress by experiencing muscle
soreness caused by muscle tension. Emotional depression can also stem

from stress, leading to feelings of worthlessness, self-reproach, and/or excessive and inappropriate guilt.

Injuries and illness can cause chronic stress in the athlete. Often the athlete who is removed from sports participation for an extended period of time experiences the psychological reaction of loss. The five phases of loss psychology are denial or disbelief, anger, bargaining, depression, and acceptance.

The coach is the first person to recognize that an athlete is overtraining or becoming stale. Staleness can result because the athlete has overtrained or because the coach teaches through negative reinforcement. The athletic trainer is also in a position to recognize subtle signs of an overstressed athlete. The physician may also become aware of an athlete who is "pushing too hard" or for other reasons is becoming "stressed out."

REVIEW QUESTIONS AND CLASS ACTIVITIES

1. What is meant by good and bad stress?
2. How may a coach or an athlete cause the problems of overtraining and staleness?
3. What are the signs of conflict adjustment?
4. What does an athlete's reaction to pain have to do with psychological stress?
5. Depression can occur from chronic negative stress. What are depression's major signs?
6. Describe the GAS theory. Why may it be a factor in an athlete who is overstressed?
7. What is the psychology of loss? How may it relate to an athlete who becomes injured or ill?
8. Put yourself in place of a coach. What indicators would reveal that the athlete is overstressed?
9. As an athletic trainer, how would you help an athlete reduce muscle tension caused by overstress?
10. Discuss the symptoms of pregame anxiety and what can be done to alleviate some of them.
11. How can a coach or athletic trainer recognize staleness in athletes?

REFERENCES

1. Benson HH: *Beyond the relaxation response,* New York, 1984, Times Books.
2. Costill DL: Detection of overtraining, *Sports Med Dig* 8:4, 1986.
3. Dychtwald K: *Body-mind,* New York, 1984, Jove.
4. Fairs GJ: Psychological aspects of athletic rehabilitation, *Clin Sports Med* 4:65, 1985.
5. Hafen BQ: *First aid for health emergencies,* ed 4, St Paul, Minn, 1988, West Publishing.
6. Jacobson E: *Progressive relaxation,* ed 2, Chicago, 1938, University of Chicago Press.
7. Johnson RJ: Help your athletes heal themselves, *Phys Sports Med* 19:107, 1991.
8. May JR: Psychological sequelae and rehabilitation of the injured athlete, *Sports Med Digest* 12:1, 1990.
9. Monat A, Lazarus RS, eds: *Stress and coping: an anthology,* New York, 1977, Columbia University Press.
10. Partin N: Sport psychology and physical therapy, *Ath Train* 24:159, 1989.
11. Pearsall P: *Superimmunity,* New York, 1987, McGraw-Hill.
12. Pelletier KR: *Mind as healer, mind as*

slayer, New York, 1977, Dell Publishing.

13. Rotella RJ: Psychological care of the injured athlete. In Kulund DN, ed: *The injured athlete,* Philadelphia, 1988, JB Lippincott.
14. Samples P: Mind over muscle: returning the injured athlete to play, *Phys Sportsmed* 15:172, 1987.
15. Selye H: *Stress without distress,* New York, 1974, JB Lippincott.
16. Silva JM, Hardy CJ: The sport psychologist. In Mueller FO, Ryan AJ, eds: *Prevention of athletic injuries: the role of the sportsmedicine team,* Philadelphia, 1991, FA Davis.
17. Weiss MR, Troxel RK: Psychology of the injured athlete, *Ath Train* 21:104, 1986.
18. Willmer P: *Depression: a psychobiological synthesis,* New York, 1985, John Wiley & Sons.
19. Wolpe J: *The practice of behavior therapy,* ed 2, New York, 1973, Pergamon Press.

ANNOTATED BIBLIOGRAPHY

Garhammer J: *Strength training,* New York, 1986, Harper & Row.
  Provides an excellent presentation on the basics of strength training and conditioning.
May JR, Sieb GE: Athletic injuries: psychological factors in the onset, sequelae, rehabilitation, and prevention. In *Sports psychology: the psychologic health of the athlete,* Great Neck, NY, 1987, PMA Publishing.
  Excellently detailed coverage about what stress is and how to cope with it.
Pearsall P: *Superimmunity,* New York 1987, McGraw-Hill.
  An in-depth look at the relationship of emotions to health.
Pelletier KR: *Mind as healer, minds as slayer,* New York, 1977, Dell Publishing.
  Provides an in-depth discussion of the relationship of the mind to the cause and healing of disease.
Selye H: *Stress without distress,* New York, 1974, JB Lippincott.
  A practical guide to understanding the role of stress in life.

Nutrition

When you finish this chapter, you will be able to:

- Explain the importance of good nutrition in enhancing performance and preventing injuries
- Identify the correct foods for a balanced diet
- Explain the necessity of fluid in the athlete's diet
- Describe the advantages and disadvantages of supplementary nutrients in the athlete's diet
- Explain the advantages and disadvantages of carbohydrate loading
- Identify foods that should be included in preevent meals
- Discuss the principles of weight management and the effect of weight gain and weight loss on athletic performance
- Identify the signs of bulimia and anorexia nervosa

NUTRITIONAL CONSIDERATIONS

A very important component of injury prevention is the athlete's diet. If the physical stresses that are imposed by hard training and competition are not adequately replenished by good nutrition, proper physical restoration cannot be achieved (Figure 4-1). In many cases an athlete follows the nutritional patterns of elite performers, whether they are sound or not, in hopes of emulating his or her achievements. The coach must consider nutrition education as a means to optimal performance and injury prevention or, when injuries do occur, to optimal healing.

Nutrition education is a means to optimal performance and maximum injury prevention.

Basic Nutritional Guidelines

Exercise often makes severe metabolic demands on the body. Keeping the body's tissues strong, repairing damaged tissues, recuperating fatigued muscles, and regenerating lost energy necessitate a proper diet.

The Athlete's Training Diet

In general, the athlete's daily diet should consist of 70% carbohydrates, 23% fat, and 10% to 15% protein. Adhering to the suggestions in Figure 4-2 will provide these percentages for the most part.

Carbohydrates Carbohydrates are organic compounds composed of carbon, hydrogen, and oxygen. They make up the starches and sugars found in foods such as breadstuffs, pasta, potatoes, candy, and pastries. During digestion, complex sugars are broken down into simple sugars to be absorbed into the blood and other tissues. Sugars are carried to the

Carbohydrates are found in foods such as bread, pasta, and potatoes.

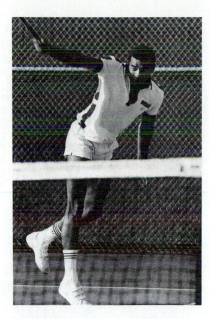

Figure 4-1
The nutritional demands of most athletes are major, requiring an increase in the daily number of calories.

liver to be converted into glycogen. Glycogen can be stored in the liver, muscle cells, and other cells. Excess glycogen that is not used as energy and has not been converted into glucose is converted into fat. If the athlete's diet consists of less than 50% of the total energy requirement of carbohydrates, muscle glycogen may not be fully restored. An athlete in training who wishes to reduce body fat should cut down on fat rather than carbohydrates.

Fats Fats and carbohydrates are composed of the same elements—carbon, hydrogen, and oxygen—but in fat the hydrogen content is higher. Fats represent a concentrated source of reserve energy. Fats are used when carbohydrate stores are depleted. Examples of high-fat foods are butter, cream, mayonnaise, meat gravy, and lard. In terms of training, fats require more oxygen than carbohydrates for digestion. Fats are burned during prolonged exercise of low intensity. Carbohydrates available in the body help to burn fat. Fats are slower to digest and may cause gastric distress leading to diarrhea.

Butter, cream, mayonnaise, and meat gravy are foods high in fat.

Protein Proteins are nitrogenous organic compounds that are composed of amino acids. Amino acids are made of carbon, nitrogen, and oxygen atoms and are considered the building blocks of the body. As with fats, many athletes overingest proteins, thinking proteins will automatically make them stronger. In fact, it is only when an individual engages in an extremely high level of muscle overload that the 10% to 15% protein in daily intake may be slightly increased (Figure 4-3). Overeating protein can displace carbohydrates from the diet and in the case of animalprotein can introduce undesirable fats. Digesting an excessive amount of protein can require extra water for urinary excretion and consequently can increase urination.

Foods such as peanuts and meat are high in protein.

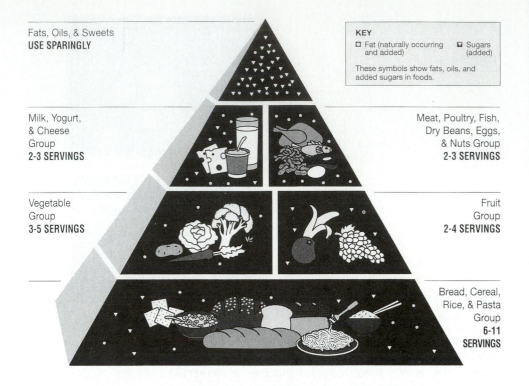

Fats, Oils, & Sweets
USE SPARINGLY

KEY
□ Fat (naturally occurring and added)   ☑ Sugars (added)

These symbols show fats, oils, and added sugars in foods.

Milk, Yogurt,
& Cheese
Group
2-3 SERVINGS

Meat, Poultry, Fish,
Dry Beans, Eggs,
& Nuts Group
2-3 SERVINGS

Vegetable
Group
3-5 SERVINGS

Fruit
Group
2-4 SERVINGS

Bread, Cereal,
Rice, & Pasta
Group
**6-11
SERVINGS**

Figure 4-2

The Food Guide Pyramid assists the athlete in making proper food choices.

Vitamin requirements do not increase during exercise.

Vitamins   More misinformation has been disseminated about vitamins than about any other nutritional factor. Vitamins are essential for maintaining good health. A lack of vitamins in the diet leads to deficiency conditions, which express themselves in a variety of ways. The problem of vitamin deficiency is rarely caused by the lack of a single vitamin. It is, rather, the result of a multiple vitamin deficiency. A good, varied diet that includes a balance of the basic four food categories will supply all vitamin requirements.

Several vitamins can be made synthetically and, according to the available research, the body is unable to distinguish between the natural and the synthetic vitamins; either is used equally well. The body, however, cannot manufacture any of the vitamins except D, which is derived from sunshine. Thus it must obtain its requirements from the diet. Supplementary vitamins are of considerable value during postoperative

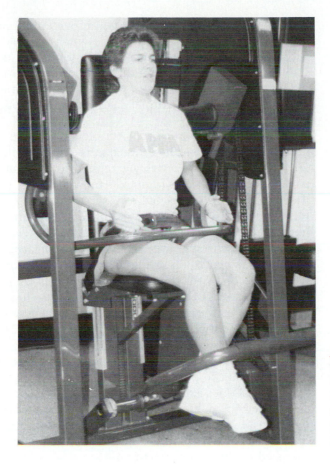

Figure 4-3

Only when the athlete engages in an extremely high-level muscle overload should the 10% to 15% daily protein intake be slightly increased.

or recuperative periods after illness or injury and are often prescribed by the physician to aid in the healing process.

Vitamins are usually identified as either fat soluble or water soluble. Fat-soluble vitamins usually persist in the diet in a reasonably intact state; they are found in butter, fortified margarines, and liver and are not usually destroyed in cooking. Vitamins A, D, E, and K are fat soluble. Little information is currently available concerning the biochemical role each of the fat-soluble vitamins plays, and there is some concern about their toxicity, since the amount of vitamin in excess of body needs is stored in the body. Vitamins A and K are present in a rather large variety of foods, whereas D and E are present in a limited number. Water-soluble vitamins grouped together as the B complex and vitamin C are often lost through cooking vitamin-containing foods in water and then disposing of the water in which they were cooked.

Minerals and electrolytes Essential to good health and life itself are inorganic salts known as minerals. They aid in metabolism and formation of tissue such as bone and teeth and maintain the balance of the body's internal environment. In most cases a wide variety of fresh foods,

Essential minerals are found in fresh fruits and vegetables.

especially fruits and vegetables, will provide the proper amount of minerals (with the exception of iron, which will be discussed in dietary supplementation). The principal dietary mineral elements are calcium, sodium, potassium, magnesium, phosphorus, chlorine, and sulfur. In addition, there are a number of essential trace elements such as iron, iodine, cobalt, copper, fluorine, manganese, molybdenum, selenium, vanadium, and zinc.

Electrolyte requirements Electrolytes, such as sodium chloride and potassium, are electrically charged salts. They maintain the balance of water outside the cell. Electrolyte replenishment may be needed when a person is not fit, suffers from extreme water loss, participates in a marathon, or has just completed an exercise period and is expected to perform at near-maximal effort within the next few hours. In most cases, however, there must be water replacement instead of electrolyte supplementation. Electrolytes can be sufficiently replaced with a balanced diet.

Fluids in sports It should be noted by the coach and athlete that a weight loss of 2% or more of body weight from sweating can cause fatigue and a loss of concentration, can increase heart rate, and may even lead to a circulatory collapse. Urine should be monitored as indication of adequate hydration. Ideally urine should show as being clear or light colored. Dark-colored urine may indicate a concentration of metabolic waste. Adequate fluid must be present in the blood to transport oxygen to the muscles. In general, the athlete requires 4 glasses of fluid per every 1,000 calories expended in exercise. Two glasses of cold water should be digested 15 to 30 minutes before exercise and two glasses after. During exercise 1 glass of fluid every 20 minutes can help to avoid dehydration. The coach must remember that thirst alone is not an indicator of the need for hydration (Figure 4-4).

Exercise longer than 1 hour requires the addition of 120 to 240 calories per hour along with fluid. Energy can stem from glucose, sucrose, polymers, or solid carbohydrates such as fruit or candy. For every pound of sweat loss, two glasses of fluid replacement are needed. Fluid replacement after exercise should continue until the urine is clear.

Sports drinks should provide rapid gastric emptying, return normal body fluid balance, restore minerals lost through sweat, and provide adequate carbohydrate replacement. The three types of sports drinks are fluid replacers for activities engaged in for less than 2 hours, carbohydrate loaders for the ultraendurance athlete, and drinks containing a nutrient balance. In general, potassium and sodium do not need to be supplemented when the athlete engages in ultraendurance activities.

Water is necessary for the various metabolic chemical reactions to occur within the body. It forms about 75% of all living matter; it dilutes the toxic by-products of metabolism; and it helps to regulate body temperature by dissipating excess heat through perspiration. A water balance must be maintained at all times. Deprivation of water leads to more rapid dehydration, with subsequent impairment of performance.

Even during cold weather, dehydration can occur. When dehydra-

All athletes should have unlimited access to water before and after exercise.

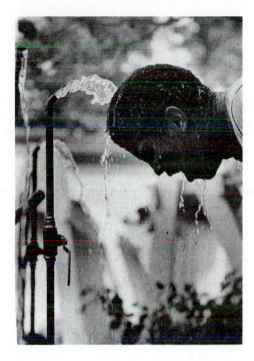

Figure 4-4

Athletes must have unlimited access to water, especially in hot weather.

tion does occur, blood volume is lessened, making warming of the hands, toes, and face more difficult.[5]

Dietary Supplementation and Manipulation

Vitamins and minerals   If a variety of fresh foods are eaten daily, there is little reason for the athlete to supplement his or her diet with vitamins or minerals, other than with iron (this is particularly important for the menstruating female). Taking vitamins in excess quantities (megavitamin dosage, see Appendix B) can have adverse effects and lead to toxicity from the storage of fat-soluble vitamins such as A, D, and E with a megadose of 10 times the RDA. Even for those athletes who sweat profusely, salt supplementation is unnecessary since salt is inherent in the usual Western diet.

Even water-soluble vitamins, if taken in doses that saturate the body, can lead to physical problems. For example, B-complex vitamins can lead to limb numbness, movement difficulties, and even paralysis. Niacin in particular, if taken in large quantities, can cause extreme vasodilation, resulting in itching and bright red skin. Thiamin in megadoses can produce anaphylactic shock. Too much vitamin C, often thought completely safe in large doses, can lead to gastroenteritis, diarrhea, colitis, and kidney stones.

Overingestion of minerals can also cause physical problems for the athlete. Megadoses of sodium (salt tablets) and potassium can irritate the gastrointestinal tract and cause dehydration and muscle cramping. Too

Salt supplementation is seldom necessary since most athletes already eat a high-sodium diet.

much chromium, a trace mineral, can cause damage to the liver and the kidneys. Selenium can produce fatigue and skin problems; zinc, another trace mineral, can produce nausea, diarrhea, and dizziness, as well as interfere with the body's immune response.

Calcium supplementation Calcium is by far the largest mineral amount present in the human body. Most dietary calcium comes from dairy products and some green leafy vegetables and grains. Calcium and phosphorus work closely together in bone and tooth formation, blood clotting, nerve transmission, muscle contraction and relaxation, cell membrane permeability, and enzyme activation. Although not specifically important for sports performance, calcium is essential to the female athlete for bone health.

Iron supplementation Iron deficiency, which is much more prevalent than usually thought, can affect muscular performance. Not infrequently, teenaged boys will exhibit an iron deficiency as the result of an inadequate diet and the demands of a rapid growth rate. Among female athletes, iron deficiency is not at all uncommon; borderline anemia may occur as a result of not getting enough dietary iron and blood loss from menstruation. The loss may be further compounded, particularly in the initial phases, by a strenuous training program wherein a temporary drop in plasma and hemoglobin results in so-called sports anemia, which is caused by the increased destruction of red blood cells. Should an iron deficiency be detected, iron supplementation should be introduced under medical supervision. The recommended daily dietary allowance for girls and women from age 10 up through the reproductive years is 18 mg. Recent surveys have indicated that an average daily intake of only 11 to 12 mg over a period of several years results in an iron store depletion, with the hemoglobin levels falling below the anemia borderline. Adolescent female athletes apparently become more iron depleted than do nonathletes. This deficiency decreases their ability to work effectively, thus decreasing performance.

Protein Protein supplementation with the idea of stimulating muscle strength and size is a waste of the athlete's money. Only proper exercise can increase muscle mass, and adequate protein intake can increase performance and strength.

Nutritional Readiness for Competition

It has often been said that the most important meal prior to competition is the one eaten the night before. This is especially true if the contest is to require 60 minutes or more of hard, sustained exercise.

Carbohydrate feeding and loading Events that call for sudden bursts of all-out energy are not particularly affected by preevent nutrition modification. However, endurance activities may be positively affected by carbohydrate manipulation. In some cases the amount of stored glycogen can be doubled through a loading process by increasing the ingestion of carbohydrates.[2]

Extra helpings of breads, cereals, and potatoes should be the rule.

Female athletes may have an increased need for iron and protein, especially when they are menstruating.

Endurance athletes should consume extra portions of breads, cereal, and potatoes before competition.

Bread and potatoes do not deserve their reputation as fattening foods. Potatoes should be eaten plain, that is, baked or boiled without the addition of milk, cream, or butter, which are the fattening agents. Bread preferably should be constituted from the less-refined flours or enriched by the restoration of the vitamins and minerals lost through refining. Since carbohydrates are most readily available and most easily absorbed in terms of metabolic demands, they are the first elements used for muscular work.

To maximize the absorption of glycogen, the athlete should gradually taper the work intensity 1 week before the event. This work reduction should be followed by increased ingestion of carbohydrate foods 3 days before the competition. Increasing preevent ingestion of carbohydrates is of no particular use unless activity is sustained for 90 minutes or more, since events of short duration are not affected or modified by such loading. Indeed, dehydration may develop.

Marathon runners have shown no difference in carbohydrate stores during the first half of the race, but carbohydrate feeding exercise can postpone fatigue as much as 15 to 30 minutes, which was 2 to 3 hours into the exercise session. Taking sweetened drinks during the latter part of the race seems to be of some help, but the explanation is open to question, since physiological evidence is unclear. The apparent lift may be psychological; perhaps the fluid itself may have some bearing. It should be noted that carbohydrate ingestion has some risk. Depositing glycogen in the muscles this way also deposits three times as much water as glycogen, causing the athlete to feel heavy and stiff.

Preevent nutrition   Too often athletic trainers and coaches concern themselves principally with the meal immediately preceding competition, seeming not to realize that preevent nutrition begins some time before that. Events that call for sudden bursts of all-out energy rather than endurance or sustained effort do not appear to be particularly affected by preevent nutrition. However, preparing for moderate or sustained effort that requires endurance includes consideration for nutrition approximately 48 hours preceding competition. Precompetitive tensions such as abdominal cramps, dry mouth, acidosis, and other metabolic symptoms can be reduced or eliminated by careful attention to diet. It is wise to taper off the training program starting approximately 48 hours before competition. This enables the body to replenish certain essential stores

Preevent nutrition begins at the start of the season, not just before a big game.

THE PREGAME MEAL

The athlete should:
1. Eat 3 to 4 hours before competition
2. Avoid foods that are high in animal fat, protein, and sugar
3. Avoid coffee and tea
4. Eat a meal that primarily contains complex carbohydrates
5. Drink water

and to reduce or eliminate various metabolites that might reduce performance.

The liquid meal—which is nutritionally sound and contains the recommended daily dietary proportions of nutrients—is widely used as the meal immediately before performance and is recommended as a means of eliminating or reducing the pregame syndrome. Foods of high cellulose content such as lettuce should be avoided because they tend to increase the need for defecation. The elimination of highly spiced and fatty or fried foods is also desirable because of the likelihood of gastrointestinal irritation. Sugars should be avoided because they retard stomach emptying. Liquids should be low in fat and readily absorbable. Fruit juices should be avoided. Drinks that contain caffeine induce a period of stimulation of the central nervous system that is followed by a period of depression and therefore are not advisable. Tea and coffee are also diuretics; that is, they stimulate the flow of urine and thus may cause additional discomfort during the competitive period. Water intake should be normal. Cocoa, whether made from milk or water, is an excellent beverage to provide some variety.

It is generally accepted that the preevent meal should be consumed approximately 3 to 4 hours before competition. Eating just before activity can cause acute discomfort when attempting to perform physically. Also, the increase in portal circulation required for digestion is achieved by withdrawing from the systemic circulation blood that would otherwise be readily available for the performance of physical work.

Alternative Eating Patterns

There is no scientific evidence that performance can generally be improved through the athlete's diet. Improvement in performance may be attributed to a balanced diet if there have been previous dietary deficiencies. The main value of proper nutrition lies in preventing the deleterious effects of improper or inadequate nutrition.

Food fads are rampant among athletes. No food, vitamin, supplement, or hormone will substitute for sound nutrition and hard work. Dietary abuses are sometimes condoned by parents and coaches in the mistaken belief that they will help, whereas in reality many of them are deleterious.

The vegetarian athlete   Some athletes opt to eat a vegetarian diet. This decision can be based on religious, philosophical, ecological, or health reasons. Types of vegetarian diets differ according to what animal products are ingested. For example, vegans eat only plant food, lactovegetarians ingest dairy products plus plant food, and ovolactovegetarians consume eggs, dairy products, and plant food.

The primary concern in the vegetarian diet is whether or not enough protein is being consumed, because the essential amino acids are balanced better in animal products than in plant foods. The vegetarian athlete, therefore, must carefully plan his or her diet to include all the essential amino acids.

Foods to avoid immediately preceding competition:
Lettuce
Spicy foods
Fatty or fried foods
Sugars
Fruit juices
Caffeine drinks
Coffee and tea

WEIGHT MANAGEMENT

The need for gain or loss of weight in an athlete often poses a problem because the individual's ingrained eating habits are difficult to change. The inability to supervise the athlete's meal program for balance and quantity further complicates the problem. It is sometimes difficult to determine whether a person is overweight. Some athletes who appear overweight or who tip the scales above average standards are not overweight at all; they usually possess greater musculature and larger bones. In such situations, knowledge of somatotyping is valuable to the coach or athletic trainer.[8]

The three basic somatotypes are the ectomorph, the mesomorph, and the endomorph (Figure 4-5). Ectomorphs are slender, tall individuals having long thin bones and narrow chest, head, and fingers. Mesomorphs have large bones, well-defined musculature, long neck, broad shoulders, slender waist, broad hips, and long extremities. Endomorphs usually have little muscle definition, small bones, large heads, long trunks, short necks, short arms, and legs tapered to the ends. A fourth somatotype is the mixed type. Ectomorphs tend to be thin and to have higher-than-average fuel needs in contrast to endomorphs, who tend toward fatness. Mesomorphs usually fall between endomorphs and ectomorphs in body weight.

Somatotypes:
ectomorph
mesomorph
endomorph

Weight Control

The energy requirements of individuals vary with age, sex, weight, health status, and occupation. Body weight is determined in part by build, or

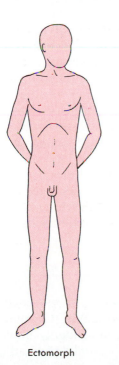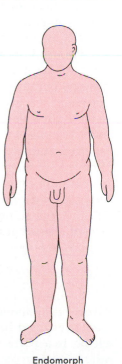

Figure 4-5

The three somatotypes are ectomorph, mesomorph, and endomorph.

Ectomorph   Mesomorph   Endomorph

Intense, rapid weight reduction always has negative consequences on performance.

Weight reduction can be particularly harmful to high school–aged athletes because they are still growing.

somatotype. Because of these many variables, there is no shortcut or magic formula to weight control. If an increase in weight is desirable, it is better achieved through a gain in muscle bulk than through a gain in fat. To lose weight one must increase physical activity and maintain a proper diet; only in this way can caloric expenditure exceed intake.

Intense weight reduction during a short time may seriously impair performance. Ordinarily, weight reduction is produced within 2 to 7 days. Weight loss during this time may range from 2 to 4½ pounds. Individuals who need to lose weight should do so gradually over as long a period as is feasible under the circumstances.

Publicity in recent years has charged that certain coaches were requiring some of their athletes to achieve excessive weight loss so that they could make a certain weight for competition. Such practices cannot be condoned. They are not only undesirable from the standpoint of maintaining physical effectiveness but also potentially harmful. A rapid decrease in weight caused by extreme restriction of caloric intake is contraindicated immediately before and during periods of maximum physical effort. Also, weight reduction by high school athletes poses a serious problem because of the growth and maturation factors.[8]

Some coaches advocate dryout and *total fasting* at the beginning of a program of weight reduction. Usually they suggest elimination of at least carbohydrates and salt. Such an approach has serious implications for health because salt loss incurred through perspiration greatly increases the possibility of a clinically identified sodium deficiency. When vigorous physical activity is performed, these features not only are magnified but also may lead to a renal shutdown. During total fast a decrease in heart size accompanies these hydrodynamic changes.

Weight loss during training should not exceed 2 to 3 pounds a week, and the conditioning program should be started at least 5 to 6 weeks before competition. It should be noted that weight fluctuations impair physical performance. Healthy weight loss should consider that athletes consume at least 1,200 calories per day to include proper nutritional need. Daily calorie reduction can range from 500 to 1,000 calories per day (Coleman 1990). A reduction of 3,500 calories (calorie per lb of fat) per week along with 20 to 30 minutes of moderate-intensity exercise 3 times per week should lead to fat reduction.

Gaining muscle weight consists of eating 350 extra calories per day along with engaging in proper exercise. Eating nutrient-rich higher-calorie foods along with heavy resistance training should develop muscle weight instead of fat. It is to be remembered that the percent of body fat is more important than body weight.[5]

EATING DISORDERS
Bulimia

The typical bulimic person is a girl or woman, adolescent to middle-aged, Caucasian, and belonging to a middle- or upper-class family. The individual is a perfectionist who is obedient, overcompliant, highly motivated, very successful academically, well-liked by peers, and a good ath-

---

RECOGNIZING THE ATHLETE WITH AN EATING DISORDER

Signs to look for:
1. Social isolation and withdrawal from friends and family
2. A lack of confidence in athletic abilities
3. Ritualistic eating behavior (e.g., organized food on plate)
4. An obsession with counting calories
5. An obsession with exercising, especially just before a meal
6. An obsession with weight
7. A constant overestimation of body size
8. Patterns of leaving the table directly after eating to go into the restroom
9. Problems related to eating disorders (e.g., malnutrition, menstrual irregularities, or chronic fatigue)

---

lete. The bulimic individual typically gorges on thousands of calories after a period of starvation and then purges the body through induced vomiting and further fasting or with laxatives or diuretics.

Anorexia Nervosa

It has been estimated that 30% to 50% of all individuals diagnosed as having anorexia nervosa also develop some symptoms of bulimia. Anorexia nervosa is characterized by a distorted body image and a major concern about weight gain. As with bulimia, anorexia nervosa affects mostly girls and women. It usually begins in adolescence and can be mild, without major consequences, or can be life threatening. As many as 15% to 21% of individuals diagnosed as anorexic will ultimately die of this disorder.[1] Anorexia nervosa is prevalent in sports such as gymnastics and wrestling where weight is important.

Despite being extremely thin, anorexic athletes see themselves as too fat. These individuals deny hunger and are hyperactive, engaging in abnormal amounts of exercise such as aerobics or distance running.[4] In general, the anorexic individual is highly pliant.

The coach and athletic trainer must be sensitive to eating problems. A coach can sometimes, by a critical action or word, cause the athlete to develop a distorted self-image leading to anorexia nervosa.

Early intervention is essential. Any athlete with signs of bulimia or anorexia nervosa must be confronted in a kind, empathetic manner by the coach, athletic trainer, or school nurse. When an eating disorder is detected, the individual must be referred for psychological or psychiatric treatment.

Coaches must be alert to the signs and causes of eating disorders.

SUMMARY

The athlete requires proper nutrition to recover promptly from fatigue and to repair damaged tissue. Eating the correct amounts of nutrients in the basic food categories is extremely important to the athlete. Most athletic endeavors require that the athlete eat a diet consisting of 55% or more carbohydrates, 10% to 15% proteins, and 25% to 30% fats.

Vitamins and minerals are metabolic regulators that transform energy. Vitamins are classified as water soluble or fat soluble. A good, varied diet, including a balance of the basic four food categories, will supply all the essential vitamins. Minerals, like vitamins, are essential for good health and are provided by a good diet.

Water is one of the three prime necessities of life and comes from several sources to meet the body's needs. The athlete should drink at least 500 ml of water before competition and 600 ml per hour when exercising.

Athletes traditionally supplement their daily diets in many ways. In most cases they have found that doing so does not improve their performance significantly. In some cases supplementation can hinder performance and even predispose the athlete to eventual injury. However, iron supplementation may be of value for some teenaged boys and girls. Iron deficiency is not uncommon among female athletes.

The practice of increasing the amount of carbohydrates ingested helps the endurance athlete. Although carbohydrate loading may help some athletes, it may hinder others. Fat loading should be avoided.

Preevent nutrition varies according to the athlete. As a general rule, athletes should eat 3 to 4 hours before competition. Foods high in cellulose, meat proteins, fat, and sugar, as well as coffee and tea, should be avoided. Meals containing complex carbohydrates should be eaten along with water for hydration.

There is no scientific evidence to support the idea that performance can be generally improved through alternative eating patterns such as the vegetarian diet. The athlete who avoids eating animal flesh or all animal products must monitor his or her diet carefully to ensure that all essential nutrients are eaten daily.

Extreme care must be taken when weight management is required for a specific sport. Severe weight loss can lead to serious illnesses or injuries. The best means to a healthy weight loss is eating from the basic four food categories daily in the correct percentages while reducing the amount of overall calories.

Eating disorders are a problem among many participants in sports and dance. The obsession with weight loss can cause the eating disorders bulimia and anorexia nervosa to emerge. Bulimia's basic pattern is one of secretive binge eating and purging. Anorexia nervosa is a weight obsession characterized by a distorted body image. Anorexia sufferers see themselves as overweight when in reality they are markedly underweight.

REVIEW QUESTIONS AND CLASS ACTIVITIES

1. What are the three energy sources in the body? Which is the first one used? The last? The most efficient?
2. What are the daily dietary requirements of the food pyramid food groups? Should the requirements of the typical athlete's diet differ from them? If so, in what ways?

3. What nutrients cannot be stored in the body and must be replenished regularly?
4. Do so-called electrolyte beverages replenish the water and electrolyte level in the body better and faster than plain water?
5. How can dehydration affect performance?
6. Do dietary supplements enhance athletic performance? If so, which ones?
7. What is carbohydrate loading and how can it help an athlete?
8. What are some basic guidelines for preevent nutrition for high school athletes who may not have a supervised training table?
9. Have students prepare a pregame menu for an athletic team, keeping in mind the time frame and the nutrients needed for maximum energy.
10. How much weight loss per week is safe off season? In season?
11. Have students prepare a listing of their food intake for 1 week to determine whether they are eating a balanced diet.
12. Do female athletes have any special nutritional needs?
13. How can one recognize an eating disorder in an athlete? What should be done to help?
14. Invite a nutritionist, psychologist, or psychiatrist to class to discuss eating disorders and how the coach or athletic trainer can handle these problems.

REFERENCES

1. Arnheim D, Prentice W: *Principles of athletic training*, ed 8, St Louis, 1994, Times Mirror/Mosby–Year Book.
2. Clark N: Fluid facts, *Phys Sportsmed* 20:33, 1992.
3. Coggan AR, Coyle EF: Effect of carbohydrate feeding during high intensity exercise, *Appl Physiol* 65: 1703, 1988.
4. Coleman E: Sports drink update, Gatorade Sports Science Exchange, *Sports Nutr* 1, 1988.
5. Coleman E: *Nutrition to maximize your athletic performance*, Van Nuys, Calif, 1990, PM.
6. Overdorf VG: Conditioning for thinness: the dilemma of the eating disordered female athletes, *JO-PHERD* 58:62, 1987.
7. Replacing body fluids is vital during winter, *First Aider*, Gardner, Kan, 1987, Cramer Products.
8. Sherman WM: Carbohydrate, muscle glycogen, and improved performance, *Phys Sportsmed* 15: 157, 1987.
9. Slavin JL: Calorie supplements for athletes, *Phys Sportsmed* 15:157, 1987.
10. Smith J: A look at the components and effectiveness of sports drinks, *J Ath Train* 27:123, 1992.
11. Tipton CM: Commentary: physicians should advise wrestlers about weight loss, *Phys Sportsmed* 15: 160, 1987.

ANNOTATED BIBLIOGRAPHY

Berming JR, Steen SN: *Sports nutrition for the 90's. The health professional's handbook.*
   This text is written for health professionals consulting athletes on nutrition.
Brooks M et al: *Pocket picture guides: sports injuries,* ed 2, New York, 1992, Gower Medical Publishing.
   Show pictures of the most common sports-related injuries emphasizing recognition of pathology by sight, palpitation, signs, and symptoms.
Browns F et al eds: *Advances in nutrition and top sport.* A text covering major topics in athletic nutrition focusing on peak performance.

Coleman E: *Nutrition to maximize your athletic performance*, Van Nuys, Calif, 1990, PM.

An easy-to-understand nutritional guide for the coach and athlete.

Frankle RT, Yang MV, eds: *Obesity and weight control: the health professional's guide to understanding and treatment*, 1988, Aspen Publishers. A multidisciplinary approach to understanding and treatment of weight control.

Guthrie HA: *Human nutrition*, St Louis, 1995, Mosby–Year Book.

A foundation text in all aspects of human nutrition.

Hamilton EMN et al: Nutrition: concepts and controversies, ed 4, St Paul, Minn, 1988, West.

A comprehensive text on nutrition. Chapter 12 discusses nutrition and exercise and specifically addresses children and teens.

Peterson M, Peterson K: *Eat to compete: a guide to sports nutrition*, St Louis, 1988, Mosby-Year Book.

A nutritional guide for the athlete and coach.

Thompson RA, Sherman RT: *Helping athletes with eating disorders*, Champaign, Ill, 1992, Human Kinetics.

Accurate and concise information sports personnel on eating disorders.

Williams C, Devlin JT, eds: *Foods, nutrition and sports performance*, New York, 1992, Routledge, Chapman & Hall.

A compendium of papers from 1991 conference of recommendations by international for optimum sport performance.

PART II

Sports Injury Causation, Response, and Management

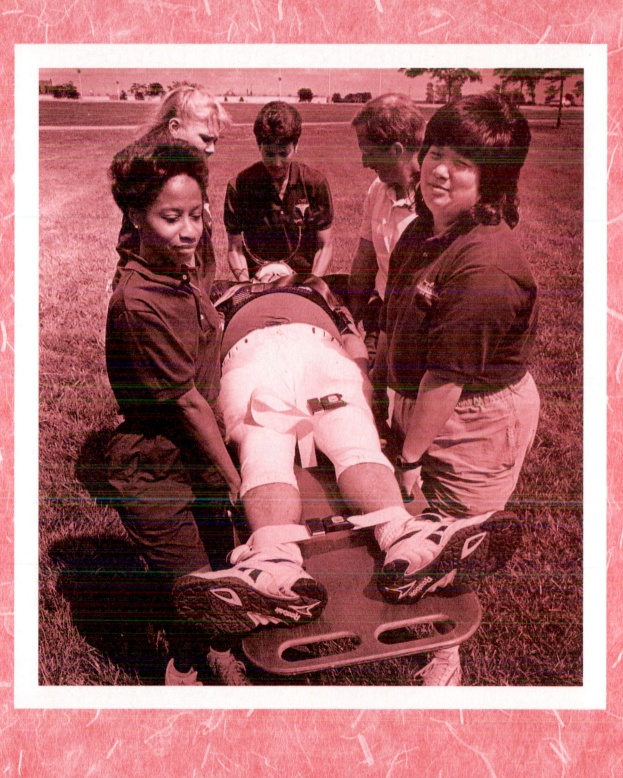

Protective Sports Devices

When you finish this chapter, you will be able to:

- Identify the major legal ramifications related to manufacturing, buying, and issuing commercial protective equipment
- Fit selected protective equipment properly (e.g., football helmets, shoulder pads, running shoes)
- Differentiate between good and bad features of selected protective devices
- Compare the advantages and disadvantages of customized versus commercial foot and ankle protective devices
- Describe the controversies surrounding the use of certain protective devices—are they in fact weapons against opposing players, or do they really work?
- Rate the protective value of various materials used in sports to make pads and orthotic devices

prophylactic
Pertaining to prevention, preservation, or protection

Modifications and improvements in sports equipment are continually being made, especially for sports in which injury is common. In this chapter, commercial and **prophylactic** techniques are discussed.

COMMERCIAL EQUIPMENT

The proper selection and fit of sports equipment are essential in the prevention of many sports injuries. This is particularly true in direct-contact and collision sports such as football, hockey, and lacrosse, but it can also be true in indirect-contact sports such as basketball and soccer. Whenever protective sports equipment is selected and purchased, a major decision in the safeguarding of the athletes' health and welfare is being made.[14]

Currently there is serious concern about the standards for protective sports equipment, particularly material durability standards—concerns that include who should set these standards, mass production of equipment, equipment testing methods, and requirements for wearing protective equipment. Some people are concerned that a piece of equipment that protects one athlete may be used as a weapon against another athlete.

Standards are also needed for protective equipment maintenance, both to keep it in good repair and to determine when to throw it away. Too often old, worn-out, and ill-fitting equipment is passed down from the varsity players to the younger and often less-experienced players, compounding their risk of injury. Coaches must learn to be less concerned with the color, look, and style of a piece of equipment and more concerned with its ability to prevent injury.

A major step toward the improvement of sports equipment has been achieved through such groups as the American Society for Testing and Materials (ASTM). Its Committee on Sports Equipment and Facilities, established in 1969, has been highly active in establishing standardization of specifications, test methods, and recommended practices for sports equipment and facilities to minimize injury, and promotion of knowledge as it relates to protective equipment standards. Engineering, chemistry, biomechanics, anatomy, physiology, physics, computer science, and other related disciplines are applied to solve problems inherent in safety standardization of sports equipment and facilities.

Old, worn-out, ill-fitting equipment should never be passed down to younger, less-experienced players; it compounds their risk of injury.

Legal Concerns

As with other aspects of sports participation, there is increasing litigation related to equipment. Manufacturers and purchasers of sports equipment must foresee all possible uses and misuses of the equipment and must warn the user of any potential risks inherent in the use or misuse of that equipment.

To decrease the possibilities of sports injuries and litigation stemming from equipment, the practitioner should do the following:

1. Buy sports equipment from reputable manufacturers.
2. Buy the safest equipment that resources will permit.
3. Make sure that all equipment is assembled correctly. The person who assembles equipment must be competent to do so and must follow the manufacturer's instructions to the letter.
4. Maintain all equipment properly, according to the manufacturer's guidelines.
5. Use equipment only for the purpose for which it was designed.
6. Warn athletes who use the equipment about all possible risks that using the equipment could entail.
7. Use great caution in the construction or customizing of any piece of equipment.
8. Use no defective equipment. All equipment must routinely be inspected for defects, and all defective equipment must be rendered unusable.

Commercial stock and custom protective devices differ considerably. Stock devices are premade and packaged and are for immediate use. Customized devices are constructed according to the individual characteristics of an athlete. Stock items may have problems with their sizing. In contrast, a custom device can be specifically sized and made to fit the protection and support needs of the individual.

HEAD PROTECTION

Direct-collision sports such as football and hockey require special protective equipment, especially for the head. Football involves more body contact than does hockey, but hockey players generally move faster and therefore create greater impact forces. Besides direct head contact stemming from hitting the boards, hockey has the added injury elements of swinging sticks and fast-moving pucks. Other sports using fast-moving projectiles are baseball, with its pitched ball and swinging bat, and track and field, with the javelin, discus, and heavy shot, which can also produce serious head injuries.

Football Helmets

A major influence on football helmet standardization in the United States has been the research of Hodgson and Thomas and the National Operating Committee on Standards for Athletic Equipment (NOCSAE) for football helmet certification. To be NOCSAE approved, a helmet must be able to tolerate forces applied to many different areas of it. Football helmets typically must withstand repeated blows and high-mass–low-velocity impacts such as running into a goalpost and hitting the head on the ground.

Schools must provide the athlete with quality equipment. This especially is true of the football helmet. All helmets must have a NOCSAE certification. The fact that a helmet is certified does not mean that it is completely fail-safe. Athletes, as well as their parents, must be apprised of the dangers that are inherent in any sport, particularly football. To make this especially clear, the NOCSAE has adopted the following recommended warning to be placed on all football helmets:

> Warning: Do not strike an opponent with any part of this helmet or face mask. This is a violation of football rules and may cause you to suffer severe brain or neck injury including paralysis or death. Severe brain or neck injury may also occur accidentally while playing football. NO HELMET CAN PREVENT ALL SUCH INJURIES. USE THIS HELMET AT YOUR OWN RISK.

Each player's helmet must have a visible exterior warning label ensuring that players have been made aware of the risks involved in the game of American football. The label must be attached to each helmet by both the manufacturer and the reconditioner.

Many types of helmets are in use today. They currently fall into two categories: (1) padded, and (2) air- and fluid-filled (Figure 5-1). There are also helmets that are combinations of the two types.

When fitting helmets, always wet the player's hair to simulate playing conditions; this will make the initial fitting easier. Then closely follow the manufacturer's directions for a proper fit. In general, the helmet should adhere to the following fit standards:

1. The helmet should fit snugly around all parts of the player's head (front, sides, and crown), and there should be no gaps between the pads and the head or face.
2. It should cover the base of the skull. The pads placed at the back of the neck should be snug but not to the extent of discomfort.
3. It should not come down over the eyes. It should sit (front edge) ¾ inch (1.91 cm) above the player's eyebrows.

Football helmets must withstand repeated blows that are of high mass and low velocity.

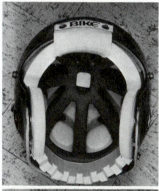

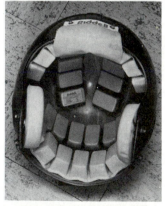

Figure 5-1

Football helmets fall into two basic categories, padded and air- and fluid-filled.

4. The ear holes should match.
5. It should not shift when manual pressure is applied.
6. It should not recoil on impact.
7. The chin strap should be an equal distance from the center of the helmet. Straps must keep the helmet from moving up and down or side to side.
8. The cheek pads should fit snugly against the sides of the face.
9. The face mask should be attached securely to the helmet, allowing a complete field of vision.
10. Coaches must remember to follow the manufacturer's suggested guidelines.

Whichever football helmet is used, it must be routinely checked for proper fit, especially in the first few days that it is worn (Figure 5-2). A check for snugness should be made by inserting a tongue depressor between the head and the liner. Fit is proper when the tongue depressor firmly resists being moved back and forth. If air bladder helmets are used by a team that travels to a different altitude and air pressure, the helmet fit must be routinely rechecked.

Chin straps are also important in maintaining the proper head and helmet relationship. Two basic types of chin straps are in use today—a two-snap and a four-snap strap. Many coaches prefer the four-snap chin strap because it keeps the helmet from tilting forward and backward.

Even high-quality helmets are of no use if not properly fitted or maintained.

Figure 5-2

Fitting a football helmet. **A,** Pull down on face mask; helmet must not move. **B,** Turn helmet to position on the athlete's head. **C,** Push down on helmet; there must be no movement. **D,** Try to rock helmet back and forth; there must be no movement. **E,** Check for a snug jaw pad fit. **F,** Proper adjustment of the chin strap is necessary to ensure proper helmet fit.

A   B   C

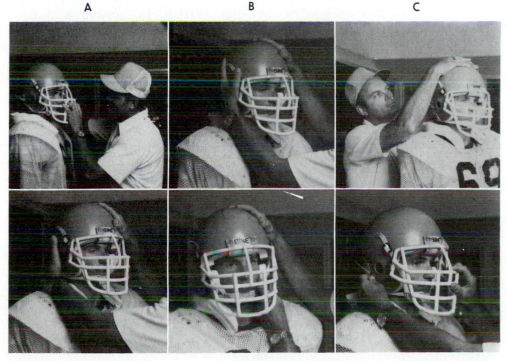

D   E   F

Jaw pads are also essential to keep the helmet from rocking laterally. They should rest snugly against the player's cheekbones. Even if a helmet's ability to withstand the forces of the game is certified, it is of no avail if the helmet is not properly fitted or maintained.

Ice Hockey Helmets

Ice hockey helmets must withstand the high-velocity impact of a stick or puck and the low-velocity forces of falling or hitting a sideboard.

As with football helmets, there has been a concerted effort to upgrade and standardize ice hockey helmets. In contrast to football, blows to the head in ice hockey are usually singular rather than multiple. An ice hockey helmet must withstand both high-velocity impacts (e.g., being hit with a stick or a puck, which produces low mass and high velocity), as well as the high-mass–low-velocity forces produced by running into the sideboard or falling on the ice. In each instance, the hockey helmet, like the football helmet, must be able to spread the impact over a large surface area through a firm exterior shell and at the same time be able to decelerate forces that act on the head through a proper energy-absorbing liner. It is essential for all hockey players to wear protective helmets that carry the stamp of approval from the Canadian Standards Association (CSA).

Baseball/Softball Batting Helmets

Like ice hockey helmets, the baseball/softball helmet must withstand high-velocity impacts. Unlike football and ice hockey, baseball and softball have not produced a great deal of data on batting helmets. It has been suggested, however, that baseball/softball helmets do not adequately dissipate the energy of the ball during impact (Figure 5-3). A possible answer is to add external padding or to improve the helmet's suspension. The use of a helmet with an ear flap can afford some additional protection to the batter. Each on-deck batter and runner is required to wear a baseball/softball head protector that carries a NOCSAE stamp similar to that on football helmets.

FACE PROTECTION

Devices that provide face protection fall into four categories: full face guards, mouth guards, ear guards, and eye protection devices.

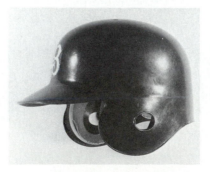

Figure 5-3

There is some question about how well baseball batting helmets protect against high-velocity impacts.

Face Guards

Face guards are used in a variety of sports to protect the face from flying or carried objects during a collision with another player (Figure 5-4).Since the adoption of face guards and mouth guards for use in football, mouth injuries have been reduced more than 50% (Figure 5-5), but the incidenceof neck injuries has increased significantly. The catcher in baseball, hockey players, lacrosse players, and football players should all be adequately protected against facial injuries, particularly lacerations and fractures (Figure 5-6).

A great variety of face masks and bars is available to the player, depending on the position played and the protection needed. In football no face protection should have fewer than two bars. Proper mounting of

In sports, the face may be protected by:
Face guards
Mouth guards
Ear guards
Eye-protection devices

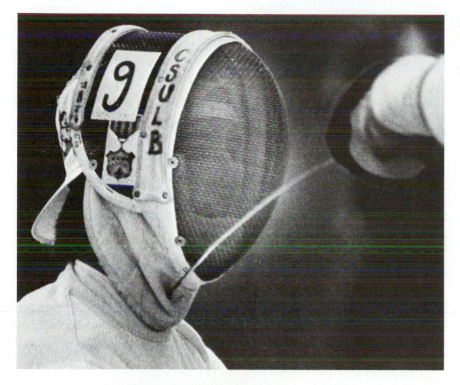

Figure 5-4

Sports such as fencing require complete face protection.

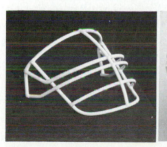 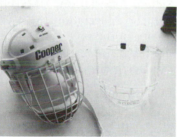

Figure 5-5

A variety of face guards used in sports.

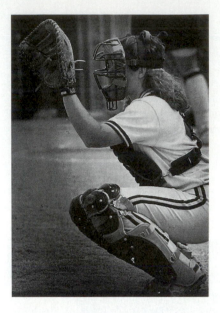

Figure 5-6

A catcher's face mask
protects the player against
facial injury; the addition of
the chin flap provided
additional protection to the
throat region.

the face mask and bars is imperative for maximum safety. All mountings should be made in such a way that the bar attachments are flush with the helmet. A 3-inch (7.62 cm) space should exist between the top of the face guard and the lower edge of the helmet. No helmet should be drilled more than one time on each side, and this must be done by a factory-authorized reconditioner. Attachment of a bar or face mask not specifically designed for the helmet can invalidate the manufacturer's warranty.

Ice hockey face masks have been shown to reduce the incidence of facial injuries. In high school they are required for all players, not just the goalkeeper. The rule stipulates that helmets be equipped with commercial plastic-coated wire-mesh guards, which must meet standards set by the Hockey Equipment Certification Council (HECC) and the American Society for Testing Materials (ASTM).[7] The openings in the guard must be small enough to prevent a hockey stick from penetrating. Plastic guards such as polycarbonate face shields have been approved by the NECC/ASTM and the CSA Committee on Hockey Protective Equipment. The rule also requires that in addition to face protectors, goalkeepers must wear commercial throat protectors. The National Federation of High School Associations (NFSHSA) rule is similar to the National Collegiate Athletic Association (NCAA) rule requiring players to wear face guards. There should be a space of 1 to 1½ inches (3.81 cm) between the player's nose and the face guard. As with the helmet shell, pads, and chin strap, the face guard must be checked daily for defects.

Mouth Guards

The majority of dental traumas can be prevented if the athlete wears a correctly fitted intraoral mouth guard, as compared with an extraoral type (Figure 5-7). In addition to protecting the teeth, the intraoral mouth

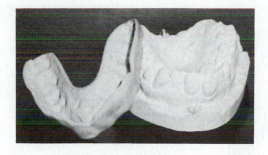

Figure 5-7

Customized intraoral mouth protector.

guard absorbs the shock of chin blows and helps to prevent cerebral concussion. The mouth protector should give the athlete proper and tight fit, comfort, unrestricted breathing, and unimpeded speech during competition. The athlete's air passages should not be obstructed in any way by the mouthpiece. It is best when the mouthpiece is retained on the upper jaw and projects backward only as far as the last molar, thus permitting speech.

Cutting down mouth guards to cover only the front four teeth should never be condoned. It invalidates the manufacturer's warranty against dental injuries, and a cut-down mouth guard can easily become dislodged and lead to an obstructed airway, which poses a serious life-threatening situation for the athlete. Maximum protection is afforded when the mouth guard is composed of a flexible, resilient material and is form fitted to the teeth and upper jaw.[16]

The types of mouth guards generally used in sports include the ready-made, a commercial mouth guard formed after submersion in boiling water, and the custom-fabricated type, which is formed over a model made from an impression of the athlete's maxillary arch.

High schools and colleges now require that mouth guards be worn at all times during football playing, and they must be visible to the officials. To assist enforcement, official mouth guards are increasingly made in the most visible color, yellow.[16] The NCAA mandates that a time out be charged a team if a player fails to wear the mouth guard. In a recent study to determine if mouth-formed mouth guards are large enough to meet the mandated NCAA rule, researchers at one Division I institution determined that a large percentage of the university football players (85%) did not receive adequate protection from the standard mouth-formed guard. At another university with a predominantly black football team, only 5.5% of the players received adequate protection. It is important that coaches and athletic trainers measure the arch length of the mouth guards to ensure adequate protection for the athlete and to be in compliance with the NCAA rule. Other sport governing bodies also require the use of mouth guards to reduce dental injuries and concussions in their sports.[1]

> A properly fitted mouth guard protects the teeth, absorbs blows to the chin, and can prevent concussion.

Ear Guards

With the exception of boxing and wrestling, most contact sports do not make a special practice of protecting the ears. Both boxing and wrestling

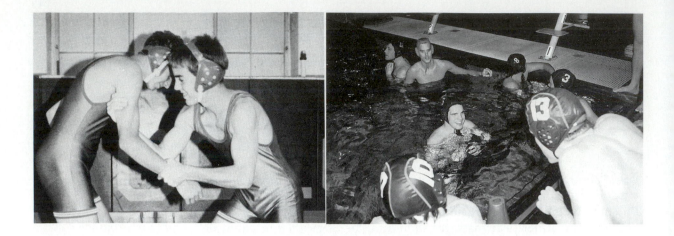

Figure 5-8

Ear protection. **A**, Wrestler's ear guard. **B**, Water polo player's ear protection.

can cause irritation of the ears to the point that permanent deformity can ensure. To avoid this problem special ear guards should be routinely worn. Recently a very effective ear protection has been developed for the water polo player (Figure 5-8).

Eye Protection Devices

The athlete who wears glasses must be protected during sports activities. Glasses broken during the heat of competitive battle can pose considerable danger. The eyes of the athlete can be protected by glass guards, case-hardened lenses, plastic lenses, or contact lenses.

Spectacles

For the athlete who must wear corrective lenses, spectacles can be both a blessing and a nuisance. They may slip on sweat, get bent when hit, fog from perspiration, detract from peripheral vision, and be difficult to wear with protective headgear. Even with all these disadvantages, properly fitted and designed spectacles can provide adequate protection and withstand the rigors of the sport. If the athlete has glass lenses, they must be case-hardened to prevent them from splintering on impact. When a case-hardened lens breaks, it crumbles, eliminating the sharp edges that may penetrate the eye. The cost of this process is relatively low. The only disadvantages involved are that the glasses are heavier than average, and they may be scratched more easily than regular glasses.

Another possible sports advantage of glass-lensed spectacles is a process through which the lenses can become color tinted when

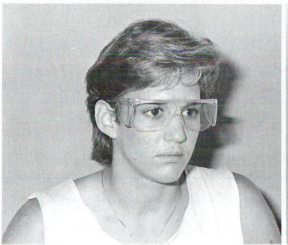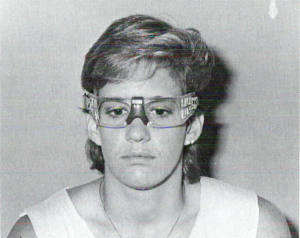

exposed to ultraviolet rays from the sun and then return to a clear state when removed from the sun's rays. They are known as *photochromic lenses*.

Plastic lenses for spectacles are popular with athletes. They are much lighter in weight than glass lenses and they can be made scratch-resistant with a special coating.

Contact Lenses

The athlete who is able to wear contact lenses without discomfort can avoid many of the inconveniences of spectacles. Their greatest advantage is probably the fact that they "become a part of the eye" and move with it.

Contact lenses come mainly in two types: the corneal type, which covers just the iris of the eye, and the scleral type, which covers the entire front of the eye, including the white. Peripheral vision, astigmatism, and corneal waviness are improved through the use of contact lenses. Unlike regular glasses, contact lenses do not normally cloud during temperature changes. They also can be tinted to reduce glare. For example, yellow lenses can be used against ice glare and blue ones against glare from snow. There is currently a trend toward athletes' preferring the soft, hydrophilic lenses to the hard type. Adjustment time for the soft lenses is shorter than for the hard, they can be more easily replaced, and they are more adaptable to the sports environment.

Eye and Glasses Guards

It is essential that athletes take special precautions to protect their eyes, especially in sports that use fast-moving projectiles and implements (Figure 5-9). Besides the more obvious sports of ice hockey, lacrosse, and baseball, the racquet sports also cause serious eye injury. Athletes not

Eye protection must be worn by all athletes who play sports that use fast-moving projectiles.

wearing spectacles should wear closed eye guards to protect the orbital cavity. Athletes who normally wear spectacles with plastic or case-hardened lenses are to some degree already protected against eye injury from an implement or projectile; however, greater safety is afforded by the metal-rimmed frame that surrounds and fits over the athlete's glasses. The protection the guard affords is excellent, but it does hinder vision in some planes. Polycarbonate eye shields that have recently been developed can be attached to football face masks, hockey helmets, and baseball/softball helmets.

TRUNK AND THORAX PROTECTION

Trunk and thorax protection is essential in many contact and collision sports. Areas that are most exposed to impact forces must be properly covered with some material that offers protection against soft-tissue compression. Of particular concern are the exposed bony protuberances of the body that have insufficient soft tissue for protection such as shoulders, ribs, and spine, as well as external genitalia (Figures 5-10, 5-11, 5-12 and 5-13).

As discussed earlier, the problem that arises in the wearing of protective equipment is that, although it is armor against injury to the athlete wearing it, it can also serve as a weapon against all opponents. Standards must become more stringent in determining what equipment is absolutely necessary for body protection without being itself a source of trauma.

Shoulder

Manufacturers of shoulder pads have made great strides toward protecting the football player against direct force on the shoulder muscle complex (Figures 5-11 and 5-12). There are two general types of pads, flat and cantilevered. The player who uses the shoulder a great deal in blocking and tackling requires the bulkier cantilevered type as compared with the quarterback and ball receiver, who use the flat type. Over the years the shoulder pad's front and rear panels have been extended along with the cantilever. The following are rules for fitting the football shoulder pad:

1. The width of the shoulder is measured to determine the proper size of pad.
2. The inside shoulder pad should cover the tip of the shoulder in a direct line with the lateral aspect of the shoulder.
3. The epaulets and cups should cover the deltoid muscle and allow movements required by the athlete's specific position.
4. The neck opening must allow the athlete to raise the arm over the head without placing undue pressure on the neck yet must not allow the pad to slide back and forth.
5. If a split-clavicle shoulder pad is used, the channel for the top of the shoulder must be in the proper position.
6. Straps underneath the arm must hold the pads firmly in place, but not so they constrict soft tissue. A collar and drop-down pads may be added to provide additional protection.

Protection is essential in bony areas such as the shoulders, ribs, and spine.

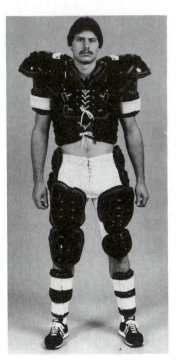

Figure 5-10

Top of the line football protective pads. This system uses open cell foam and air management to disperse a direct impact over the entire surface area of the pad, minimizing the blow to the athlete.

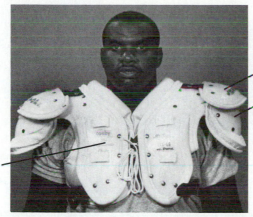

Epaulet

Shoulder
cup

Breastplate

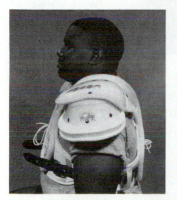
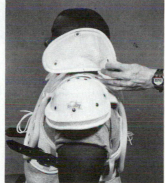
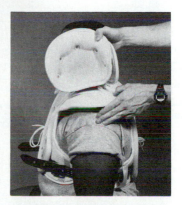

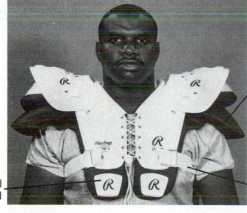
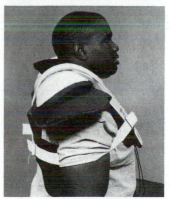

Extended
deltoid
pad

Pectoral
pad

Belt strap

Figure 5-11

Football shoulder pads
should be made to protect
the player against direct
force to the entire shoulder
complex.

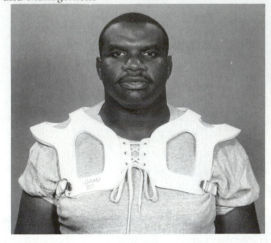

A

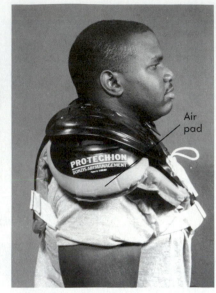

B

Figure 5-12

Customized foam is placed
on the underside of the
shoulder pad to provide
additional protection.

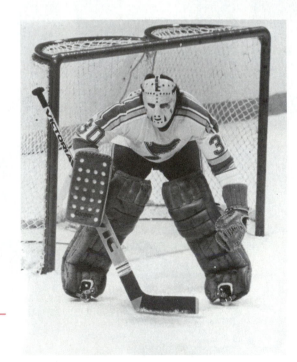

Figure 5-13

An ice hockey goalie's
equipment represents the
ultimate in body protection.

Some coaches use a combination of football and ice hockey shoulder
pads to prevent injuries to high on the upper arm and shoulder. A pair
of Jofa hockey shoulder pads are placed under the football pads. The deltoid cap of the hockey pad is connected to the main body of the hockey
pad by an adjustable lace. The distal end of the deltoid cap is held in place

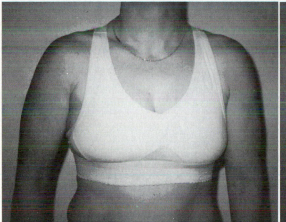 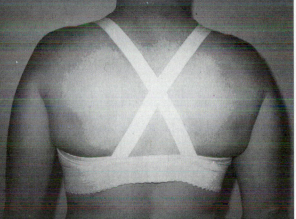

Figure 5-14

Large-breasted women often prefer bras with good upwards support made of nonelastic material.

by a Velcro strap. The chest pad is adjustable to ensure proper fit for any size athlete. The football shoulder pads are placed over the hockey pads. The coach should observe for a proper fit. Larger football pads may be needed.[1]

Breast Support

In the past the primary concern for female breast protection had focused on preventing contusions or bruising. With the continued increase in the number of physically active women, concern has been redirected to protecting the breasts against unwanted movement as the result of running and jumping. This is a particular problem for large-breasted women. Many girls and women in the past may have avoided vigorous physical activity, especially in public, because of the discomfort of uncontrolled movement of their breasts. Manufacturers have made a concerted effort to develop specialized bras for women who participate in all types of physical activity. The athletic clothing industry has produced an array of stylish, comfortable, and supportive sports bras. Women today have a variety of choices in their sport bras: style, support, fabric, and color. Some of the designs are stylish enough that the sports bras are sometimes worn as an outer garment.

Sport bras fall into three categories:

1. Bras with good upward support with nonelastic material have wide bands under the breasts with wide shoulder straps that are attached close to the hooks in the back (Figure 5-14, *A* and *B*).
2. Compressive bras are like wide elastic bandages binding the breasts to the chest wall (Figure 5-15).
3. Bras with slight modification of standard styles, usually with less elasticity, do not afford good protection.

Most regular bras do not provide support sufficient to prevent excessive breast motion, and many are poorly designed. To be effective a bra should hold the breasts to the chest and prevent stretching of the

To be effective a bra should hold the breasts tightly to the chest.

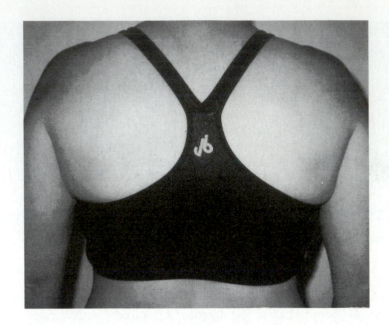

Figure 5-15

Compressive bras hold the breasts close to the chest wall.

Suspensory ligaments of Cooper

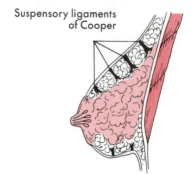

Figure 5-16

Stretching of Cooper's ligament causes premature sagging.

Cooper's ligament, which causes premature sagging (Figure 5-16). Metal parts (snaps, fasteners, underwire support) rub and abrade the skin. They lack sufficient padding. Seams over the nipples compound the rubbing of the bra on the nipple, leading to irritation.

For women with small breasts no special type of bra is required except to protect the nipple area. Women with medium-sized breasts seem to prefer the compressive bras, but women with a size C cup or larger should wear a firm supportive bra. Fabric, fabric weight, and firmness of construction will depend on the intensity of activity, support needed, sensitivity to the fabric, and climate. In contact sports additional padding may be placed inside the cup if needed. Women competing in ice hockey, for example, wear protective plastic chest pieces that attach to their shoulder pads to protect the breast tissue from contusions. Women should look for a bra with these features:

1. No irritating seams or fasteners next to the skin
2. Nonslip straps
3. Good supports or compression that holds the breasts close to the body
4. Firm, durable construction.

Thorax

Manufacturers such as Bike Company and Casco provide equipment for thorax protection. Many of the thorax protectors and rib belts can be

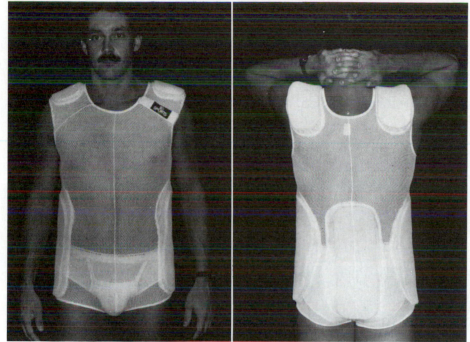

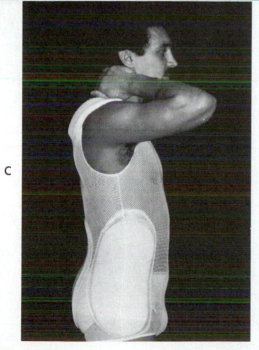

Figure 5-17

Bennet 34 Body Guard.
A, Front view. **B**, Back view.
C, Side view.

modified, replacing stock pads with customized thermomoldable plastic protective devices. A relatively recent item developed by a football player is the mesh body suit that has protective pads sewn into various areas (Figure 5-17). It is marketed as the Bennett 34 Body Gard. Recently many lightweight pads have been developed to protect the athlete against external forces. A jacket for the protection of a rib injury incorporates a pad composed of air-inflated, interconnected cylinders that protect against severe external forces. This same principle has been used in the development of other protective pads (Figure 5-18).

Hips and Buttocks

Pads in the region of the hips and buttocks are often needed by athletes in collision and high-velocity sports such as hockey and football. Other athletes needing protection in this region are amateur boxers, snow skiers, equestrians, jockeys, and water skiers. Two popular commercial pads are the girdle and belt types (Figure 5-19).

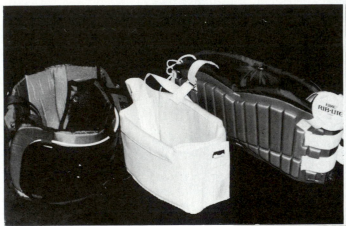
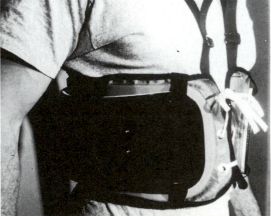
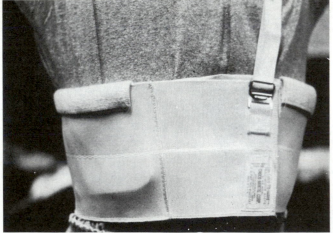

Figure 5-18

A, Donzis, Cosco, and Bike rib protectors. **B,** Donzis flak jacket. **C,** Cosco rib belt worn with insert molded to the body.

Groin and Genitalia

Sports involving high-velocity projectiles (e.g., hockey, lacrosse, and base-ball) require cup protection for male participants. The cup comes as a stock item that fits into place in a jockstrap, or athletic supporter.[15]

LIMB PROTECTION

Limbs, like other areas of the body, can be exposed a great deal to sports injuries and can require protection or, where there is weakness, support. Compression and mild soft-tissue support can be provided by neoprene sleeves, and hard bony areas of the body can be protected by commercial pads (Figure 5-20). In contrast, the athlete with a history of injury that needs special protection and support may require a commercial brace.

Footwear

Footwear can mean the difference between success, failure, and injury in competition. It is essential that the coach and equipment personnel make every effort to fit their athletes with proper shoes and socks.

Socks

Poorly fitted socks can cause abnormal stresses on the foot. For example, socks that are too short crowd the toes, especially the fourth and fifth ones. Socks that are too long can cause skin irritation because of wrinkles. All athletic socks should be clean, dry, and without holes to avoid irritations. Manufacturers are now providing a double-knit tubular sock without heels that decreases friction considerably within the shoe. The heel-less tubular sock is especially good for the basketball player. The sock's material also should be noted. Cotton socks can be too bulky; a combination of materials such as cotton and polyester is less bulky and dries faster.

All athletic socks should be clean and dry and without holes. Socks of the wrong size can irritate the skin.

Figure 5-19

Girdle style hip and coccygeal (tail-bone) pad.

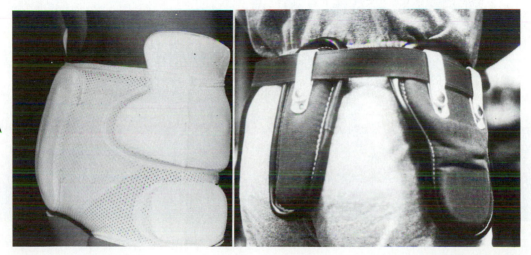

A   B

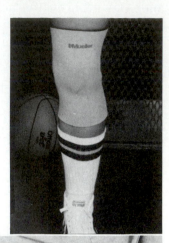

Figure 5-20

Types of neoprene sleeves.

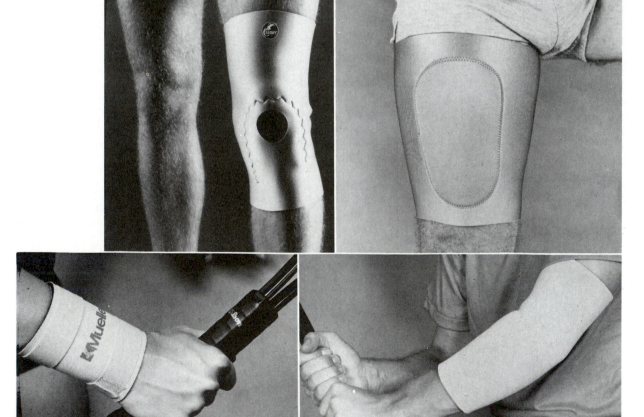

RUNNING SHOE DESIGN AND CONSTRUCTION

For the athlete to avoid injury, the running shoe should[3]:
1. Have a strong heel counter that fits well around the foot and locks the shoe around the foot
2. Always have good flexibility in the forefoot where toes bend
3. Preferably have a fairly high heel for the athlete with a tight Achilles tendon
4. Have a midsole that is moderately soft but does not flatten easily
5. Have a heel counter that is high enough to surround the foot but still allows room for an orthotic insert if needed
6. Have a counter that is attached to the sole to avoid the possibility of its coming loose
7. Always be of quality construction

Shoes

Even more damaging than improperly fitted socks are improperly fitted shoes. Chronic abnormal pressures to the foot often cause permanent structural deformities, as well as potentially dangerous calluses and blisters. Besides these local problems, improperly fitted shoes result in mechanical disturbances that affect the body's total postural balance and may eventually lead to pathological conditions of the muscles and joints. It also should be noted that shoes that are worn and/or broken down predispose the athlete to injuries of the foot and leg.

Shoe composition   The bare human foot is designed to function on uneven surfaces. Shoes were created to protect against harmful surfaces, but they should never interfere with natural functioning. Sports shoes, like all shoes, are constructed of different parts, each of which is designed for function, protection, and durability. Each sport places unique stresses and performance demands on the foot. In general, all sport shoes, like street shoes, are made of similar parts—a sole, uppers, heel counter, and toe box. The sole or bottom of a shoe is divided into an outer, middle, and inner section, each of which must be sturdy and flexible and provide a degree of cushioning, depending on the specific sport requirements. A heel counter should support and cushion the heel, and the toe box should protect without crowding.[3] The uppers must give the foot support and freedom to withstand a high degree of stress (Figure 5-21).

Shoe fitting   Fitting sports footgear is always difficult, mainly because the individual's left foot varies in size and shape from the right foot. Therefore measuring both feet is imperative. To fit the sports shoe properly, the athlete should approximate the conditions under which he or she will perform, such as wearing athletic socks, jumping up and down, and running. It is also desirable to fit the athlete's shoes at the end of the day to accommodate the gradual increase in size that occurs from the time of awakening. The athlete must carefully consider this choice because he or she will be spending countless hours in those shoes.

Always wear shoes appropriate for the sport.

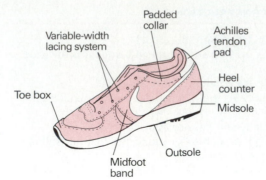

Variable-width
lacing system

Padded
collar

Achilles
tendon
pad

Toe box

Heel
counter

Midsole

Midfoot
band

Outsole

Figure 5-21

Properly fitted and
constructed shoes can
prevent foot injuries.

A properly fitted shoe will
bend where the foot bends.

During performance conditions the new shoe should feel snug but not too tight. The sports shoe should be long enough that all toes can be fully extended without being cramped. Its width should permit full movement of the toes, including flexion, extension, and some spreading. A good point to remember is that the wide part of the shoe should match the wide part of the foot to allow the shoe to crease evenly when the athlete is on the balls of the feet. The shoe should bend (or "break") at its widest part; when the break of the shoe and the ball joint coincide, the fit is correct. However, if the break of the shoe is in back or in front of the normal bend of the foot (metatarsophalangeal joint), the shoe and the foot will be opposing one another, causing abnormal skin and structural stresses to occur. Two measurements must be considered when fitting shoes: (1) the distance from the heel to the bend in the foot and (2) the distance from the heel to the end of the longest toe. An individual's feet may be equal in length from the heels to the balls of the feet but different between heels and toes. Shoes, therefore, should be selected for the longer of the two measurements. Other factors to consider when buying the sports shoe are the stiffness of the sole and the width of the shank, or narrowest part of the sole. A shoe with a too rigid, nonyielding sole places a great deal of extra strain on the foot tendons. A shoe with too narrow a shank also places extra strain because it fails to adequately support the athlete's inner, longitudinal arches. Two other shoe features to consider are innersoles to reduce friction and built-in arch supports.

The cleated or specially soled sports shoe presents some additional problems in fitting. For example, American football uses the multishort–cleated polyurethane sole and the five-in-front and two-in-back cleat arrangement with the soccer-type sole, both of which have cleats no longer than ½ inch (1.27 cm) (Figure 5-22). Special-soled shoes are also worn when playing on a synthetic surface. If cleated shoes are used, no matter which sport, the cleats must be properly positioned under the two major weight-bearing joints and must not be felt through the soles of the shoes.

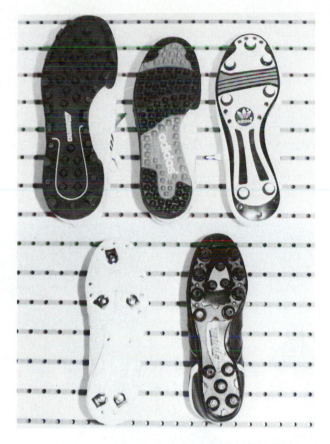

Figure 5-22

Variations in cleated
shoes—the longer the cleat,
the higher the incidence of
injury.

Commercial Foot Pads

Commercial foot pads are intended for use by the general public and are
not usually designed to withstand the rigors of sports activities. Those
commercial pads that are suited for sports are generally not durable
enough for hard, extended use. If money is no object, the ready-made
commercial pad has the advantage of saving time. Commercial pads are
manufactured for almost every type of common structural foot condition, ranging from corns and bunions to fallen arches and pronated feet.
In general, excessive foot pronation often eventually leads to overuse injuries. Available to the athlete commercially are preorthotic and arch supports (Figure 5-23). Scholl 610.2, Spenco arch supports, Shea devices,
and Foothotics Ready to Dispense orthotics are commonly used before
more formal customized orthotic devices are made (see p. 126). They offer a compromise to the custom-made foot orthotics, providing some biomechanical control. Indiscriminate use of these aids, however, may in-
tensify the pathological condition and encourage the athlete to delay seeing the team physician or team podiatrist for evaluation.

Indiscriminate use of
commercial foot orthotics
may give the athlete a false
sense of security.

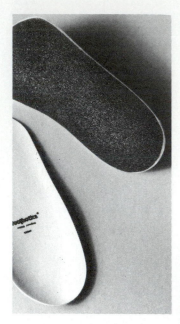

For the most part, foot devices are fabricated and customized from a variety of materials such as foam, felt, plaster, aluminum, and spring steel (see Customizing Protective and Supportive Devices in this chapter). One item that began as a custom-fabricated device but now is commercial is the heel cup, designed to reduce tissue shearing and shock (Figure 5-24).

Commercial Ankle Supports

Most commercial ankle supports are either the *elastic,* or *spat* splint types (Figure 5-25). The elastic type is a flexible, fibered sheath that slides over the foot and the ankle, purportedly giving mild support to a weak ankle. It has little use either as a strong support or as a protection to the post-acute or chronically weakened ankle in sports. The spat type is usually

Figure 5-23

Ready-to-dispense orthotic devices.

Figure 5-24

Heel cups and pads, including lifts of orthotic felt.

Figure 5-25

Commercial ankle supports.
A, Spat ankle support.
B, Ankle splints.

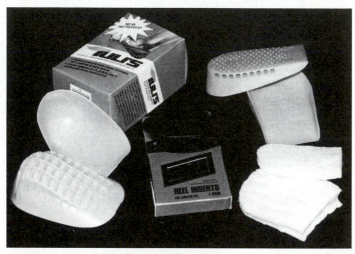

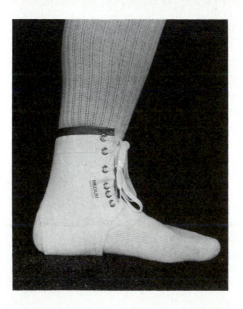

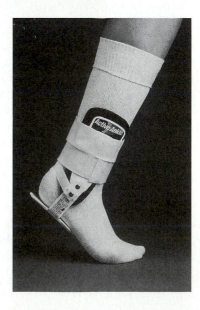

less resilient than the elastic type and has an open front that permits it to fit directly over the ankle and then tie snugly like a shoe. Some spats have vertical ribs to add inversion or eversion. Although providing some assistance, no commercial ankle support affords as much protection as does adhesive tape properly applied directly to the skin surface. Prophylactic ankle taping is superior to lace-on braces for the first 20 minutes of inversion activity. After 20 minutes they are equal in their ability to support the ankle. The decrease in support from the tape after 20 minutes is based on conservative measurements done in a laboratory setting. On the practice field the lace-on braces may be considered equal to or better than tape for ankle support. A fabricated orthoplast strip brace cut 3 or 4 inches (7.62 or 10.16 cm) wide is an effective semirigid support for a sprained ankle. An air cast or gel cast also provide support for a sprained ankle.

Shin and Lower Leg

The shin is commonly neglected in contact and collision sports. Commercially marketed hard-shelled, molded shin guards are used in field hockey and soccer (Figure 5-26).

Thigh and Upper Leg

Thigh and upper leg protection is necessary in collision sports such as hockey and football. Generally, pads slip into ready-made pockets in the sports suit or uniform (Figure 5-27). To avoid abnormal slipping within the pocket or to protect from injury, customized pads are constructed.

Knee Supports and Protective Devices

Knees are next in order to ankles and feet in terms of incidence of sports injury. As a result of the variety and rather high frequency of knee afflictions, many protective and supportive devices have been devised. The devices most frequently used in sports today are sleeves, pads, and braces.

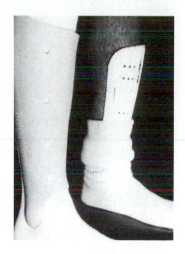

Figure 5-26
Full shin guard.

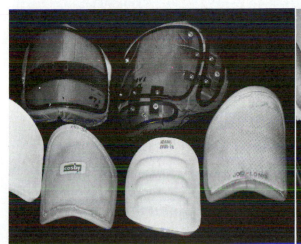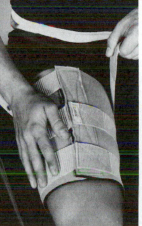

Figure 5-27
Commercial protective thigh braces.

Elastic knee pads or guards are extremely valuable in sports in which the athlete falls or receives a direct blow to the anterior aspect of the knee (Figure 5-28). An elastic sleeve containing a resilient pad may help to dissipate an anterior striking force but fails to protect the knee against lateral, medial, or twisting forces.

Knee Braces and Protective Devices

There are a number of different knee braces on the market. Some consist of vertical rigid strips held in an elastic sleeve or an elastic sleeve containing rigid hinges to be placed on either side of the knee joint. These braces are extremely questionable as to their ability to act as a protection against initial or recurrent injury. Braces of the wrap-around type with rigid strips contained in less elastic material hold the knee more firmly in place (Figure 5-29).

The prophylactic knee brace   Currently, prophylactic knee bracing has become increasingly popular in high school, college, and professional football. The braces are usually worn by players who are at greatest risk— offensive and defensive linemen, linebackers, and tight ends.[4,6] The braces vary depending on the manufacturer but commonly consist of a single-sided strut made of metal or heavy plastic having a dual axis with a dual hinge. To date, anecdotal reports are divided, with some indicating a decrease in knee injuries and others reporting no difference or an increase in injuries.[5,8] More specifically, studies indicate that the effectiveness of prophylactic knee braces is highly controversial. The American Academy of Orthopaedic Surgeons (AAOS) in 1987 pre-

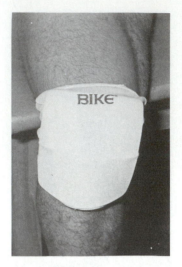

Figure 5-28

Bike knee pad.

Figure 5-29

Commercial lateral stabilizing knee brace.

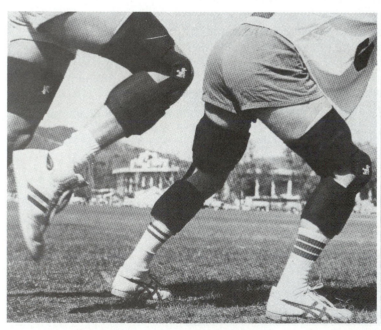

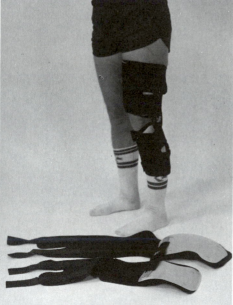

sented a position statement that warns, "routine use of prophylactic knee braces currently available has not been proved effective in reducing the number and severity of knee injuries." The AAOS has approved the use of rehabilitative and functional knee braces, saying that those braces have been scientifically shown to be effective in treating knee injuries.[2]

More studies need to be conducted concerning the relative strength of braces, whether they prestress the knee joint and produce injuries, whether in fact they actually can reduce injuries, and whether performance is adversely affected in any way.[9,11] Braces that are constructed based on surrogated limb testing apparently have a higher level of credibility in acting as a prophylactic knee device.[7,13]

The fitted knee brace   Following serious knee joint injury that produces chronic instability or necessitates surgery, a customized orthopedic knee brace may be prescribed for the athlete. The Lenox Hill and Pro Am braces are examples of braces that help stabilize the joint with rotary problems (Figures 5-30 and 5-31).

Other popular knee devices are sleeves composed of elastic or neoprene material. Sleeves of this type provide mild soft-tissue support and to some extent retain body heat and help to reduce edema caused by tissue compression.

Hand, Wrist, and Elbow Protection

As with the lower limbs, the upper limbs require initial protection from injury, as well as prevention of further injury following a trauma. One of the finest physical instruments, the human hand, is perhaps one of the most neglected in terms of protection, especially in sports. Special attention must be paid to protecting the integrity of all aspects of the hand

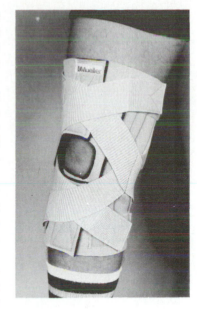

Figure 5-30

A preventive knee brace designed to protect the knee from a lateral force and to distribute lead away from joint.

Figure 5-31

Postinjury knee braces.

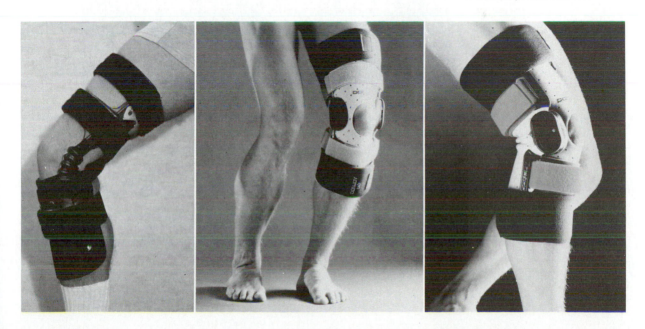

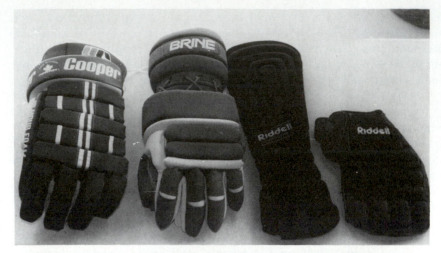

Figure 5-32

The hand is an often
neglected area of the body in
sports.

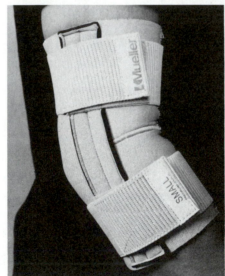

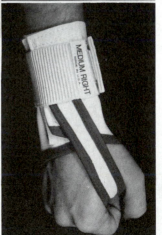

Figure 5-33

Commercial pads and braces.

when encountering high-speed projectiles or receiving external forces that contuse or shear. Constant stress to the hand, as characterized by the force received by the hand of the baseball catcher, can lead to irreversible damage in later life (Figure 5-32). The wrist and the elbow are also vulnerable to sports trauma and often need compression or support for protection (Figure 5-33).

Construction of Protective and Supportive Devices

Being able to construct protective and supportive devices is of considerable value in sports. The primary materials used are sponge rubber, felt, adhesive felt, adhesive sponge rubber, gauze pads, cotton, lamb's wool, and plastic. All these have special uses in athletic training (Figure 5-34).

Prophylactic Taping in Sports

The use of adhesive substances in the care of external lesions of the skin goes back to ancient times. The Greek civilization is credited with formulating a healing paste composed of lead oxide, olive oil, and water, which was used for a wide variety of skin conditions. This composition was only recently changed by the addition of resin and yellow beeswax and, even more recently, rubber. Since its inception, adhesive tape has developed into a vital therapeutic adjunct.[10]

Two types of tape are generally used in athletic training; one has a linen type backing and the other has an elastic backing. Linen tape provides little or no "give" when applied. Elastic tape, in comparison, is designed to stretch. Linen tape generally costs less than elastic tape.

Adhesive Tape and Injury Prophylaxis

Adhesive tape as a prophylaxis has been routinely applied to ankles for many years; recently, however, there has been controversy about the real benefits, if any, ankle taping provides.

Tape as an Adjunct to Conditioning and Rehabilitation

Ankle taping to prevent injury should be used only as an adjunct to proper and extensive exercise. Tape should never be applied indiscriminantly, but only under highly controlled conditions. The primary muscles

Figure 5-34

Types of sports orthoses.
A, Orthoplast with a foam rubber doughnut.
B, Orthoplast splint.
C, Orthoplast rib protector with a foam rubber pad.
D, Fiberglass material for splint construction. **E,** Plaster of paris material for cast construction. **F,** Foam rubber pad. **G,** Aloplast foam moldable material for protective pad construction.

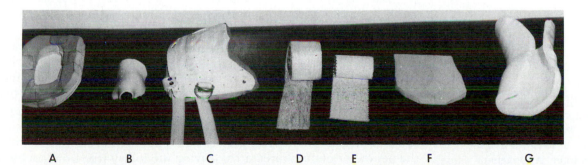

A   B   C   D   E   F   G

of concern are those that point the foot (plantar muscles) and those that evert the foot (peroneal group and the gastrocnemius-soleus complex). Special attention should be paid to stretching the heel cord. If the heel cord is tight, the foot tends to point downward making it more susceptible to inversion sprain.

Athletes with normal or near-normal ankles should rely more on strengthening exercises than on artificial aids. When prophylaxis is needed in a high-risk sport, wraps may be preferable to rigid taping. Ankle taping should not become routine unless an honest effort at reconditioning has failed to adequately restore function to the ankle. An improperly applied wrap or taping can compound an injury and may even create postural imbalances that could adversely affect other parts of the body. NOTE: Proper tape application is discussed in Chapter 10, Taping and Bandaging.

Soft Pad Materials

Sponge rubber (foam rubber) is resilient, nonabsorbent, and able to protect the body against shock. It is particularly valuable for use as a protective padding for bruised areas, and it can also serve as a supportive pad. Newly formulated foam rubber is currently being used extensively as innersoles in sports shoes. Covered by a synthetic leather sheet, this new material prevents blisters and calluses by absorbing vertical, front-to-back, and rotary forces. Sponge rubber generally ranges from ⅛ to ½ inch (0.3 to 1.25 cm) in thickness.

Felt is a material composed of matted wool fibers pressed into varying thicknesses that range from ¼ to 1 inch (0.6 to 2.5 cm). Its benefit lies in its comfortable, semiresilient surface, which gives a firmer pressure than most sponge rubbers. Because felt will absorb perspiration, it clings to the skin, and it has less tendency to move about than sponge rubber. Because of its absorbent qualities it must be replaced daily.

Adhesive felt (moleskin) or *sponge rubber* is a felt or sponge rubber material containing an adhesive mass on one side, thus combining a cushioning effect with the ability to be held in a specific spot by the adhesive mass. It is a versatile material that is useful on all body parts.

Gauze padding is less versatile than other pad materials. It is assembled in varying thicknesses and can be used as an absorbent or protective pad.

Cotton is probably the cheapest and most widely used material in sports. It has the ability to absorb, to hold emollients, and to offer a mild padding effect.

Lamb's wool is a material commonly used on and around the athlete's toes when circular protection is required. In contrast to cotton, lamb's wool does not pack but keeps its resiliency over a long period of time.

Protective pads can be of varying shapes and sizes, cut to fit the body contours. In addition to the flat and variously shaped compression pads, pads of two other distinct shapes, the *doughnut* and the *horseshoe,* are often used (Figure 5-35). Each is adapted so that pressure is placed around the perimeter of an injured area, leaving the injury free from additional pressure or trauma.

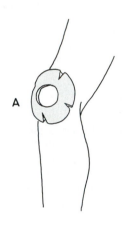

A

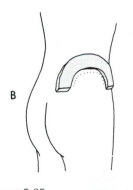

B

Figure 5-35

Protective pads can be of varying shapes and sizes and are cut to fit the body contours. **A,** Doughnut shape. **B,** Horseshoe shape.

Rigid Materials

A number of plastic materials are becoming widely used in sports medicine for customized orthoses. They can brace, splint, and protect a body area. They may provide casting for a fracture, support for a foot defect, or a firm, nonyielding surface to protect a severe contusion.[15]

Plastics used for these purposes differ in their chemical composition and reaction to heat. The three major categories are heat-forming and heat-setting plastics and heat-plastic foams.

Heat-forming plastics are of the low-temperature variety and the most popular in athletic training. When heated to between 140° and 180° F (60° and 82.2° C), depending on the material, the plastic can be accurately molded to a body part. Aquaplast (polyester sheets) and Orthoplast (synthetic rubber thermoplast) are popular types.

Heat-setting plastics require relatively higher temperatures for shaping. They are rigid and difficult to form, usually requiring a mold rather than being formed directly to the body part. High-impact vinyl (polyvinyl chloride), Kydex (polyvinyl chloride acrylic), and Nyloplex (heat-plastic acrylic) are examples of the more commonly used heat-forming plastics.

Heat-plastic foams are plastics that have differences in density as a result of the addition of liquids, gas, or crystals. They are commonly used as shoe inserts and other body padding. Aloplast (polyethylene foam) and Plastazate (polyethylene foam) are two commonly used products.

> Heatforming plastics of the low-temperature variety are the most popular in athletic training.

SUMMARY

The proper selection and fitting of sports equipment are essentials in the prevention of many sports injuries. Because of the number of current litigations, sports equipment standards are of serious concern regarding the durability of the material and the fit and wear requirements of the equipment. Manufacturers must foresee all of the possible uses and misuses of their equipment and warn the user of any potential risks.

Head protection in many collision and contact sports is of concern to sports professionals. A major concern is that the helmet be used as intended and not as a weapon. To avoid unwarranted litigation, make sure there is a warning label on the outside of the helmet indicating that it is not fail-safe and must be used as intended. Proper fit is also a major requirement.

Face protection is of major importance in sports that have fast-moving projectiles, use implements that come in close proximity to other athletes, and are characterized by body collisions. Protecting teeth and eyes is of particular significance. The customized mouth guard, fitted to individual requirements, provides the best protection for the teeth and also protects against concussions. Eyes must be protected against projectiles and sports implements. The safest eye guard for the athlete not wearing contact lenses or spectacles is the closed type that completely protects the orbital cavity.

Many sports require protection of various parts of the athlete's body. American football players, ice hockey players, and baseball/softball catchers are examples of players who require body protection. Commonly, the protection is for the shoulders, chest, thighs, ribs, hips, buttocks, groin, genitalia (male athletes), and breasts (female athletes).

Quality sportswear, properly fitted, is essential to prevent injuries. Socks must be clean, without holes, and made of appropriate materials. Shoes must be suited to the sport and must be fitted to the larger foot. The wide part of the foot must match the wide part of the shoe. If the shoe has cleats, they must be positioned at the metatarsophalangeal joints.

Currently, there are many stock pieces of specialized, protective equipment on the market. They may be be designed to support ankles, knees, or other body parts. In addition to stock equipment, athletic trainers often construct customized equipment out of a variety of materials to pad injuries or support feet. Professionals such as orthopedists and podiatrists may devise orthopedic footwear and orthotic devices to improve the biomechanics of the athlete's foot.

REVIEW QUESTIONS AND CLASS ACTIVITIES

1. What are the legal responsibilities of the equipment manager, coach, and athletic trainer in terms of protective equipment?
2. Invite an attorney to discuss product liability and its impact on the athletic trainer, coach, and equipment manager.
3. What are the various sports with high-risk factors that require protective equipment?
4. How can the athletic trainer or coach select and use safety equipment so as to decrease the possibility of sports injuries and litigation?
5. Why are continual inspection and/or replacement of used equipment important?
6. What are the standards for fitting football helmets? Are there standards for any other helmets?
7. Invite your school equipment manager or athletic trainer to demonstrate to the class all the protective equipment and how to fit it to the athlete.
8. Why are mouth guards important and what are the advantages of custom-made mouth guards over the stock type?
9. What are the advantages and disadvantages of glasses and contact lenses in athletic competition?
10. How do you fit shoulder pads for the different-sized players and their positions?
11. Why is breast protection necessary? Which types of sport bras are available and what should the athlete look for when purchasing one?
12. How do you properly fit shoes? What type of shoes should you use for the various sports and the different floor and field surfaces?
13. What type of commercial pads and braces are on the market today? Do they provide adequate support and protection from injury?
14. What types of custom material are on the market to prevent injuries and protect injured areas? How would you use each of them?

REFERENCES

1. Carrier D: Alternative to shoulder girdle protection, *Ath Train* 21:228, 1986.
2. Erickson AR et al: An in vitra dynamic evaluation of prophylactic knee braces during lateral impact

loading, *Am J Sports Med* 21:26,
1993.

3. Frederick EC et al: The running
   shoe: dilemmas and dichotomies
   design. In Segesser B, Phorringer
   W, ed: *The shoe in sport,* Chicago,
   1989, Mosby-Year Book.

4. Haycock CE: How I manage breast
   problems in athletes, *Phys Sports
   Med* 15:89, 1987.

5. Hewson GF, Jr et al: Prophylactic
   knee bracing in college football,
   Am J Sports Med 14:262, 1986.

6. Lorentzen D, Lawson L: Selected
   sports bras: a biomechanical analysis of breast motion while jogging,
   Phys Sports Med 5:128, 1987.

7. Nash HL: AAOS: braces may not
   prevent knee injuries, *Phys Sports
   Med* 16:57, 1988.

8. Paulos L et al: Biomechanics of lateral bracing, phase II. Review presented at the AAOS annual meeting, San Francisco, Jan 22, 1987.

9. Potera C: Knee braces, questions
   raised about performance, *Phys
   Sports Med* 13:153, 1985.

10. Reese RC, Jr et al: Athletic taping
    and protective equipment. In Ni-
    cholas JA, Hershman EB, ed: *The
    upper extremity in sports medicine,* St
    Louis, 1990, Mosby-Year Book.

11. Rovere GD et al: Prophylactic knee
    bracing in college football, *Am J
    Sports Med* 15:111, 1987.

12. Schootman M, Van Mechelen W:
    Efficiency of preventive knee
    braces in football: epidemiology as-
    sessment, *Clin J Sports Med* 3:166,
    1993.

13. Sforzo GA et al: Knee bracing
    wearing during exercise, *Med Sci
    Sports Exerc* 19(suppl):5, 1987.

14. The National Collegiate Athletic
    Association. *Sports medicine hand-
    book,* ed 6, Overland Park, Kan,
    1993 NCAA Sports Science.

15. Torg JS: Orthotic devices fabrica-
    tions. In Torg JS et al, ed: *Current
    therapy in sports medicine,* ed 2,
    Toronto, 1990, BC Decker.

16. Wilkinson EE, Powers JM: Proper-
    ties of custom-made mouth pro-
    tection materials, *Phys Sports Med*
    14:77, 1986.

ANNOTATED BIBLIOGRAPHY

Nicholas JA, Hershman EB, eds: *The upper extremity in sports medicine,* St Louis,
1990, Mosby-Year Book.
  Includes a special chapter on protective equipment for the shoulder, elbow,
  wrist, and hand.

Nicholas JA, Hershrom EB, eds: *The lower extremity and spine in sports medicine,*
vol 1, St Louis, 1986, Mosby–Year Book.
  Contains two excellent chapters on protective devices: Chapter 9 (RC Reese,
  TP Burross), Athletic training techniques and protective equipment, and Chapter 20 (LJ Micheli et al), Athletic footwear and modifications.

Segesser B, Pjorringer W, eds: *The shoe in sports,* St Louis, 1989, Mosby-Year Book.
  An excellent detailed text on different types of sport shoes and their unique
  features.

Wu K: *Foot orthoses: principles and clinical applications,* Baltimore, 1990, Williams &
Wilkins.
  A complete text on examination, fabrication, and application of foot orthoses.

Mechanisms, Characteristics, and Classifications of Sports Injuries

When you finish this chapter, you will be able to:

- Identify the most common exposed skin injuries
- Explain the specific mechanical forces that cause skin, internal soft-tissue, synovial joint, and bone injuries
- Define the terms that describe the major injuries incurred during sports participation
- Recognize the different types of fractures
- Describe how epiphyseal injuries occur
- Explain how body mechanics can predispose an individual to injury

Chapter 6 is concerned with defining the key factors related to trauma in sports and is designed to provide the coach with foundation to characteristics and classification of sports injuries.

GENERAL INJURY CAUSATIONS

Injuries related to sports participation can be caused primarily by the sport itself or can occur as a secondary event (Figure 6-1).

Direct Injury

A *direct injury* is one that results primarily from the damage imposed by a particular sport. The injury can be externally caused, as by body contact or use of a piece of equipment. The use of some implement such as a racquet or gymnastics equipment can also produce an instantaneous injury.

Indirect Injury

In comparison to a direct injury, secondary problems can arise from an injury, especially if it has not been properly treated initially with rest, ice, compression, and elevation (RICE) or if the athlete has been allowed to return to competition too soon. An example of an early secondary problem after injury may be chronic swelling and weakness in a joint. An example of later occurrence is arthritis that has developed in a joint many years after repeated joint injuries that were improperly treated.

Injuries or other problems that are not directly related to a specific stress in a sport can also adversely influence performance or the athlete's health and safety. An example of this is an asthma attack that can adversely affect performance and may result in death.

SKIN WOUNDS

Generally, trauma to the skin is visually exposed and is categorized as a skin wound. A *wound* is defined as a break in the continuity of the soft parts of body structures caused by a trauma to tissues.

Figure 6-1

Many sports place severe stress on major joints.

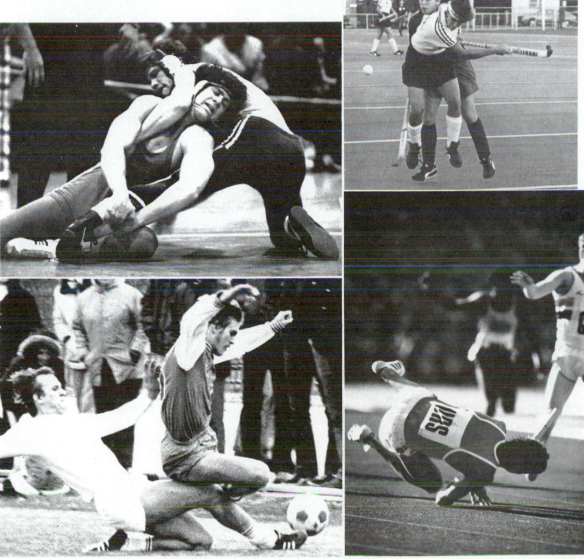

Continued.

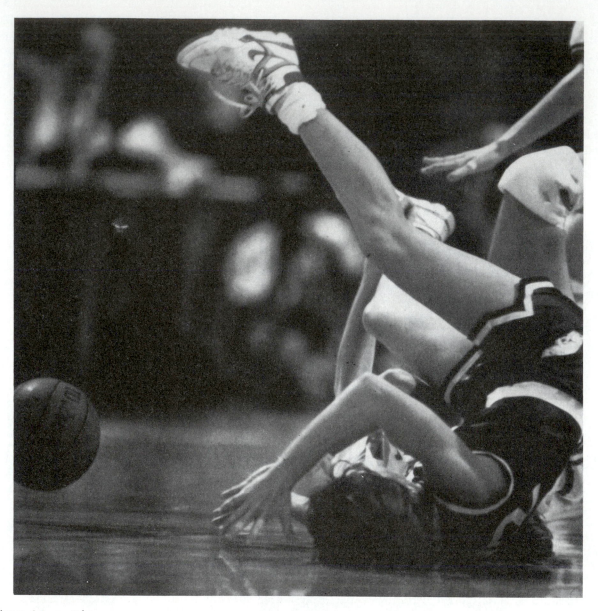

Figure 6-1, cont'd

For legend see p. 137.

Anatomical Characteristics

The skin, or integument, is the external covering of the body. It is the body's largest organ and essentially consists of two layers, the epidermis and the dermis (corium). Because of the soft, pliable nature of skin, it can be easily traumatized.

Injurious Mechanical Forces

Numerous mechanical forces can adversely affect the skin's integrity. These forces are friction or rubbing, scraping, compression or pressure, tearing, cutting, and penetration.

TABLE 6-1 Soft-tissue trauma

Primary Tissue	Type	Mechanical Forces	Condition
Skin	Acute	Rubbing, friction	Blister
		Compression, contusion	Bruise
		Tearing	Laceration
		Tearing, ripping	Avulsion
		Penetration	Puncture
Muscle, tendon	Acute	Compression	Contusion
		Tension	Strain
	Chronic	Tension, shear	Myositis, fasciitis
		Tension	Tendinitis, tenosynovitis
		Compression, tension	Bursitis
			Ectopic calcification— myositis ossificans, calcific tendinitis

Wound Classification

Wounds are classified according to the mechanical force that causes them (Table 6-1, Figure 6-2).

Blister Continuous rubbing over the surface of the skin causes a collection of fluid below or within the epidermal layer called a blister.

Abrasion Abrasion is a common condition in which the skin is scraped against a rough surface. The epidermis and dermis are worn away, exposing numerous blood capillaries (Figure 6-2, *A*).

Skin bruise When a blow compresses or crushes the skin surface and produces bleeding under the skin, the condition is identified as a bruise, or contusion.

Laceration A laceration is a wound in which the flesh has been irregularly torn (Figure 6-2, *B*).

Skin avulsion Skin that is torn by the same mechanism as a laceration to the extent that tissue is completely ripped from its source is an avulsion injury (Figure 6-2, E_1 and E_2).

Incision An incision wound is one in which the skin has been sharply cut (Figure 6-2, *D*).

Puncture wound Puncture wounds, as the name implies, are penetrations of the skin by a sharp object (Figure 6-2, *C*).

SKELETAL MUSCLE TRAUMA

Skeletal muscles have an extremely high percentage of sports injuries.

Anatomical Characteristics

Muscles are composed of contractile cells, or fibers, that produce movement. Of major concern in sports medicine are conditions that affect striated, or skeletal muscles.

muscle
Tissue that when stimulated
contracts and produces
motion

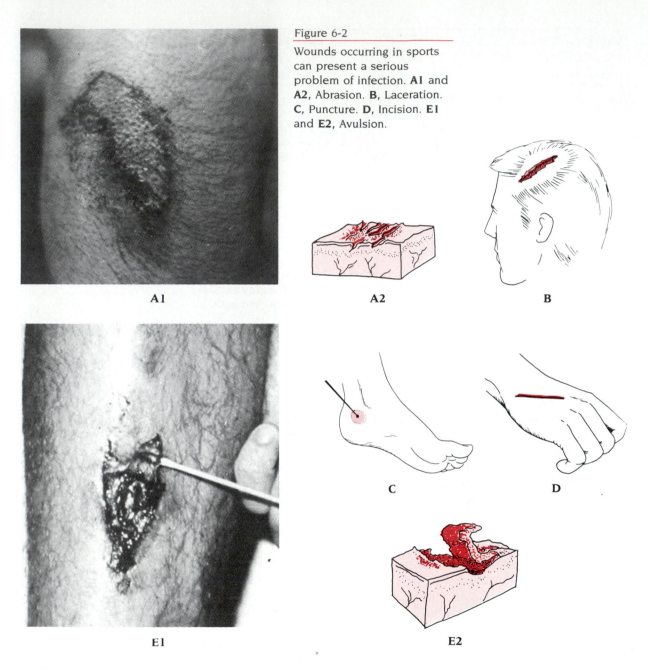

Figure 6-2

Wounds occurring in sports can present a serious problem of infection. **A1** and **A2**, Abrasion. **B**, Laceration. **C**, Puncture. **D**, Incision. **E1** and **E2**, Avulsion.

A1

A2

B

C

D

E1

E2

tendon

Tough cord or band of white fibrous connective tissue that attaches muscle to bone

A muscle **tendon** attaches a muscle to a bone and concentrates a pulley force in a limited area. A tendon is commonly twice the strength of the muscle it serves. When a force is great enough to tear tendinous tissue, the tear usually occurs at the muscle belly, musculotendinous junction, or bony attachment. Constant, abnormal, prolonged tension on a tendon causes a gradual infiltration of scar tissue into the tendon, weakening it over time.[2]

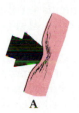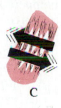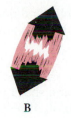

A   B   C

Figure 6-3

Mechanical forces that can injure soft tissue. **A,** Compression. **B,** Tension. **C,** Shear.

Injurious Mechanical Forces

Muscle tissue can be traumatized by three major mechanical forces: compression, tension, and shear (Figure 6-3).

Compression Force

Compression is a force that with enough energy crushes tissue. Soft tissue can withstand and absorb compression forces; however, when the force is excessive and can no longer be absorbed, a contusion, or bruise, occurs. Where constant submaximum compression exists over a period of time, the contacted tissue begins to develop abnormal wear.

Tension Force

Tension is the force that pulls and stretches tissue. Soft tissue that is suddenly stretched beyond its yield point will tear or rupture. When tissue containing a preponderance of connective tissue such as fascia, tendons, ligaments, and muscle is placed in constant tension, collagen fibers weaken and are subject to injuries.

Shearing Force

A shearing force is one that moves across the parallel organization of connective tissue. Like compression and tension, once shearing has exceeded the inherent strength of the tissue, injury occurs.

Muscle Injury Classification

Acute Muscle Injuries

The two categories of acute muscle injuries are contusions and strains.

Contusions   A bruise or contusion occurs because of a sudden crushing blow to the body. The intensity of a contusion can range from superficial to deep-tissue compression and hemorrhage (Figure 6-4).

Interrupting the continuity of the circulatory system results in a flow of blood and lymph into the surrounding tissues. A hematoma (blood tumor) is formed by the localization of the extravasated blood into a clot, which becomes encapsulated by a connective tissue membrane. The speed of healing, as with all soft-tissue injuries, depends on the extent of tissue damage and internal bleeding.

Contusion or the crushing of soft tissue can penetrate to the skeletal structures, causing a bone bruise. The extent to which an athlete may be

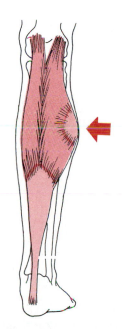

Figure 6-4

A contusion can range from a superficial to a deep-tissue compression (arrow), injuring cells and causing hemorrhage.

hampered by this condition depends on the location of the bruise and the force of the blow. Typical in cases of severe contusion are the following:

1. The athlete reports being struck a hard blow.
2. The blow causes pain and a temporary paralysis caused by pressure on and shock to the motor and sensory nerves.
3. Palpation often reveals a hard area of internal hemorrhage.
4. Tissue discoloration may also take place.

Muscle contusions are usually rated by the extent the muscle is able to produce range of motion in a part after injury. For example, a first-degree contusion will cause little movement restriction, a second-degree contusion will restrict some range of movement, and a third-degree injury usually severely restricts motion. It is noteworthy that a blow to a muscle can be so great that the associated fascia is ruptured, allowing muscle tissue to protrude through it.

Muscle strains   A strain is a stretch, tear, or rip in the muscle or adjacent tissue such as the fascia or muscle tendons (Figure 6-5). The cause of muscle strain is often obscure. Most often a strain is produced by an abnormal muscular contraction. The cause of this abnormality has been attributed to many factors. One popular theory suggests that a disruption in the reciprocal coordination of the opposite muscles takes place. The cause of this disruption or incoordination is more or less a mystery. However, some possible explanations are (1) a mineral imbalance caused by profuse sweating, (2) fatigue metabolites collected in the muscle itself, and (3) a strength imbalance between agonist and antagonist muscles.

A strain may range from a minute separation of connective tissue and muscle fibers to a complete tendinous avulsion or muscle rupture (graded as *first, second,* or *third degree*). The resulting tissue response is similar to that of the contusion or sprain, with capillary or blood vessel hemorrhage. The first-degree strain is accompanied by local pain, which is increased by tension of the muscle, and a minor loss of strength. There is mild swelling, tissue discoloration (ecchymosis), and local tenderness.[2] The second-degree strain is similar to the mild strain but has moderate signs and symptoms and impaired muscle function. A third-degree strain has signs and symptoms that are severe, with a loss of muscle function and commonly a palpable defect in the muscle.

Healing takes place in a similar fashion, with the organization of a collection of blood (hematoma), absorption of the hematoma, and, finally, the formation of a scar by connective tissue (fibroblastic) repair.

The muscles that have the highest incidence of strains in sports are the hamstring group, calf (gastrocnemius), quadriceps group, hip flexors, hip adductor group, spinalis group of the back, deltoid, and rotator cuff group of the shoulder.

Tendon injuries   In tendons, connective tissue fibers will break if their physiological limits have been reached. A breaking point occurs after a 6% to 8% increase in length. Because a tendon is usually double the strength of the muscle it serves, tears commonly occur at the muscle

A strain is a stretch, tear, or rip in the muscle of adjacent tissue.

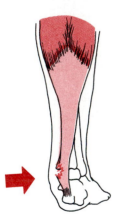

Figure 6-5

A strain can occur to any aspect of the musculotendinous unit. Depending on the amount of force, a strain can stretch or tear (arrow) or even avulse a tendon from a bone.

belly, musculotendinous junction, or bony attachment. A constant abnormal tension on tendons can cause infiltration of connective tissue.[7] Repeated small injuries can evolve into chronic muscle strain that eventually weakens the tendon. It also should be noted that a tendon's connecting tissue fibers are weakened in the beginning of a sport session, making it vulnerable to injury. When a gradually paced conditioning program is conducted, tendons increase in strength.[2]

Muscle cramps and spasms   Leading to muscle and tendon injuries are muscle cramps and spasms. A cramp is usually a painful involuntary contraction of a skeletal muscle or muscle group. Cramps have been attributed to a lack of salt or other minerals and to muscle fatigue. A reflex reaction caused by injury to a muscle is commonly called a **spasm.** The two types of cramps or spasms are the clonic type, with alternating involuntary muscular contraction and relaxation in quick succession, and the tonic type, with rigid muscle contraction that lasts over a period of time.

Overexertional muscle problems   One ever-present problem in physical conditioning and training stems from overexertion. Even though the gradual pattern of overloading the body is the best way for ultimate success, many athletes and even coaches believe that if there is no pain, there is no gain.

Exercise "overdosage" is reflected in muscle soreness, decreased joint flexibility, and general fatigue 24 hours after activity. Any one or all of the above can be present. Specific indicators of possible overexertion are acute muscle soreness, muscle stiffness, and delayed muscle soreness. The first, occurring immediately after exercise, is acute soreness, which is resolved when exercise has ceased. The second and more serious problem is delayed soreness, which is related mainly to early-season or unaccustomed work. Severe muscular discomfort occurs 24 to 48 hours after exercise.

Acute-onset muscle soreness   Acute-onset muscle soreness is related to an impedance of circulation, causing muscular ischemia. Lactic acid and potassium collect in the muscle and stimulate pain receptors.

Delayed-onset muscle soreness   Compared with acute-onset soreness, delayed-onset muscle soreness **(DOMS)** increases in intensity for 2 to 3 days until it has completely disappeared within 7 days.

The cause of DOMS apparently is sublethal and lethal damage to a small group of recruited muscle fibers. The perception of soreness is caused by the activation of free nerve endings around selected muscle fibers. The type of activity that causes the most soreness is eccentric exercise. Muscle fibers may take as long as 12 weeks to repair; therefore, athletes need abundant recovery time.

There are many ways to reduce the possibility of delayed muscle soreness. One is a gradual and complete warm-up before and after activity. If there is extreme soreness, the application of ice packs or ice massage to the point of numbness (approximately 5 to 8 minutes) followed by a static stretch will often provide relief.

muscle cramps
Clonic: involuntary muscle contraction with alternating relaxation
Tonic: rigid muscle contraction with no relaxation

spasm
Muscular contraction producing a cramp

Indicators of overexertion:
acute muscle soreness
delayed muscle soreness
muscle stiffness

DOMS
Delayed onset muscle soreness

Sports Injury Causation,
Response, and Management

Muscle stiffness Muscle stiffness is contrasted to muscle soreness because it does not produce pain. It occurs when a group of muscles have been worked hard for a long period of time. The fluids that collect in the muscles during and after exercise are absorbed into the bloodstream at a very slow rate. As a result, the muscle becomes swollen, shorter, and thicker and therefore resists stretching. Light exercise, massage, and passive mobilization assist in reducing stiffness.

Muscle cramps Like muscle soreness and stiffness, muscle cramps can be a problem related to hard conditioning. The most common cramp is tonic, in which there is continuous muscle contraction. It is caused by the body's depletion of essential electrolytes or an interruption of synergism between opposing muscles. **Clonic,** or intermittent, contraction stemming from nerve irritation rarely occurs.

clonic muscle contraction
Alternating involuntary muscle contraction and relaxation in quick succession

Chronic Muscle Injuries

As discussed previously, chronic injuries usually come about by a slow progression of many small injuries over a long period of time. A constant irritation caused by poor performance techniques or a constant stress beyond physiological limits can eventually result in a chronic condition. Another way to describe a chronic muscle injury is that it is attributable to a repetitive overuse syndrome resulting in numerous microtraumas.

Chronic muscle injuries:
Myositis and fasciitis
Tendinitis
Tenosynovitis
Bursitis
Ectopic calcification
Atrophy and contracture

Chronic muscle injuries are representative of a low-grade inflammatory process with an increase in connective tissue and scarring. The acute injury that is properly managed or that allows an athlete to return to activity before healing has completely occurred can cause chronic injury. Coaches should be knowledgeable about six chronic muscle conditions: myositis, tendinitis, tenosynovitis, bursitis, ectopic calcification, and muscle atrophy and contracture.

The suffix *-itis* means "inflammation of. . ."

Myositis/fasciitis In general, the term **myositis** means inflammation of muscle tissue. More specifically, it can be considered as a fibrositis or connective tissue inflammation. Fascia that supports and separates muscle can also become chronically inflamed following injury. A typical example of this condition is plantar fasciitis.

myositis
Inflammation of muscle tissue

Tendinitis Tendinitis has a gradual onset, general tenderness because of repeated microtraumas, and degenerative changes. Obvious signs of tendinitis are swelling and pain that move with the tendon. Tendinitis commonly can be seen in the Achilles and patellar tendons.

Tenosynovitis Tenosynovitis is inflammation of the sheath covering a tendon. In its acute state there is rapid onset, **crepitus** or movement, and general swelling. In chronic tenosynovitis the tendons become thickened, with pain and crepitus present during movement of the part (Figure 6-6). Swelling from tenosynovitis can be seen on the backs of hands and feet in athletes who have been bruised in these areas or who have sustained a severe strain.

crepitus
Crackling sound, e.g., broken bones rubbing together

Bursitis The bursa is a closed sac or envelope lined with synovia-

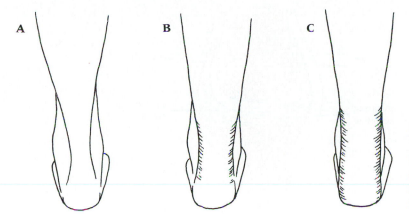

Figure 6-6

Tenosynovitis is an
inflammation of the sheath
covering a tendon. **A**, Normal.
B, Strained. **C**, Chronic
tenosynovitis.

secreting tissue found in places where friction might occur within body
tissues. Bursae are predominantly located between bony prominences
and muscles or tendons. Bursitis can be caused by overuse of muscles or
tendons, as well as from an external compression to the part. The signs
and symptoms of bursitis include swelling, pain, and some loss of function. Repeated trauma may lead to a calcification of the internal lining of
the bursa. In athletes who kneel a great deal, such as wrestlers or athletes who receive repeated blows to various parts of their body, bursitis
may develop.

Ectopic calcification   The word **ectopic** refers to faulty positioning.
In terms of ectopic calcification, calcium and other minerals are collected
in unusual areas of the body. Injury to a muscle causing an inflammation may result in a myositis ossificans or in a tendon calcific tendinitis.
Two common sites for this condition are the thigh region and the elbow
following a dislocation. In myositis ossificans, mineral material that resembles bone rapidly accumulates. If there is no repeated injury, the
growth may subside completely in 9 to 12 months, or it may mature into
a calcified area, at which time surgical removal can be accomplished with
little fear of recurrence.

ectopic calcification
Calcification located in a
place different from normal

Muscle atrophy and contracture   Two complications of muscle and
tendon conditions are atrophy and contracture. *Muscle atrophy* is the wasting away of muscle tissue. Its main cause in athletes is immobilization of
a body part or loss of nerve stimulation. A second complication to sport
injuries is *muscle contracture,* an abnormal shortening of muscle tissue in
which there is a great deal of resistance to stretch. Commonly associated
with muscle injury, a contracture is associated with a joint that has developed scar tissue.

SYNOVIAL JOINTS

The **joint** of the human body is defined as the point at which two bones
join together. A joint must transmit forces between participating bones.
It consists of cartilage and fibrous connective tissue.

joint
Point at which two bones
join together

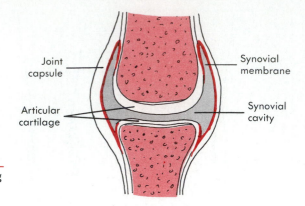

Figure 6-7

Anatomy of the freely moving
joint.

Constant compression or
tension will cause ligaments
to deteriorate; intermittent
compression and tension will
increase strength and
growth.

Roux's law states that an
organ will structurally adapt
itself in response to an
alteration of function.

synovia
A transparent viscid
lubricating fluid found in
joints, bursae, and tendons

Examples of synovial joints:
Shoulder
Hip
Elbow
Wrist
Vertebrae

Anatomic Characteristics

Joint Capsule

In the freely moving joint (Figure 6-7), a cuff of fibrous tissue known as the capsule (or capsular ligament) functions primarily to hold the bones together. Parts of the capsule become slack or taut, depending on the joint movements.

Ligaments

Ligaments are sheets or bundles of connective tissue that form a connection between two bones. Ligaments fall into two categories: ones that are considered intrinsic and ones that are extrinsic to the joint. Intrinsic ligaments occur where the articular capsule has become thickened in some places. Extrinsic ligaments are separate from the capsular thickening.

Constant compression or tension will cause ligaments to deteriorate, whereas intermittent compression and tension increase strength and growth, especially at the bony attachment. Chronic inflammation of ligamentous, capsular, and fascial tissue causes a shrinkage of connective tissue; therefore, repeated microtraumas over time make capsules and ligaments highly susceptible to major acute injuries.

Ligaments act as protective backups for the joint. Primary protection occurs from the dynamic aspect of muscles and their tendons.[1] Capsular and ligamentous tissues are highly sensitive to the deprivation caused by normal stress through joint immobilization. Capsular and ligamentous tissue respond to Roux's law of functional adaptation: an organ will adapt itself structurally to an alteration, quantitative or qualitative, of function.[12]

Synovial Membrane and Synovial Fluid

Lining the **synovial** articular capsule is a synovial membrane that is composed of connective tissue and fluid secretory cells. Synovial fluid has the consistency of egg white and acts as a joint lubricant. It has the ability to vary its thickness. During slow movement, the fluid becomes thick, whereas during fast movement, it thins.

Articular Cartilage

The ends of the bones in a freely moving joint are covered with hyaline cartilage, which acts as a cushion for the bone ends. Its general appearance is smooth and pearly. Hyaline cartilage acts like a sponge in relation to synovial fluid. As movement occurs, it absorbs and squeezes out the fluid as pressures vary between the joint surfaces. Because of its great strength, the cartilage can be deformed without damage and can still return to its original shape. However, cartilaginous degeneration, caused by repetitive microtraumas, may occur during the abnormal compressional forces that occur over a period of time.

Hyaline cartilage has no direct blood supply but receives its nourishment from the synovial fluid—more specifically, from the synovial membrane located at its edges. Deeper aspects of the cartilage are fed by spaces (lacunae) in the adjacent bone.

articulation
A joint

Joint Fat

In some joints such as the knee and elbow, there are pads of fat that lie between the synovial membrane and the capsule. They tend to fill in the spaces between the bones that form joints. As movement occurs, they move in and out of these spaces.

Articular Disks

Some freely moving joints are provided with an additional fibrocartilaginous disk. These disks vary in shape and are connected to the capsule. They are found in joints where two planes of movement exist and may act as spreaders of the synovial fluid between the joint surfaces.

Joint Nerve Supply

The articular capsule, ligaments, outer aspects of the synovial membrane, and fat pads of the synovial joint are well supplied with nerves. The inner aspect of the synovial membrane, cartilage, and articular disks, if present, have nerves as well. These nerves, called *mechanoreceptors*, provide information about the relative position of the joint and are found in the fibrous capsule and ligaments.

Synovial Joint Strength

Synovial joints differ in their ability to withstand trauma, depending on their skeletal, ligamentous, and muscular organization. Table 6-2 provides a general guide to the relative strength of selected articulations in terms of sports participation.

Muscle tension is important in limiting joint movement. When the joint capsule is overstretched, a reflex contraction of muscles in the area occurs to prevent overstretching. Ligaments can be minimally stretched based on their fiber arrangement.

In terms of stability, ligaments and capsular structures are highly important to joints. Characteristically, joints that are shallow and relatively poor fitting must depend on their capsular structures and/or muscles for

TABLE 6-2 General relative strength grades in selected articulations

Articulation	Skeleton	Ligaments	Muscles
Ankle	Strong	Moderate	Weak
Knee	Weak	Moderate	Strong
Hip	Strong	Strong	Strong
Lumbosacral	Weak	Strong	Moderate
Lumbar vertebrae	Strong	Strong	Moderate
Thoracic vertebrae	Strong	Strong	Moderate
Cervical vertebrae	Weak	Moderate	Strong
Sternoclavicular	Weak	Weak	Weak
Acromioclavicular	Weak	Moderate	Weak
Glenohumeral	Weak	Moderate	Moderate
Elbow	Moderate	Strong	Strong
Wrist	Weak	Moderate	Moderate
Phalanges (toes and fingers)	Weak	Moderate	Moderate

major support. The knee is an example of an articulation that depends mainly on muscles and ligaments for its support rather than on bony pocket.

Besides moving limbs, muscles provide joint stabilization to a greater or lesser extent and absorb the forces applied to the body.

Joint Capsules and Ligaments

Joint capsules and ligaments maintain the structural alignment of synovial joints. Attaching bone to bone, ligaments are generally strongest in the middle and weakest at the ends.[2] In comparison with the fast, protective response of ligaments and capsular tissues, muscles respond much more slowly. For example, a muscle begins to develop protective tension within just a few hundredths of a second when overly stretched but will not fully respond until approximately one tenth of a second has elapsed.[3] Articular cartilage helps freely moving joints in three ways: motion control, stability, and consistent transmission of forces.

Motion control   The shape of the articular surface determines what motion will occur. A ball-and-socket joint such as the hip is considered a universal joint, allowing movement in all planes. In contrast, a hinge joint allows movement in only one plane.

Stability   In general, bones that form a joint normally closely match with one another and produce varying degrees of stability, depending on their particular shape.

Load Transmission   The articular cartilage assists in transmitting a joint load smoothly and uniformly.

Three major mechanical forces, when exceeding a synovial joint's normal protective response, can result in acute or chronic injuries. They

Functions of articular cartilage:
Control of joint motion
Control of joint stability
Force or load transmission

TABLE 6-3 Synovial joint trauma

Primary Tissue	Type	Mechanical Forces	Condition
Capsule	Acute	Tension, compression	Sprains Dislocation, subluxation Synovial swelling
	Chronic	Tension, compression, shear	Capsulitis Synovitis Bursitis
Articular cartilage (hyaline)	Chronic	Compression, shear	Osteochondrosis Traumatic arthritis

include tension, including twisting (torsional), shearing, and compression (Table 6-3).

Synovial Joint Injury Classification

Acute Joint Injuries

The major injuries that happen to synovial joints are sprains, subluxations, and dislocations.

Sprains   The sprain, one of the most common and disabling injuries seen in sports, is a traumatic joint twist that results in stretching or total tearing of the stabilizing connective tissues such as capsules and ligaments that stabilize joints (Figure 6-8). When a joint is forced beyond its normal anatomical limits, adverse tissue changes occur. Specifically, there is injury to ligaments, to the articular capsule and synovial membrane, and to the tendons crossing the joint. According to the extent of injury, sprains are graded in three degrees

A *first-degree* sprain is characterized by some pain, minimum loss of function, mild point tenderness, little or no swelling, and no abnormal motion when tested for stability. With a *second-degree* sprain, there is pain, moderate loss of function, swelling, and, in some cases, slight-to-moderate joint instability. A *third-degree,* or severe, sprain is very painful, with major loss of function, marked instability, tenderness, and swelling. A third-degree sprain may also represent a subluxation that has spontaneously been reduced.

Blood and synovial fluid collection in the joint cavity during a sprain can produce joint swelling, local temperature increase, pain or point tenderness, and skin discoloration. As with tendons, ligaments and capsules can experience forces that completely rupture or produce an avulsion fracture (pulling of muscle away from bone).

Ligaments and capsules heal slowly because of a relatively poor blood supply; however, their nerves are plentiful and often produce a great deal of pain when injured.

The joints that are most vulnerable to sprains in sports are the ankles,

A sprain is a stretch or total shearing of connective tissue.

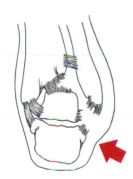

Figure 6-8

A sprain mainly involves ligamentous and capsular tissue (arrow); however, tendons can also be secondarily involved. Forcing a joint beyond its anatomical limits can stretch and tear tissue and on occasion avulse ligaments from the bony attachments.

FUNCTIONAL MUSCLE/JOINT TEST

A simple procedure for the coach to determine whether an injury is to the muscle or joint is as follows:

1. To rule out the possibility of fracture the coach has the athlete move the part through a full range of motion. Pain may indicate muscle injury.
2. Coach passively moves the relaxed part through a range of motion. Pain may indicate a joint condition.
3. Coach applies a resistance against the moving extremity. Pain may suggest a muscle injury.

knees, and shoulders. Sprains occur least often to the wrists and elbows. Since it is often difficult to distinguish between joint sprains and tendon sprains, the examiner should expect the worst possible condition and manage it accordingly. Repeated joint twisting can eventually result in chronic inflammation, degeneration, and arthritis.

Acute synovitis   The synovial membrane of a joint can be acutely injured by a contusion or a sprain. Irritation of the membrane causes an increase in lubrication production, and swelling occurs. As a result, joint pain occurs during motion, along with skin sensitivity from pressure at certain points. In a few days, with proper care, blood collected in the joint is absorbed, and swelling and pain diminish.

Subluxations and dislocations   Dislocations are second to fractures in terms of disabling the athlete. The highest incidence of dislocations involves the fingers and, next, the shoulder joint (Figure 6-9). Dislocations, which result primarily from forces causing the joint to go beyond its normal anatomical limits, are divided into two classes: **subluxations and luxations**. Subluxations are partial dislocations, in which an incomplete separation between two articulating bones occurs. Luxations are complete dislocations, presenting a total disunion of bone apposition between the articulating surfaces.

Several important factors are important in recognizing and evaluating dislocations:

1. There is a loss of limb function. The athlete usually complains of having fallen or of having received a severe blow to a particular joint and then suddenly being unable to move that part.
2. Deformity is almost always apparent; however, it may be obscured by heavy musculature, making it important for the examiner to routinely palpate the injured site to determine the loss of normal contour. Comparison of the injured side with its normal counterpart often reveals physical distortions.
3. Swelling and point tenderness are immediately present.

At times, as with a fracture, x-ray examination is the only absolute diagnostic measure. First-time dislocations or joint separations may result in a rupture of the stabilizing ligamentous and tendinous tissues sur-

subluxation
Partial dislocation

luxation
Total dislocation

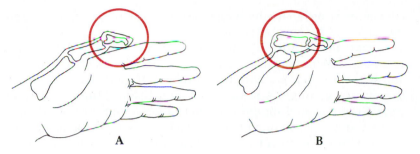

Figure 6-9

A joint that is forced beyond
its anatomical limits can
become partially dislocated
(subluxated; **A**) or completely
dislocated (luxated; **B**).

rounding the joint and an avulsion, or pulling away from the bone. Forces
are often so violent that small chips of bone are torn away with the supporting structures, or the force may separate growth plates or cause a
complete fracture of the neck of a long bone. These possibilities indicate
the importance of administering complete and thorough medical attention to first-time dislocations. It has often been said, "Once a dislocation,
always a dislocation." In most cases this statement is true, since once a
joint has been either subluxated or completely dislocated, the connective tissues that bind and hold it in its correct alignment are stretched to
such an extent that the joint will be extremely vulnerable to subsequent
dislocations.

A first-time dislocation should always be considered and treated as a
possible fracture. Once it has been ascertained that the injury is a dislocation, a physician should be consulted for further evaluation. However,
before the athlete is taken to the physician, the injury should be properly splinted and supported to prevent any further damage.

A first-time dislocation
should always be considered
a possible fracture.

Chronic Joint Injuries

As with other chronic physical injuries or problems occurring from sports
participation, chronic synovial joint injuries stem from microtraumas and
overuse. The two major categories in which they fall are **osteochondrosis** and **traumatic arthritis**. Another general expression for the chronic
synovial conditions of the child or adolescent is articular epiphyseal injury.

Osteochondrosis   Osteochondrosis is a category of conditions in
which the causes are not well understood. One suggested cause of osteochondrosis is aseptic necrosis, in which circulation to the epiphysis has
been disrupted. A synonym for this condition in a joint such as the knee
is *osteochondritis dissecans* and at a tubercle or tuberosity, *apophysitis*. Apophyseal conditions are discussed in the section Bone Trauma in this
chapter.

Another suggestion is that trauma causes particles of the articular cartilage to fracture, eventually resulting in fissures that penetrate to the
subchondral bone. If trauma to a joint occurs, pieces of cartilage may be
dislodged and cause joint locking, swelling, and pain. If the condition oc-

osteochondrosis
Disease state of bone and its
cartilage

traumatic arthritis
Osteoarthritis and/or
inflammation of surrounding
soft tissues, such as the bursal
capsule and the synovium.

Sports Injury Causation,
Response, and Management

apophysis
Bony outgrowth to which
muscles attach

Athletes who have
improperly immobilized joint
injuries or who are allowed
to return to activity before
proper healing has occurred
may eventually be afflicted
with arthritis.

bursae
Closed sacs, or envelopes,
lined with synovia and
containing fluid

curs in an **apophysis,** there may be an avulsion-type fracture and fragmentation of the epiphysis, along with pain, swelling, and disability.

Traumatic arthritis   Traumatic arthritis is usually the result of microtraumas. With repeated trauma to the articular joint surfaces, the bone
and synovium thicken, and there are pain, muscle spasms, and articular
crepitus, or grating, on movement. Joint insult leading to arthritis can
come from repeated sprains that leave a joint with weakened ligaments.
There can be malalignment of the skeleton, which stresses joints, or it
can arise from an irregular joint surface that stems from repeated articular chondral injuries. Loose bodies that have been dislodged from the articular surface can also irritate and produce arthritis. Athletes who have
joint injuries that are improperly immobilized or who are allowed to return to activity before proper healing has occurred may eventually be
afflicted with arthritis.

Chronic soft tissue conditions   The soft tissues of the synovial joint
can develop chronic problems. **Bursae** provide protection between tendons and bones, between tendons and ligaments, and between other
structures where there is friction. Bursae located in and around synovial
joints can be acutely or, over a period of time, chronically inflamed. *Bursitis* in the knee, elbow, and shoulder is common among athletes, After
repeated joint sprains or microtraumas, a chronic inflammatory condition, *capsulitis,* may occur. Usually associated with capsulitis is synovitis.
Synovitis also occurs acutely, but with repeated joint injury or with joint
injury that is improperly managed, a chronic condition can arise. Chronic
synovitis involves active joint congestion with edema. As with the synovial lining of the bursa, the synovium of a joint can undergo degenerative tissue changes. The synovium becomes irregularly thickened, exudation is present, and a fibrous underlying tissue is present as well. Several movements may be restricted, and there may be joint noises such as
grinding or creaking.[4]

BONE TRAUMA

Bone provides shape and support for the body. As with soft tissue, it can
be traumatized during sports participation (Figure 6-10).

Anatomical characteristics

Bone is a specialized type of dense connective tissue made up of cells
(osteocytes) that create semirigid structures that provide body support,
organ protection, movement (through joints and levers), a reservoir for
calcium, and the formation of blood cells (hemopoiesis) (Figure 6-11).

Types of Bone

Bones are classified according to their shapes: flat, irregular, short, and
long. Examples of flat bones are the ribs, the scapulae, and some skull
bones; irregular bones are the vertebrae and some skull bones. Short
bones are primarily in the wrist and the ankle. Long bones are the most
commonly injured in sports. They consist of the humerus, ulna, femur,
tibia, fibula, and phalanges.

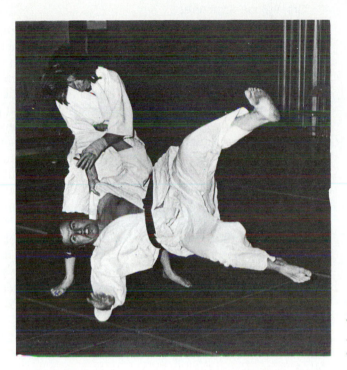

Figure 6-10

The spine and pelvis may be
at risk in many collision and
contact sports.

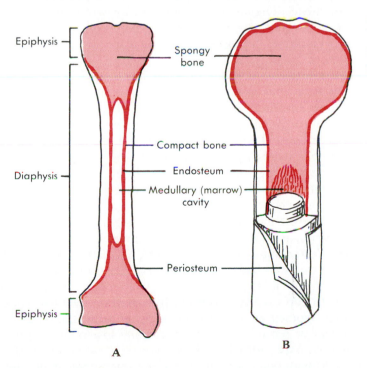

Epiphysis

Diaphysis

Epiphysis

Spongy
bone

Compact bone

Endosteum

Medullary (marrow)
cavity

Periosteum

A

B

Figure 6-11

Anatomical characteristics of
bone. **A,** Longitudinal
section. **B,** Cutaway section.

Gross Bone Structures

The gross structures of bone that are visible to the naked eye include the diaphysis, epiphysis, articular cartilage, periosteum, medullary (marrow) cavity, and endosteum. The *diaphysis* is the main shaft of the long bone. It is hollow, cylindrical, and covered by compact bone. The *epiphysis* is located at the ends of long bones. It is bulbous in shape, providing space for the muscle attachments. The epiphysis is composed primarily of cancellous bone, giving it a spongelike appearance. The ends of long bones are covered with a layer of *hyaline cartilage* that covers the joint surfaces of the epiphysis. This cartilage provides protection during movement and cushions jars and blows to the joint. A dense white fibrous membrane, the *periosteum,* covers long bones except at joint surfaces. Interlacing with the periosteum are fibers from the muscle tendons. Throughout the periosteum on its inner layer exist countless blood vessels and osteoblasts (bone-forming cells). The blood vessels provide nutrition to the bone, and the osteoblasts provide bone growth and repair. The *medullar cavity,* which is a hollow tube in the long bone diaphysis, contains a yellow, fatty marrow in adults. Lining the medullar cavity is the *endosteum* (Figure 6-11).

Bone Growth

In general, bone ossification occurs from the synthesis of bone's organic matrix by **osteoblasts,** followed immediately by the calcification of this matrix.

osteoblasts
Bone-forming cells

Growth of the long bones takes place at the epiphyseal growth plate.

The epiphyseal growth plate is a cartilagenous disk located near the end of each long bone (Figure 6-12). Growth of the long bones depends on these plates. Ossification in long bones begins in the diaphysis and in both epiphyses. It proceeds from the diaphysis toward each epiphysis and from each epiphysis toward the diaphysis.[7] The growth plate has layers of cartilage cells in different stages of maturity, with the more immature cells at one end and mature ones at the other end. As the cartilage cells mature, immature osteoblasts replace them later to produce solid bone. Epiphyseal growth plates are often less resistant to deforming forces than are ligaments of nearby joints or the outer shaft of the long bones; therefore, severe twisting or a blow to an arm or leg can result in disruption in growth. Injury can prematurely close the growth plate, causing a loss of length in the bone. Growth plate dislocation can also cause deformity of the long bone.

osteoclasts
Cells that absorb and remove osseous tissue

Once a bone has reached its full size, there occurs a balance of bone formation and bone destruction, produced by osteoblastic and **osteoclastic** cellular response. An interesting fact is that the resorption of bony tissue by osteoclast may exceed osteoblast bone growth when the athlete is out of shape or fatigued from overtraining. Conversely, bone growth can exceed resorption in a gradual overload conditioning program. Women whose estrogen is decreased as the result of training, anorexia, or secondary amenorrhea may lose bone density, predisposing them to **osteoporosis** and an increase in stress fractures.

osteoporosis
Loss of the quantity of bone or atrophy of skeletal tissue

As with other structures in the human body, bones are highly sensi-

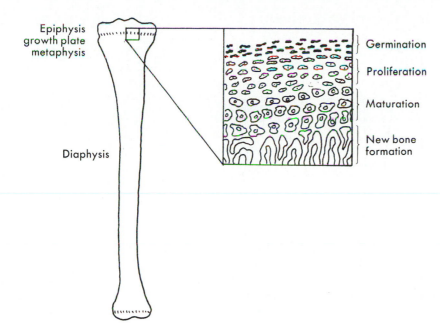

Epiphysis
growth plate
metaphysis

Germination

Proliferation

Maturation

New bone
formation

Diaphysis

Figure 6-12

The epiphyseal growth plate
is the cartilaginous disk
located near the end of each
long bone.

tive to both stress and stress deprivation. With this in mind, bone's functional adaptation follows Wolff's law[13]: *Every change in the form and function of a bone, or of its function alone, is followed by certain definite changes in its internal architecture and equally definite secondary alterations in its mathematical laws.*

Wolff's law states that
changes in bone form and/or
function will lead to changes
in bone architecture and
bone mathematical laws.

Injurious Mechanical Forces to the Skeleton

Because of its viscoelastic properties, bone will bend slightly. However, bone is generally brittle and is a poor shock absorber because of its mineral content. This brittleness increases under tension forces as opposed to compression forces.

Many factors of bone structure affect its strength. Anatomical strength or weakness can be affected by a bone's shape and its changes in shape or direction (Figure 6-13). A hollow cylinder is one of the strongest structures for resisting both bending and twisting as compared with a solid rod, which has much less resistance to such forces.[7] This may be why bones such as the tibia are primarily cylinders. Most spiral fractures of the tibia occur at its middle and distal third, where the bone is most solid.

Anatomical Long Bone Weak Points

Stress forces become concentrated where a long bone suddenly changes shape and direction. Long bones that change shape gradually are less prone to injury than those that change suddenly. The clavicle, for example, is prone to fracture because it changes from round to flat at the same time it changes direction.

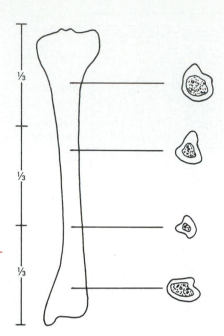

Figure 6-13

Anatomical strengths and
weaknesses of a long bone
can be affected by its shape,
changes of direction, and
hollowness.

Figure 6-14

Mechanisms, patterns, and
appearance of bone fractures.

MECHANISM	PATTERN	APPEARANCE
Bending	Transverse	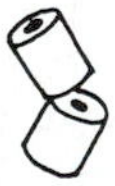
Torsion	Spiral	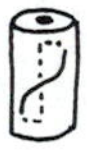
Compression plus bending	Oblique-transverse or butterfly	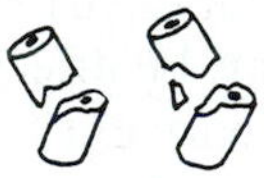
Compression plus bending plus torsion	Oblique	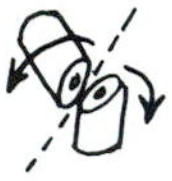
Variable	Comminuted	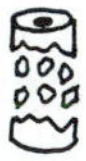
Compression	Metaphyseal compression	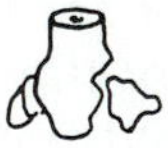

Injury Forces

Long bones can be stressed or forced to fail by *tension, compression, bending, twisting* (torsion), and *shear*. These forces, either singly or in combination, can cause a variety of fractures. For example, spiral fractures are caused by twisting, whereas oblique fractures are caused by the combined forces of axial compression, bending, and torsion. Transverse fractures occur because of bending (Figure 6-14). Along with the type of stress, the amount of the forces must be considered. The more complex the fracture, the more energy is required. External energy can be used to deform and then actually fracture the bony tissues. Some energy can be dispersed to soft tissue adjacent to the bone. When a bone fractures, the rate of energy applied has been such that the bony tissue fails, which is sometimes called the *yield point*.

Long bones can be stressed by tension, compression, bending, torsion, and shearing.

Bone Injury Classification

Bone trauma can generally be classified as periostitis, acute fracture, stress fracture, and epiphyseal damage.

Periostitis

An inflammation of the bone covering the periosteum can result from various sports traumas, mainly contusion. Periostitis often appears as rigidity of the overlying muscles. It can occur as an acute episode or can become chronic.

Acute Bone Fractures

A bone fracture can be a partial or complete interruption in a bone's continuity and can occur without external exposure **(closed fracture)** or can extend through the skin, creating an external wound (compound or **open fracture**). Fractures can result from direct trauma; in other words, the bone breaks directly at the site where a force is applied. When the fracture occurs some distance from where force is applied, it is called an indirect fracture. A sudden, violent muscle contraction or repetitive abnormal stress to a bone can also cause a fracture. Fracture must be considered one of the most serious hazards of sports and should be routinely suspected in musculoskeletal injuries. The following pages include detailed descriptions of acute fractures.

closed fracture
Fracture does not penetrate superficial tissue

open fracture
Overlying skin has been lacerated by protruding bone fragments

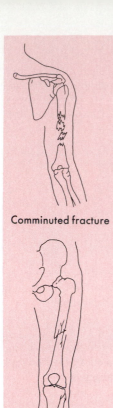

Comminuted fracture

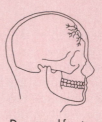

Greenstick fracture

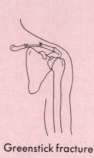

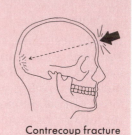

Depressed fracture

Contrecoup fracture

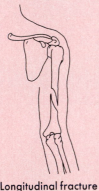

Impacted fracture

Comminuted fractures consist of three or more fragments at the fracture site. They can be caused by a hard blow or a fall in an awkward position. From the physician's point of view, these fractures impose a difficult healing situation because of the displacement of the bone fragments. Soft tissues are often interposed between the fragments, causing incomplete healing. Such cases may need surgical intervention.

Depressed fractures occur most often in flat bones such as those found in the skull. They are caused by falling and striking the head on a hard, immovable surface or by being hit with a hard object. Such injuries also result in gross pathology of soft areas.

Greenstick fractures are incomplete breaks in bones that have not completely ossified. They occur most frequently in the convex bone surface, keeping the concave surface intact. The name is derived from the similarity of such fractures to the break in a green twig taken from a tree.

Impacted fractures can result from a fall in height, which causes a long bone to receive directly on its long axis a force of such magnitude that the osseous tissue is compressed. This telescopes one part of the bone on the other. Impacted fractures require immediate splinting by the athletic trainer and traction by the physician to ensure a normal length of the injured limb.

Longitudinal fractures are those in which the bone splits along its length. They are often the result of jumping from a height and landing in such a way as to apply force or stress to the long axis.

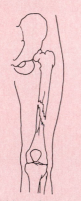

Longitudinal fracture

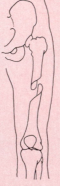

Oblique fracture

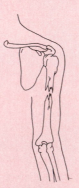

Serrated fracture

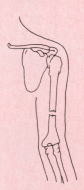

Spiral fracture

Transverse fracture

Oblique fractures are similar to spiral fractures. They occur when one end receives sudden torsion or twisting and the other end is fixed or stabilized.

Serrated fractures are sawtooth, sharp-edged fracture lines of the two bony fragments. They are usually caused by a direct blow. Because of the sharp and jagged edges, extensive internal damage such as the severance of vital blood vessels and nerves often occurs.

Spiral fractures have an S-shaped separation. They are fairly common in football and skiing, in which the foot is firmly planted and the body is suddenly rotated.

Transverse fractures occur in a straight line, more or less at right angles to the bone shaft. A direct outside blow usually causes this injury.

Contrecoup fractures occur on the side opposite to the part where trauma was initiated. Fracture of the skull is at times an example of the contrecoup. An athlete may be hit on one side of the head with such force that the brain and internal structures compress against the opposite side of the skull, causing a fracture.

Avulsion fracture An avulsion fracture is the separation of a bone fragment from its cortex at an attachment of a ligament or tendon. This fracture usually occurs as a result of a sudden, powerful twist or stretch of a body part. An example of a ligamentous episode is the sudden eversion of the foot that causes the deltoid ligament to avulse bone from the medial malleolus. An example of a tendinous avulsion is one that causes a patellar fracture, which occurs when an athlete falls forward while suddenly bending a knee. The stretch of the patellar tendon pulls a portion of the inferior patellar pole apart (Figure 6-15).

Blow-out fracture Blow-out fracture occurs to the wall of the eye orbit as the result of a blow to the eye.

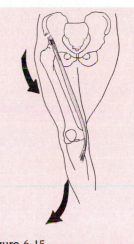

Figure 6-15

Mechanism of a tendinous avulsion fracture caused by abnormal stretching of the sartorius muscle.

Stress Fractures

Stress fractures have been variously called march, fatigue, and spontaneous fractures, although stress fracture is the most commonly used term. There are a number of likely possibilities as to the cause of a stress fracture such as an overload caused by muscle contraction, an altered stress distribution in the bone accompanying muscle fatigue, a change in the ground reaction force such as going from a wood surface to a grass surface, and performing a rhythmically repetitive stress leading up to a vibratory summation point. Rhythmic muscle action performed over a period of time at a subthreshold level causes the stress-bearing capacity of the bone to be exceeded, hence a stress fracture. A bone may become vulnerable to stress fracture during the first few weeks of intense physical activity or training. Weight-bearing bones undergo bone resorption and become weaker before they become stronger. The four fractures, in increasing order of severity, are focal microfractures, periosteal and endosteal response (stress fractures), linear fractures (stress fractures), and displaced fractures.

Typical causes of stress fractures in sports are as follows:

1. Coming back into competition too soon after an injury or illness
2. Going from one event to another without proper training in the second event
3. Starting initial training too quickly
4. Changing habits or the environment (e.g., running surfaces, the bank of a track, or shoes). The chances of receiving a stress fracture also increase where there are postural deviations. Increased susceptibility occurs when the athlete has a deviation such as flat feet, pronated feet, or a rigid high arch.

Early detection of a stress fracture may be difficult. Because of their frequency in a wide range of sports, stress fractures must be suspected in body areas that fail to respond to usual management. Until there is an obvious reaction in the bone, which may take several weeks, x-ray examination may fail to reveal usual fracture.

The major signs of a stress fracture are swelling, local tenderness, and pain. In the early stages of the fracture the athlete complains of pain when active but not at rest. Later the pain is constant and becomes more intense at night. Percussion, or light tapping on the bone at a site other than the suspected fracture, will produce pain at the fracture site.

The most common sites of stress fracture are the tibia, fibula, metatarsal shaft, calcaneus, femur, pars interarticularis of the lumbar vertebrae, ribs, and humerus (Figure 6-16).

Epiphyseal Conditions

A musculoskeletal injury to a child or adolescent should always be considered a possible epiphyseal condition.

Three types of epiphyseal growth-site injuries can be sustained by children and adolescents performing sports activities. They consist of injury to the epiphyseal growth plate, articular epiphyseal injuries, and apophyseal injuries. The most prevalent age range for these injuries is from 10 to 16 years.

Apophyseal Injuries

The young, physically immature athlete is particularly prone to apophyseal injuries. The apophyses are *traction epiphyses,* in contrast to the *pressure epiphyses* of the long bones. These apophyses serve as origins or insertions for muscles on growing bone; they provide bone shape but not length. Common traction epiphyses conditions in sports are Sever's disease and Osgood-Schlatter disease. Sever's disease is located on the calcaneal tuberosity where the Achilles tendon attaches. Osgood-Schlatter disease is a condition of the tibial tuberosity where the patellar tendon attaches.

NERVE TRAUMA

A number of abnormal nerve responses can be attributed to athletic participation or injury.

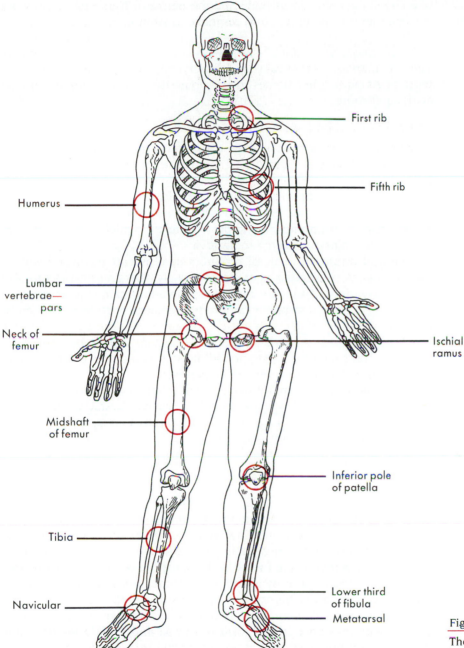

First rib

Fifth rib

Humerus

Lumbar
vertebrae—
pars

Neck of
femur

Ischial
ramus

Midshaft
of femur

Inferior pole
of patella

Tibia

Lower third
of fibula

Navicular

Metatarsal

Figure 6-16

The most common stress
fracture sites.

Anatomical Characteristics

The tissue that makes up the nervous system is throughout the body. It
is composed of *neurons, interstitial tissues* including *neuroglia* (supporting
elements), *neurilemma* cells (the membranous sheath enveloping a nerve
fiber), and *satellite cells* (flat epithelium-like cells forming the inner aspect

of a double-layered capsule covering the neuron). Nerve tissue provides the body with its reception and response to stimuli.

Injurious Mechanical Forces

The two main forces that cause major nerve injuries are compression and tension. As with other tissues in the body, the injurious forces may be acute or chronic.

Nerve Injury Classification

Some of the more common nerve conditions are those that distort sensation or produce pain. Conditions that cause sensation distortion are as follows:

Hypoesthesia—a diminished sense of feeling

Hyperesthesia—an increased sense of feelings such as pain or touch

Paresthesia—numbness, prickling, or tingling, which may occur from a direct blow or stretch to an area

Physical trauma in general produces pain as part of the inflammatory process. Any number of traumas directly affecting nerves can also produce a variety of sensory responses, including pain. For example, a sudden nerve stretch or pinch can produce a sharp burning pain that radiates down a limb along with muscle weakness. *Neuritis,* a chronic nerve problem, can be caused by a variety of forces that usually have been repeated or continued for a long period of time. Symptoms of neuritis can range from minor nerve problems to paralysis.

Pain that is felt at a point of the body other than at its actual origin is commonly known as *referred pain.* Another manifestation of referred pain is a trigger point, which occurs in the muscular system but originates in some other distant body part.

BODY MECHANICS AND INJURY SUSCEPTIBILITY
Body Efficiency

If we carefully study the mechanical structure of the human body, we see how amazing it is that humans can move so effectively in the upright posture. Even more amazing are the complex movements that humans accomplish when engaged in sport. Not only must constant gravitational force be overcome by the athlete, but the body also must be manipulated through space by a complex system of somewhat inefficient levers, fueled by a machinery that operates at an efficiency level of approximately 30%. The bony levers that move the body must overcome considerable resistance in the form of inertia and muscle viscosity and must work in most instances at an extremely unfavorable angle of pull. All these factors mitigate the effectiveness of lever action to the extent that most movement is achieved at an efficiency level of less than 25%.

Despite these seeming inefficiencies, the body can compensate by making modifications or adjustments that depend on the task at hand. For example, the center of gravity may be lowered by widening the stance, the segmented body parts may function either as a single unit or as a series of finely coordinated units, or an increase in muscle power may be elicited in an effort to offset certain mechanical ineptitudes. Structural changes in bones that result from stresses placed on them afford broader and more secure muscle anchorage and consequently aid in the development of more power.

Shock Absorption

Although the bones of the body are not primarily designed to withstand shock, the musculature serves as a shock absorber by absorbing impact and distributing it over a relatively large area, thereby lessening the concentration of the force on a small area of bone. Bones such as the shin and skull, however, which have little or no overlying musculature and thus are more susceptible to injury, should be afforded protection, especially in sports activities in which they are particularly vulnerable to blows.

The musculature serves as a shock absorber for the body.

Repetitive and Overuse Conditions

Sports injuries as a result of repetition and overuse can produce stress microtraumas. Such stress injuries frequently result in either limitation or curtailment of sports performance. Most of these injuries in athletes are directly related to the dynamics of running, throwing, or jumping. The injuries may result from constant and repetitive stresses placed on bones, joints, or soft tissues; from forcing a joint into an extreme range of motion; or from prolonged strenuous activity. Some of the injuries falling into this category may be relatively minor; still, they can prove to be quite disabling. Chapters on specific sports injuries will discuss many of the injuries stemming from microtrauma.

Upright Posture

In the upright posture human legs are long and straight, and the feet are adaptable for support and propulsion. The spine has three curves in the anteroposterior plane that help maintain balance. However, along with the invaluable advantages gained through an upright posture and an increased range of movement, there are some disadvantages. The constant gravitational pull and the weight of the supported organs make humans somewhat prone to have a protruded abdomen unless the abdominal muscles maintain sufficient tonicity to withstand these forces. The head, weighing close to 14 pounds, is balanced almost precariously on top of the seven small cervical vertebrae, which are sustained by the cervical neck ligaments and neck muscles.[1]

Postural Deviations

Postural deviations are often a major underlying cause of sports injuries. Postural malalignment may be the result of unilateral muscle and soft-tissue asymmetries or bony asymmetries. As a result, the athlete engages in poor mechanics of movement *(pathomechanics)*. Many sports activities are one sided, which leads to asymmetries in body development. The resulting imbalance is manifested by a postural deviation as the body seeks to reestablish itself in relation to its center of gravity. Often such deviations are a primary cause of injury. For example, a consistent pattern of knee injury may be related to asymmetries within the pelvis and the legs. The coach, although not usually expert in postural deviations, should be able to identify obvious asymmetrics of the body and make a referral to an athletic trainer or physician. It should be noted that a number of postural conditions offer genuine hazards to athletes by making them prone to specific acute and overuse injuries. Some of the most important conditions are indicated in the following discussions.

Knock-Knee (Genu Valgum)

Knock-knee (genu valgum) is an orthopedic disorder that presents a serious hazard to the knee joints (Figure 6-17, *A*). The weight-bearing line passes to the lateral side of the center of the knee joint as a result of the inward angling of the thigh and lower leg. This causes the body weight to be borne principally on the medial aspects of the articulating surfaces, thereby subjecting the medial knee ligaments to considerable strain.

Bowleg (Genu Varum)

Bowleg is the opposite to knock-knee (Figure 6-17, *B*). The extra stress is placed on the fibular collateral ligament. In extreme cases of either of these conditions, athletes should be directed into a noncontact activity in which they are not subjected to the conditions of stress and force encountered in contact sports.

Spinal Deviations

Round back (kyphosis)   The condition of round back or **kyphosis** as a rule is accompanied by a forward-thrust head, winged scapulae, and a flat chest (Figure 6-18). Usually activities that make great demands on

kyphosis

exaggeration of the normal curve of the thoracic spine

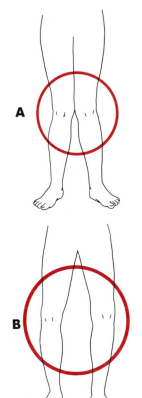

Figure 6-17

A, Genu valgum (knock knees). **B,** Genu varum (bowleg).

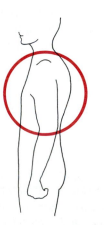

Figure 6-18

Kyphosis.

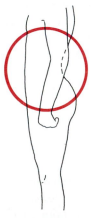

Figure 6-19

Lumbar lordosis.

the chest (pectoral) muscles are a primary cause of this condition among athletes. Kyphotic athletes who have strong and well-developed but shortened chest muscles (such as are found frequently among basketball players, gymnasts, weightlifters, and—as a product of football stances— football players) are quite susceptible to shoulder dislocations, particularly when the arm is forced into an abducted and external position accompanied by outward rotation.

Sway back (lumbar lordosis)   Sway back is an abnormal anterior curvature of the low back, commonly called swayback or hollow back (Figure 6-19). A tightening of the lower back muscles and corresponding weakening of the abdominal muscles are involved. Among football linemen this condition is aggravated by the postural demands of the offensive stance. Gymnasts, particularly female gymnasts, are also subject to swayback as the result of repeated arching of the low back with subsequent lordosis, which can also place abnormal strain on the pelvic joints. In addition, the sport demands exceptional spinal flexibility, which also can be a factor. Stress fracture and displacement of the vertebrae can result as the low back's response to the excessive and strenuous physical demands being made on it. The hamstring muscle strain, sometimes suffered by runners, may be attributed to a swayback.

Scoliosis   Scoliosis is defined as a lateral rotary curvature of the spine (Figure 6-20). Many of our sports are unilateral, and others have certain phases that tend to develop or aggravate this postural-orthopedic condition. Baseball pitching and high jumping using a one-foot takeoff are examples. Athletes with scoliosis may be subject to a variety of joint and muscle problems stemming from the stress of sport. Commonly, athletes with unequal leg length may be prone to scoliosis.

Running, Throwing, and Jumping

Many stress injuries in sports can be attributed to improper form carried out repetitively. It is essential that coaches become aware of sports techniques performed incorrectly and their injury outcomes.

Running

Since many of the abnormal or continued stress syndromes bear a direct relationship to the act of running, the coach should have an understanding of what is involved in this activity (Figure 6-21). The action of the

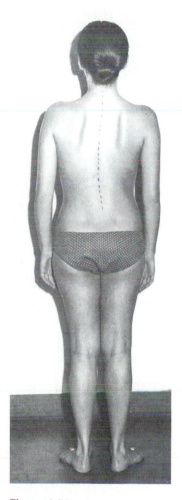

Figure 6-20

Scoliosis

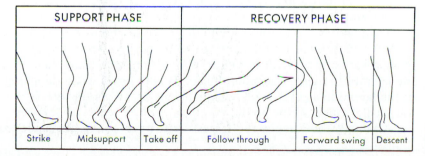

SUPPORT PHASE			RECOVERY PHASE		
Strike	Midsupport	Take off	Follow through	Forward swing	Descent

Figure 6-21

Running gait cycle.

lower extremity during a complete stride in running can be divided into two phases. The first is the stance or support phase, which starts with initial contact at heel strike and ends at toe-off. The second is the swing or recovery phase. This represents the time immediately after toe-off in which the leg is moved from behind the body to a position in front of the body in preparation for heel strike.

The foot's function during the support phase of running its twofold. At heel strike, the foot acts as a shock absorber to the impact forces and then adapts to the uneven surfaces. At push-off, the foot functions as rigid lever to transmit the explosive force from the lower extremity to the turning surface.

Locomotion of any kind, but especially that kind imposed by sports activities, places great stress on the foot as it makes contact with a surface. If the foot is abnormally structured, pathological conditions may develop over time. A foot that functions normally will place no undue stress on itself or the other joints of the lower limb. A foot with a structural malformation may eventually lead to overuse problems. Continued overuse of the foot, particularly as encountered in distance running, leads to syndromes that are relatively common in activities in which repetitive pounding of the foot occurs in the foot-strike and the takeoff thrust phases of the gait.[2]

Jumping

Jumping such as high jumping and long jumping in track and field and long horse jumping are events unto themselves or can be one aspect of a sport such as basketball or volleyball. In jumping activities the shock of takeoff and landing is transmitted to the lower limb or limbs, as well as to the pelvis and spine. Improper takeoff or landing is responsible for a great many joint injuries. The force of the takeoff can cause a stress fracture to the foot or the ankle. The shock of an improper landing is frequently the cause of injury to the ankle, knee, hip joint, or spine.

Severe torque results when the takeoff foot is either toed in or out. In either case, the ligaments, particularly in the ankle or the knee joint, are subjected to an intense rotational shear force that usually results in torn ligaments, cartilages, or bone fracture. Improper landings from either the high jump or the long jump can cause lower limb injury, but the arms and neck are also vulnerable. The flop style of high jumping, wherein the bar is cleared by going over backward and the landing is on the back, can result in a cervical injury, especially to young and inexperienced jumpers (Figure 6-22).

Traumatic forces to the ankle joint frequently occur during jumping. Such twisting or shearing action can be damaging. Approximately 85% of all ankle injuries result from forced inversion, which causes tearing of the lateral ligaments. Eversion injuries usually result in the breaking off of the lateral malleolus, with some damage to the connective tissues on the medial aspect of the ankle.

Although the knee is the largest joint in the body, its shallowness

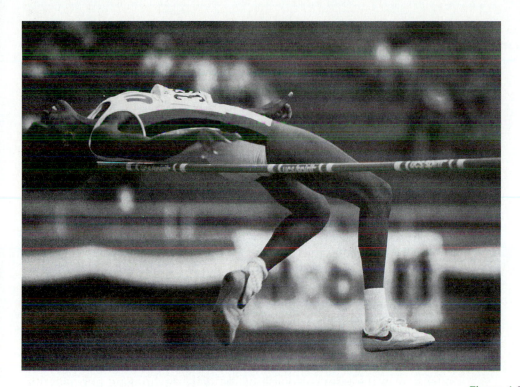

Figure 6-22

The flop style of high jumping can result in cervical injury.

renders it extremely vulnerable to injury. Medial, lateral, and twisting forces, such as encountered in most sports, subject the supportive ligamentous bands to severe strains. These injuries may occur after one violent traumatic incident, or they may result from the cumulative effects of repeated microtrauma. Such strain can result in the stretching or tearing of the supporting connective tissue. This can happen when the foot is firmly fixed and the body and leg rotate. Hyperextension of the knee, wherein the knee is forced into a position beyond the normal 180-degree position, can result in severe joint trauma that may involve the synovial membrane or the deeper periosteal tissue. This commonly occurs in take-off but can occur on landing, especially in gymnastics.

Throwing

Throwing activities account for many overuse injuries among athletes. Throwing here is considered to be any sports movements that use one or both arms in a throwing-type motion. This action can be seen in free-style and butterfly swimmers, as well as in volleyball spiking, tennis serving, and all other overhand throwing skills. Baseball pitching is used here to best represent the overhead dynamics of the throwing mechanism.

Pitching is a unilateral action that subjects the arm to repetitive stresses of great intensity. Should the thrower use incorrect techniques, the joints are affected by atypical stresses that result in trauma to the shoulder joint and its surrounding tissues. Pitching is a sequential pattern of movements in which each part of the body must perform a number of carefully executed acts.[5]

In throwing, the arm acts as a sling or catapult, transferring and imparting momentum from the body to the ball. There are various types of throwing, with the overhand, sidearm, and underarm styles being the most common. The act of throwing is fairly complex and requires considerable coordination and timing if success is to be achieved.

Overhead throwing or pitching involves three distinct phases: a preparatory or cocking phase, the delivery or acceleration phase, and the follow-through or terminal phase (Figure 6-23). Specific injuries appear peculiar to each phase. In throwing, the most powerful muscle groups are brought into play initially, progressing ultimately to the least powerful but the most coordinated (i.e., the legs, trunk, shoulder girdle, arm, forearm, and finally the hand). The body's center of gravity is transported in the direction of the throw as the leg opposite the throwing arm is first elevated and then moved forward and planted on the ground, thus stopping the forward movement of the leg and permitting the body weight to be transferred from the supporting leg to the moving leg. Initially the trunk rotates backward as the throwing arm and wrist are cocked, then rotates forward, continuing its rotation beyond the planted foot as the throwing arm moves forcibly from a position of extreme external rotation, abduction, and extension through flexion to forcible and complete extension in the terminal phase of the delivery, bringing into play the powerful internal rotators and adductors. These muscles exert a tremendous force and, over a period of time, create cumulative microtraumas that can result in shoulder problems or the so-called pitcher's or tennis elbow and eventually traumatic arthritis.

Figure 6-23

Phases of the pitch from left to right: wind-up, early cocking, late cocking, acceleration, follow-through.

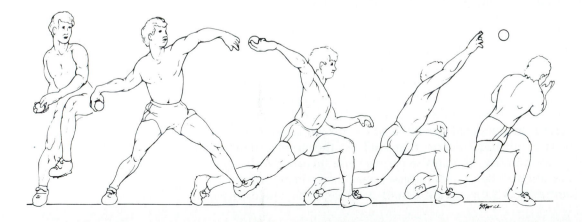

In throwing, the shoulder and the elbow seem particularly vulnerable to trauma. Uncoordinated or stress movements can subject either articulation to a considerable amount of abnormal force or torque. In pitching, with considerable speed being engendered, the forearm is the crucial element. The inward or outward rotation that is used to impart additional speed and action to the ball subjects the elbow and the shoulder to appreciable torque, which may become traumatizing if the action is improperly performed over a considerable period of time. The rotator cuff muscles, long head of the biceps brachii, pronator teres, anconeus, and deltoid are the muscles that are most affected in throwing.[2]

SUMMARY

Skin trauma can occur from a variety of forces (e.g., friction, scraping, compression, tearing, cutting, and penetration) that produce, in order, blisters, skin bruises, lacerations, skin avulsions, incisions, and puncture wounds.

Skeletal muscle trauma from sports participation can involve any aspect of the muscle-tension unit. Forces that injure muscles are compression, tension, and shear. Acute muscle injuries include contusions and strains. Avulsion fractures and muscle ruptures can occur from an acute episode. Chronic muscle conditions are myositis, fasciitis, tendinitis, tenosynovitis, and bursitis. Chronic muscle irritation can cause ectopic calcification; muscle disuse can cause atrophy; and immobilization can cause joint contracture.

Sports injuries to the synovial joints are common. Anatomically, synovial joints have relative strengths or weaknesses based on their ligamentous and capsular type and their muscle arrangements. Forces that can injure synovial joints are tension, compression, torsion, and shear. Sprains involve acute injury to ligaments or the joint capsule. A third-degree sprain may go so far as to cause ligament rupture or an avulsion fracture. Acute synovial joint injuries that go beyond the third degree may result in a dislocation. Two major chronic synovial joint conditions are osteochondrosis and traumatic arthritis. Other chronic conditions are bursitis, capsulitis, and synovitis.

Long bones can be anatomically susceptible to fractures because of their shape and as a result of changes in direction of the force applied to them. Mechanical forces that cause injury are compression, tension, bending, torsion, and shear. Bending and torsional forces are forms of tension. Acute fractures may include avulsion, blow-out, comminuted, depressed, greenstick, impacted, longitudinal, oblique, serrated, spiral, transverse, and contrecoup types. Stress fractures are commonly the result of overload to a given bone area. Stress fractures are apparently caused by an altered stress distribution or by the performance of a rhythmically repetitive action that leads to a vibratory summation and thus to a fracture. Three major epiphyseal injuries in sports occur to the growth plate, the articular cartilage, and the apophysis.

Nerve trauma can be produced by overstretching or compression. As with other injuries, it can be acute or chronic. The sudden stretch of a nerve can cause a burning sensation. Abnormal pressure on a nerve can produce hypoesthesia, hyperesthesia, or paresthesia. A variety of traumas to nerves can produce acute pain or a chronic pain such as neuritis.

An athlete who has faulty body mechanics has a potential for injury. Postural deviations can increase the chances for pathomechanics. Improper use of the body in such activities as running, throwing, and jumping can predispose the athlete to an overuse injury.

REVIEW QUESTIONS AND CLASS ACTIVITIES

1. What is the difference between a primary injury and a secondary injury? Can you give examples of both?
2. Define strains, muscle spasms, sprains, dislocations, and types of fractures. What signs or symptoms would the athlete have for each one, and what immediate care would you give the athlete?
3. What structures are found at a joint? What are their functions?
4. Bones have certain characteristics that make them prone to injuries. What are they? Are women more susceptible to bone problems?
5. Describe various types of fractures and the mechanisms that cause them. Why and how do stress fractures occur?
6. Invite an orthopedist to class to discuss common injuries to the musculoskeletal system for the adolescent athlete, epiphyseal fractures, and early recognition and management of these injuries.
7. Postural deviations are often a primary cause of injuries as a result of either unilateral asymmetries, bone anomalies, abnormal skeletal alignments, or poor mechanics of movement. What are some of these deviations and how do they put on athlete at risk for injury? Which deviations are congenital, and which may be acquired?
8. With the help of one of your students (dressed appropriately), point out where common postural deviations occur and show how to evaluate the back for kyphosis, lordosis, and scoliosis.
9. Discuss what body structures are prone to injury with each anomaly and what activities are contraindicated.
10. Discuss how overuse injuries can result from faulty running, throwing, and jumping movements.

REFERENCES

1. Anthony CP, Thibodeau GA: *Textbook of anatomy and physiology,* ed 13, St Louis, 1989, Mosby-Year Book.
2. Arnheim D, Prentice W: *Principles of athletic training,* ed 8, St Louis, 1992, Mosby-Year Book.
3. Bone loss in amenorrheic athletes, *Sports Med Dig* 9:6, 1987.
4. Blauvelt CT, Nelson FRT: *A manual of orthopaedic terminology,* ed 4, St Louis, 1990, Mosby-Year Book.
5. Bratz JH, Gogia PP: The mechanics of pitching, *Orthop Sports Phys Ther* 9:56, 1987.
6. Byrnes WB, Clarkson PM: Delayed onset muscle soreness and training, *Clin sports med* 5:1986.
7. Cailliet R: *Soft tissue pain and disability,* Philadelphia, 1988, FA Davis.
8. Cavanaugh RR: The biomechanics of lower extremity action in distance running, *Foot Ankle* 7:197, 1987.
9. Evans WJ: Exercise-induced skeletal muscle damage, *Phys Sportsmed* 15:89, 1987.

10. Markey KL: Stress fractures, *Clin sports med* 6:1987.
11. Radin EL et al: Joint use and misuse, *Int J Sports Med* 10:585, 1989.
12. Roux W: *Die Entwickiungsmechanic,* Leipzig, 1905, W Englemann.
13. Williams JGP: *Color atlas of injury in sport,* Chicago, 1990, Mosby-Year Book.
14. Wolff J: *Das Geset der Transformation der Knockan,* Berlin, 1892, A Hirschwald.

ANNOTATED BIBLIOGRAPHY

Blauvelt CT, Nelson RRT: *A manual of orthopaedic terminology,* ed 4, St Louis, 1990, Mosby-Year Book.
A resource book for all individuals who need to identify medical words or their acronyms.

Booher JM, Thibodeau GA: *Athletic injury assessment,* St Louis, 1994, Mosby-Year Book.
An excellent guide to the recognition, assessment, classification, and evaluation of athletic injuries.

Bruce R, ed: *Sports medicine—the school age athlete,* Philadelphia, 1991, WB Saunders.
Text aimed at musculoskeletal sports injuries occurring in the young athlete.

Calliet R: *Soft tissue pain and disability,* Philadelphia, 1988, FA Davis.
An excellent in-depth reference on soft tissue injuries throughout the various joints of the body. Chapter 1 discusses the types of connective tissue, common disorders, joint motion, and posture concepts.

Dyment PG, ed: *Sports and the adolescent,* Philadelphia, 1991, Hanley & Belfus.
A book directed to the specific concerns of adolescents. An easy-to-read small text covering most aspects of sports medicine.

Garrick JG, Webb DR: *Sports injuries: diagnosis and management,* Philadelphia, 1990, WB Saunders.
An overview of musculoskeletal injuries that are unique to sports and exercise.

Standard nomenclature of athletic injuries, Monroe, Wis, 1976, American Medical Association.
An in-depth list of conditions in the fields of athletic training and sports medicine. Each condition is described in terms of its cause, symptoms, signs, complications, laboratory finding, x-ray findings, and pathology.

Williams JGP: *Color atlas of injury in sport,* Chicago, 1990, Mosby-Year Book.
An excellent visual guide to the area of sports injuries. It covers the nature and incidence of sport injury, types of tissue damage, and regional injuries caused by a variety of sports activites.

Selected Emergency Procedures

When you finish this chapter, you will be able to:

- Establish an emergency system for a school sports program
- Explain the importance of knowing cardiopulmonary resuscitation (CPR) and how to manage an obstructed airway
- Describe the types of hemorrhage and their management
- Assess the types of shock and their management
- Describe the emergency management of musculoskeletal injuries

Time is critical in an emergency.

Most sports injuries do not result in life-or-death emergency situations, but when such situations do arise, prompt care is essential. Emergency is defined as "an unforeseen combination of circumstances and the resulting state that calls for immediate action."[5] Time becomes the critical factor, and assistance to the injured individual must be based on knowledge of what to do and how to do it—how to provide effective aid immediately. There is no room for uncertainty, indecision, or error.

Coaches without direct and immediate access to an emergency technician (EMT), athletic trainer, or physician must have a basic knowledge of emergency care related to his or her sport. Every coach should be certified in both first aid and cardiopulmonary resuscitation (CPR).[2]

The athletic training team, consisting of the coach, the athletic trainer, and the team physician, must at all times act in a reasonable and prudent manner. This behavior is especially important during emergencies.

THE EMERGENCY PLAN

The prime concern of emergency aid is to maintain cardiovascular function and, indirectly, central nervous system function, since failure of any of these systems may lead to death. The key to emergency aid in the sports setting is the initial evaluation of the injured athlete. Time is of the essence, so this evaluation must be done rapidly and accurately so that proper aid can be rendered without delay. In some instances these

first steps not only will be lifesaving but also may determine the degree
and extent of permanent disability.

All sports programs must have an emergency plan that when called
on can immediately be set in place. The following issues must be ad-
dressed when developing the emergency system:

1. Are location of phones and emergency telephone numbers well
known? (Use 911 if available.)
2. Who is designated to make the telephone call? Who has the key
to gates or padlocks, and who will open them?
3. What information should be given over the telephone?
   a. Type of emergency
   b. Type of suspected injury
   c. Present condition of the athlete
   d. Current assistance being given (e.g., cardiopulmonary resuscitation)
   e. Location of telephone being used
   f. Exact location of emergency (give names of streets and cross
streets) and how to enter facility
4. Is there a separate emergency plan for each sport's field, courts,
and gymnasiums?
5. Have coaches, athletic trainers, athletic director, and other school
personnel been apprised of the emergency plan? Do these individuals know their responsibilities in an emergency?

It is essential that individuals providing emergency care to the injured athlete cooperate and act professionally. Too often, the rescue squad
personnel, the physician, and the athletic trainer disagree over exactly
how the injured athlete should be handled and transported. The coach
or athletic trainer is usually the first individual to deal with the emergency situation. The athletic trainer has generally had more training and
experience in moving and transporting an injured athlete than the coach
or physician. If the rescue squad is called and responds, it should have
the final say on how that athlete is to be transported.

To alleviate potential conflicts, the athletic department, with input
from coaches and the athletic trainer, should establish procedures and
guidelines and arrange practice sessions with all parties concerned with
handling the injured athlete. The rescue squad may not be experienced
in dealing with someone who is wearing a helmet. The athletic trainer
should make sure before an incident occurs that the EMTs understand
the importance of leaving the helmet in place. When dealing with the
injured athlete, all egos should be put aside. Certainly the most important consideration is what is the best for the athlete.

PRINCIPLES OF ASSESSMENT

The athletic trainer cannot deliver appropriate medical care to the injured
athlete until some systematic assessment of the situation has been made.
This assessment (Figure 7-1) helps to determine the nature of the injury
and provides direction in the decision-making process concerning the

*All sports programs must
have an emergency plan.*

*The rescue squad makes the
final decision on how to
transport an injured athlete.*

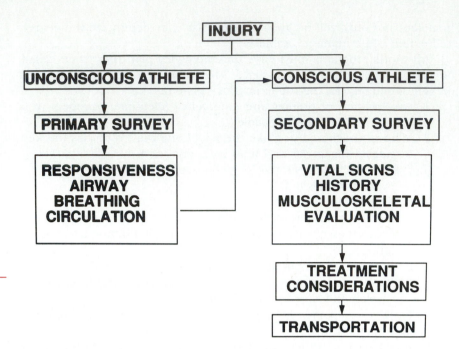

Figure 7-1

Flow chart showing the
appropriate emergency
procedures for the injured
athlete.

emergency care that must be rendered. The *primary survey* refers to assessment of life-threatening problems including airway, breathing, circulation (ABCs), and severe bleeding. It takes precedence over all other aspects of victim assessment and should be used to correct life-threatening situations.[8] Once the condition of the victim is stabilized, the *secondary survey* takes a closer look at the injury sustained by the athlete. The secondary survey gathers specific information about the injury from the athlete, systematically assesses vital signs and symptoms, and allows a more detailed evaluation of the injury. The secondary survey is done to uncover problems that do not pose an immediate threat to life but that may do so if they remain uncorrected.[8]

An injured athlete who is conscious and stable will not require a primary survey. However the unconscious athlete must be monitored for life-threatening problems throughout the assessment process.

Use a secondary survey when the athlete is conscious.

The Unconscious Athlete

The state of unconsciousness provides one of the greatest dilemmas in sports. Whether it is advisable to move the athlete and allow the game to resume or to await the arrival of a physician is a question that too often is resolved hastily and without much forethought. Unconsciousness may be defined as a state of insensibility in which there is a lack of conscious awareness. This condition can be brought about by a blow to either the head or the solar plexus, or it may result from general shock. It is often difficult to determine the exact cause of unconsciousness (Table 7-1).

TABLE 7-1 Evaluating the unconscious athlete

Functional Signs		Selected Conditions					
	Fainting	Concussion	Grand Mal Epilepsy	Brain Compression and Injury	Sunstroke	Diabetic Coma	Stroke
Onset	Usually sudden	Usually sudden	Sudden	Usually gradual	Gradual or sudden	Gradual	Gradual
Mental	Complete unconsciousness	Confusion or unconsciousness	Unconsciousness	Unconsciousness gradually deepening	Delirium or unconsciousness	Drowsiness, later unconsciousness	Listlessness, later unconsciousness
Pulse	Feeble and fast	Feeble and irregular	Fast	Gradually slower	Fast and feeble	Fast and feeble	Fast and very feeble
Respiration	Quick and shallow	Shallow and irregular	Noisy, later deep and slow	Slow and noisy	Difficult	Deep and sighing	Rapid and shallow, with occasional deep sigh
Skin	Pale, cold, and clammy	Pale and cold	Livid, later pale	Hot and flushed	Very hot and dry	Livid, later pale	Pale, cold, and clammy
Pupils	Equal and dilated	Equal	Equal and dilated	Unequal	Equal	Equal	Equal and dilated
Paralysis	None	None	None	May be present in leg and/or arm	None	None	None
Convulsions	None	None	None	Present in some cases	Present in some cases	None	None
Breath	NA	NA	NA	NA	NA	Acetone smell	NA
Special features	Giddiness and sway before collapse	Signs of head injury, vomiting during recovery	Bites tongue, voids urine and feces, may injure self while falling	Signs of head injury, delayed onset of symptoms	Vomiting in some cases	In early stages, headache, restlessness, and nausea	May vomit; early stages: shivering, thirst, defective vision, and ear noises

The unconscious athlete must always be considered to have a life-threatening injury that requires an immediate primary survey. The following guidelines should be followed when dealing with the unconscious athlete:

1. Body position should immediately be noted, and the level of consciousness and unresponsiveness should be determined.
2. Airway, breathing, and circulation (ABC) should be established immediately.
3. Injury to the neck and spine is always a possibility in the unconscious athlete.
4. If the athlete is wearing a helmet, it should never be removed until neck and spine injury have been unequivocally ruled out. However, the face mask must be cut away and removed to allow CPR.
5. If the athlete is supine and not breathing, establish ABC immediately.
6. If the athlete is supine and breathing, do nothing until consciousness returns.
7. If the athlete is prone and not breathing, log roll him or her carefully to supine position and establish ABC immediately.
8. If the athlete is prone and breathing, do nothing until consciousness returns, then carefully log roll him or her onto a spine board because CPR could be necessary at any time.
9. Monitor and maintain life support for the unconscious athlete until emergency medical personnel arrive.
10. Once the athlete is stabilized the athletic trainer should begin a secondary survey.

PRIMARY SURVEY
Treatment of Life-Threatening Injuries

Life-threatening injuries take precedence over all other injuries sustained by the athlete. Situations that are considered life-threatening include those that will require cardiopulmonary resuscitation (i.e., obstruction of the airway, no breathing, no circulation) and those that have profuse bleeding.

Overview of Emergency CPR

It is essential that a careful evaluation of the injured person be made to determine whether cardiopulmonary resuscitation (CPR) should be conducted. The following is an overview of adult CPR and is not intended to be used by persons who are not certified in CPR. It should also be noted that, because of the serious nature of CPR, updates should routinely be studied through the American Red Cross and the American Heart Association.

All coaches and athletic trainers should be certified in CPR.

First, establish unresponsiveness of the athlete by tapping or gently shaking his or her shoulder and shouting, "Are you okay?" Note that shaking should be avoided if there is a possible neck injury. If the athlete is unresponsive, call out for help, position the athlete for assistance, and then proceed with the ABCs of CPR.[8] The ABC mnemonic of CPR is easily remembered and indicates the sequential steps used for basic life support:

*A*irway opened
*B*reathing restored
*C*irculation restored

Frequently, when A is restored, B and C will resume spontaneously, and it is then unnecessary to perform them. In some instances, the restoration of A and B obviates the necessity for step C. If the athlete is in a position other than supine, he or she must be carefully rolled over as a unit, avoiding any twisting of the body, because CPR can be administered only with the athlete lying flat on the back with knees straight or slightly flexed. When performing CPR on an adult victim, the following sequence should be followed.

Opening the Airway

1. **NOTE:** A face mask may have to be cut away before CPR can be rendered (Figure 7-2). Open the airway by using the head-tilt/chin-lift method. Lift chin with one hand while pushing down on

Figure 7-2

A face mask and shoulder pads have to be removed before CPR is given. Throughout this process, the head and neck are stabilized. **A**, Cutting support to release mask. **B**, Carefully lifting the mask away from the face. **C**, Cutting away shirt. **D**, Cutting shoulder pad laces.

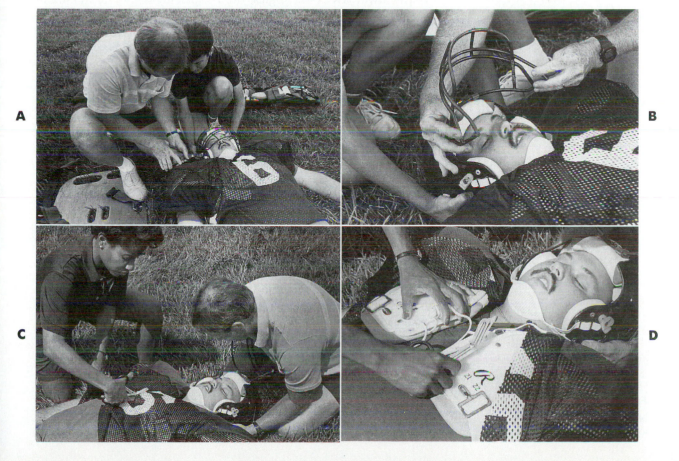

victim's forehead with the other, avoiding the use of excessive force. The tongue is the most common cause of respiratory obstruction; the forward lift of the jaw raises the tongue away from the back of the throat, thus clearing the airway. NOTE: On victims with suspected head or neck injuries, perform a modified jaw maneuver. In this procedure displace the jaw forward only, keeping the head in a fixed, neutral position.

2. In an unconscious individual, because the tongue often acts as an impediment to respiration by blocking the airway, it is necessary to use the chin-lift maneuver. Lift the chin by placing the fingers of one hand under the lower jaw near the chin, lifting and bringing the chin forward, thus supporting the jaw and lifting the tongue. Avoid compressing the soft tissue under the jaw, because this could obstruct the airway. Avoid completely closing the mouth. The teeth should be slightly apart. *Look* to see if the chest rises and falls. *Listen* for air passing in or out of the nose or mouth. *Feel* on your cheek whether is being expelled; this procedure should take 3 to 5 seconds.

3. If neither of the foregoing is sufficiently effective, additional forward displacement of the jaw can be affected by grasping each side of the lower jaw at the angles, thus displacing the lower mandible forward as the head is tilted backward. In executing this maneuver both elbows should rest on the same surface as that on which the victim is lying. Should the lips close, they can be opened by retracting the lower lip with a thumb. This is the maneuver that should be used on individuals with suspected neck injuries because it can be performed effectively without extending the cervical spine.

Establishing Breathing

1. To determine if the victim is breathing, maintain the open airway, place your ear over the mouth, observe the chest, and look, listen, and feel for breath sounds.

2. With the hand that is on the athlete's forehead, pinch the nose shut, keeping the heel of the hand in place to hold the head back (if there is no neck injury) (Figure 7-3). Taking a deep breath, place your mouth over the athlete's mouth to provide an airtight seal and give two slow full breaths at a rate of 1 to 1½ seconds per inflation. NOTE: To avoid the possibility of becoming contaminated by bloodborne pathogens, the rescuer should wear a disposable physical barrier before initiating mouth to mouth resuscitation.[10] Observe the chest rise. Remove your mouth, and listen for the air to escape through passive exhalation.

NOTE: If the airway is obstructed, reposition the victim's head and try again to ventilate. If still obstructed, give 6 to 10 subdiaphragmatic abdominal thrusts followed by a finger sweep to clear objects from the mouth. Continue to repeat this sequence until ventilation occurs.

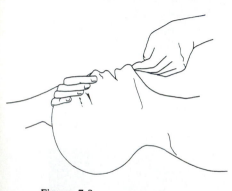

Figure 7-3

Head-tilt/chin-lift technique for establishing an airway.

A   B

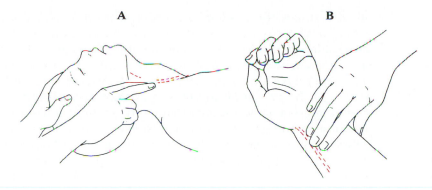

Figure 7-4

Pulse rate taken at the carotid artery, **A,** and radial artery, **B.**

Establishing Circulation

1. To determine pulselessness, feel the carotid pulse with two fingers of one hand while maintaining head-tilt with the other (Figure 7-4).
2. If there is no pulse, activate the Emergency Medical System (EMS) by having someone dial 911.
3. Maintain open airway. Position yourself close to the side of the athlete's chest. With the middle and index fingers of the hand closest to the waist, locate the lower margin of the athlete's rib cage on the side next to you (Figure 7-5).
4. Run the fingers up along the rib cage to the notch where the ribs meet the sternum.
5. Place the middle finger on the notch and the index finger next to it on the lower end of the sternum.
6. Next, the hand closest to the athlete's head is positioned on the lower half of the sternum next to the index finger of the first hand that located the notch; then the heel of that hand is placed on the long axis of the breastbone.
7. The first hand is then removed from the notch and placed on top of the hand on the sternum so that the heels of both hands are parallel and the fingers are directed straight away from the coach or athletic trainer (Figure 7-6).
8. Fingers can be extended or interlaced, but they must be kept *off* the chest wall.
9. Elbows are kept in a locked position with arms straight and shoulders positioned over the hands, enabling the thrust to be straight down.
10. In a normal-sized adult, enough force must be applied to depress the sternum 1½ to 2 inches (4 to 5 cm). After depression, there must be complete release of the sternum to allow the heart to refill. The time of release should equal the time of compression. For one or two operators, compression must be given at the rate of 80 to 100 times per minute, maintaining a rate of 15 chest compressions to two full breaths.
11. CPR techniques involving two rescuers are no longer recom-

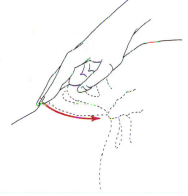

Figure 7-5

With the middle and index fingers of the hand closest to the waist, the lower margin of the victim's rib cage is located. The fingers are then run along the rib cage to the notch where the ribs meet the sternum. The middle finger is placed on the notch with the index finger next to it on the lower end of the sternum.

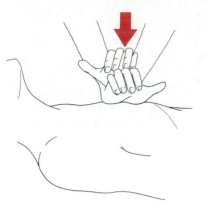

Figure 7-6

The heel of the headward
hand is placed on the long
axis of the lower half of the
sternum, next to the index
finger of the first hand. The
first hand is removed from
the notch and placed on top
of the hand on the sternum,
with fingers interlaced.

Figure 7-7

Cardiac compression, using
two rescuers, interposes one
breath for every five chest
compressions. This technique
is recommended only for
individuals who have been
specifically trained.

mended unless the rescuers are EMTs or more qualified than
EMTs. However, when two qualified rescuers are available, they
are positioned at opposite sides of the athlete (Figure 7-7). The
one providing the breathing does so by giving a breath after every five chest compressions, which are administered by the other
rescuer at the rate of 80 to 100 compressions per minute. The
carotid pulse must be checked frequently by the ventilator during chest compression to ascertain the effectiveness of the compression. In the beginning, check after 10 sets of 15:2 have been
completed, after which ventilation and compression should be
interrupted during every few minutes of ventilation to determine
whether spontaneous breathing and pulse have occurred. With
the exception of inserting an airway and transporting, *never interrupt CPR for more than 5 seconds.* Adequate circulation must be
maintained. Any interruption in compression permits the blood
flow to drop to zero.

Number of Rescuers	Ratio of Compressions to Breaths	Rate of Compressions
1	15:2	80-100 times/min
2	5:1	80-100 times/min

Obstructed Airway Management

Choking on foreign objects claims close to 2,000 lives every year. Choking is a possibility in many sports activities; for example, an athlete may

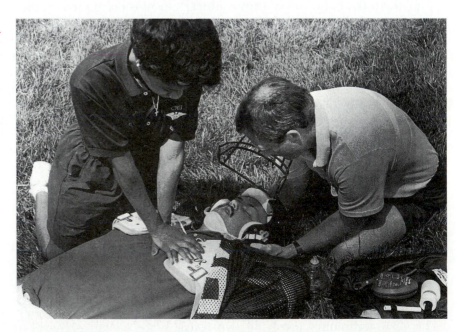

choke on a mouth guard, a broken bit of dental work, chewing gum, or even a "chaw" of tobacco. When such emergencies arise, early recognition and prompt, knowledgeable action are necessary to avert a tragedy. An unconscious person can choke also—the tongue may fall back in the throat, thus blocking the upper airway. Blood clots resulting from head, facial, or dental injuries may impede normal breathing, as may vomiting. When complete airway obstruction occurs, the individual is unable to speak, cough, or breathe. If the athlete is conscious, there is a tremendous effort made to breathe, the head is forced back, and the face initially is flushed and then becomes cyanotic as oxygen deprivation is incurred. If partial airway obstruction is causing the choking, some air passage can be detected, but during a complete obstruction no air movement is discernible.

Athletes can choke on mouth guards, gum, or "chaw."

To relieve airway obstruction caused by foreign bodies, two maneuvers are recommended: (1) the Heimlich maneuver and (2) finger sweeps of the mouth and throat.

Heimlich maneuver   As with CPR, the Heimlich maneuver (subdiaphragmatic abdominal thrusts) requires practice before proficiency is acquired. There are two methods of obstructed airway management, depending on whether the victim is in an erect position or has collapsed and is either unconscious or too heavy to lift. For the conscious victim the Heimlich maneuver is performed until he or she is relieved or becomes unconscious. In cases of unconsciousness, 6 to 10 abdominal thrusts are applied, followed by a finger sweep with an attempt at ventilation.

Method A   Stand behind and to one side of the athlete. Place both arms around the waist just above the belt line, and permit the athlete's head, arms, and upper trunk to hang forward (Figure 7-8, A). Grasp one of your fists with the other, placing the thumb side of the grasped fist immediately below the xiphoid process of the sternum, clear of the rib cage. Now sharply and forcefully thrust the fists into the abdomen, inward and upward, several times. This "hug" pushes up on the diaphragm, compressing the air in the lungs, creating forceful pressure against the blockage, and thus usually causing the obstruction to be promptly expelled. Repeat the maneuver until successful.

Method B   If the athlete is on the ground or on the floor, place him or her on the back and straddle the thighs, keeping your weight fairly centered over your knees. Place the heel of your left hand against the back of your right hand and push sharply into the abdomen just above the belt line (note the position, Figure 7-8, B). Repeat this maneuver 6 to 10 times, then repeat the finger sweep. Care must be taken in either of these methods to avoid extreme force or applying force over the rib cage because fractures of the ribs and damage to the organs can result.

Finger sweeping   If a foreign object such as a mouth guard is lodged in the mouth or the throat and is visible, it may be possible to remove or release it with the fingers. Care must be taken that the probing does not drive the object deeper into the throat. It is usually impossible to open

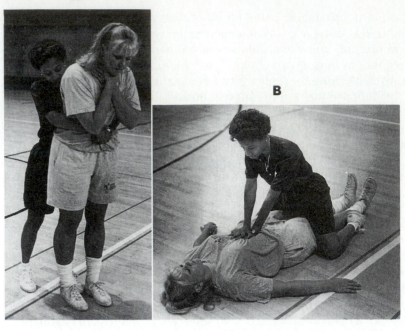

Figure 7-8

The Heimlich maneuver for
an obstructed airway. **A,**
Manual thrust maneuver for
the conscious athlete. **B,**
Manual thrust maneuver for
the unconscious athlete.

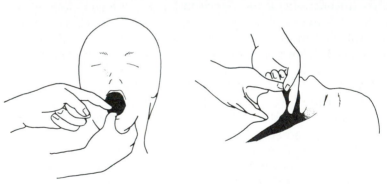

Figure 7-9

Finger sweeping of the
mouth is essential in
attempting to remove a
foreign object from a choking
victim.

the mouth of a conscious victim who is in distress, so the Heimlich maneuver technique should be put to use immediately. In the unconscious
athlete, turn the head either to the side or face up, open the mouth by
grasping the tongue and the lower jaw, hold them firmly between the
thumb and fingers, and lift—an action that pulls the tongue away from
the back of the throat and from the impediment. If this is difficult to do,
the crossed finger method can usually be used effectively. The index finger of the free hand (or if both hands are used, an assistant can probe)
should be inserted into one side of the mouth along the cheek, deeply
into the throat; using a hooking maneuver, attempt to free the impediment, moving it into a position from which it can be removed (Figure
7-9). Attempt to ventilate after each sweep until the airway is open. Once
the object is removed, if the athlete is not already breathing, an attempt
is made to ventilate him or her.

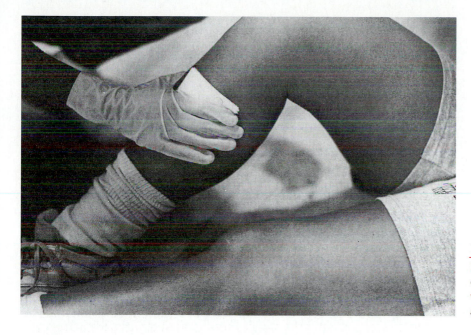

Figure 7-10

Direct pressure for the
control of bleeding is applied
with the hand over a sterile
gauze pad.

Control of Hemorrhage

An abnormal external or internal discharge of blood is called a hemorrhage. The hemorrhage may be venous, capillary, or arterial and may be external or internal. Venous blood is characteristically dark red with a continuous flow, capillary bleeding exudes from tissue and is a reddish color, and arterial bleeding flows in spurts and is bright red.

External Bleeding

External bleeding stems from open skin wounds such as abrasions, incisions, lacerations, and punctures, or avulsions. The control of external bleeding includes the use of direct pressure, elevation, and pressure points.

Direct pressure Pressure is directly applied with the hand over a sterile gauze pad. The pressure is applied firmly against the resistance of a bone (Figure 7-10).

Elevation Elevation, in combination with direct pressure, provides an additional means for the reduction of external hemorrhage. Elevating a hemorrhaging part against gravity reduces blood pressure and, consequently, slows bleeding.[11]

Pressure points When direct pressure combined with elevation fails to slow hemorrhage, the use of pressure points may be the method of choice. Eleven points on each side of the body have been identified for controlling external bleeding; the two most commonly used are the brachial artery in the upper limb and the femoral artery in the lower limb. The brachial artery is compressed against the medial aspect of the hu-

External bleeding can usually be managed by using direct pressure, elevation, or pressure points.

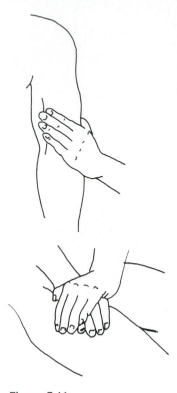

Figure 7-11

The two most common sites for direct pressure are the brachial artery and the femoral artery.

merus, and the femoral artery is compressed as it is detected within the femoral triangle (Figure 7-11).

Internal Hemorrhage

Internal hemorrhage is invisible to the eye unless manifested through some body opening or identified through x-ray studies or other diagnostic techniques. Its danger lies in the difficulty of diagnosis. When internal hemorrhaging occurs, either under the skin such as in a bruise or contusion, intramuscularly, or in joints, the athlete may be moved without danger in most instances. However, the detection of bleeding within a body cavity such as the skull or thorax is of the utmost importance because it could mean the difference between life and death. Because the symptoms are obscure, internal hemorrhage is difficult to diagnose properly. As a result of this difficulty, athletes with internal injuries require hospitalization under complete and constant observation by a medical staff to determine the nature and extent of the injuries. All severe hemorrhaging will eventually result in shock and should therefore be treated on this premise. Even if there is no outward indication of shock, the athlete should be kept quiet and body heat should be maintained at a constant and suitable temperature (see section on shock for the preferred body position).

Shock

In any injury, shock is a possibility, but when severe bleeding, fractures, or deep internal injuries are present, the development of shock is certain. Shock occurs when there is a diminished amount of blood available to the circulatory system. As a result there are not enough oxygen-carrying blood cells available to the tissues, particularly those of the nervous system. This situation occurs when the vascular system loses its capacity to hold the fluid portion of the blood within its system because of dilation of the blood vessels within the body and disruption of the osmotic fluid balance (Figure 7-12). When this occurs, a quantity of plasma is lost from the blood vessels to the tissue spaces of the body, leaving the solid blood particles within the vessels and thus causing stagnation and slowing the blood flow. With this general collapse of the vascular system there is widespread tissue death, which will eventually cause the death of the individual unless treatment is given.

Certain conditions such as extreme fatigue, extreme exposure to heat or cold, extreme dehydration of fluids and minerals, or illness predispose an athlete to shock.

In a situation in which there is a potential shock condition, there are other signs by which the athletic trainer or coach should assess the possibility of the athlete's lapsing into a state of shock as an aftermath of the injury. The most important clue to potential is the recognition of a severe injury. It may happen that none of the usual signs of shock is present.

Figure 7-12

During shock, blood vessels dilate, causing the osmotic fluid balance to be disrupted and allowing plasma to become lost into tissue spaces.

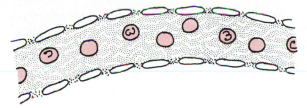

Normal capillary   Dilated capillary

Symptoms and Signs

The major characteristic of shock is marked paleness of the skin that may lead to cyanosis. As the condition progresses, the face takes on a pinched expression with staring of the eyes, which often lose their luster and become dilated. The pulse becomes weak and rapid, with the breathing rate increased and shallow. Blood pressure decreases, and in severe situations there is urinary retention and fecal incontinence. If conscious, the athlete may display a disinterest in his or her surroundings or may display irritability, restlessness, or excitement. There may also be extreme thirst.[7]

Management

Depending on the causative factor for the shock, the following emergency care should be given:

1. Maintain body heat, using warm but not hot blankets.
2. Elevate the feet and legs 8 to 12 inches for most situations.

However, shock management does vary according to the type of injury.[7] For example, for a neck injury, the athlete should be immobilized as found; for a head injury, his or her head and shoulders should be elevated; and for a leg fracture, his or her leg should be kept level and should be raised after splinting.

Shock can also be compounded or initially produced by the psychological reaction of the athlete to an injury situation. Fear or the sudden realization that a serious situation has occurred can result in shock. In the case of a psychological reaction to an injury, the athlete should be instructed to lie down and avoid viewing the injury. This athlete should be handled with patience and gentleness, but firmness as well. Spectators should be kept away from the injured athlete. Reassurance is of vital concern to the injured athlete. The person should be given immediate comfort through the loosening of clothing. Nothing should be given

Signs of shock
Blood pressure is low
Systolic pressure is usually below 90 mm Hg
Pulse is rapid and very weak
Athlete may be drowsy and appear sluggish
Respiration is shallow and extremely rapid
Skin is pale, cool, clammy

TYPES OF SHOCK

The main types of shock are hypovolemic, respiratory, neurogenic, psychogenic, cardiogenic, septic, anaphylactic, and metabolic.[7]

Hypovolemic shock stems from trauma in which there is blood loss. Without enough blood in the circulatory system, organs are not properly supplied with oxygen.

Respiratory shock occurs when the lungs are unable to supply enough oxygen to the circulating blood. Trauma that produces a pneumothorax or injury to the breathing control mechanism can produce respiratory shock.

Neurogenic shock is caused by the general dilation of blood vessels within the cardiovascular system. When it occurs, the typical 6 L of blood can no longer fill the system. As a result the cardiovascular system can no longer supply oxygen to the body.

Psychogenic shock refers to what is commonly known as fainting (syncope). It is caused when there is temporary dilation of blood vessels, reducing the normal amount of blood in the brain.

Cardiogenic shock refers to the inability of the heart to pump enough blood to the body.

Septic shock occurs from a severe, usually bacterial, infection. Toxins liberated from the bacteria can cause small blood vessels in the body to dilate.

Anaphylactic shock is the result of a severe allergic reaction caused by foods, insect stings, drugs, or inhaling dusts, pollens, or other substances.

Metabolic shock happens when a severe illness such as diabetes goes untreated. Another cause is an extreme loss of bodily fluid (e.g., through urination, vomiting, or diarrhea).

by mouth until a physician has determined that no surgical procedures are indicated.

Secondary Survey

Once the life-threatening injuries have been dealt with, the athletic trainer should conduct a secondary survey to assess the existing injury more precisely.

Recognizing Vital Signs

Vital signs to observe
  Pulse
  Respiration
  Blood pressure
  Temperature
  Skin color
  Pupils
  State of consciousness
  Movement
  Abnormal nerve response

The ability to recognize physiological signs of injury is essential to the proper handling of potentially critical injuries. When evaluating the seriously ill or injured athlete, the coach, athletic trainer, or physician must be aware of nine response areas; heart rate, breathing rate, blood pressure, temperatures, skin color, pupils of the eye, movement, the presence of pain, and unconsciousness.

Pulse

The pulse is the direct extension of the functioning heart. In emergency situations it is usually determined at the carotid artery at the neck or the radial artery in the wrist (Figure 7-4). A normal pulse rate per minute for adults ranges between 60 and 80 beats and in children from 80 to 100 beats; however, it should be noted that trained athletes usually have slower pulses than the typical population.

An alteration of a pulse from the normal may indicate the presence of a pathological condition. For example, a rapid but weak pulse could mean shock, bleeding, diabetic coma, or heat exhaustion. A rapid and strong pulse may mean heatstroke or severe fright, a strong but slow pulse could indicate a skull fracture or stroke, whereas no pulse means cardiac arrest or death.[3]

Respiration

The normal breathing rate per minute is approximately 12 breaths in adults and 20 to 25 breaths in children. Breathing may be shallow (indicating shock), irregular, or gasping (indicating cardiac involvement). Frothy blood from the mouth indicates a chest injury, such as a fractured rib, that has affected a lung. Look, listen, and feel: *look* to ascertain whether the chest is rising or falling, *listen* for air passing in and out of the mouth or nose or both; and *feel* where the chest is moving.

Blood Pressure

Blood pressure indicates the amount of force that is produced against the arterial walls. It is indicated at two pressure levels: systolic and diastolic, **Systolic blood pressure** occurs when the heart pumps blood, whereas **diastolic blood pressure** is the residual pressure present in the arteries when the heart is between beats. The normal systolic pressure for 15- to 20-year-old males ranges from 115 to 120 mm Hg. The diastolic pressure, on the other hand, usually ranges from 75 to 80 mm Hg. The normal blood pressure of females is usually 8 to 10 mm Hg lower than in males for both systolic and diastolic pressures. Between the ages of 15 and 20, a systolic pressure of 135 mm Hg and above may be excessive; also, 110 mm Hg and below may be considered too low. The outer ranges for diastolic pressure should not exceed 60 and 85 mm Hg, respectively. A lowered blood pressure could indicate hemorrhage, shock, heart attack, or internal organ injury.

systolic blood pressure
The pressure caused by the heart's pumping

diastolic blood pressure
The residual pressure when the heart is between beats

Temperature

Body temperature is maintained by water evaporation and heat radiation. It is normally 98.6° F (37° C). Temperature is measured with a thermometer, which is placed under the tongue, in the armpit, or, in case of unconsciousness, in the rectum. Changes in body temperature can be reflected in the skin. For example, hot dry skin might indicate disease, infection, or overexposure to environmental heat. Cool, clammy skin could reflect trauma, shock, or heat exhaustion, whereas cool, dry skin is possibly the result of overexposure to cold.

A rise or fall of internal temperature may be caused by a variety of

To convert Fahrenheit to centigrade (Celsius)
$$°C = (°F - 32) ÷ 1.8$$
To convert centigrade to Fahrenheit
$$°F = (1.8 × °C) + 32$$

circumstances such as the onset of a communicable disease, cold exposure, pain, fear, or nervousness. Characteristically, with the lowered temperature there may be chills with chattering teeth, blue lips, goose bumps, and pale skin.

Skin Color

For individuals who are lightly pigmented, the skin can be a good indicator of the state of health. In this instance, three colors are commonly identified in medical emergencies: red, white, and blue. A red skin color may indicate heatstroke, high blood pressure, or carbon monoxide poisoning. A pale, ashen, or white skin can mean insufficient circulation, shock, fright, hemorrhage, heat exhaustion, or insulin shock. Skin that is bluish in color (cyanotic), primarily noted in lips and fingernails, usually means that circulating blood is poorly oxygenated. This may indicate an airway obstruction or respiratory insufficiency.

Assessing a dark-skinned athlete is different from assessing a light-skinned athlete. These individuals normally have pink coloration of the nail beds and inside the lips, mouth, and tongue. When a dark-skinned person goes into shock, the skin around the mouth and nose will often have a grayish cast, whereas the tongue, the inside of the mouth, the lips, and nail beds will have a bluish cast. Shock resulting from hemorrhage will cause the tongue and inside of the mouth to become a pale, grayish color instead of blue. Fever in these athletes can be noted by a red flush at the tips of the ears.[4]

Pupils

Some athletes normally have irregular and unequal pupils.

The pupils are extremely sensitive to situations affecting the nervous system. Although most persons have pupils of regular outline and equal size, some individuals normally have pupils that may be irregular and unequal. This disparity requires the coach or athletic trainer to know which of their athletes deviates from the norm.

A constricted pupil may indicate that the athlete is using a central nervous system–depressant drug. If one or both pupils are dilated, the athlete may have sustained a head injury, may be experiencing shock, heatstroke, or hemorrhage, or may have ingested a stimulant drug (Figure 7-13). The pupils' response to light should also be noted. If one or both pupils fail to accommodate to light, there may be brain injury, or alcohol or drug poisoning. When examining an athlete's pupils, the examiner should note the presence of contact lenses or an artificial eye. Pupil response is more critical in evaluation than pupil size.

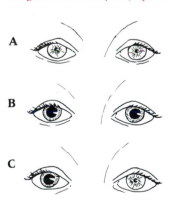

Figure 7-13

The pupils of the eyes are extremely sensitive to situations affecting the nervous system. **A,** Normal pupils. **B,** Dilated pupils. **C,** Irregular pupils.

State of Consciousness

When recognizing vital signs, the examiner must always note the athlete's state of consciousness. Normally the athlete is alert, aware of the environment, and responds quickly to vocal stimulation. Head injury, heatstroke, and diabetic coma can vary an individual's level of conscious awareness.

Movement

The inability to move a body part can indicate a serious central nervous system injury that has involved the motor system. An inability to move one side of the body could be caused by a head injury or cerebrovascular accident (stroke). Paralysis of the upper limb may indicate a spinal injury, inability to move the lower extremities could mean an injury below the neck, and pressure on the spinal cord could lead to limited use of the limbs.[4]

Abnormal Nerve Response

The injured athlete's pain or other reactions to adverse stimuli can provide valuable clues to the coach or athletic trainer. Numbness or tingling in a limb with or without movement can indicate nerve or cold damage. Blocking of a main artery can produce severe pain, loss of sensation, or lack of a pulse in a limb. A complete lack of pain or of awareness of serious but obvious injury may be caused by shock, hysteria, drug usage, or a spinal cord injury. Generalized or localized pain in the injured region probably means there is no injury to the spinal cord.[2]

Musculoskeletal Assessment

A logical process must be used to evaluate accurately the extent of a musculoskeletal injury. One must be aware of the major signs that reveal the site, nature, and, above all, severity of the injury. Detection of these signs can be facilitated, as is true with all trauma, (1) *by understanding the mechanism of traumatic sequence* and (2) *methodically inspecting the injury.* Knowledge of the mechanism of an injury is extremely important in determining which area of the body is most affected. When the injury mechanism has been determined, the examiner proceeds to the next phase: physical inspection of the affected region. At this point information is gathered by what is seen, what is heard, and what is felt.

In an attempt to understand the mechanism of injury, a brief history of the complaint must be taken. The athlete is asked, if possible, about the events leading up to the injury and how it occurred. The athlete is further asked what was heard or felt when the injury took place. The athletic trainer makes a *visual observation* of the injured site, comparing it to the uninjured body part. The initial visual examination can disclose obvious deformity, swelling, and skin discoloration.

Next, *auditory observation* of what was heard at the time of the injury is determined. Sounds occurring at the time of injury or during manual inspection yield pertinent information about the type and extent of pathology present. Such uncommon sounds as grating or harsh rubbing may indicate fracture. Joint sounds may be detected when either arthritis or internal derangement is present. Areas of the body that have abnormal amounts of fluid may produce sloshing sounds when gently palpated or moved. Such sounds as a snap, crack, or pop at the moment of injury often indicate bone breakage.

Finally, the region of the injury is gently palpated. Feeling, or palpating, a part with trained fingers can, in conjunction with visual and audible signs, indicate the nature of the injury. Palpation is started away from the injury and gradually moves towards it. As the examiner gently feels the injury and surrounding structures with the fingertips, several factors can be revealed: the extent of point tenderness, the extent of irritation (whether it is confined to soft tissue alone or extends to the bony tissue), and deformities that may not be detected by visual examination alone.

Assessment Decisions

After a quick on-site injury inspection and evaluation, the athletic trainer makes the following decisions:

1. The seriousness of the injury
2. The type of first aid and immobilization necessary
3. Whether the injury warrants immediate referral to a physician for further assessment
4. The manner of transportation from the injury site to the sidelines, training room, or hospital.

All information about the initial history, signs, and symptoms of the injury must be documented, if possible, so that they may be described in detail to the physician.

Immediate Treatment

Because musculoskeletal injuries are extremely common in sports, a knowledge of their immediate care is necessary. Three areas of first aid are highly important: (1) control of hemorrhage and management of early inflammation, muscle spasm, and pain; (2) splinting; and (3) handling and transportation.

Hemorrhage, Inflammation, Muscle Spasm, and Pain Management

Of major importance in musculoskeletal injuries is the initial control of hemorrhage, early inflammation, muscle spasm, and pain. The acronym for this process is ICE (ice, compression, and elevation). Added to this is the important factor of rest.

Rest, Ice, Compression, and Elevation (RICE)

Rest Rest is essential for musculoskeletal injuries. This can be achieved by not moving the part or can be guaranteed by the application of tape, wraps, splints, casts, and the assistance of a cane or crutches. Immobilization of an injury for the first 2 or 3 days after injury helps to ensure healing of the wound without complication. Moving too early will only increase hemorrhage and the extent of disability, prolonging recovery.

Ice (cold application) Cold, primarily ice in various forms, is an effective first aid agent. It is not clear exactly how cold acts physiologically. It is known to reduce pain and spasm and to minimize enzyme activity, thus reducing tissue necrosis.[10] Cold application thus decreases the

---

Decisions that can be made from the secondary survey
Seriousness of injury
Type of first aid required
Whether injury warrants physical referral
Type of transportation needed

RICE (rest, ice, compression, and elevation) are essential in the emergency care of musculoskeletal injuries.

chance of swelling, which can occur for 4 to 6 hours following injury. There is some uncertainty about what extent vasoconstriction plays in the reduction of swelling. Cold makes blood more viscous, lessens capillary permeability, and decreases the blood flow to the injured area.[5] Cold applied to a recent injury will lower metabolism and the tissue demands for oxygen and reduce hypoxia. This benefit extends to uninjured tissue, preventing injury-related tissue death from spreading to adjacent normal cellular structures.[5] It should be noted however, that prolonged application of cold can cause tissue damage.[5]

For best results, ice packs (crushed ice and towel) should be applied directly to the skin. Frozen gel packs should not be used directly against the skin, because they reach much lower temperatures than ice packs. A good rule of thumb is to apply a cold pack to a recent injury for a 20-minute period and repeat every 1 to 1½ hours throughout the waking day. Depending on the severity and site of the injury, cold may be applied intermittently for 1 to 72 hours. For example, a mild strain will probably require one or two 20-minute periods of cold application, whereas a severe knee or ankle sprain might need 3 days of intermittent cold. If in doubt about the severity of an injury, it is best to extend the time RICE is applied.

Compression In most cases immediate compression of an acute injury is considered an important adjunct to cold and elevation and in some cases may be superior to them.[13] Placing external pressure on an injury assists in decreasing hemorrhage and hematoma formation. Fluid seepage into the interstitial spaces is retarded by compression, and absorption is facilitated. However, application of compression to some conditions such as the anterior compartment syndrome, may be contraindicated.

Many types of compression are available. An elastic wrap that has been soaked in water and frozen in a refrigerator can provide both compression and cold when applied to a recent injury. Pads can be cut from felt or foam rubber to fit difficult-to-compress body areas. A horseshoe-shaped pad, for example, placed around the malleolus in combination with an elastic wrap and tape, provides an excellent way to prevent or reduce ankle edema (Figure 7-14). Although cold is applied intermittently, compression should be maintained throughout the day and, if possible, throughout the night. At night it is best to remove the wrap completely and elevate the body part above the heart to avoid pooling of fluids when the body processes slow down.

Elevation Along with cold and compression, elevation reduces internal bleeding. By elevating the affected part above the level of the heart, bleeding is reduced, and venous return is encouraged, further reducing swelling.

RICE schedule
1. Evaluate the extent of injury.
2. Apply crushed ice in a moist towel pack to the injury.
3. Hold ice pack firmly against the injury site with an elastic wrap.

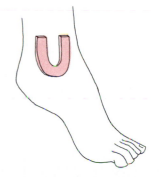

Figure 7-14

A horseshoe-shaped pad can be placed around the malleolus to reduce edema.

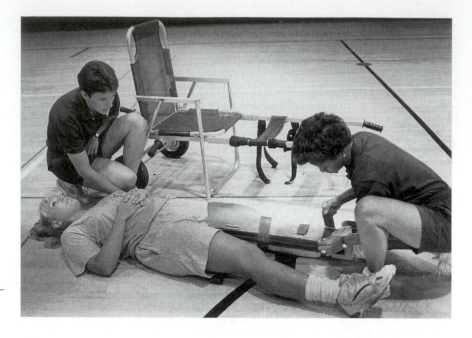

Figure 7-15

Any suspected fracture
should routinely be splinted.

4. Elevate injured body part above the level of the heart.
5. After 20 minutes, remove ice pack.
6. Replace ice pack with a compress wrap and pad.
7. Elevate injured body part.
8. Reapply ice pack in 1 to 1½ hours and, depending on degree of injury, continue this rotation until injury resolution has taken place and healing has begun.
9. If possible, leave compression wrap in place overnight.
10. Elevate injured part above the heart.
11. When rising the next day, RICE is begun again and carried on throughout the day.
12. With second- or third-degree injury, continue this same process for 2 or 3 days.

Emergency Splinting

A suspected fracture must be splinted before the athlete is moved.

Any suspected fracture should always be splinted before the athlete is moved. Transporting a person with a fracture without proper immobilization can result in increased tissue damage, hemorrhage, and shock. Conceivably a mishandled fracture could cause death. Therefore, a thorough knowledge of splinting techniques is important (Figure 7-15).

The application of splints should be a simple process through the use of emergency splints. In most instances the coach or athletic trainer does not have to improvise a splint, because such devices are readily available in most sports settings. The use of padded boards is recommended. They are easily available, can be considered disposable, and are easy to apply.

Figure 7-15 cont'd.

Knee, thigh, or hip splint

Ankle and leg splint

Forearm splint

Hand and finger splint

Gauze roll splint

Upper arm and elbow splint

Commercial basswood splints are excellent, as are disposable cardboard and clear plastic commercial splints.

Air splints   An air splint is a clear plastic splint that is inflated with air around the affected part and can be used for extremity splinting, but its use requires some special training (Figure 7-16). This splint provides support and moderate pressure to the body part and affords a clear view of the site for x-ray examination. The inflatable splint should **not** be used if it will alter a fracture deformity.

Rapid form immobilizers   The rapid form immobilizer is a relatively new type of splint. It consists of styrofoam chips contained inside an air-tight cloth sleeve that is pliable. It can be molded to the shape of any joint or angulated fracture using velcro straps. A hand-held pump sucks the air out of the sleeve, giving it a cardboardlike rigidity. This splint is most useful for injuries that must be splinted in the position in which they are found (Figure 7-17).

Half-ring splint   For fractures of the femur the half-ring type of traction splint offers the best support and immobilization but takes considerable practice to master. An open fracture must be carefully dressed to avoid additional contamination.

Whatever the material used, the principles of good splinting remain the same. Two major concepts of splinting are (1) to splint from one joint above the fracture to one joint below the fracture and (2) to splint where

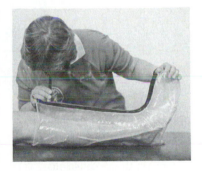

Figure 7-16

The air splint provides excellent support, as well as a clear site for x-ray examination.

Figure 7-17

Rapid form immobilizers
allow angulated fractures to
be splinted.

the athlete lies. If at all possible, do not move the athlete until he or she
has been splinted.

Splinting of lower-limb fractures Fractures of the ankle or leg require immobilization of the foot and knee. Any fracture involving the
knee, thigh, or hip needs splinting of all the lower-limb joints and one
side of the trunk.

Splinting of upper-limb fractures Fractures around the shoulder
complex are immobilized by a sling and swathe bandage, with the upper

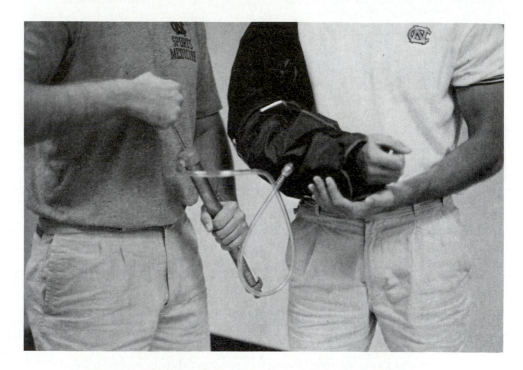

Figure 7-18

The spine board. **A,** When
moving the unconscious
athlete, first establish
whether the athlete is
breathing and has a pulse.
NOTE: *The unconscious athlete
must always be treated as having
a serious neck injury.* **A**

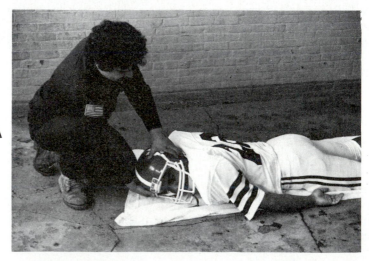

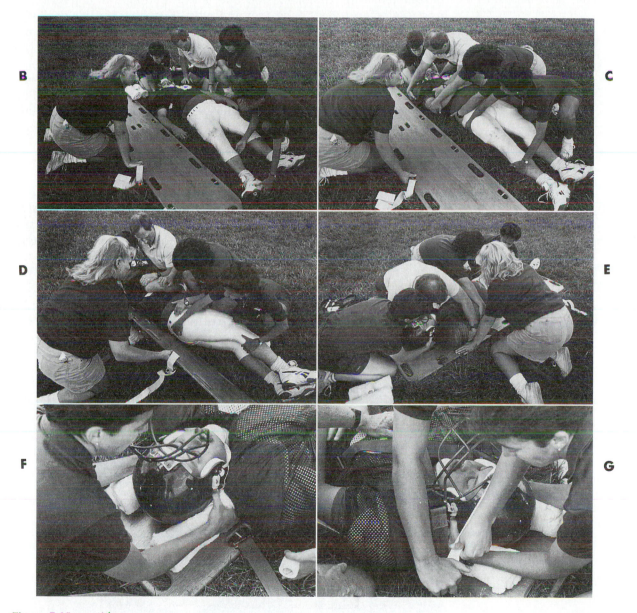

Figure 7-18, cont'd

B, Spine board is placed as close to the athlete as possible. **C,** Each assistant is responsible for one of the athlete's segments. **D,** When the command "roll" is given, the board is carefully slid under the athlete. **E,** Great care is given to move the athlete as a unit, always keeping the head and neck stabilized. **F,** The head is stabilized by sandbags. **G,** The athlete is secured to the spine board through the use of straps.

limb bound to the body securely. Upper-arm and elbow fractures must be splinted, with immobilization effected in a straight-arm position to lessen bone override. Lower-arm and wrist fractures should be splinted in a position of forearm flexion and should be supported by a sling. Hand and finger dislocations and fractures should be splinted with tongue depressors, gauze rolls, or aluminum splints.

Splinting of the spine and pelvis Injuries involving a possible spine or pelvic fracture are best splinted and moved using a spine board (Figures 7-18 and 7-19). When such injuries are suspected, *the coach or athletic trainer should not, under any circumstances, move the injured athlete except under the express direction of a physician.*

HANDLING THE INJURED ATHLETE

Moving, lifting, and transporting the injured athlete must be executed so as to prevent further injury. Emergency aid authorities have suggested that improper handling causes more additional insult to injuries than any other emergency procedure.[4,7] There is no excuse for poor handling of the injured athlete.

Moving the Injured Athlete

It is very important that an athlete believed to have a spinal fracture be moved like a "log." The athlete who is unconscious and unable to describe the injury in terms of sensation and site *must be treated as having a severe cervical injury.*

Suspected Spinal Injury

A suspected spinal injury requires extremely careful handling and is best left to properly trained ambulance attendants or certified paramedics who

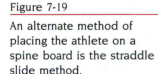

Figure 7-19

An alternate method of placing the athlete on a spine board is the straddle slide method.

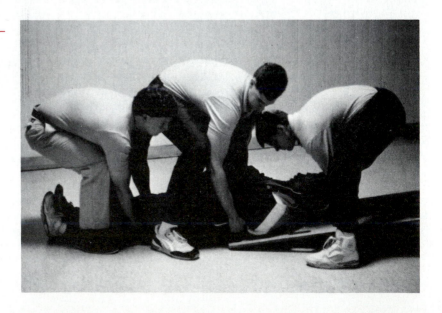

are more skilled and have the proper equipment for such transport. If such personnel are not available, moving should be done under the express direction of a physician or athletic trainer, and a spine board should be used (see Figure 7-18, *A-G*). One danger inherent in moving an athlete with a suspected spinal injury, in particular a cervical injury, is the tendency of the neck and head to turn because of the victim's inability to control his or her movements. Torque so induced creates considerable possibility of spinal cord or root damage when small fractures are present. The most important principle in transporting an individual on a spine board is *to keep the head and neck in alignment with the long axis of the body.* In such cases it should be best to have one individual whose sole responsibility is to ensure and maintain proper positioning of the head and neck until the head is secured to a backboard.

> The head and neck of an unconscious athlete are prone to movement that can cause spinal damage.

Placing the Athlete on a Spine Board

Once an injury to the neck has been recognized as severe, a physician and an ambulance should be summoned immediately. Primary emergency care involves maintaining normal breathing, treating for shock, and keeping the athlete quiet and in the position found until medical assistance arrives. Ideally, transportation should not be attempted until the physician has examined the athlete and has given permission to move him or her. The athlete should be transported while lying on the back, with the curve of the neck supported by a rolled-up towel or pad or encased in a stabilization collar. Neck stabilization must be maintained throughout transportation—first to the ambulance, then to the hospital, and throughout the hospital procedure. If stabilization is not continued, additional cord damage and paralysis may ensue.

These steps should be followed when moving an athlete with suspected neck injury:

1. Establish whether the athlete is breathing and has a pulse (Figure 7-18, *A*).
2. Plan to move the athlete on a spine board.
3. If the athlete is lying prone, he or she must be turned over for CPR or to be secured to the spine board. *An athlete with a possible cervical fracture is transported face up. An athlete with a spinal fracture in the lower trunk area is transported face down.*[2]
   a. Place all extremities in an axial alignment (see Figure 7-18, *A*).
   b. To roll the athlete over requires four or five persons, with the "captain" of the team protecting the athlete's head and neck. The neck must be stabilized and must not be moved from its original position, no matter how distorted it may appear.
   c. The spine board is placed close to the side of the athlete (see Figure 7-18, *B*).
   d. Each assistant is responsible for one of the athlete's body segments. One assistant is responsible for turning the trunk, another the hips, another the thighs, and the last the lower legs (Figure 7-18, *C*).
4. With the spine board close to the athlete's side, the captain gives

the command to roll him or her onto the board as one unit (see Figure 7-18, *D*).

5. On the board, the athlete's head and neck continue to be stabilized by the captain (see Figure 7-18, *E*).

6. If the athlete is a football player, the helmet is *not* removed; however, the face guard is removed or lifted away from the face for possible CPR. NOTE: To remove the face guard, the plastic fasteners holding it to the helmet are cut.

7. The head and neck are next stabilized on the spine board by a chin strap secured to metal loops. Finally, the trunk and lower limbs are secured to the spine board by straps (see Figure 7-18, *F* and *G*).

An alternate method of moving the athlete onto a spine board, if he or she is face up, is the *straddle slide method*. Five persons are used—a captain stationed at the athlete's head and three or four assistants. One assistant is in charge of lifting the athlete's trunk, one the hips, and one the legs. On the command "lift" by the captain, the athlete is lifted while the fourth assistant slides a spine board under the athlete between the feet of the captain and assistants (Figure 7-19).

Transporting the Injured Athlete

Great caution must be taken when transporting the injured athlete.

As with moving, transporting the injured athlete must be executed so as to prevent further injury. There is no excuse for the use of poor transportation techniques in sports. Planning should take into consideration all the possible transportation methods and the necessary equipment to execute them. Capable persons, stretchers, and even an ambulance may

Figure 7-20

The ambulatory aid method of transporting a mildly injured athlete.

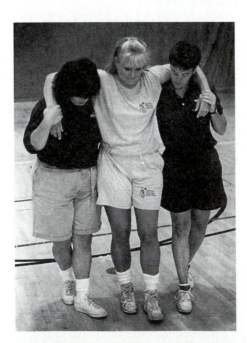

be needed to transport the injured athlete. Four modes of assisting in travel are used: ambulatory aid, manual conveyance, stretcher carrying, and vehicular transfer.

Ambulatory Aid

Ambulatory aid (Figure 7-20) is that support or assistance given to an injured athlete who is able to walk. Before the athlete is allowed to walk, he or she should be carefully scrutinized to make sure that the injuries are minor. Whenever serious injuries are suspected, walking should be prohibited. Complete support should be given on both sides of the athlete. The athlete's arms are draped over the assistants' shoulders, and their arms encircle his or her back.

Manual Conveyance

Manual conveyance (Figure 7-21) may be used to move a mildly injured individual a greater distance than could be walked with ease. As with the use of ambulatory aid, any decision to carry the athlete must be made only after a complete examination to determine the existence of potentially serious conditions. The most convenient carry is performed by two assistants.

Stretcher Carrying

Whenever a serious injury is suspected, the best and safest mode of transportation for a short distance is by stretcher. With each segment of the body supported, the athlete is gently lifted and placed on the stretcher, which is carried adequately by four assistants, two supporting the ends

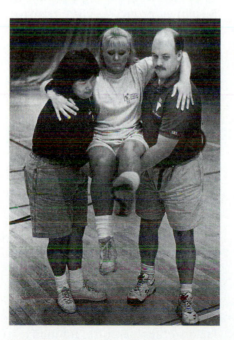

Figure 7-21
Manual conveyance method for transporting a mildly injured athlete.

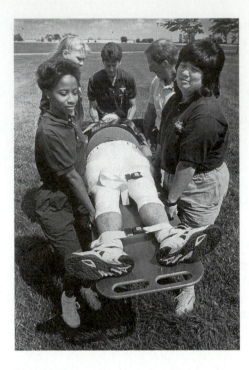

Figure 7-22

Whenever a serious injury is suspected, a stretcher is the safest method of transporting the athlete.

of the stretcher and two supporting either end (Figure 7-22). Any person with an injury serious enough to require the use of a stretcher must be carefully examined before being moved.

When transporting a person with a limb injury, be certain the injury is splinted properly before transport. Athletes with shoulder injuries are more comfortably moved in a semi-sitting position, unless other injuries preclude such positioning. If injury to the upper extremity is such that flexion of the elbow is not possible, the individual should be transported on a stretcher with the limb properly splinted and carried at the side, with adequate padding placed between the arm and the body.

OSHA

Occupational Safety and Health Administration (OSHA) Blood-borne Pathogen Standard

Blood-borne pathogens Coaches and other personnel working directly with the athlete must be concerned with blood-borne pathogens. Two blood-borne infections that have an increased incidence are hepatitis B virus (HBV) and the human immunodeficiency virus (HIV). Both of these diseases are discussed in more detail in the box on p. 202 and in chapter 20.

ENVIRONMENTAL STRESS

People concerned with sports are increasingly aware of the impact of environmental stress on the performer. One not only must be aware of the factors of temperature, humidity, and wind but must also be prepared to make appropriate changes in the types of uniforms and equipment to be worn, the length and number of practice sessions, and the weight loss of each athlete.

Heat Illness

Concern is rising at the increase in causes of heat exhaustion and heatstroke in sports. Among football players and distance runners there have been a number of deaths in high school and college, all of which were directly attributable to heatstroke. Uniforms and helmets have been found to be major causative factors in the deaths of players.

In the United States, heat illness is the second most frequent cause of sports death.

It is vitally important to have knowledge of temperature and humidity in planning practice and game uniforming and procedures. The coach should become familiar with the use of the sling psychrometer or the instrument used in establishing the WBGT Index (wet-bulb, globe temperature index). The coach should be able to determine not only relative humidity but also the danger zones; then he or she can advise the athletes with authority. In addition, the coach should become familiar with the clinical signs and treatment of heat stress.

Body temperature regulation results almost entirely from cutaneous cooling, or the evaporation of sweat. During exercise there is some respiratory heat loss, but the amount is relatively small. The effectiveness of sweat evaporation is strongly influenced by relative humidity and wind velocity and under the most ideal conditions does not exceed 70% to 80%. When temperature exceeds 80° F (26.6° C), sweating is the body's only effective means of heat dissipation. However, when a high temperature is accompanied by high humidity, a condition with serious implication exists, since high humidity reduces the rate of evaporation *without*

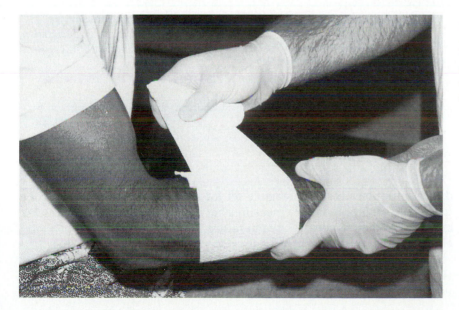

Figure 7-23

Any bleeding athlete must have the bleeding stopped and the wounds covered with a dressing that blocks fluid seepage.

ATHLETIC-CARE RESPONSIBILITIES

The following list of athletic-care responsibilities are adapted from the 1993-94 NEAA guidelines in Sports Medicine and the Occupational Safety and Health Administation (OSHA).[3]

1. Before athletic participation any of the athlete's existing wounds must be covered with a dressing that blocks incoming or outgoing contamination.
2. Sterile latex gloves, disinfectant bleach, antiseptics, a special separate receptacle is available for any sorted equipment, uniforms, bandages and/or dressings, and a separate container for used needles, syringes and scalpels.[3]
3. Any athlete bleeding must have that bleeding stopped and the wounds covered with a dressing that blocks fluid seepage (Figure 7-23). The wound dressing must be held securely in place. Any athlete who is bleeding must be removed from play as soon as possible. Clothing or other pieces of equipment saturated with blood must be evaluated for potential infectivity (NCAA). If deemed dangerous, clothing and/or other equipment must be changed before returning to participation.[3]
4. It is the responsibilities of officials, athletes, coaches, and medical personnel to recognize and report as early as possible a bleeding situation.[3]
5. Coaches or other personnel caring for a bleeding situation must wear sterile latex gloves when contacting bodily fluids containing blood (Figure 7-24). Following care, gloves are disposed of and hands thoroughly washed.[3]
6. Athletic personnel must be sure that blood or other bodily fluids containing blood are removed and cleaned. It should be removed while wearing gloves. Following removal the area is cleaned with a proper decontaminant such as a disinfectant bleach.[3]
7. Sharp devices used in caring for wounds such as needles or scalpels must be disposed of in such a way as to avoid any danger of injuring someone else.[3]
8. Following a practice or game all blood-soiled uniforms and equipment should be handled and laundered with extreme care. There must be avoidance of any possible contamination of individuals, clothing, and/or equipment.[3]
9. All sports personnel should be educated in basic first aid and infection prevention and control.[3]
10. A visiting athlete may require care of an injury having exposed blood by the host institution. Therefore all host school teams should agree on standards to be carried out in the area of care and prevention of blood-borne pathogens.[3]

diminishing sweating. The stage is set for heat exhaustion or heatstroke unless certain precautionary measures have been observed (see Tables 7-2 and 7-3). When a person's temperature reaches 106° F (41.1° C), the chances of survival are exceedingly slim.

An average runner may lose 1.5 to 2.5 liters of water per hour through active sweating; much greater amounts can be lost by football players in warm weather activity. Seldom is more than 50% of this fluid

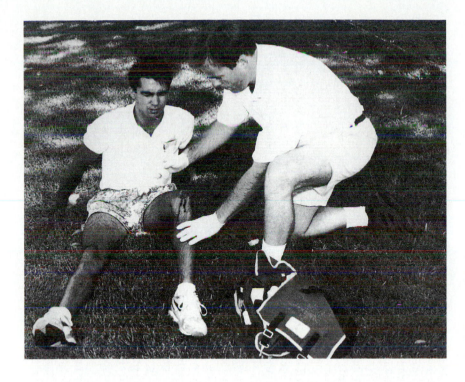

Figure 7-24

Coaches or other personnel caring for a bleeding athlete must wear sterile latex gloves when contacting bodily fluids containing blood.

TABLE 7-2 Contrasting heatstroke and heat exhaustion

	Heatstroke	**Heat Exhaustion**
Cause	Inadequacy or failure of heat loss	Excessive fluid loss
Symptoms	Headache, weakness, sudden loss of consciousness	Gradual weakness, nausea, anxiety, excess sweating, light-headedness
Signs	Hot, red, dry skin, little sweating, strong pulse; very high temperature	Pale, grayish, clammy skin; weak, rapid pulse; low blood pressure; faintness; fast, shallow respiration
Management	Rapid cooling by full body immersion in cold water, ice packs, fanning; immediate hospitalization	For syncope, head down, replace lost water and salt

loss replaced, even though replacement fluids are taken **ad libitum** since athletes usually find it uncomfortable to exercise vigorously with a full stomach, which can interfere with the respiratory muscles. The problem in fluid replacement is how rapidly the fluid can be eliminated from the stomach into the intestine, from which it can enter the bloodstream. Cold drinks (45° to 55° F [7.2° to 12.8° C]) tend to empty more rapidly from the stomach than do warmer drinks and offer no particular threat to a normal heart nor induce cramps.

water ad libitum
Unlimited access to water

TABLE 7-3 Heat disorders: treatment and prevention

Disorders	Cause	Clinical Features and Diagnosis	Treatment	Prevention
Heat cramps	Hard work in heat; sweating heavily; salt intake inadequate	Muscle twitching and cramps, usually after midday; spasms in arms, legs, abdomen; low serum sodium chloride (salt)	Ingesting fluids and foods containing sodium chloride (salt)	Proper acclimatization, eating foods containing sodium chloride (salt)
Heat exhaustion	Prolonged sweating; inadequate replacement of body fluid losses; diarrhea; intestinal infection; predisposes to heatstroke	Excessive thirst; dry tongue and mouth; weight loss; fatigue; weakness; incoordination; mental dullness; small urine volume; elevated body temperature; high serum protein and sodium; reduced swelling	Bed rest in cool room, IV fluids if drinking is impaired; increase fluid intake to 6 to 8 L/day; sponge with cool water; keep record of body weight; keep fluid balance record; provide semiliquid food until salivation is normal	Supply adequate water and other liquids Provide adequate rest and opportunity for cooling
Heatstroke	Thermoregulatory failure of sudden onset	Abrupt onset, preceded by headache, vertigo, and fatigue, absence of sweating; hot, flushed dry skin; pulse rate increases rapidly and may reach 160 to 180; respiration increases; blood pressure seldom rises; temperature rises rapidly to 105° or 106° F (40° to 41° C), athlete feels as if he or she is burning up; diarrhea, vomiting, circulatory collapse may produce death; may lead to permanent brain damage	Heroic measures to reduce temperature must be taken immediately (e.g., full body immersion in cold water, air fan over body, massage limbs, etc.); temperature must be taken every 10 minutes and not allowed to fall below 101° F (38.5° C) to avoid converting hyperpyrexia to hypotherapy; remove to hospital as soon as possible	Ensure proper acclimatization, proper hydration Educate those who supervise activities conducted in the heat Adapt activities to environment Screen participants with history of heat illness

Sweating occurs whether or not the athlete drinks water, and if the sweat losses are not replaced by fluid intake over a period of several hours, dehydration results.[2] Therefore, athletes must have unlimited access to water. Failure to permit *ad libitum* access will not only undermine their playing but also may permit a dangerous situation to develop that could conceivably have fatal consequences.

Women are apparently more physiologically efficient in body temperature regulation than men. Although they possess as many heat-activated sweat glands as men, they sweat less and manifest a higher heart rate when working in heat.[10] Although slight differences exist, the same precautionary measures apply to both genders.

Body build must be considered when determining individual susceptibility to heat stress. Overweight individuals may have as much as 18% greater heat production than an underweight individual, since metabolic heat is produced proportionately to surface area. It has been found that heat victims tend to be overweight.

Prevention and Management

The following should be considered when planning a training-competitive program that is likely to take place during hot weather:

1. *Gradual acclimatization.* This is probably the single most effective method of avoiding heat stress. Acclimatization should involve not only becoming accustomed to heat but also becoming acclimatized to exercise in hot temperatures. A good preseason conditioning program, started well before the advent of the competitive season and carefully graded as to intensity, is recommended.[3]
2. *Uniforms.* Select uniforms on the basis of temperature and humidity. Initial practices should be conducted in short-sleeved T-shirts, shorts, and socks, moving gradually into short-sleeved net jerseys, lightweight pants, and socks as acclimatization proceeds.
3. *Weight records.* Keep careful weight records of all players. Weights should be taken both before and after practice. A loss of 3% to 5% of body weight will reduce blood volume and could be a serious health threat.
4. *Prevent hydration.* Drinking 8 to 12 ounces of water before competition may help to prevent heat illness.
5. *Fluid replacement.* Intake of water should be carefully observed. Athletes should have unlimited access to cold water at all times. This means before, during, and after activity.
6. *Salt intake and electrolyte beverages.* In maintaining an adequate salt content, 1 tablespoon per day will satisfy most sports needs. It should be noted that excessive salt intake along with limited water intake causes cellular dehydration. Many commercial electrolyte drinks have high concentrations of salt that cause a fluid retention within the stomach and small intestines, producing upper abdominal distress.
7. *Diet.* A well-balanced diet is essential. Fat intake should be minimized.

The prevention of heat illness involves the following:
Gradual acclimatization
Lightweight uniforms
Routine weight record keeping
Unrestricted fluid replacement
Well-balanced diet
Routine temperature and humidity readings

8. *Temperature and humidity readings.* Dry-bulb and wet-bulb readings should be taken on the field before practice. The purchase of a sling psychrometer for this purpose is recommended. It is relatively inexpensive and uncomplicated to use. The relative humidity should be calculated. The suggestions in the following box regarding temperature and humidity will serve as a guide.

Temp (°)	Humidity	Procedure
80°-90° F (26.7°-32.2° C)	Under 70%	Watch athletes who tend toward obesity.
80°-90° F (26.7°-32.2° C)	Over 70%	Athletes should take a 10-minute rest every hour, and T-shirts should be changed when wet. All athletes should be under constant and careful supervision.
90°-100° F (32.2°-37.8° C)	Under 70%	
Over 100° F (37.8° C)	Over 70%	Under these conditions it would be well to suspend practice. A shortened program conducted in shorts and T-shirts could be established.

Cold Stress

Many sports played in cold weather do not require heavy protective clothing; thus weather becomes a factor in injury susceptibility.

Cold weather is a frequent adjunct to many outdoor sports in which the sport itself does not require heavy protective clothing; consequently, the weather becomes a pertinent factor in injury susceptibility. In most instances the activity itself enables the athlete to increase the metabolic rate sufficiently to function physically in a normal manner and dissipate the resulting heat and perspiration through the usual physiological mechanisms. An athlete may fail to warm up sufficiently or may become chilled because of relative inactivity for varying periods demanded by the particular sport during competition or training; consequently, the athlete is exceedingly prone to injury. Low temperatures alone can pose some problems, but when such temperatures are further accentuated by wind, the chill factor becomes critical. For example, a runner proceeding at 10 mph directly into a wind of 5 mph creates a chill factor equivalent to that of a 15-mph headwind.

Low temperatures accentuated by wind can pose major problems for athletes.

During strenuous physical activity in cold weather, as muscular fatigue builds up, the rate of exercise begins to drop and may reach a level wherein the body heat loss to the environment exceeds the metabolic heat protection, resulting in definite impairment of neuromuscular responses and exhaustion. A relatively small drop of body core temperature can induce shivering sufficient to affect one's neuromuscular coordination materially. Shivering ceases below a body temperature of 85° to 90° F (29.4° to 32.2° C). Death is imminent if the core temperature rises to 107° F (41.6° C) or drops to between 77° and 85° F (25° and 29° C).

Apparel for competitors must be geared to the weather. The function of such apparel is to provide a semitropical microclimate for the body and to prevent chilling. Such clothing should not restrict movement,

ENVIRONMENTAL CONDUCT OF SPORTS, PARTICULARLY FOOTBALL

I. General warning
   A. Most adverse reactions to environmental heat and humidity occur during the first few days of training.
   B. It is necessary to become thoroughly acclimatized to successfully compete in a hot or humid environment.
   C. Occurrence of a heat injury indicates poor supervision of the sports program.
II. Athletes who are most susceptible to heat injury:
   A. Individuals unaccustomed to working in the heat.
   B. Overweight individuals, particularly large linemen.
   C. Eager athletes who constantly compete at capacity.
   D. Athletes having an infection, fever, or gastrointestinal disturbance.
   E. Athletes who receive immunization injections and subsequently develop temperature elevations.
III. Prevention of heat injury
   A. Take complete medical history and provide physical examination:
      1. History of previous heat illnesses or fainting in the heat.
      2. Inquiry about sweating and peripheral vascular defects.
   B. Evaluate general physical condition.
      1. Type and duration of training activities for previous month.
         a. Extent of work in the heat.
         b. General training activities.
   C. Measure temperature and humidity on the practice or playing fields.
      1. Make measurements before and during training or competitive sessions.
      2. Adjust activity level to environmental conditions.
         a. Decrease activity if hot or humid.
         b. Eliminate unnecessary clothing worn when hot or humid.
   D. Acclimatize athletes to heat gradually
      1. Acclimatization to heat requires work in the heat
         a. Recommend type and variety of warm-weather workouts for preseason training.
         b. Provide graduated training program for first 7 to 10 days—and other abnormally hot or humid days.
      2. Train in early morning or evening.
      3. Provide adequate rest intervals and water replacement during the acclimatization period.
   E. Watch body weight loss during activity in the heat.
      1. Body water should be replaced as it is lost.
         a. Allow additional water as desired by player.
         b. Provide salt on training tables (no salt tablets should be taken).
         c. Weigh each day before and after training or competition.
            (1) Treat athlete who loses excessive weight each day.
            (2) Treat well-conditioned athlete who continues to lose weight for several days.

Continued.

ENVIRONMENTAL CONDUCT OF SPORTS, PARTICULARLY FOOTBALL—cont'd

 F. Clothing and uniforms
  1. Provide lightweight clothing that is loose-fitting at the neck, waist, and sleeve. Use shorts and T-shirt at beginning of training.
  2. Avoid excessive padding and taping.
  3. Avoid use of long stockings, long sleeves, double jerseys, and other excessive clothing.
  4. Avoid use of rubberized clothing and sweatsuits.
  5. Provide clean clothing daily—all items.
 G. Provide rest periods to dissipate accumulated body heat.
  1. Rest in cool, shaded area with some air movement.
  2. Avoid hot brick walls and hot benches.
  3. Loosen or remove jerseys and other garments.
  4. Take water during the rest period.
IV. Trouble signs: stop activity!

Headache	Collapse	Pallor
Nausea	Unconsciousness	Flush
Mental slowness	Vomiting	Faintness
Incoherence	Diarrhea	Chill
Visual disturbance	Cramps	Cyanotic appearance
Fatigue	Seizures	
Weakness	Rigidity	
Unsteadiness	Weak, rapid pulse	

should be as lightweight as possible, and should consist of material that will permit the free passage of sweat and body heat that would otherwise accumulate on the skin or the clothing and provide a chilling factor when activity ceases. Clothing should be layered, and outwear should have zippers for ease of removal. Before exercise, during activity breaks and rest periods, and at the termination of exercise, a warm-up suit should be worn to prevent chilling. Because a major heat loss can occur from the head and hands, wearing a warm cap and mittens is important. Activity in cold, wet, and windy weather poses a problem, since such weather reduces the insulative values of clothing and, consequently, the individual may be unable to achieve an energy level equal to the body heat loss. Runners who wish to continue outdoor work in cold weather should use lightweight insulative clothing and, if breathing cold air seems distressful, should use ski goggles and a ski face mask or should cover the mouth and nose with a free-hanging cloth. Contrary to common belief, the breathing of cold air is not harmful to pulmonary tissues.

Overexposure to Cold

Severe overexposure to cold is less common than heat illness; however, it is still a major risk of winter sports, long-distance running in cold weather, and swimming in cold water.[9]

General body cooling   A core temperature below 80° F (26.7° C) leads to unconsciousness. With a rectal temperature of 86.4° F (30.2° C), the athlete displays slurring of speech, clumsy movement, pupils that respond sluggishly, shallow respiration, and a heartbeat that may be irregular and slow.[1] The skin appears pale; the tissue of the lips, around the nose, and underneath the fingernails is a bluish hue (cyanosis).[2] Muscle tonus increases, causing the neck and limbs to become stiff and rigid. Metabolic pH changes also occur and lead to acidosis, liver necrosis, uremia, renal failure, and seizures.

Severe exposure to cold is a major medical emergency. The first concern is the maintenance of an airway. If the heart has stopped and the athlete's temperature is approximately 84° F (29° C) or less, it may be difficult to reestablish a heart rhythm. External rewarming should take place if the condition ranges from mild to moderate. Emergency rewarming at the site includes immersing the athlete's hands and forearms in water that is between 113° and 118° F (45° and 48° C). If the athlete is conscious, a hot drink may help in rewarming. Alcohol of any kind must be avoided because it vasodilates peripheral capillaries. In cases of severe cold exposure, rewarming too rapidly can cause the peripheral capillaries to become dilated, pulling blood and warmth from the core of the body. In a hospital setting, the athlete may be given warm enemas and warm intravenous solutions.

> Alcohol may make you feel warm, but it actually makes you more susceptible to cold.

Local body cooling   Local cooling of the body can result in tissue damage ranging from superficial to deep. Exposure to a damp, freezing cold causes mild or superficial frostbite (frostnip). In contrast, exposure to dry temperature well below freezing will more commonly produce a deep freezing type of frostbite.

Prevention   The primary preventive measures for local cold injuries are obvious but often disregarded. The athlete should wear nonconstricting, multilayered clothing, including warm gloves and socks. Because so much heat is lost via an unprotected head, warm headgear is essential in cold weather. Local cold injuries that may be seen in athletes are frostnip, superficial frostbite, deep freezing frostbite, and chilblains.

Frostnip affects ears, nose, cheeks, fingers, and toes. It is commonly seen when there is a high wind, severe cold, or both. The skin initially appears very firm, with cold, painless areas that may peel or blister in 24 to 72 hours. Affected areas can be treated early by firm, sustained pressure of the hand (without rubbing), by blowing hot breath on the spot, or if the injury is to the fingertips, by placing them in the armpits.

> Cold injuries in sports include:
>   Frostnip
>   Superficial frostbite
>   Deep frostbite
>   Chilblains

Superficial frostbite affects only the skin and subcutaneous tissue. It appears pale, hard, cold, and waxy. Touching the injured area will reveal a sense of hardness but with yielding of the underlying deeper tissue structures. When rewarming, the superficial frostbite will at first feel numb, then will sting and burn. Later the area may produce blisters and be painful for a number of weeks.

Deep frostbite is a serious injury indicating that tissues are frozen. This is a medical emergency requiring immediate hospitalization. As with

REWARMING METHODS FOR COLD STRESS

Rewarming methods are usually listed under the headings of passive rewarming and active external rewarming.
1. Passive rewarming
   a. Remove from environmental exposure (e.g., wind and cold).
   b. Replace wet clothing with dry.
   c. Cover body with insulating material (e.g., blanket).
2. Active external rewarming
   a. Gradually rewarm body part by immersion in heated water not to exceed 110° F (43° C).
   b. Do not rub affected area.

frostnip and superficial frostbite, the tissue is initially cold, hard, pale or white, and numb. Rapid rewarming is required and should include hot drinks and heating pads or hot water bottles that are 100° to 110° F (38° to 43° C). On rewarming, the tissue will become blotchy red, swollen, and extremely painful. Later the injury may become gangrenous, causing a loss of tissue.

Chilblains result from prolonged and constant exposure to cold for many hours. In time there is skin redness, swelling, tingling, and pain in the toes and fingers. This adverse response is caused by problems of peripheral circulation and can be avoided by preventing further cold exposure.

SUMMARY

An emergency is defined as ". . . an unforeseen combination of circumstances and the resulting state that calls for immediate action."[9] The prime concern of emergency aid is to maintain cardiovascular function and, indirectly, central nervous system function. All sports programs should have an emergency system that is activated anytime an athlete is seriously injured.

Primary assessment may include determining if the ABCs of life support procedures are required and thoroughly understanding an athlete's vital signs. Other situations in which primary assessment procedures are performed are in cases of musculoskeletal injury and when an athlete is unconscious.

The mnemonic for cardiopulmonary resuscitation is ABC: *A*—airway opened; *B*—breathing restored; *C*—circulation restored. When using one rescuer, the ratio of compression to breaths is 15:2, with 80 to 100 compressions per minute. To relieve an obstructed airway the manual thrust maneuver and/or the finger sweep of the throat should be performed.

Rest, ice, compression, and elevation (RICE) should be used for the immediate care of a musculoskeletal injury. Ice should be applied for 10 to 20 minutes every 1 to 1½ hours throughout the waking day. A severe injury may require this procedure for 3 days.

Hemorrhage can occur externally and internally. External bleeding can be controlled either by direct pressure, or by elevation. Internal hemorrhage can occur subcutaneously, intramuscularly, or within a body cavity.

Shock can arise from a variety of situations. Shock can be hypovolemic, respiratory, neurogenic, psychogenic, cardiogenic, septic, anaphylactic, and metabolic. Symptoms may include skin paleness, dilated eyes, weak and rapid pulse, and rapid, shallow breathing. Management might include keeping the body warm and level but elevating the feet.

Any suspected fracture should be splinted before the athlete is moved. The clear plastic air splint provides support, pressure, and a clear view for x-ray examination. Two major concepts of splinting are to splint from one joint above to one joint below the fracture. Do not move the athlete until the fracture has been splinted.

Great care must be taken in moving the seriously injured athlete. The unconscious athlete must be handled as though he or she has a cervical fracture. Moving an athlete with a suspected serious neck injury must be performed only by persons specifically trained to do so. A spine board should be used, avoiding any movement of the cervical region. Environmental stress can adversely affect an athlete's performance and pose a serious health problem. Hyperthermia is one of sport's major concerns. In times of high temperatures and humidity, the wet-bulb, globe temperature index should be routinely determined using the sling psychrometer. Losing 3% of more of body weight because of fluid loss may pose a health problem.

Cold weather requires athletes to wear the correct apparel and to warm up properly before engaging in sports activities. The wind chill factor must always be considered when performing. As is true in a hot environment, the athlete must ingest adequate fluids when in cold conditions. Alcohol must be avoided at all times. Extreme cold exposure can cause conditions such as frostnip, chilblains, and frostbite.

REVIEW QUESTIONS AND CLASS ACTIVITIES

1. What items and procedures should be included in an emergency care plan at a high school?
2. What are the vital signs to watch for and what is normal for each? What does each variance indicate?
3. Demonstrate an evaluation of an unconscious athlete. How can you determine if the athlete has a spinal injury with nerve damage? Have the class pair up and practice this evaluation.
4. Demonstrate the proper procedures for adult CPR. If you do not have adequate manikins for the class to practice on, have the students use a folded towel to mimic the athlete's thorax so they can practice the procedure.
5. Demonstrate the proper procedures to remove an airway obstruction from a conscious athlete and from an unconscious athlete. Have the class practice these procedures, but do not have them actually do the manual thrusts. How does care for a partial airway obstruction differ from care for a total obstruction?

6. What are the major steps in a primary musculoskeletal assessment?
7. Explain the principles of rest, ice, compression, and elevation.
8. Demonstrate how to care for external hemorrhaging.
9. What are the signs and symptoms of shock? How can shock be prevented? How is it managed?
10. How should you care for an athlete with a suspected spinal injury? Have the class practice how to roll an injured athlete onto his or her back and how to immobilize the athlete on a long spine board.
11. How does the body handle external and internal temperature changes?
12. How can hyperthermia and hypothermia be prevented?
13. What immediate treatment is necessary if you suspect a problem involving heat or cold?
14. Demonstrate the use of a sling psychrometer and discuss how it can be used to determine when to practice and how to dress for practice so that heat illnesses can be avoided.

REFERENCES

1. American Red Cross CPR: *Basic life support for the professional rescuer,* Washington, 1989, American Red Cross.
2. American Red Cross: *First aid: responding to emergencies,* St Louis, 1991, Mosby-Year Book.
3. Arnheim DD, Prentice WE: *Modern principles of athletic training,* ed 8, St Louis, 1992, Times Mirror/Mosby College Publishing.
4. *Basic guidelines for heating the heart, The first order,* Gardner, Kan, 1985, Cramer Products.
5. Drowatzky JM: Legal duties and liability in athletic training, *Ath Train* 20:11, 1985.
6. Hafen BQ: *First aid for health emergencies,* ed 4, St Paul, Minn, 1988, West Publishing.
7. Hafen BQ, Karren KJ: *Prehospital emergency care,* ed 3, Englewood, Colo, 1989, Morton Publishing.
8. National Collegiate Athletic Association: *Sports medicine handbook, 1993-94,* ed 6, Overland Park, Kan.
9. National Safety Council: *Bloodborne pathogens,* Boston, 1993, Jones & Bartlett Publishers.
10. Parcel GS, Rinear CE: *Basic emergency care of the sick and injured,* ed 4, St Louis, 1990, Times Mirror/Mosby College Publishing.

ANNOTATED BIBLIOGRAPHY

Flegel M: *Sport first aid leisure press,* Champaign, Ill., 1992, A basic on-the-field first aid book for coaches.

Hafen BQ: *First aid for health emergencies,* ed 5, St Paul, Minn, 1992, West Publishing. Presents in-depth coverage of emergency care.

National Safety Council: *Bloodborne pathogens,* Boston, 1993, Jones & Barlett Publishers. An in-depth guide to prevention, immunization, exposure control and transmission to blood-borne pathogens such as Hepatitis B infection and human immunodeficiency virus (HIV).

National Safety Council: *First aid and CPR,* ed 2, Boston, 1993, Jones & Bartlett Publishers. A well-illustrated guide to care of health emergencies.

The Musculoskeletal Healing Process: An Appreciation

When you finish this chapter, you will be able to:

- List the major events in healing of acute soft tissue injuries
- List the major events in healing of bone fractures
- Describe the implications of pain for sports injuries
- Identify the basic values and procedures in the use of superficial cold and heat therapy
- Explain the various factors of exercise rehabilitation, including exercise and crutch walking

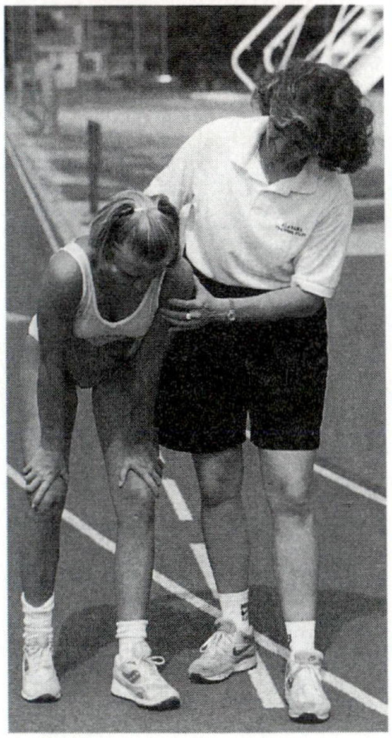

I t is very important that coaches have an appreciation of tissue damage inherent in various sports injuries. They are not to become expert in the healing response and rehabilitation but should appreciate the work of the athletic trainer and physician and understand that healing takes time and cannot be rushed. The health care personnel and the coach should work closely together to maximize the athlete's healing response (Figure 8-1).

In general the coach should have a basic knowledge of how tissue responds to trauma and the need for proper immediate and follow-up care. In order to effectively communicate with the health care personnel, the coach must understand healing and know what questions to ask.

In this chapter the focus is primarily on healing in the musculoskeletal system. Soft tissue, bony tissue, and pain perception are discussed separately.

SOFT TISSUE HEALING

Soft tissue is considered to be all bodily tissues other than bone. The healing responses of soft tissue fall into three phases: the inflammatory phase, the repair phase, and the remodeling phase.

Inflammatory Phase

Inflammation is the body's reaction to disease or injury. As the first phase of the healing response, it is present during the first 3 or 4 days after an injury takes place. The major outward signs are redness, heat, swelling,

Figure 8-1

The coach and health care professional must work together to maximize the athlete's healthy response.

pain, and, in some cases, a loss of function. In general, inflammation is designed to protect the body and localize and get rid of some injurious agent in preparation for tissue repair.

Acute Inflammation

When trauma occurs and before inflammation begins, the intact blood vessels in the region of the injury decrease in their diameter (vasoconstriction) and as a result decrease blood flow in the area. This lasts up to 10 minutes. At the moment blood vessels constrict, blood coagulation begins to seal broken blood vessels. Key chemicals that will influence the next reactions are also activated.

Vasoconstriction is replaced by an increase in the diameter of the small blood vessels **(vasodilation)** in the area of injury. Associated with dilation is an increase in blood stickiness or gumminess (viscosity), which leads to a slowing of blood flow and swelling. With dilation also comes serum seepage through the intact blood vessel lining in the injury area. This seepage lasts from a few minutes to 15 to 30 minutes, depending on the severity of the injury. In more severe trauma, seepage may be delayed.

When circulation is slowed, white cells (leukocytes) become concentrated mainly on the inner walls of the venules. The white cells then move through the walls of the venules through a process of **ameboid action.** These white cells then move to the injured body part and carry out the process of cleaning the area of debris. This process is known as **phagocytosis.**

Internal Bleeding and Swelling

The amount of swelling associated with an injury is dependent on the extent of damaged vessels and hemorrhage and the amount of **serum** seepage that occurs through intact blood vessels (Figure 8-2). As stated earlier, blood begins to coagulate almost immediately after injury. Blood coagulation occurs in three stages: first, thromboplastin is formed; second, under the influence of thromboplastin plus calcium, prothrombin is converted into thrombin; third, thrombin changes from fibrinogen into the final fibrin clot.

Repair Phase

In the beginning an injury is associated with tissue death from the initial trauma. Because circulation has been disrupted following trauma, cellular death may continue because of lack of oxygen. Tissue death also is increased by white cells spilling over their digestive enzymes to kill normal cells. The coach should be aware that properly applied immediate care of the injury, including rest, ice, compression, and elevation, serves to decrease the potential of continued cellular death.

Repair is synonymous with initial healing and **regeneration,** the restoration of lost tissue. The healing period normally ranges from the inflammatory phase to about 3 weeks following injury.

Coaches working closely with health care personnel can maximize athletes' healing.

Inflammatory phase:
   Redness
   Heat
   Swelling
   Pain
   Loss of function

vasoconstriction
Decrease in the diameter of a blood vessel

vasodilation
Increase in the diameter of a blood vessel

ameboid action
White cell moves through blood vessel wall by means of extending a protoplasmic foot, a process called *diapedisis*

phagocytosis
Process of investing microorganisms, other cells, and foreign particles, commonly by monocytes, white blood cells

serum
Watery portions after coagulation

Cellular death continues after initial injury because:
   Disruption of circulation causes lack of oxygen
   Digestive enzymes of engulfing phagocytes spill over to kill normal cells

regeneration
Regrowth of lost cells

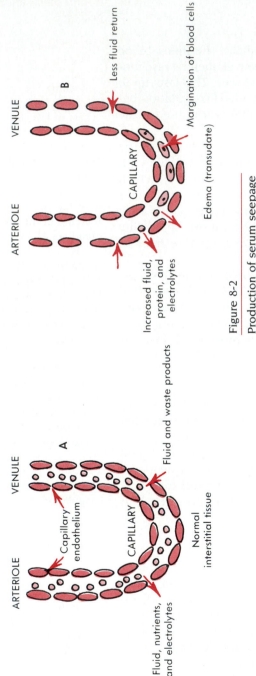

VENULE B

Less fluid return

Margination of blood cells

CAPILLARY

ARTERIOLE

Edema (transudate)

Increased fluid, protein, and electrolytes

Fluid and waste products

VENULE A

Capillary endothelium

CAPILLARY

ARTERIOLE

Normal interstitial tissue

Fluid, nutrients, and electrolytes

VENULE C

Less fluid return

CAPILLARY

ARTERIOLE

Edema (exudate)

Increased fluid, protein, and cells

Figure 8-2

Production of serum seepage and edema. **A,** Normal fluid, mineral, and electrolyte exchange. **B,** Pressure balance is disrupted due to injury and there is oozing of fluids, proteins, and electrolytes through the blood vessel walls. Blood cells are pushed against capillary walls, causing a margination. **C,** Edema and exudate—as inflammation continues, neutrophils and other blood cells migrate to the surrounding tissue to form an exudate.

During this stage two types of healing occur. *Primary healing* takes place in an injury that has even and closely opposed tissue edges, such as a cut or incision. With this type of injury, if the edges are held in very close approximation, a minimum of scar tissue is produced. *Secondary healing* results when there is a gaping lesion with large tissue loss that becomes replaced by scar tissue. External wounds such as lacerations and internal musculoskeletal injuries commonly engage in secondary healing.

It is always hoped that maximum restoration of destroyed tissue or regeneration takes place without undue scarring. This is dependent on the extent of injury, application of proper immediate care, and the type of tissue that predominates. For example, voluntary muscle tissue has limited regeneration capabilities, while bone and connective tissue readily regenerate.

Remodeling Phase

Remodeling of the traumatized area overlaps that of repair and regeneration. Normally in acute injuries the first 3 weeks are characterized by increased production of scar tissue and the strength of its fibers. Strength of scar tissue continues to increase from 3 months to 1 year following injury. Ligamentous tissue has been found, in some cases, to take as long as a year to become completely remodeled. To avoid a rigid, nonyielding scar, there must be a physiological balance between **synthesis** and **lysis.** If excessive strain is placed on the injury or if strain occurs too early, the healing process is extended. For proper healing of muscle and tendons, there must be careful consideration as to when to mobilize the site. Early mobilization can assist in producing a more viable injury site; too long a period of immobilization can delay healing. The coach should always consult the athletic trainer or physician regarding the time to begin activity.

synthesis
Buildup

lysis
Breakdown

Chronic Inflammation

The chronic muscle and joint problem is an ever-present concern in sports. It often results from repeated acute microtraumas and overuse. A prominent feature is constant low-grade inflammation, causing the development of scar tissue and tissue degeneration.

Chronic inflammation can stem from repeated acute microtraumas and overuse.

FRACTURE HEALING

Those concerned with sports must fully realize the potential seriousness of a bone fracture. Coaches often become impatient for the athlete with a fracture to return to competition before healing is complete. Time is required for proper bone union to take place. Like soft tissue healing, bone healing must go through a number of phases.

Phases of bone healing:
Inflammatory
Repair
Soft and hard callus
Remodeling

Inflammatory Phase

Acute inflammation with proper immobilization usually lasts about 4 days. When a bone fractures, there is injury to bony tissue and also to the surrounding tissue. There is hemorrhage and hematoma development. It is also accompanied by a destruction of some uninjured bone related to a disruption of the intact blood circulation.

Repair Phase

As with a soft tissue injury, the hematoma begins to organize into a highly vascular granulated mass. This will gradually form a connective tissue junction between the fractured bone ends.

Soft and Hard Callus

Gradually the connective tissue junction forms into a soft callus. The soft callus is composed mostly of connective tissue and a network of woven bone. Beginning 3 to 4 weeks after injury and lasting 3 or 4 months, a hard callus forms. The hard callus is then replaced with mature bone. If the immobilization is unsatisfactory, cartilage tissue will be formed instead of mature bone.

Remodeling

When the hard callus has been resorbed and replaced with mature bone, the remodeling process begins. It should be noted that remodeling may take years. Remodeling is considered finished when a fractured bone has been restored to its former shape or has developed a shape that can withstand major stresses.

Proper Fracture Care

Conditions that interfere
with fracture healing:
  Poor blood supply
  Poor immobilization
  Infection

In the treatment of fractures the bones must be immobilized completely until x-ray studies reveal that the hard callus has been replaced with mature bone. It is up to the physician to know the various types of fractures and the best form of immobilization for each specific fracture. During healing, fractures can keep an athlete out of participation for his or her particular sport for several weeks or months, depending on the nature, extent, and site of the fracture. During this period certain conditions can seriously interfere with the healing process. Three such conditions are discussed below.

1. If there is a *poor blood supply to the fractured area* and one of the parts of the broken bone is not properly supplied by the blood, that part will die, and union or healing of the fracture will not take place. This condition is known as *aseptic necrosis* and can often be seen in the head of the femur, the navicular bone in the wrist, the talus in the ankle, and isolated bone fragments. The condition is relatively rare among vital, healthy young athletes except in the navicular bone of the wrist.

2. *Poor immobilization of the fracture site* resulting from poor casting that permits motion between the bone parts may not only prevent proper union but may also, in the event that union does transpire, cause deformity to develop.

3. *Infection* can materially interfere with the normal healing process,

particularly in the case of a compound fracture, which offers an ideal situation for development of a severe streptococcal or staphylococcal infection. The closed fracture is not immune to contamination because infections within the body or a poor blood supply can cause bone infection. Infection of the fracture site may interfere with the proper union of the bone. If soft tissue parts get caught between the severed ends of the bone—such as muscle, connective tissue, or other soft tissue immediately adjacent to the fracture—proper bone union may be unable to occur, often necessitating surgical cleansing of the area of soft tissues by a surgeon.

PAIN PERCEPTION

Pain is one of the major indicators of the inflammatory process. Receptors associated with pain are found in meninges, periosteum, skin, teeth, and some internal organs. Some pain receptors are stimulated by mechanical stresses such as in direct tissue injury and receptors that respond to chemicals that are given off by the injury. Chemicals associated with tissue injury—bradykinin, serotonin, histamine, and prostaglandin—can produce pain. Pain is often described subjectively as burning, sharp, dull, crushing, or piercing.

Deep pain is contrasted to superficial pain because of its poor localization. Pain in the visceral structures is often associated with the autonomic system of sweating, blood pressure changes, and nausea. Deep internal organ pain often also radiates to unrelated external body areas. If this occurs, the pain becomes referred to a body structure that was developed from the same embryonic segment or dermatome as the structure in which the pain originated (dermatomal rule).

A number of theories on how pain is produced and perceived by the brain have been advanced. Only in the last few decades has science demonstrated that pain is both a psychological and physiological phenomenon and therefore is unique to each individual. Sports activities demonstrate this fact clearly. Through conditioning, an athlete learns to endure the pain of rigorous activity and to block the sensations of a minor injury (Figure 8-3).

As understanding of pain increases, there is a growing distinction between chronic and acute pain.[1] Acute pain is the body's protection against something harmful. On the other hand, chronic pain is a paradox that apparently serves no useful purpose. As discussed earlier, pain is both physical and perceptive.

Psychological Aspects of Pain

Pain, especially chronic pain, is a subjective psychological phenomenon. When painful injuries are treated, the total athlete must be considered, not just the pain or condition. Even in the most well-adjusted person, pain will create emotional changes. Constant pain often causes self-centeredness and an increased sense of dependency.

> Deep pain is contrasted to superficial pain because of its poor localization.

> When dealing with pain, the whole athlete must be considered, not just the injury.

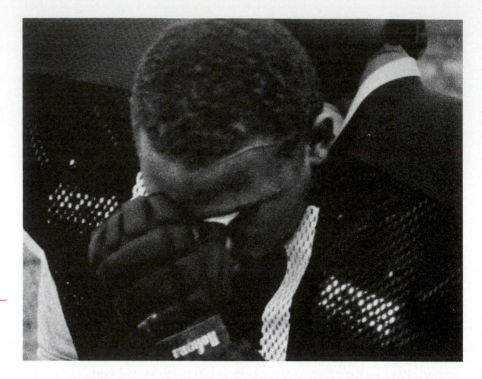

Figure 8-3

An athlete learns through
conditioning to block the
pain of minor injuries during
rigorous activity.

Athletes, like nonathletes, vary in their pain thresholds. Some can tolerate enormous pain, while others find mild pain almost unbearable. Pain appears to be worse at night because persons are alone, more aware of themselves, and devoid of external diversions.[1] Personality differences can also cause differences in pain tolerance. For example, athletes who are anxious, dependent, and immature have less tolerance for pain than those who are relaxed and emotionally in control (Figure 8-4).

Referred Pain

One of the major areas of pain of which coaches and athletic trainers must be aware is that produced from visceral injury. *Gray's Anatomy* states:

> Although most physiological impulses carried by visceral afferent fibers fail to reach consciousness, pathological conditions or excessive stimulation (e.g., trauma and inflammation) may bring into action those which carry pain. The central nervous system has a poorly developed power of localizing the source of such pain, and by some mechanism not clearly understood, the pain may be referred to the region supplied by the somatic afferent fibers whose central connections are the same as those of the visceral afferents.

Visceral pain has a tendency to radiate and give rise to pain that becomes referred to the skin's surface.[1]

OVERVIEW OF THERAPY IN ATHLETICS

Coaches are not specifically trained or certified to manage their athletes' sports injuries. This falls under the heading of treatment that must be directed by a licensed physician. This is particularly true of the definitive use of penetrating therapeutic modalities and exercise rehabilitation. The following material is an overview of therapy in athletics. Coaches, although not therapists themselves, should have enough knowledge to ask logical questions of the health care giver on the status of the injured athlete.

Cold and Heat

It has been known for centuries that cold and heat, when applied to the skin, have therapeutic capabilities. Both are currently used in athletic training in various ways depending on their availability and the philosophy of the user.

Cold as Therapy (Cryotherapy)

As discussed in Chapter 7, the application of cold for the first aid of trauma to the musculoskeletal system is a well-accepted practice. *Cryotherapy* is cold therapy. It applies to the use of ice or cold applications to withdraw heat from the body and lower tissue temperature.[3] When an ice pack is applied intermittently for 20 minutes every 1½ waking hours, it reduces many of the adverse aspects of the initial inflammatory phase that lasts for 3 to 4 days. Depending on the severity of the injury, 3 to 4 days are usual.

A major therapeutic value of cold following the inflammatory phase is to produce anesthesia and allow the athlete to engage in pain-free exercise.[7,8] Another major factor is that cold applications can reduce the muscle pain-spasm-pain cycle. When a muscle is injured, it may go into spasm as a means of protecting itself against further injury. Spasm places pressure on nerve endings and produces more pain. With increased pain there is more spasm, hence the expression *pain-spasm-pain cycle*. Breaking this cycle allows more range of motion in a joint; muscles can be stretched more easily; and movement can be pain-free.[7] See the box on physiological variables of cryotherapy on the following page.

Techniques for application of cold   Cold as a first aid medium has been discussed in Chapter 7. It should be applied when hemorrhaging is under control and repair has started, usually 1 to 3 days after injury, based on the nature and extent of the condition. Depending on the body site and thickness of the subcutaneous fat, the following neuromuscular response has been suggested.[1]

The major therapeutic value of cold is its ability to produce anesthesia, allowing pain-free exercise.

Cold therapy can begin 1 to 3 days after injury.

The extent of cooling depends on the thickness of the subcutaneous fat layer.

Stage	Response	Time after Initiation
1	Cold sensation	0 to 3 min
2	Burning, aching	2 to 7 min
3	Local numbness, anesthesia; pain, reflex impulses stopped; pain-spasm-pain cycle interrupted	5 to 12 min

PHYSIOLOGICAL VARIABLES OF CRYOTHERAPY	
Condition	Response to therapy
Muscle spasm	Decreases
Pain perception	Decreases
Blood flow	Decreases to 10 min
Metabolic rate	Decreases
Connective tissue elasticity	Decreases
Joint stiffness	Increases
Capillary permeability	Increases
Edema	Controversial

Cryotherapy becomes uncomfortable during stage 2, when burning or aching occurs. This requires encouragement, especially during the first experience. When the athlete experiences the comfort of stage 3, little further encouragement is necessary.[7]

Cryokinetics   Cryokinetics is the technique of using intermittent cold applications along with passive and active exercise. Cold should be combined with passive or active movement for the treatment of painful musculoskeletal conditions. At stage 3, cold has depressed the excitability of free nerve endings and peripheral nerve fibers, with a subsequent increase in the pain threshold. With the pain diminished, greater pain-free motion is allowed. Although passive movement in the early stages of healing assists in developing more viable connective tissue, voluntary active movement is preferred whenever possible. Commonly, cryokinetics is repeated three times. The athlete performs movement until pain returns; the cold is reapplied until stage 3 is again reached. Activity is again performed.[1]

Ice massage   Ice massage has been used in sports to some advantage. The technique calls for massaging the affected part with an ice cylinder obtained from freezing water in a styrofoam cup, which insulates the hand against the cold. Grasping the ice cylinder with a towel, move it in a circular manner over the affected area, continuing until the part progresses from an uncomfortable chill sensation to an ache and then numbness. This should take about 5 to 10 minutes. When the body part is numb, gradual stretching and mobilization can be executed (Figure 8-5). This technique is simple and inexpensive, and it can be carried out at home.

Ice water immersion   Immersion in water 50° to 60° F (10° to 15° C) is a simple means of treating a distal part. After analgesia, which occurs rapidly, the athlete is encouraged to move the part in a normal manner. A combination of cold water and the hydromassage action of a whirlpool has been found to reduce initial swelling and encourage healing.

Ice pack   There are a number of different ice packs. The most common are plastic bags filled with ice, cold gel packs, chemical cold packs, and ice towels. Ice packs are useful for approximately 15 to 20 minutes.

Cryotherapeutic techniques:
  Cryokinetics
  Ice massage
  Immersion in ice water
  Ice blanket or ice pack

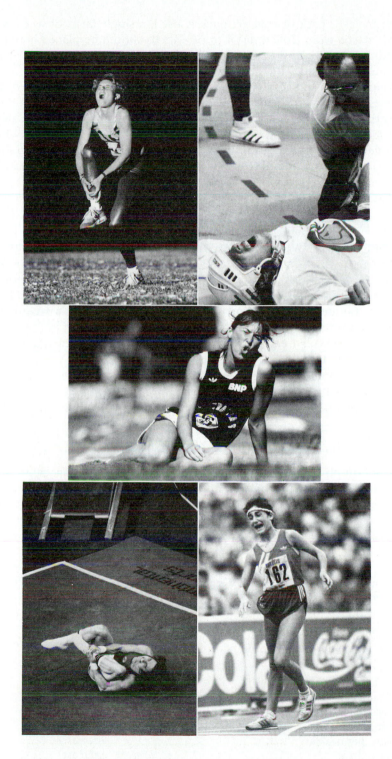

Figure 8-4

Severe pain can be the
outcome of serious sports
injuries.

When a plastic pack or cold gel pack is used, a single layer of wet towel or wet elastic wrap (rolled distal to proximal) should be placed between the skin and pack. Besides toweling, a dry elastic wrap should be available and used to hold the pack firmly in place.

Vapocoolant   Increasingly, vapocoolant sprays are being used for treatment of musculoskeletal problems attributed to sports activity. Currently the vapocoolant of choice is fluori-methane, a nonflammable, nontoxic substance. Under pressure in a bottle, it gives off a fine spray when it is inverted and an emitter is pressed. The major value of a vapocoolant spray is its ability to reduce muscle spasm and increase range of motion. Care must be taken not to frost the skin.

Adverse cold reactions and contraindications   Even though superficial cold when carefully applied is usually safe, some individuals have adverse reactions. Some athletes are allergic to cold and react with hives and joint pain or swelling. A few may have *Raynaud's phenomenon*, in which there are intermittent attacks of pallor followed by a bluish skin discoloration (cyanosis), then redness of the fingers and/or toes, before a return to normal. There may also be numbness, tingling, and burning of the skin. Besides this, a secondary reaction may result in a vasospasm disease and other serious organ dysfunctions.

Paroxysmal cold hemoglobinuria (**hemoglobin** in urine), a rarer disease, may lead to kidney dysfunction.

If cold is applied to the athlete in any form, care must be taken to avoid the possibility of peripheral nerve injury. Peripheral nerves close to the skin surface and skin areas with little subcutaneous fat are subject to cold injury.

Heat as Therapy

The application of heat for disease and traumatic injuries has been used for centuries. Recently, however, its use in the immediate treatment phase of a musculoskeletal injury has been replaced with cold. As with cryotherapy, there are many unanswered questions as to how heat produces physiological responses, when it is best applied, and what types of

hemoglobin

Pigment in red blood cells containing iron

TABLE 8-1 Physiological variables of thermotherapy

Condition	Response to Therapy
Muscle spasm	Decreases
Pain perception	Decreases
Blood flow	Increases
Metabolic rate	Increases
Connective tissue elasticity	Increases
Joint stiffness	Decreases
Capillary permeability	Increases
Edema	Increases

heat therapy are most appropriate for a given condition. The desirable therapeutic effects of heat include (1) increasing the extensibility of connective tissues, (2) decreasing joint stiffness, (3) reducing pain, (4) relieving muscle spasm, (5) reducing inflammation, edema, and exudates, and (6) increasing blood flow (Table 8-1).[9]

Heat affects the extensibility of connective tissue by increasing the viscous flow of collagen fibers and subsequently relaxing the tension. From a therapeutic point of view, heating-contracted connective tissue permits an increase in muscle extensibility through stretching. Muscle contractions, a contracted joint capsule, and scars can be effectively stretched while being heated or just after the heat is removed.[9] An increase in extensibility does not occur unless the heat treatment is associated with stretching exercises.

Heat, like cold, can relieve pain, but for different reasons. Whereas cold numbs the area, heat stimulates the nerves on the skin and stimulates key chemicals that aid in blocking pain sensations. Muscle spasm due to a reduction of blood supply can be relieved by heat. Heat is also believed to assist inflammation and swelling by a number of related factors, such as raising temperature, increasing metabolism, reducing oxygen tension, lowering the pH level, increasing the flow of fluids through the intact capillary walls, and releasing key hormones that cause the capillary dilation.

Heat treatments can be categorized as moist (e.g., from a whirlpool or water packs) or dry (e.g., from a heat lamp). Heat is provided through conduction, convection, or conversion. **Conduction** refers to heat transfer by direct contact from a warmer object to a cooler object. **Convection** is indirect heat, or transfer of heat, caused by air or fluid circulating around the body. **Conversion** is the production of heat by other forms of energy. An example is diathermy, which produces heat from shortwave radio frequencies.

Contraindications for the use of heat for therapy Superficial heat mainly affects the surface of the skin. It is generally contraindicated to apply heat over a numb skin area. It is also contraindicated to apply heat over skin areas that have an inadequate blood supply. Such a situation can result in tissue death. Avoid applying heat over a hemorrhaging region, to gonads, or to a pregnant abdomen. Important contraindications and precautions regarding the use of heat from any source are as follows:

1. Never apply heat when there is a loss of sensation.
2. Never apply heat immediately after an injury.
3. Never apply heat when there is decreased arterial circulation.
4. Never apply heat directly over the eyes or genitals.
5. Never heat the abdomen during pregnancy.

General applications of heat therapy Examples of superficial heat include moist hot packs, water soaks, whirlpool baths, contrast baths, paraffin baths, and analgesic balms and liniments.[9]

Moist heat therapies Heated water is one of the most widely used therapeutic modalities in sports medicine. It is readily available for use

Heat has the capacity to increase the extensibility of connective tissue.

conduction
Heat transfer by direct contact from a warmer object to a cooler object

convection
Heating indirectly through another medium, such as air or liquid

conversion
Heating by other forms of energy

in any sports medicine program. The greatest disadvantage of hydrotherapy is the difficulty in controlling the therapeutic effects. This is primarily caused by the rapid dissipation of heat, which makes maintaining a constant tissue temperature difficult.

For the most part moist heat aids the healing process in some local conditions by causing higher superficial tissue temperatures; however, joints and muscles increase little in temperature. Superficial tissue is a poor thermal conductor, and temperature rises quickly on the skin surface as compared with the underlying tissues.

Hydrotherapy is best applied to postacute conditions of sprains, strains, and contusions. It produces mild healing qualities with a general relaxation of tense, spasmed muscles.[11]

General precautions   The contraindications to and precautions for hydrotherapy are the same as for other types of heat devices. The following precautions must be considered:

1. Avoid overheating sensitive skin, the eyes, and the genitals.
2. Never apply heat to a recent injury until hemorrhage has subsided.
3. Use caution when the athlete is submerged in heated water, since light-headedness and even unconsciousness may result as blood is withdrawn from the head and centralized in other body areas.

Moist heat packs   Commercial moist heat packs fall into the category of conductive heating. Each pad retains water and a constant heat level for 20 to 30 minutes. The usefulness of the moist heat pack lies in its adaptability; it can be positioned anywhere on the body (Figure 8-6).

The major value of the moist heat pack is in the general relaxation it brings and reduction of the pain-spasm-pain cycle. There are limitations of the moist heat pack and all other superficial heating modalities: "the deeper tissues, including the musculature, are usually not significantly heated because the heat transfer from the skin surface into deeper tissues is inhibited by the subcutaneous fat, which acts as a thermal insu-

Moist heat packs afford body part relaxation and reduction of the pain-spasm-pain cycle.

Figure 8-5

Ice massage is an excellent therapeutic modality in sports medicine.

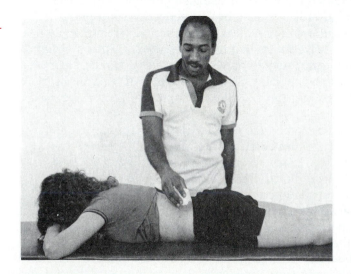

lator, and by the increased skin flow, which cools and carries away the heat externally applied."[11]

Water immersion baths Water is a reasonably good conductor of heat with little heat loss to an immersed part. The most commonly used methods in sports are the whirlpool hydromassage bath and contrast bath.

Whirlpool bath A whirlpool bath is a combination therapy, giving the athlete both a massaging action and a hot or cold water bath (Table 8-2, Figure 8-7). It has become one of the most popular heat therapies used in sports medicine. Through water agitation and the heat transmitted to

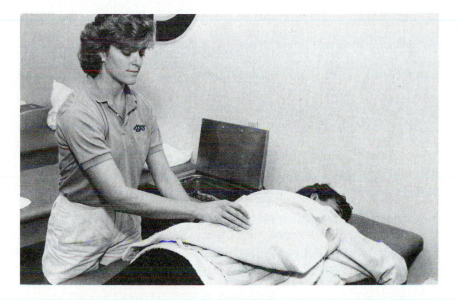

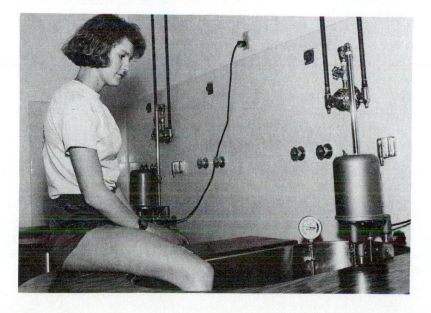

The whirlpool bath provides both heated water and massaging action.

Figure 8-6

A protective layer of cloth must be applied between the skin and the moist heat pack.

Figure 8-7

A whirlpool bath provides therapy through heat conduction and convection.

TABLE 8-2 Whirlpool temperatures

Descriptive Terms	Temperature
Very cold	55° F (12.8° C)
Cold	55°-65° F (12.8°-18.3° C)
Tepid	80°-90° F (27°-32.2° C)
Neutral	92°-96° F (33.5°-35.5° C)
Warm	96°-98° F (35.5°-36.5° C)
Hot	98°-104° F (36.5°-40° C)

TABLE 8-3 Sample whirlpool routine

Injury Progress	Water Temperature	Duration of Treatment
Step 2	55° F (12.8° C)	5 minutes
Step 3	65° F (18.3° C)	10 minutes
Step 4	90° F (32.2° C)	10 minutes
Step 5	98° F (36.5° C)	10-20 minutes
Chronic injury	102° F (38.9° C)	10-20 minutes
Full body immersion	92° F (35° C)	5-10 minutes

the injured area, local circulation can be increased, which is usually followed by a reduction in congestion, spasm, and pain. Table 8-3 describes a general treatment approach when using the whirlpool in sports. When using the whirlpool soon after an injury, the water jet should be directed toward the sides of the tank. Directing the stream of water on the injury will only aggravate the condition and perhaps cause additional bleeding.

Great care should be taken when an athlete undergoes full-body immersion because of the possibility of light-headedness. Constant supervision is a must. To avoid the possibility of passing on infection from one athlete to another, the tank should be emptied after each use and scrubbed with a commercial disinfectant, rinsed, and dried. Safety is of major importance in the use of the whirlpool. All electrical outlets should have a ground fault circuit interrupter. At no time should the athlete turn the motor on or off. Ideally, the on-off switch should be a considerable distance from the machine.[11]

hyperemia
An unusual amount of blood in a body part

Contrast baths Contrast baths produce **hyperemia** in feet, ankles, hands, and wrists of individuals who have a chronic inflammatory condition.

The athlete is submerged for 10 minutes in water that is between 105° and 110° F (40.6° C and 43.3° C). After the initial soak, the athlete is submerged for 1 minute in water that is between 59° and 68° F (15° and 20° C) and then is shifted to the hot water for 4 minutes, alternating temperatures for a period of 30 minutes.[1,5]

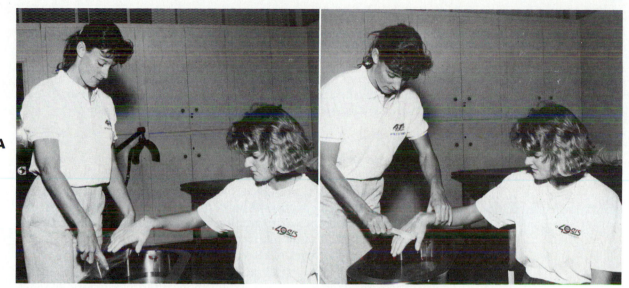

A

B

Figure 8-8

A paraffin bath is an excellent application of therapeutic heat for the distal extremities. **A,** After paraffin coating has been accomplished, the part is covered by a plastic material. **B,** When heat is no longer generated, the paraffin is scraped back into the container.

Paraffin bath is a popular method of applying heat to the distal extremities (Figure 8-8). The paraffin bath is a thermostatically controlled unit that keeps a temperature of 126° C to 130° F (52° to 50° C). The paraffin mixture consists of a ratio of 2 pounds of wax to 1 gallon of mineral oil, which lowers the paraffin's melting point.

Paraffin mixture provides six times the heat of water. Paraffin bath is especially effective in heating chronic injuries of the hand, wrist, elbow, ankle, and foot.

PENETRATING HEAT THERAPIES

As with other therapeutic modalities, a coach should have an appreciation of the penetrating type of heat therapies. Of all therapies found in the athletic medicine setting, penetrating heat therapies constitute the greatest danger if misapplied. Because of the dangers of misuse of the penetrating heat therapies, only properly licensed and certified individuals who have received adequate training should ever attempt to use them. Three types of penetrating heat are currently used for therapy. All heat by means of conversion. They consist of *shortwave diathermy, microwave diathermy,* and *ultrasound therapy.* Of the three, ultrasound therapy is most commonly used.

A certified athletic trainer can administer penetration therapies.

Shortwave Diathermy

Shortwave diathermy heats deeper tissues by introducing a high-frequency electrical current. Shortwave diathermy is highly effective in cases of bursitis, capsulitis, osteoarthritis, deep muscle spasm, and strains. The depth of the technique can be as much as 2 inches (5 cm).[9]

Microwave Diathermy

The heat from microwave diathermy is more easily absorbed in tissue with higher water content such as muscle and blood than is heat from shortwave diathermy. In the unit the alternating current (AC) is changed into direct current (DC). Microwave diathermy is highly effective in treating conditions such as fibrositis, myositis, osteoarthritis, bursitis, calcific tendinitis, sprains, strains, and posttraumatic joint stiffness.[1]

Ultrasound Therapy

For soft-tissue healing, ultrasound uses high-frequency sound waves beyond the audible range. Sound energy causes molecules in the tissues to vibrate, producing heat and mechanical energy. Tissue penetration depends on impedance or acoustical properties of the media, which are proportional to tissue density. The greatest heat is developed between bone and the adjacent soft-tissue interface (Figure 8-9).

In general, three types of effects occur during the application of ultrasound: thermal, mechanical, and chemical. Heat developed by ultrasound increases connective tissue extensibility, alters blood flow, changes nerve conduction velocity, elevates pain threshold, raises enzymatic activity, and changes muscle contractility.[9] The mechanical effect is from vibration.

Ultrasound is used in treating joint contractures, scar tissue, tendinitis, bursitis, skeletal muscle spasm, and pain. Conditions that develop an undesirable calcification are also often treated with ultrasound. These may include calcific bursitis, calcific tendinitis, myositis ossificans, and exostosis.

Figure 8-9

An athletic trainer performing ultrasound therapy.

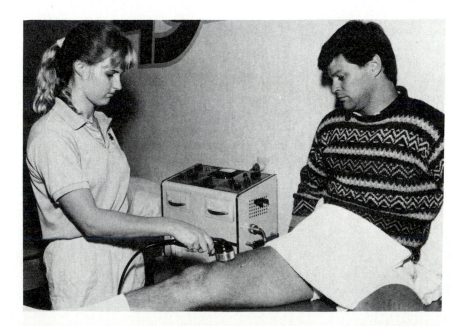

ELECTROTHERAPY

In recent years the use of electrotherapy has significantly increased in sports medicine (Figure 8-10). Electricity is a form of energy that displays magnetic, chemical, mechanical, and thermal effects on tissue. It is a flow of electrons between two points. The human body has electrical conductivity because of positive and negative ions in tissue fluids. A tissue's conductivity varies according to the amount of fluid it contains. Muscle tissue provides excellent conduction, but denser tissues such as tendons and fascia are poor conductors. Fat acts as an insulator against electrical conduction. Because of complexity and the danger of misuse, only licensed and/or certified individuals who have been adequately trained should ever attempt to use electrotherapy.[9]

Electrical Muscle Stimulation

Electrical stimulation as therapy for athletes is used to reduce muscle atrophy, swelling, and pain; to reeducate movement; to introduce antiinflammatory and analgesic drugs through iontophoresis; and to treat trigger points. In electrotherapy two types of current are used: direct (DC), or galvanic, and alternating (AC), or faradic. In DC muscle stimulation an *active* pad and a *dispersal* pad are affixed directly to the skin. The current flows between the two pads. The physiological effects can occur anywhere between the pads, but they usually occur at the active electrode, since current density is greatest at this point. AC muscle stimulation can deliver the electrical energy in a variety of ways, including interrupted, surging, and continuous. It is highly effective in causing muscle contractions.[9]

Iontophoresis

In iontophoresis, chemical ions are transported through the intact skin by an electrical current. Medications of choice for treating musculoskel-

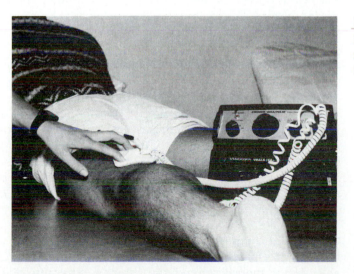

Figure 8-10

Electrotherapy is being used more and more in sports medicine.

etal inflammatory conditions are pain relievers such as lidocaine (Xylocaine) and antiinflammatory agents such as hydrocortisone and dexamethasone. This treatment is most often used for tendinitis, bursitis, myositis, and arthritis.[9]

Transcutaneous Electrical Nerve Stimulation (TENS)

In recent years TENS has become popular for treating both acute and chronic pain. Based on Melzack and Wall's gate-control theory of pain, some researchers theorize that TENS produces inhibition of spinal cord neurons, direct peripheral blockage of nerve fibers, and activation of endogenous opiates such as endorphins. Because TENS does not cause muscle contraction, it can be used immediately after injury. TENS apparatus does not have to be worn continuously; ½ to 1 hour of application will often relieve pain hours after it is removed. Another major value of TENS is that it allows pain-free exercise.[1]

Low-Power Laser

Laser is an acronym that stands for light amplification of stimulated emissions of radiations.[5] The low-power laser is a relatively new device whose applications in an athletic setting may include acceleration of connective tissue synthesis, control of microorganisms, increased vascularization, and reduction of pain and inflammation.[10]

Additional Therapies

Many other therapy modalities may be used in sports medicine. Some that the coach may hear about or observe firsthand are massage, traction, and intermittent compression, as well as the oriental approaches of acupressure and acupuncture.[1]

Massage

Massage is one of the oldest treatment modalities, going back before recorded history. It is defined as the systematic manipulation of the soft tissue of the body. The hand movements of the athletic trainer or therapist of gliding, compressing, stretching, percussing, and vibrating the skin are regulated to create specific responses in the athlete.[1]

Traction

Traction can be defined as a drawing tension applied to a body segment. It is most commonly used in the cervical and lumbar regions of the spine.[6] In general, traction is employed to cause a separation of vertebral bodies by stretching ligaments and joint capsules. Stretching is designed to relieve pressure on nerves and nerves roots.[1] Traction can be accomplished manually, by machine, or by an apparatus (Figure 8-11).

Intermittent Compression Devices

Intermittent compression units are used for the purpose of controlling or reducing swelling. Intermittent compression utilizes a pneumatic inflatable sleeve applied around the injury's extremity (Figure 8-12). The

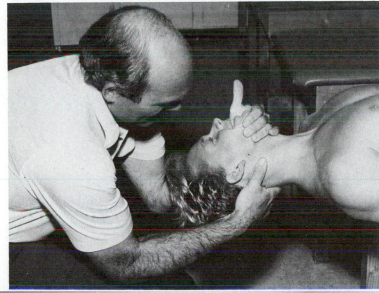

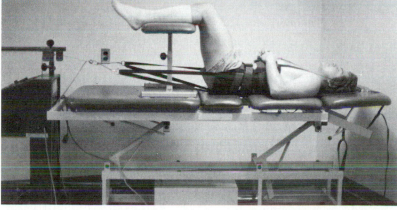

Figure 8-11

Traction to stretch ligaments
and joint capsule can be
performed manually or
mechanically.

sleeve is inflated to a specific pressure that forces excess fluid rate vascular and lymphatic channels.[1]

Acupressure and Acupuncture

Both acupressure and acupuncture have been found beneficial in treating some sports injuries. Acupuncture, using very fine needles, penetrates
points that lie along series meridians that run throughout the body. According to acupuncture theory, stimulation of specific meridian points can
reduce pain and thus bring about a cure. Acupressure is a type of oriental massage that is applied to acupuncture points. Massage on a point
may range from 1 to 5 minutes.[1]

EXERCISE RECONDITIONING

Although it is often neglected, exercise is one of the most important
therapeutic tools available to the area of sports injuries. Through a care-

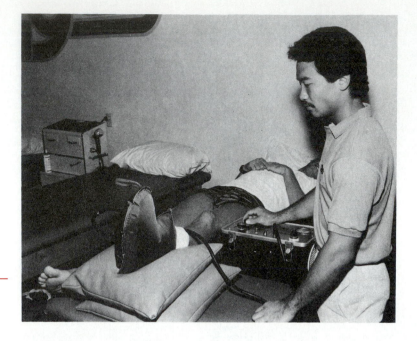

Figure 8-12

Intermittent compression
devices are designed to
reduce edema after injury.

fully applied exercise program in conjunction with other therapies and
directed by a physician, an athlete often can safely return to competition
after injury. The two major categories of exercise reconditioning are conditioning and rehabilitation. *Exercise rehabilitation* is the restoration of an
athlete to the level of preinjury fitness through a carefully planned and
carried out program of therapeutic exercise. It is essential that the athlete return to competition with function fully restored. Too often athletes fail to regain full function and as a result perform at a subpar level,
thereby risking permanent disability.

An injured athlete should be monitored throughout the entire con-
valescent and reconditioning periods. At no time should the immediate
or future health of the athlete be endangered as a result of hasty decisions; at the same time the dedicated athlete should be given every possible opportunity to compete, provided such competition does not pose
undue risk. A coach must be aware that the final decision in this matter

*The physician makes the
final decision about whether
an athlete returns to
competition.*

must rest with the team physician. The team physician must decide at
what point the athlete can reenter competition without the danger of
reinjury, as well as when the use of supportive taping or other aids is
necessary to prevent further injury. It has been said that *a good substitute
is always more valuable than an injured star.* There must be full cooperation
between coach, athletic trainer, and team physician in helping to restore
the athlete to the proper level of competitive fitness. Rehabilitation
through exercise is one factor in the total therapy regimen.[1]

Exercise rehabilitation after a sports injury is the combined responsibility of all individuals connected with a specific sport. To devise a program that is most conducive to the good of the athlete, basic objectives

HELPING INJURED ATHLETES TO RECONDITION

The following are some tips that the coach should follow when his or her athlete is in the process of reconditioning:

1. Help the athlete to trust that every effort is being made to recondition the injury without jeopardizing its ultimate recovery.
2. Help the athlete to understand that the coach, athletic trainer, and physician are cooperating in every way possible to have the athlete gain a full recovery as soon as possible.
3. Help the athlete to become educated in every way possible on the injury sustained and the care procedure being taken to help in the recovery process.
4. Help the athlete understand that success in recovery depends on how well he or she becomes actively involved in the healing process.

that consider his or her needs must be developed. In addition to maintaining a good psychological climate, the objectives are to *(1) prevent deconditioning of the total body and (2) rehabilitate the injured part without hampering the healing process.*

Preventing deconditioning involves keeping the body physically fit while the injury heals. Both the coach and athletic trainer and/or team physician should work together to provide the injured athlete with a safe reconditioning program. In establishing a conditioning program, emphasis should be placed on maintaining strength, flexibility, endurance, and coordination of the total body. Whenever possible, athletes should engage in activities that will aid them in their sport but will not endanger recovery from the injury. When one limb is immobilized in a sling or cast, the opposite limb should be exercised if it can be done without pain or stress to the injured body part. In fact, all uninvolved body parts and joints should be exercised daily so as to maintain a reasonable degree of general strength and endurance.

Restoring the injured part to a preinjury state is so important that an exercise rehabilitation program must be started as soon as possible. It is essential that the person setting up and directing exercise rehabilitation be specifically trained in this area. An injured body part must be prevented from developing disuse degeneration. Disuse produces atrophy, muscle contractures, inflexibility, and healing delay as a result of circulatory impairment. This is not to imply that sports injuries should be run off or worked through. Rather, a proper balance between resting and exercise should be maintained.

In addition to restoring the injured part, rehabilitation must also prevent the athlete from deconditioning.

Muscular Strength and Endurance
Muscle Strength

Muscular strength allows the athlete to overcome a given resistance. It is one of the essential factors in restoring function after injury. Muscle size and strength can be increased with use and can decrease in cases of dis-

Muscle strength refers to a
muscle's ability to overcome
a given resistance. Muscle
endurance refers to a
muscle's ability to perform
repetitive movements.

use. Both isotonic and isometric muscle contractions are used to advantage in rehabilitation. All movements and exercises should be carefully controlled and initially should be guided by pain. Pain-free motion should be a goal. Every effort should be made to prevent atrophy and the loss of muscle tone when a body part or joint is immobilized. As strength is slowly regained, weight bearing may be introduced when the joint is deemed capable of support. Isotonic and isokinetic exercises are preferable because they increase function of a part through a range of movement (Figure 8-13). Isometric exercises involve no movement of the joints, but they develop strength primarily in the position exercised.

Immobilized parts may initially be carefully exercised through isometrics, while using a submaximal effort. Such exercise assists in preventing atrophy and reduces loss of muscular strength until free movement can be executed. When at all possible, a program designed to maintain cardiovascular endurance should accompany the program of musculoskeletal reconditioning.

After initial isometric exercises, as pain and swelling diminish or disappear, the athlete should begin a program of movement using either isotonic or isokinetic exercises to assist in the development of strength, endurance, and range of motion. Isokinetic exercises provide one of the best means of developing strength and endurance in the rehabilitative process, since they demand uniform strength and resistance throughout the full range of movement at a prescribed level of resistance. Isokinetic exercises assist the training experience by increasing the muscular force

Figure 8-13

Isokinetic exercise is often
preferable in the early stages
of limb rehabilitation
because it develops function
through a full range of
motion.

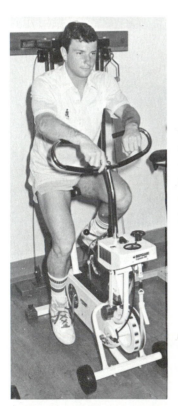

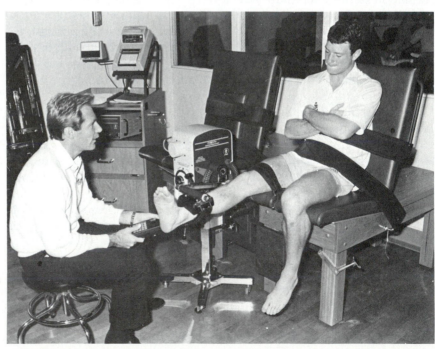

at all speeds of contraction. Rehabilitation is enhanced when the injured athlete is able to perform an exercise set at a specific speed and contractive force equal to the demands of his or her sport.

Flexibility

Flexibility must be present if a part is to be functional. A part that is immobilized in a cast or brace or is not moved regularly through a full range of movement will eventually become inflexible. Important aspects of the athletic rehabilitation regimen are the stretching and muscle release techniques. These techniques are instituted only if they will not aggravate the injury.

Muscle Endurance

Muscle endurance, which is important to the restoration of the injured part, is the ability to sustain muscle contractions at a submaximal effort over a period of time. Muscle strength and endurance are indivisible parts of a continuum. For example, exercises employing progressive resistance at or near maximal effort for four to six repetitions mainly affect strength; decreasing the resistance and increasing the number of repetitions require the ability to sustain a movement, thus increasing muscle endurance.

Proprioception

It is essential that an injured athlete redevelop the feel or awareness of where the body part is located at all times. Depending on the injury, this can be accomplished in many ways. The wobble or tilt board may be used for leg injuries. Other balance activities, such as standing on one foot and springing upward on a bouncer, can help proprioception. It is necessary that proprioception be restored before coordination, agility, and speed activities are attempted.

Coordination, Agility, and Speed of Movement

Exercise rehabilitation is concerned with reestablishing coordination and speed of movement. Before returning to a sport ready to resume full activity, an athlete must be able to perform at the same level of proficiency and have the same potential for delaying fatigue as before he or she became hurt. An athlete who is not at full capacity or who favors an injured part will most likely be reinjured or develop associated problems. Examples of coordination and agility exercises are zig-zag running, figure-8 running, and running and cutting.

To avoid further injury, it is essential that an athlete be fully rehabilitated before returning to the sport.

Psychological Aspects of Rehabilitation

The highly motivated injured athlete may begrudge time spent out of action. The coach and athletic trainer must establish the fact that every person is unique as to healing and that everything is being done to assist the athlete's healing process. When an injury is serious, false hope should not be put forth for a fast comeback. There should be a spirit of cooperation established between the athlete, coach, athletic trainer, and physician.

Exercise Overdosage

Engaging in exercise that is too intense or prolonged can be extremely detrimental to the progress of the athlete. The most obvious sign of overdosage is increased pain or discomfort lasting more than 3 hours. Other signs are decreased range of motion and decreased strength of the injured part. In most situations early rehabilitation involves submaximal exercise performed in short bouts that are repeated many times daily. Exercise rehabilitation in the early stages of recovery is performed two or three times a day. As recovery increases, the intensity of exercise also increases, and the exercise is performed less often during the day and, ultimately, the week.

Rehabilitative Exercise Phases

Rehabilitative exercise in sports medicine can generally be categorized into six phases. A unique phase that comes before elective surgery is the presurgical phase. After the presurgical exercise phase, five additional phases can be identified: postsurgical or acute (phase 1), early (phase 2), intermediate (phase 3), advanced (phase 4), and initial sports reentry (phase 5). Not all injured athletes experience all phases to achieve full rehabilitation. Depending on the type of injury and individual response to healing, phases may sometimes overlap.

Presurgical Exercise Phase

Exercise performed in the presurgical phase often assists in recovery after surgery.

If surgery can be postponed, exercise may be used as a means to improve its outcome. By maintaining and in some cases increasing muscle tone and improving kinesthetic awareness, the athlete is prepared to continue the exercise rehabilitative program after surgery.

Postsurgical or Acute Injury Exercise Phase (Phase 1)

The postsurgical exercise phase should start 24 hours after surgery.

Exercise is often encouraged after surgery to the musculoskeletal system. The optimal time for commencement of therapeutic exercise is approximately 24 hours after surgery or injury. Exercise is employed to avoid muscle atrophy and to ensure return to sports participation as quickly as possible. Postsurgical exercise often repeats what was done presurgically. Commonly, the body part that was surgically repaired is immobilized by a cast, dressing, or sling. When immobilized, muscle tension or isometrics may be employed to maintain muscle strength. Unless contraindicated, joints that are immediately adjacent (**distal** and **proximal**) to the immobilized part should be gently exercised to maintain their strength and mobility.

distal
Farthest from the point of attachment (opposite of proximal)

proximal
Closest to the point of attachment (opposite of distal)

Early Exercise Phase (Phase 2)

The early exercise phase is a direct extension of the postsurgical, or acute injury, phase. The primary goals of this phase are to restore full muscle contraction without pain and to maintain strength in muscles surrounding the immobilized part. Muscle tensing is continued. Depending on the nature of the condition, isometric exercise against resistance may be added. Joints that are close to the injury are maintained in good condition by strengthening and mobility exercises.

Intermediate Exercise Phase (Phase 3)

When pain-free full muscle contraction has been achieved, the goals are to develop up to 50% range of motion of the unaffected part and 50% strength. A third goal is to restore near-normal neuromuscular coordination and proprioception.

Advanced Exercise Phase (Phase 4)

The goal of phase 4 is to restore at least 90% of the athlete's range of motion and strength. Also the athlete is to undergo reconditioning for returning to his or her sport. The ideal goals in this phase are to fully restore power, flexibility, endurance, speed, proprioception, and agility of the injured part, as well as the entire body.

> The ideal goals of the advanced phase of exercise are to restore full power, flexibility, endurance, speed, and agility to the athlete.

Initial Sports Reentry Phase (Phase 5)

Phase 5 of the exercise rehabilitation program involves returning to sports participation. In this phase the underlying factors are gradualness and avoiding having the athlete overdo. In some cases this phase is a period in which muscle bulk is restored; in other instances the athlete carefully tests the results of the exercise rehabilitation process. It is essential that the athlete not return to competition before full range of movement, strength, and coordination have been attained and psychological readiness has been achieved.

The Exercise Rehabilitation Plan

No exercise rehabilitation program can properly take place without a carefully thought-out plan. It should contain four major elements: a clear understanding of the injury situation, an injury evaluation, an exercise plan, and criteria for recovery and returning to a specific sport.

> Essential parts of the exercise rehabilitation plan:
> Determination of injury situation
> Injury evaluation
> Exercise plan
> Criteria for full recovery
> Return to the sport

Injury Situation

Persons responsible for carrying out exercise rehabilitation must have a complete and clear understanding of the injury. This should include (1) exactly how the injury was sustained, (2) careful inspection of the injury, and (3) the medical diagnosis, consisting of the major signs, symptoms, and anatomical structures affected.

Injury Evaluation

Before an exercise program is developed, an evaluation is made. It should include range of motion, muscle strength, and functional capacity of the part. The evaluation must take into consideration swelling, pain, and movements or exercises that may be contraindicated.

Exercise Plan

When there is a clear understanding of the athlete's functional capacity, exercises are selected on a progressive basis. The exercises are grouped according to phases of rehabilitation. Criteria for progressing from one phase to another are established, as are criteria for ultimate recovery.

Criteria for Full Recovery

The athlete must successfully pass a functional evaluation before obtaining a release for competition. This means having recovered full range of motion, strength, and size of the injured body part. In addition the athlete must demonstrate full-function capabilities that are sport specific as well as a psychological readiness for returning to the sport.

SUMMARY

The healing process of soft tissue consists of the inflammatory, repair, and remodeling phases. The inflammatory phase lasts 3 to 4 days and is designed to protect and localize the injury and prepare the tissue for repair. The phase is synonymous with healing and the restoration of lost tissue. Remodeling is the phase of healing that returns the injured tissue to full strength.

Fracture healing follows many of the steps of soft tissue healing, with the exception of the development of a soft and hard callus. The soft callus is composed mostly of connective tissue. The hard callus is composed of connective tissue and a network of woven bone that will slowly be replaced by mature bone. Fracture healing can be delayed if there is improper blood supply to the fractured area and poor immobilization.

Pain is both a psychological and physiological phenomenon. Pain perception is subjective and may be described as burning, sharp, dull, crushing, or piercing. Acute pain is designed to protect the body, while chronic pain serves no useful purpose. Chronic pain is believed to be caused by a noxious stimulus that affects the high-threshold nociceptors in skin, blood vessels, subcutaneous tissue, fascia, periosteum, viscera, and other pain-sensitive structures.

Both superficial cold and heat provide therapeutic benefits. Although in different ways, they can break up the muscle pain-spasm-pain cycle and reduce swelling. Cold application produces local anesthesia while increasing local circulation. Common superficial cold therapy techniques are ice massage, ice water immersion, and ice packs. Superficial heat therapy techniques are moist heat packs, whirlpool baths, contrast baths, and paraffin baths. Other modalities used in athletic injuries by licensed and certified personnel include shortwave and microwave diathermy, ultrasound, electrical muscle stimulation, iontophoresis, and transcutaneous electrical nerve stimulation (TENS).

Exercise reconditioning is a major tool for returning the injured athlete to his or her sport. Exercise rehabilitation, like physical conditioning, follows the SAID principle. It should be designed to prevent deconditioning and restore the injured part to a preinjury state. Isometric muscle contraction is commonly used to maintain strength of an immobilized part. When mobility is allowed, flexibility and isokinetic and isotonic strengthening exercises may be employed. Proprioception activities are engaged to restore balance. Coordination, agility, and speed of movement activities follow the restoration of balance. Exercise overdosage must be avoided, with short bouts of submaximal exercise being performed in the early stages of rehabilitation. An exercise rehabilitation plan should include the injury situation, evaluation, exercise plan, and criteria for full recovery.

REVIEW QUESTIONS AND CLASS ACTIVITIES

1. How does healing occur in soft tissue? What are the outward signs of the inflammatory phase of healing?
2. How do fractures heal? What conditions can interfere with proper fracture care?
3. Contrast deep structural pain with superficial pain. How do psychological factors affect perception of pain?
4. What are the physiological effects of cold applications?
5. Why is cold so effective if used before a rehabilitation program?
6. In what situations should cold not be used?
7. Have the class try each cold application so they will understand the neuromuscular response to cold.
8. What are the physiological effects of heat?
9. Under what conditions should superficial heat not be used?
10. What are the different types of superficial heat and how are they applied?
11. What are some special considerations to keep in mind when having an athlete use the whirlpool bath?
12. What other modalities are used in sports injury care by properly licensed and certified personnel?
13. What are some consequences of inactivity?
14. What are the major components of a rehabilitation program?
15. Explain the four categories of reconditioning exercises.
16. What are the different phases of exercise? What goals should be set at each level before progressing to the next level?
17. When you are setting up a total rehabilitation program, what four elements must you clearly understand?
18. How would you determine if an athlete is ready to return to full sports participation? Who should be the final judge of this?
19. Take the class to the training room or local sports medicine clinic to see the equipment used to rehabilitate an injured athlete.

REFERENCES

1. Arnheim D, Prentice W: *Principles of athletic training*, ed 8, St Louis, 1993, Mosby-Year Book.
2. Ball AT, Horton PG: The use and abuse of hydrotherapy in athletics: a review, *Ath Train* 22:115, 1987.
3. Bassett FH et al: Cryotherapy-induced nerve injury, *Am J Sports Med* 20:516, 1992.
4. Bonica JJ: Pathophysiology in pain. In *Current concepts of postoperative pain*, New York, 1987, HP Publishing.
5. Enwemeka C: Laser biostimulation of healing wounds: specific effects and mechanisms of action, *J Orthop Sports Phys Ther* 9:333, 1988.
6. Hooker D: Traction as a specialized modality. In Prentice W, ed: *Therapeutic modalities in sports medi-*

cine, St Louis, 1995, Mosby-Year Book.

7. Knight KL: *Cryotherapy: theory, technique, and physiology,* Chattanooga, Tenn, 1985, Chattanooga Corp.

8. Michlovitz SL: Cryotherapy: the use of cold as a therapeutic agent. In Michlovitz SL, ed: *Thermal agents in rehabilitation,* Philadelphia, 1989, FA Davis.

9. Prentice WE: *Therapeutic modalities in sports medicine,* St Louis, 1990, Time Mirror/Mosby College Publishing.

10. Saliba E: Low-power laser. In Prentice W, ed: *Therapeutic modalities in sports medicine,* St Louis, 1990, Mosby-Year Book.

11. Walsh M: Hydrotherapy: the use of water as a therapeutic agent. In Michlovitz SL, ed: *Thermal agents in rehabilitation,* Philadelphia, 1986, FA Davis.

ANNOTATED BIBLIOGRAPHY

Abdenour TE, Thygerson AL: *Sports injury care,* Boston, 1993, Jones & Bartlett. A practical "how to" book on sports injury care for the coach and/or athletic trainer.

Andrews JR, Harrelson GL: *Physical rehabilitation of the injured athlete,* Philadelphia, 1991, WB Saunders. Text covering the rehabilitation of the athlete including psychological aspects, physiology, immobilization, and remobilization.

Committee on Sports Medicine and Fitness, American Academy of Pediatric Sports Medicine, eds: *Health care for young athletes,* ed 2, Elk Grove Village, Ill, 1991, American Academy of Pediatrics. A broad approach to health care for all interested in the young athlete.

Guten GN: *Play healthy, stay healthy: your guide to managing and treating 40 common sports injuries,* Champaign, Ill, 1991, Leisure Press. A self-help guide for the active athlete.

Knight KL: *Cryotherapy: theory, technique, and physiology,* Chattanooga, Tenn, 1985, Chattanooga Corp. Presents excellent coverage, both theoretical and practical, of cryotherapy, one of the most widely used therapeutic approaches in sports medicine and athletic training. It is clearly written and easily applied.

Ordet SM, Grand LS: *Dynamics of clinical rehabilitation exercise,* Baltimore, 1992, Williams & Wilkins. A "how to" and "why" of exercise.

Prentice WE: *Therapeutic modalities in sports medicine,* ed 3, St Louis, 1995, Mosby–Year Book. A complete guide to therapeutic modalities (not including exercise rehabilitation) in sports medicine and athletic training.

Pryor SR: *Getting back on your feet.* Post Mills, Vt, 1991, Chelsea Green Pub. A patient guide to crutch usage or other assistive devices following surgery in trauma.

Torg JS et al: *Rehabilitation of athletic injuries,* Chicago, 1987, Year Book Medical Publishers. Provides a systematic approach to sports injury diagnosis and rehabilitation.

Wound Dressing and Bandaging

When you finish this chapter, you will be able to:

- Demonstrate basic skills in wound dressing
- Demonstrate the application of roller bandages
- Demonstrate the application of the elastic wrap to major body parts
- Demonstrate the application of triangular and cravat bandages

A major skill in athletic training is the proper application of wound dressing and other types of bandages. Each of these skill areas requires a great deal of practice before a high level of proficiency can be attained. The following categories are basic to the athletic training and sports medicine program.

WOUND DRESSINGS

bandage
A strip of cloth or other material used to hold a dressing in place

dressing
A material, such as gauze, applied to a wound

All wounds must be considered contaminated by microorganisms.

A **bandage,** when properly applied, can contribute decidedly to recovery from sports injuries. Bandages carelessly or improperly applied may cause discomfort, allow wound contamination, even hamper repair and healing. In all cases bandages must be firmly applied—neither so tight that circulation is impaired nor so loose that the **dressing** is allowed to slip.

Skin lesions are extremely prevalent in sports; abrasions, lacerations, and puncture wounds are almost daily occurrences. It is of the utmost importance to the well-being of the athlete that open wounds be cared for immediately. All wounds, even those that are relatively superficial, must be considered to be contaminated by microorganisms and therefore must be cleansed, medicated (when called for), and dressed. Dressing wounds requires a sterile environment to prevent infections.[1]

Individuals who perform wound management in sports have often been criticized for not following good principles of cleanliness. It is obvious from the large number of athletes who acquire severe wound infections each year that this criticism is valid. To alleviate this problem one must adhere to standard procedures in the prevention of wound contamination.

Wound Description

Abrasions are common conditions in which the skin is scraped against a rough surface such as grass, artificial playing surface, floor, or mat. The top layer of skin wears away, exposing numerous blood capillaries. This general exposure, with dirt and foreign materials scraping and penetrating the skin, increases the probability of infection unless the wound is properly debrided and cleansed. (Figure 9-1 shows abrasions and the other wound descriptions listed here.)

Puncture wounds can easily occur during physical activities and can be fatal. Direct penetration of tissues by a pointed object such as a track shoe spike can introduce the tetanus bacillus into the bloodstream, possibly making the athlete a victim of lockjaw. All puncture wounds and severe lacerations should be referred immediately to a physician.

Avulsion wounds occur when skin is torn from the body and are frequently associated with major bleeding. The avulsed tissue should be placed on moist gauze, preferably saturated with saline solution.[3] It is then put into a plastic bag, immersed in cold water, and taken along with the athlete to the hospital for reattachment.[3]

Incisions are clearly cut wounds that often appear where a blow has been delivered over a sharp bone or a bone that is poorly padded. They are not as serious as the other types of exposed wounds.

Lacerations, also common in sports, occur when a sharp or pointed object tears the tissues, giving a wound the appearance of a jagged-edge cavity. As with abrasions, lacerations present an environment conducive to severe infections. The same mechanism that causes a laceration also can lead to a skin avulsion, in which a piece of skin is ripped off.

APAIL is an acronym to help remember the types of skin wounds.

Eight basic uses for dressings and bandages:
Protect wounds from infection
Protect wounds from further insult and contamination
Control external and internal hemorrhage
Act as a compress over exposed or unexposed injuries
Immobilize an injured part
Protect an unexposed injury
Support an injured part
Hold protective equipment in place

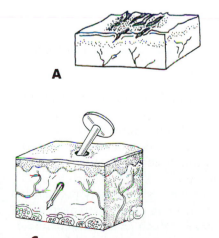

A

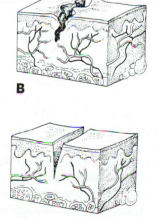

B

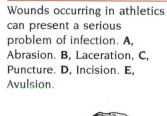

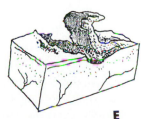

C　　　　**D**　　　　　　　　**E**

Figure 9-1

Wounds occurring in athletics can present a serious problem of infection. **A,** Abrasion. **B,** Laceration, **C,** Puncture. **D,** Incision. **E,** Avulsion.

Tetanus and Wound Infection

Tetanus (lockjaw) is an acute disease causing fever and convulsions. Tonic spasm of skeletal muscles is always a possibility for any nonimmunized athlete. The tetanus bacillus enters a wound as a spore and, depending on individual susceptibility, acts on the motor end plate of the central nervous system. After initial childhood immunization by tetanus toxoid, boosters should be given every 10 years. An athlete not immunized should receive an injection of tetanus immune globulin (Hyper-Tet) immediately after sustaining a skin wound.

Suggested Practices in Wound Care

The following are suggested procedures to use in the training room to cut down the possibility of wound infections. Table 9-1 offers more specific suggestions regarding the care of external wounds.

As discussed in Chapter 6, all persons managing sports injuries where bodily fluids, especially blood, are involved must follow the standards established by OSHA. All exposed wounds should be treated as if containing blood-borne pathogens such as **HIV** and **HBV**.[3]

HIV
Human immunodeficiency virus

HBV
Hepatitis B virus

1. Make sure all instruments used such as scissors, tweezers, and swabs are sterilized.
2. Clean hands thoroughly.
3. If there is a possibility of direct contact with any bodily fluids such as blood, wear latex gloves to avoid AIDS contamination.
4. Clean a skin lesion thoroughly.
5. Place a nonmedicated dressing on a lesion if the athlete is to be sent for medical attention.
6. Avoid touching any parts of a sterile dressing that will come in contact with a wound.
7. Place medication on a pad rather than directly on a lesion.
8. Secure the dressing with tape or a wrap.
9. If necessary, elevate the part for control of bleeding.
10. Follow the OSHA standards (see box on p.202).

Materials

Bandages used on sports injuries consist essentially of gauze, cotton cloth, and elastic wrapping. Plastics are also being used more frequently. Each material offers a specific contribution to the care of injuries.

Gauze　Gauze materials are used in three forms: as sterile pads for wounds, as padding in the prevention of blisters on a taped ankle, and as a roller bandage for holding dressings and compresses in place.

Cotton cloth　Cotton is used primarily for cloth ankle wraps and for triangular and cravat-type bandages. It is soft, is easily obtained, and can be washed many times without deterioration.

Elastic roller bandage　The elastic bandage is extremely popular in sports because of its extensibility, which allows it to conform to most parts of the body. Elastic wraps are active bandages, which let the athlete move without restriction. They also act as a controlled compression bandage,

Elastic bandages allow the athlete to move without restriction.

TABLE 9-1 Care of external wounds

Type of Wound	Action of Coach or Athletic Trainer	Initial Care	Follow-up Care
Abrasion	1. Provide initial care. 2. Wound seldom requires medical attention unless infected.	1. Cleanse abraded area with soap and water; debride with brush. 2. Apply a solution of hydrogen peroxide over abraded area; continue until foaming has subsided. 3. Apply a petroleum-based medicated ointment to keep abraded surface moist. In sports it is not desirable for abrasions to acquire a scab. Place a nonadherent sterile pad (Telfa pad) over the ointment.	1. Change dressing daily and look for signs of infection.
Laceration	1. Cleanse around the wound. Avoid wiping more contaminating agents into the area. 2. Apply dry, sterile compress pad and refer to physician.	1. Complete cleansing and suturing are accomplished by a physician; injections of tetanus toxoid may be required.	1. Change dressing daily and look for signs of infection.
Puncture	1. Cleanse around the wound. Avoid wiping more contaminating agents into the area. 2. Apply dry, sterile compress pad and refer to physician.	1. Complete cleansing and injections of tetanus toxoid, if needed, are managed by a physician.	1. Change dressing daily and look for signs of infection.
Incision	1. Clean around wound. 2. Apply dry, sterile compress pad to control bleeding and refer to physician.	1. Cleanse wound. 2. Suturing and injections of tetanus toxoid are managed by a physician, if needed.	1. Change dressing daily and look for signs of infection.
Avulsion	1. Clean around wound; save avulsed tissue. 2. Apply dry, sterile compress pad to control bleeding and refer to physician.	1. Wound is cleansed thoroughly; avulsed skin is replaced and sutured by a physician; tetanus toxoid injection may be required.	1. Change dressing daily and look for signs of infection.

in which the regulation of pressure is graded according to the athlete's specific needs; however, they can cause dangerous constriction if not properly applied. A *cohesive elastic bandage* exerts constant, even pressure. It is lightweight and contours easily to the body part. The bandage is composed of two layers of nonwoven rayon, which are separated by strands of Spandex material. The cohesive elastic bandage is coated with a substance that makes the material adhere to itself, eliminating the need for metal clips or adhesive tape for holding it in place.

Plastics Plastics are playing an increasing role in sports medicine. Spray plastic coatings are used to protect wounds. A variety of plastic adhesive tapes are also used because they are waterproof. A good practice is to use plastic food envelopes to insulate analgesic balm packs and to protect bandages and dressings from moisture. A common plastic-coated pad used for wound dressing is the Telfa pad. Plastic materials that can be formed into a desired shape when heated are also becoming an integral part of the training room list of supplies.[1]

COMMON TYPES OF BANDAGES USED IN SPORTS MEDICINE

Two common bandages used in sports are the roller and the triangular.

Roller Bandages

Roller bandages are made of many materials; gauze, cotton cloth, and elastic wrapping are predominantly used in the training room. The width and length vary according to the body part to be bandaged. The sizes most frequently used are the 2-inch (5 cm) width by 6-yard (5.5 m) length for hand, finger, toe, and head bandages; the 3-inch (7.5 cm) width by 10-yard (9 m) length for the extremities; and the 4-inch (10 cm) or 6-inch (15 cm) width by 10-yard length for thigh, groin, and trunk. For ease and convenience in the application of the roller bandage, the strips of material are first rolled into a cylinder. When a bandage is selected, it should be a single piece that is free from wrinkles, seams, and any other imperfections that may cause skin irritation.[2]

Wrinkles or seams in roller bandages may irritate skin.

Application

Application of the roller bandage must be executed in a specific manner to achieve the purpose of the wrap. When a roller bandage is about to be placed on a body part, the roll should be held in the preferred hand with the loose end extending from the bottom of the roll. The back surface of the loose end is placed on the part and held in position by the other hand. The bandage cylinder is then unrolled and passed around the injured area. As the hand pulls the material from the roll, it also standardizes the bandage pressure and guides the bandage in the proper direction. To anchor and stabilize the bandage, a number of turns, one on top of the other, are made. Circling a body part requires the operator to alternate the bandage roll from one hand to the other and back again.

To apply a roller bandage, hold it in the preferred hand with the loose end extending from the bottom of the roll.

To acquire maximum benefits from a roller bandage, it should be applied uniformly and firmly but not too tightly. Excessive or unequal pres-

sure can hinder the normal blood flow within the part. The following
points should be considered when using the roller bandage:

1. A body part should be wrapped in its position of maximum muscle
   contraction to ensure unhampered movement or circulation.
2. It is better to use a large number of turns with moderate tension
   than a limited number of turns applied too tightly.
3. Each turn of the bandage should be overlapped by at least one
   half of the overlying wrap to prevent the separation of the material while engaged in activity. Separation of the bandage turns
   tends to pinch and irritate the skin.
4. When limbs are wrapped, fingers and toes should be scrutinized
   often for signs of circulation impairment. Abnormally cold or cyanotic phalanges are signs of excessive bandage pressure.

The usual anchoring of roller bandages consists of several circular
wraps directly overlying each other. Whenever possible, anchoring
is commenced at the smallest circumference of a limb and is then
moved upward. Wrists and ankles are the usual sites for anchoring bandages of the limbs. Bandages are applied to these areas in the following
manner:

Begin anchoring bandages at
the smallest part of the limb.

1. The loose end of the roller bandage is laid obliquely on the anterior aspects of the wrist or ankle and held in this position. The
   roll is then carried posteriorly under and completely around the
   limb and back to the starting point.
2. The triangular portion of the uncovered oblique end is folded over
   the second turn.
3. The folded triangle is covered by a third turn, which finishes a
   secure anchor.

After a roller bandage has been applied, it is held in place by a *locking technique*. The method most often used to finish a wrap is that of firmly
tying or pinning the bandage or placing adhesive tape over several overlying turns.

Once a bandage has been put on and has served its purpose, removal
can be performed either by unwrapping or by carefully cutting with bandage scissors. Whatever method of bandage removal is used, extreme caution must be taken to avoid additional injury.

CLOTH ANKLE WRAP

Because tape is so expensive, the ankle wrap is an inexpensive and expedient means of mildly protecting ankles (Figure 9-2).

MATERIALS NEEDED: Each muslin wrap should be 1½ to 2 inches (3.8 to 5
cm) wide and 72 to 96 inches (180 to 240 cm) long to ensure complete
coverage and protection. The purpose of this wrap is to give mild support against lateral and medial motion of the ankle. It is applied over a
sock.

POSITION OF THE ATHLETE: The athlete sits on a table, extending the leg and
positioning the foot at a 90-degree angle. To avoid any distortion, it is
important that the ankle be neither overflexed nor overextended.

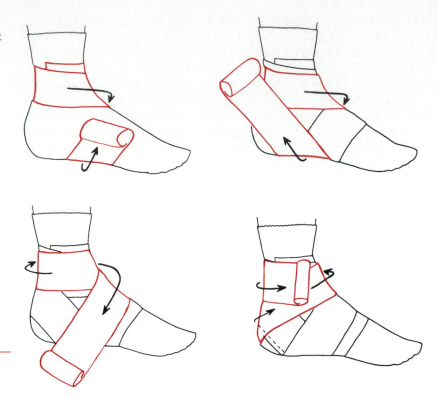

Figure 9-2

Ankle wrap.

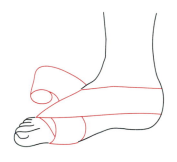

PROCEDURE

1. Start the wrap above the instep around the ankle, circle the ankle and move it at an acute angle to the inside of the foot.
2. From the inside of the foot move the wrap under the arch, coming up on the outside and crossing at the beginning point, where it continues around the ankle, hooking the heel.
3. Then move the wrap up, inside, over the instep, and around the ankle, hooking the opposite side of the heel. This completes one series of the ankle wrap.
4. Complete a second series with the remaining material.
5. For additional support, two heel locks with adhesive tape may be applied over the ankle wrap.

Elastic Wrap Techniques

Any time an elastic wrap is applied to the athlete always check for and avoid decreased circulation and blueness of the extremity and check for a blood capillary refill.

ANKLE AND FOOT SPICA

The ankle and foot spica bandage (Figure 9-3) is primarily used in sports for the compression of new injuries, as well as for holding wound dressings in place.

MATERIALS NEEDED: Depending on the size of the ankle and foot, a 2- or 3-inch wrap is used.

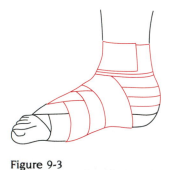

Figure 9-3

Ankle and foot spica.

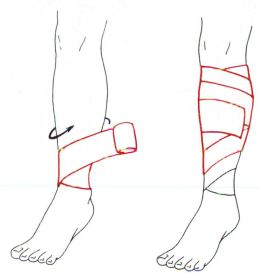

Figure 9-4

Spiral bandage.

POSITION OF THE ATHLETE: The athlete sits with ankle and foot extended over a table.

PROCEDURE

1. An anchor is placed around the foot near the metatarsal arch.
2. The elastic bandage is brought across the instep and around the heel and returned to the starting point.
3. The procedure is repeated several times, with each succeeding revolution progressing upward on the foot and the ankle.
4. Each **spica** overlaps approximately three fourths of the preceding layer.

SPIRAL BANDAGE

The spiral bandage (Figure 9-4) is widely used in sports for covering a large area of a cylindrical part.

MATERIALS NEEDED: Depending on the size of the area, a 3- or 4-inch wrap is required.

POSITION OF THE ATHLETE: If the wrap is for the lower limb, the athlete bears weight on the opposite leg.

PROCEDURE

1. The elastic spiral bandage is anchored at the smallest circumference of the limb and is wrapped upward in a spiral against gravity.
2. To prevent the bandage from slipping down on a moving extremity, two pieces of tape should be folded lengthwise and placed on the bandage at either side of the limb or tape adherent can be sprayed on the part.
3. After the bandage is anchored, it is carried upward in consecutive spiral turns, each overlapping the other by at least ½ inch.
4. The bandage is terminated by locking it with circular turns, which are then firmly secured by tape.

Check circulation after applying an elastic wrap.

spica
A figure-8 bandage, with one of the two loops being larger

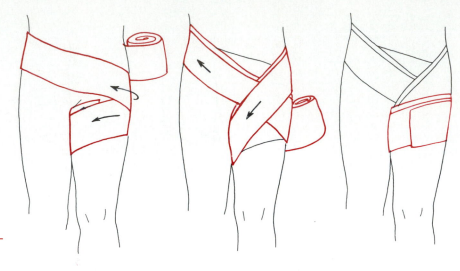

Figure 9-5
_____

Elastic groin support.

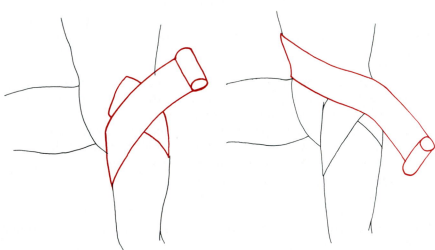

Figure 9-6
_____

Hip spica for hip flexors.

GROIN SUPPORT

The following procedure is used to support a groin strain and hip adductor strains (Figure 9-5).

MATERIALS NEEDED: One roll of extra-long 6-inch (15 cm) elastic bandage, a roll of 1½-inch (3.8 cm) adhesive tape, and nonsterile cotton.

POSITION OF THE ATHLETE: The athlete stands on a table with weight placed on the uninjured leg. The affected limb is relaxed and internally rotated. This procedure is different from that described earlier in which the wrap was used for pressure only.

PROCEDURE

1. A piece of nonsterile cotton or a felt pad may be placed over the injured site to provide additional compression and support.
2. The end of the elastic bandage is started at the upper part of the

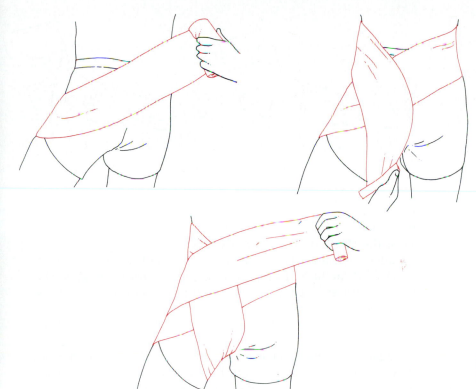

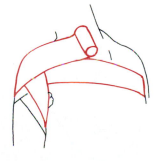

Figure 9-7

Method used to limit
movement of buttocks.

inner aspect of the thigh and is carried posteriorly around the
thigh. Then it is brought across the lower abdomen and over the
crest of the ilium on the opposite side of the body.

3. The wrap is continued around the back, repeating the same pattern and securing the wrap end with a 1½-inch (3.8 cm) adhesive tape.

NOTE: Variations of this method can be seen in Figure 9-6, used to support injured hip flexors, and Figure 9-7, used to limit the movement of
the buttocks.

SHOULDER SPICA

The shoulder spica (Figure 9-8) is used mainly for the retention of wound
dressings and for moderate muscular support.

MATERIALS NEEDED: One roll of extra-length 4- to 6-inch elastic wrap, 1½
-inch adhesive tape, and padding for axilla.

POSITION OF THE ATHLETE: Athlete stands with side toward the operator.

PROCEDURE

1. The axilla must be well padded to prevent skin irritation and constriction of blood vessels.

2. The bandage is anchored by one turn around the affected upper
arm.

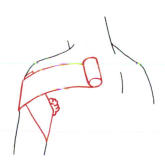

Figure 9-8

Elastic shoulder spica.

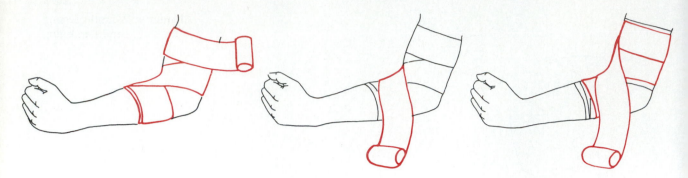

Figure 9-9

Elastic elbow figure-8 bandage.

3. After anchoring the bandage around the arm on the injured side, the wrap is carried around the back under the unaffected arm and across the chest to the injured shoulder.
4. The affected arm is again encircled by the bandage, which continues around the back. Every figure-8 pattern moves progressively upward with an overlap of at least half of the previous underlying wrap.

ELBOW FIGURE-8

The elbow figure-8 bandage (Figure 9-9) can be used to secure a dressing in the antecubital fossa or to restrain full extension in hyperextension injuries. When it is reversed, it can be used on the posterior aspect of the elbow.

MATERIALS NEEDED: One 3-inch elastic roll and 1½-inch adhesive tape.

POSITION OF THE ATHLETE: Athlete flexes elbow between 45 degrees and 90 degrees, depending on the restriction of movement required.

PROCEDURE

1. Anchor the bandage by encircling the lower arm.
2. Bring the roll obliquely upward over the posterior aspect of the elbow.
3. Carry the roll obliquely upward, crossing the antecubital fossa; then pass once again completely around the upper arm and return to the beginning position by again crossing the antecubital fossa.
4. Continue the procedure as described, but for every new sequence move upward toward the elbow one half the width of the underlying wrap.

EYE BANDAGE

When a bandage is needed to hold a dressing on an eye, the following procedure is suggested (Figure 9-10).

MATERIALS NEEDED: 2-inch gauge bandage roll, scissors, and ½ or 1-inch tape.

POSITION OF THE ATHLETE: Athlete sits in chair or on edge of table.

PROCEDURE

1. The bandage is started with three circular turns around the head and then is brought obliquely down the back of the head.

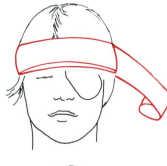

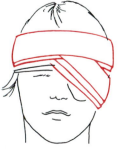

Figure 9-10

Eye bandage.

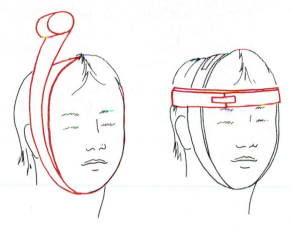

Figure 9-11

Jaw bandage.

2. From behind the head the bandage is carried forward underneath the earlobe and upward, crossing, respectively, the cheek bone, the injured eye, and the bridge of the nose; it is then returned to the original circular turns.
3. The head is encircled by the bandage, and the procedure is repeated, with each wrap overlapping at least two thirds of the underlying material over the injured eye.
4. When at least three series have been applied over the injured eye, the bandage is locked after completion of a circular turn around the head.

JAW BANDAGE

Bandages properly applied can be used to hold dressings and to stabilize dislocated or fractured jaws (Figure 9-11).

MATERIALS NEEDED: 2- or 3-inch gauze bandage roll, scissors, and 1½ - or 2-inch tape.

POSITION OF THE ATHLETE: Athlete sits in chair or on edge of table.

PROCEDURE
1. The bandage is started by encircling the jaw and head in front of both ears several times.
2. The bandage is locked by a number of turns around the head.
3. Each of the two sets of turns is fastened with tape strips.

GAUZE CIRCULAR WRIST BANDAGE

In training procedures the circular bandage (Figure 9-12) is used to cover a cylindrical area and to anchor other types of bandages.

MATERIALS NEEDED: One roll of 1- or 1½-inch gauze, 1-inch tape, and scissors.

POSITION OF THE ATHLETE: Athlete positions elbow at a 45-degree angle.

PROCEDURE
1. A turn is executed around the part at an oblique angle.
2. A small triangle of material is exposed by the oblique turn.

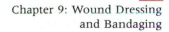

Figure 9-12

Circular wrist bandage.

3. The triangle is bent over the first turn, with succeeding turns made over the turned-down material, locking it in place.
4. After several turns have been made, the bandage is fastened at a point away from the injury.

GAUZE RECURRENT FINGER BANDAGE

This technique (Figure 9-13) is designed to hold a wound dressing on a finger.

MATERIALS NEEDED: One roll of ½ -inch gauze, ½-inch tape, and scissors.

POSITION OF THE ATHLETE: Athlete positions elbow at a 45-degree angle.

PROCEDURE

1. The gauze roll starts at the base of the finger dorsally and is extended up the full length of the finger and back down on the volar aspect. This procedure can be performed several times, depending on the thickness required.
2. After the finger has been covered vertically, a spiral pattern is started at the base, initially moved up to the distal aspect of the finger and then proximally down, continuing several times.
3. The spiral pattern is completed at the finger's distal end and is secured by a piece of tape.

GAUZE HAND AND WRIST FIGURE-8

A figure-8 bandage (Figure 9-14) can be used for mild wrist and hand support, as well as for holding dressings in place.

MATERIALS NEEDED: One roll of ½ -inch gauze, ½-inch tape, and scissors.

Figure 9-13

Recurrent finger bandage.

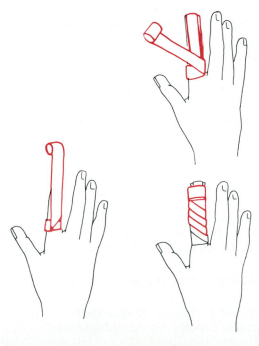

POSITION OF THE ATHLETE: Athlete positions elbow at a 45-degree angle.
PROCEDURE

1. The anchor is executed with one or two turns around the palm of the hand.
2. The roll is carried obliquely across the anterior or posterior portion of the hand, depending on the position of the wound, to the wrist, which it circles once, then it is returned to the primary anchor.
3. As many figures as needed are applied.

GAUZE FINGER BANDAGE

The finger bandage can be used to hold dressings or tongue depressor splints in place.
MATERIALS NEEDED: One roll of 1-inch gauze, ½-inch tape, and scissors.
POSITION OF THE ATHLETE: Athlete positions elbow at a 45-degree angle.
PROCEDURE: It is applied in a fashion similar to that described above, with the exception that a spiral is carried downward to the tip of the finger and then back up to finish around the wrist.

Triangular and Cravat Bandages

Triangular and cravat bandages, usually made of cotton cloth, may be used where roller types are not applicable or available.

The triangular and cravat bandages are primarily used as first aid devices. They are valuable in emergency bandaging because of their ease and speed of application. In sports the more diversified roller bandages are usually available and lend themselves more to the needs of the athlete. The principal use of the triangular bandage in athletic training is for arm slings. There are two basic kinds of slings, the cervical arm sling and the shoulder arm sling, and each has a specific purpose.

Triangular and cravat bandages allow ease and speed of application.

CERVICAL ARM SLING

The cervical arm sling (Figure 9-15) is designed to support the forearm, wrist, and hand. A triangular bandage is placed around the neck and under the bent arm that is to be supported.

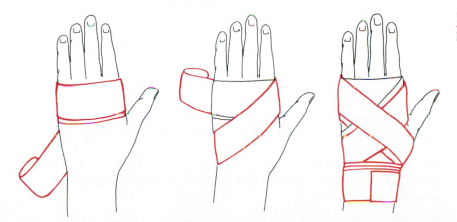

Figure 9-14

Hand and wrist figure-8.

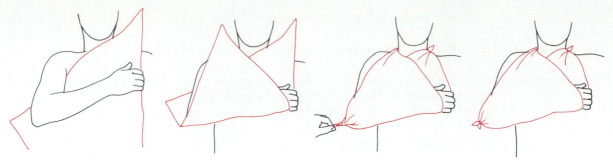

Figure 9-15

Cervical arm sling.

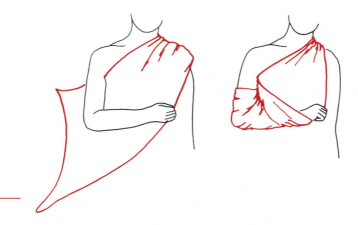

Figure 9-16

Shoulder arm sling.

MATERIALS NEEDED: One triangular bandage.

POSITION OF THE ATHLETE: The athlete stands with the affected arm bent at approximately a 70-degree angle.

PROCEDURE

1. The triangular bandage is positioned by the operator under the injured arm with the apex facing the elbow.
2. The end of the triangle nearest the body is carried over the shoulder of the uninjured arm; the other end is allowed to hang down loosely.
3. The loose end is pulled over the shoulder of the injured side.
4. The two ends of the bandage are tied in a square knot behind the neck. For the sake of comfort, the knot should be on either side of the neck, not directly in the middle.
5. The apex of the triangle is brought around to the front of the elbow and fastened by twisting the end, then tying in a knot.

NOTE: In cases in which greater arm stabilization is required than that afforded by a sling, an additional bandage can be swathed about the upper arm and body.

SHOULDER ARM SLING

The shoulder arm sling (Figure 9-16) is suggested for forearm support when there is an injury to the shoulder girdle or when the cervical arm sling is irritating to the athlete.

MATERIALS NEEDED: One triangle bandage and one safety pin.

POSITION OF THE ATHLETE: The athlete stands with his or her injured arm bent at approximately a 70-degree angle.

PROCEDURE

1. The upper end of the shoulder sling is placed over the *uninjured* shoulder side.
2. The lower end of the triangle is brought over the forearm and drawn between the upper arm and the body, swinging around the athlete's back and then upward to meet the other end, where a square knot is tied.
3. The apex end of the triangle is brought around to the front of the elbow and fastened with a safety pin.

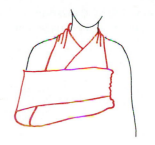

Figure 9-17

Sling and swathe.

SLING AND SWATHE

The sling and swathe combination is designed to stabilize the arm securely in cases of shoulder dislocation or fracture (Figure 9-17).

SUMMARY

Bandages, when properly applied, can contribute to recovery from sport injuries. Wounds should be properly cared for immediately. Cleanliness is of major importance at all times in the training room and on the field. Materials commonly used for bandages and dressing in sports are gauze, cotton cloth, elastic material, and plastics.

A large number of athletes each year receive severe wound infections due to improper care. Wound contamination can lead to the potentially fatal disease tetanus (lockjaw) if the athlete has not received a tetanus toxoid inoculation. The coach or athletic trainer may also be at risk in treating an AIDS-infected athlete. The wearing of latex gloves may prevent AIDS contamination. Skin wounds are categorized as abrasions, puncture wounds, lacerations, incisions, and avulsion wounds.

Common types of bandages used in sports are roller, triangular, and cravat for first aid and arm slings, of which the cervical and shoulder types are the most common. Common roller bandages are gauze for wounds, cotton cloth ankle wraps, and elastic wraps. As with taping, roller bandages must be applied uniformly, firmly but not so tightly as to impede circulation.

REVIEW QUESTIONS AND CLASS ACTIVITIES

1. What is the difference between a dressing and a bandage? What are the uses of each?
2. What are some common types of bandages used in sports medicine today? What are these bandages used for? How do you apply them?
3. Demonstrate the correct way of dressing a wound.

4. Observe the athletic trainer in dressing wounds in the training room.
5. Demonstrate proper use of the roller, triangular, and cravat bandages.

REFERENCES

1. Arnheim DD: *Modern principles of athletic training,* ed 8, St Louis, 1993, Times Mirror/Mosby College Publishing.
2. Hafen BQ: *First aid for health emergencies,* ed 4, St Paul, Minn, 1989, West Publishing.
3. National Safety Council: *Bloodborne pathogens,* Boston, 1993, Jones & Bartlett Publishers.
4. Parcel GS: *Basic emergency care of the sick and injured,* ed 4, St Louis, 1990, Times Mirror/Mosby College Publishing.

ANNOTATED BIBLIOGRAPHY

Athletic training, National Athletic Training Association, PO Box 1865, Greenville, NC 27835-1865.
    Each volume of this quarterly journal contains practical procedures for bandaging and taping as well as for orthotic application.

First aider, Gardner, Kan., Cramer Products. Published seven times throughout the school year. This periodical contains useful taping and bandaging techniques that have been submitted by readers.

National Safety Council: *First aid and CPR,* Boston, 1993, Jones & Bartlett Publishers.
    Chapter 5 provides an excellent discussion on wound care. *Sports Med Dig,* PO Box 2160, Van Nuys, CA 91404-2160.

Sports Med Guide, Mueller Sports Medicine, 1 Quench Dr, Prairie du Sac, WI 53578.
    Published four times a year, this quarterly often presents, along with discussions on specific injuries, many innovative taping and bandaging techniques.

Taping

When you finish this chapter, you will be able to:

- Demonstrate the basic skill in the use of taping in sports
- Demonstrate the skillful application of tape for a variety of musculoskeletal problems
- Demonstrate the application of the elastic wrap to major body parts

TAPING and bandaging are major skills used for the care of injuries and the protection of the athlete. This chapter presents some of the more prevalent taping techniques used in sports medicine and athletic training.

Historically, taping has been an important part of athletic training. It is one area of proficiency that the athletic trainer has, and it must be equated with other proficiency areas, such as customizing protective equipment and rehabilitation.

TAPE USAGE
Injury Care

When used for sports injuries, adhesive tape offers a number of possibilities:

- Retention of wound dressings
- Stabilization of compression-type bandages that control external and internal hemorrhaging
- Support of recent injuries to prevent additional insult that might result from the activities of the athlete

Injury Protection

Protecting against acute injuries is another major use of tape support. This protection can be achieved by limiting the motion of a body part or by securing some special device (see Chapter 5).

Linen Adhesive Tape

Modern adhesive tape has great adaptability for use in sports because of its uniform adhesive mass, adhering qualities, lightness, and the relative strength of the backing materials. All of these qualities are of value in holding wound dressings in place and in supporting and protecting injured areas. This tape comes in a variety of sizes; 1-, 1½-, and 2-inch (2.5, 3.75, and 5 cm) widths are commonly used in sports medicine. The tape also comes in tubes or special packs. Some popular packs provide greater tape length on each spool. When linen tape is purchased, factors such as cost, grade of backing, quality of adhesive mass, and properties of unwinding should be considered.

When purchasing linen tape, consider:
    Grade of backing
    Quality of adhesive mass
    Winding tension

Tape Grade

Linen-backed tape is most often graded according to the number of longitudinal and vertical fibers per inch of backing material. The heavier and more costly backing contains 85 or more longitudinal fibers and 65 vertical fibers per square inch. The lighter, less expensive grade has 65 or fewer longitudinal fibers and 45 vertical fibers.

Adhesive Mass

As a result of improvements in adhesive mass, certain essentials should be expected from tape. It should adhere readily when applied and should maintain this adherence in the presence of profuse perspiration and activity. Besides sticking well, the mass must contain as few skin irritants as possible and must be able to be removed easily without leaving a mass residue or pulling away the superficial skin.

Winding Tension

The winding tension of a tape roll is quite important to the operator. Sports place a unique demand on the unwinding quality of tape; if tape is to be applied for protection and support, there must be even and constant unwinding tension. In most cases a proper wind needs little additional tension to provide sufficient tightness.

Stretch Tape

Increasingly, tape with varying elasticity is being used in sports medicine, often in combination with linen tape. Because of its conforming qualities, stretch tape is used for the small, angular body parts, such as the feet, wrist, hands, and fingers. As with linen tape, stretch tape comes in a variety of widths.

Increasingly, tape with varying elasticity is being used in sports medicine.

Tape Storage

When storing tape, take the following steps:
1. Store in a cool place such as in a low cupboard.
2. Stack so that the tape rests on its flat top or bottom to avoid distortion.

Store tape in a cool place, and stack it flat.

Using Adhesive Tape in Sports

Preparation for Taping

Special attention must be given when applying tape directly to the skin. Perspiration and dirt collected during sport activities will prevent tape from properly sticking to the skin. Whenever tape is used, the skin surface should be cleansed with soap and water to remove all dirt and oil. Also, hair should be shaved to prevent additional irritation when the tape is removed. If additional adherence or protection from irritation is needed, a preparation containing rosin and a skin-toughening preparation should be applied. Commercial benzoin and skin toughener offer astringent action and dry readily, leaving a tacky residue to which tape will adhere firmly.

Taping directly on skin provides maximum support. However, applying tape day after day can lead to skin irritation. To overcome this problem many athletic trainers sacrifice some support by using a protective covering to the skin. The most popular is a moderately elastic commercial underwrap material that is extremely thin and fits snugly to the contours of the part to be taped. One commonly used underwrap material is polyester and urethane foam, which is fine, porous, extremely lightweight, and resilient. Proper use of an underwrap requires the part to be shaved and sprayed with a tape adherent. Underwrap material should be applied only one layer thick. It is also desirable to place a protective greased pad anterior and posterior to the ankle to prevent tape cuts and secondary infection.

Skin surface should be cleansed and hair should be shaved before applying tape.

Proper Taping Technique

The correct tape width depends on the area to be covered. The more acute the angles, the narrower the tape must be to fit the many contours. For example, the fingers and toes usually require ½- or 1-inch (1.25 or 2.5 cm) tape; the ankles require 1½-inch (3.75 cm) tape; and the larger skin areas such as thighs and back can accommodate 2- to 3-inch (5 to 7.5 cm) tape with ease. **NOTE:** *Supportive tape improperly applied can aggravate an existing injury or disrupt the mechanics of a body part, causing an initial injury to occur.*

Tearing Tape

Coaches and athletic trainers use various techniques in tearing tape (Figure 10-1). A method should permit the operator to keep the tape roll in hand most of the time. The following is a suggested procedure:

1. Hold the tape roll in the preferred hand, with the index finger hooked through the center of the tape roll and the thumb pressing its outer edge.
2. With the other hand, grasp the loose end between the thumb and index finger.
3. With both hands in place, pull both ends of the tape so that it is tight. Next, make a quick, scissorslike move to tear the tape. In tearing tape the movement of one hand is away from the body

To tear tape, move hands quickly in opposite directions.

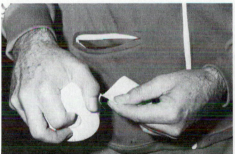

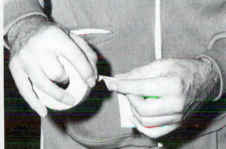

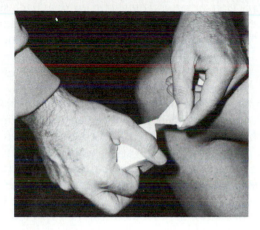

Figure 10-1

Methods of tearing
linen-backed tape.

and the other hand toward the body. Remember, do not try to
bend or twist the tape to tear it.

When tearing is properly executed, the torn edges of the linen-backed
tape are relatively straight, without curves, twists, or loose threads sticking out. Once the first thread is torn, the rest of the tape tears easily.
Learning to tear tape effectively from many different positions is essential for speed and efficiency. Many tapes other than the linen-backed type
cannot be torn manually but require a knife, scissors, or razor blade.

Rules for Tape Application

Included below are a few of the important rules to be observed in the
use of adhesive tape. In practice the athletic trainer will identify others.

1. *If the part to be taped is a joint, place it in the position in which it is to
   be stabilized.* If the part is musculature, make the necessary allowance for contraction and expansion.
2. *Overlap the tape at least half the width of the tape below.* Unless tape
   is overlapped sufficiently, the active athlete will separate it, exposing the underlying skin to irritation.
3. *Avoid continuous taping.* Tape continuously wrapped around a part
   may cause constriction. It is suggested that one turn be made at a
   time and that each encirclement be torn to overlap the starting

end by approximately 1 inch. This rule is particularly true of the nonyielding linen-backed tape.

4. *Keep the tape roll in hand whenever possible.* By learning to keep the tape roll in the hand, seldom laying it down, and by learning to tear the tape, an operator can develop taping speed and accuracy.

5. *Smooth and mold the tape as it is laid on the skin.* To save additional time, tape strips should be smoothed and molded to the body part as they are put in place; this is done by stroking the top with the fingers, palms, and heels of both hands.

6. *Allow tape to fit the natural contour of the skin.* Each strip of tape must be placed with a particular purpose in mind. Linen-backed tape is not sufficiently elastic to bend around acute angles but must be allowed to fall as it may, fitting naturally to the body contours. Failing to allow this fit creates wrinkles and gaps that can result in skin irritations.

7. *Start taping with an anchor piece and finish by applying a lock strip.* Commence taping, if possible, by sticking the tape to an anchor piece that encircles the part. This placement affords a good medium for the stabilization of succeeding tape strips, so that they will not be affected by the movement of the part.

8. *Where maximum support is desired, tape directly over skin.* In cases of sensitive skin, other mediums may be used as tape bases. With artificial bases, some movement can be expected between the skin and the base.

9. *Do not apply tape if skin is hot or cold from a therapeutic treatment.*

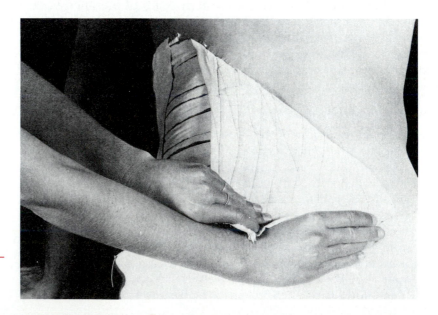

Figure 10-2

To remove tape from the body by hand, pull in a direct line with the body.

Removing Adhesive Tape

Tape usually can be removed from the skin by hand, by tape scissors or tape cutters, or by chemical solvents.

Manual removal   When pulling tape from the body, be careful not to tear or irritate the skin. Tape must not be wrenched in an outward direction from the skin but should be pulled in a direct line with the body (Figure 10-2). Remember to remove the skin carefully from the tape and not to peel the tape from the skin. One hand gently pulls the tape in one direction, and the opposite hand gently presses the skin away from the tape.

Use of tape scissors or cutters   The characteristic tape scissors have a blunt nose that slips underneath the tape smoothly without gouging the skin. Take care to avoid cutting the tape too near the site of the injury, lest the scissors aggravate the condition. Cut on the uninjured side.

Use of chemical solvents   When an adhesive mass is left on the skin after taping, a chemical agent may have to be used. Commercial cleaning solvents often contain a highly flammable agent. Take extreme care to store solvent in a cool place and in a tightly covered metal container. Extensive inhalation of benzene fumes has a toxic effect. Adequate ventilation should be maintained when using a solvent.

Peel the skin from the tape, not the tape from the skin.

COMMON TAPING PROCEDURES
The Foot
The Arch
ARCH TECHNIQUE NO. 1: WITH PAD SUPPORT

Arch taping with pad support uses the following procedures to strengthen weakened arches (Figure 10-3). NOTE: The longitudinal arch should be lifted.

MATERIALS NEEDED: One roll of 1½-inch (3.8 cm) tape, tape adherent, and a ⅛- or ¼-inch (0.3 or 0.6 cm) adhesive foam rubber pad or wool felt pad, cut to fit the longitudinal arch.

POSITION OF THE ATHLETE: The athlete lies face downward on the table with the foot that is to be taped extending approximately 6 inches (15 cm) over the edge of the table. To ensure proper position, allow the foot to hang in a relaxed position.

PROCEDURE

1. Place a series of strips of tape directly around the arch or, if added support is required, around an arch pad and the arch. The first strip should go just above the metatarsal arch (1).
2. Each successive strip overlaps the preceding piece about half the width of the tape (2 through 4).

CAUTION: Avoid putting on so many strips of tape as to hamper the action of the ankle.

ARCH TECHNIQUE NO. 2: THE X FOR THE LONGITUDINAL ARCH

When using the figure-8 method for taping the longitudinal arch, execute the following steps (Figure 10-4).

MATERIALS NEEDED: One roll of 1-inch tape and tape adherent.

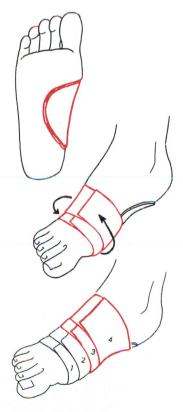

Figure 10-3

Arch taping technique no. 1, including an arch pad and circular tape strips.

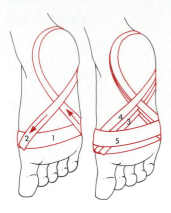

Figure 10-4

Arch taping technique no. 2 (X taping).

POSITION OF THE ATHLETE: The athlete lies face downward on a table, with the affected foot extending approximately 6 inches (15 cm) over the edge of the table. To ensure proper position, allow the foot to hang in a relaxed natural position.

PROCEDURE

1. Lightly place an anchor strip around the ball of the foot, making certain not to constrict the action of the toes (1).
2. Start tape strip 2 from the lateral edge of the anchor. Move it upward at an acute angle, cross the center of the longitudinal arch, encircle the heel, and descend. Then, cross the arch again and end at the medial aspect of the anchor (2). Repeat three or four times (3 and 4).
3. Lock the taped Xs with a single piece of tape placed around the ball of foot.

After **X** strips are applied, cover entire arch with 1½-inch circular tape strips.

ARCH TECHNIQUE NO. 3: THE X TEAR DROP ARCH AND FOREFOOT SUPPORT

As its name implies, this taping both supports the longitudinal arch and stabilizes the forefoot into good alignment (Figure 10-5).

MATERIALS NEEDED: One roll of 1-inch (2.5 cm) tape and tape adherent.

POSITION OF THE ATHLETE: The athlete lies face down on a table, with the foot to be taped extending approximately 6 inches (15 cm) over the edge of the table.

PROCEDURE

1. Place an anchor strip around the ball of the foot (1).
2. Start tape strip 2 on the side of the foot, beginning at the base of the great toe. Take the tape around the heel, crossing the arch and returning to the starting point (2).
3. The pattern of the third strip of tape is the same as the second strip except that it is started on the little toe side of the foot (3). Repeat two or three times (4 through 6).
4. Lock each series of strips by placing tape around the ball joint. A completed procedure usually consists of a series of three strips.

ARCH TECHNIQUE NO. 4: FAN ARCH SUPPORT

Fan Arch technique No. 4 supports the entire plantar aspect of the foot (Figure 10-6).

MATERIALS NEEDED: One roll of 1-inch (2.5 cm) tape and tape adherent. One roll 1½-inch tape.

POSITION OF THE ATHLETE: The athlete lies face down on a table, with the foot to be taped extending approximately 6 inches (15 cm) over the edge of the table.

PROCEDURE:

1. Place an anchor strip around the ball of the foot (1).
2. Starting at the third metatarsal head, take the tape around the heel from the lateral side and meet the strip where it began (2 and 3).
3. The next strip starts near the second metatarsal head and finishes on the fourth metatarsal head (4).

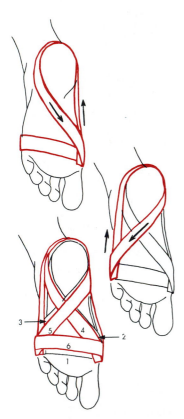

Figure 10-5

Arch taping technique no. 3, with double **X** and forefoot support.

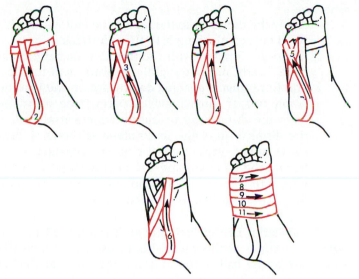

Figure 10-6

Fan arch taping technique.

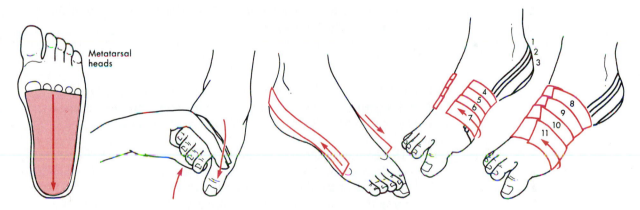

Figure 10-7

LowDye taping technique for fallen medial longitudinal arch, foot pronation, arch strains, and plantar fasciitis.

4. The last strip begins on the fourth metatarsal head and finishes on the fifth (5). The technique, when completed, forms a fan-shaped pattern covering the metatarsal region (6).
5. Lock strips (7 through 11) using 1½-inch tape encircling the complete arch.

LOWDYE TECHNIQUE

The LowDye technique is an excellent method for managing the fallen medial longitudinal arch, foot pronation, arch strains, and plantar fasciitis. Moleskin is cut in 3-inch (7.5 cm) strips to the shape of the sole of the foot. It should cover the head of the metatarsal bones and the calcaneus bone (Figure 10-7).

MATERIALS NEEDED: One roll of 1-inch (2.5 cm) and one roll of 2-inch (5 cm) tape and moleskin.

POSITION OF THE ATHLETE: The athlete sits with the foot in a neutral position with the great toe and medial aspect of the foot in plantar flexion.

PROCEDURE

1. Apply the moleskin to the sole of the foot, pulling it slightly downward before attaching it to the calcaneus.
2. Grasp the forefoot with the thumb under the distal 2 to 5 metatarsal heads, pushing slightly upward, with the tips of the second and third fingers pushing downward on the first metatarsal head. Apply two or three 1-inch (2.5 cm) tape strips laterally, starting from the distal head of the fifth metatarsal bone and ending at the distal head of the first metatarsal bone (1 through 3). Keep these lateral strips below the outer malleolus.
3. Secure the moleskin and lateral tape strip by circling the forefoot with four 2-inch (5 cm) strips (4 through 7). Start at the lateral dorsum of the foot, circle under the plantar aspect, and finish at the medial dorsum of the foot. Apply four strips of 2-inch stretch-tape strips that encircle the arch (8 through 11).

NOTE: A variation of this method is to use two 2-inch (5 cm) moleskin strips, one at the ball of the foot and the other at the base of the fifth metatarsal. Cross the strips and extend them along the plantar surface of the foot; angle them over the center of the heel and 2 inches up the back of the foot. For anchors, apply 2-inch (5 cm) elastic tape around the forefoot, lateral to medial, giving additional support.

The Toes

THE SPRAINED GREAT TOE

This procedure is used for taping a sprained great toe (Figure 10-8).

MATERIALS NEEDED: One roll of 1-inch (2.5 cm) tape and tape adherent.

POSITION OF THE ATHLETE: The athlete assumes a sitting position.

PROCEDURE

1. The greatest support is given to the joint by a half-figure-8 taping (1 through 3). Start the series at an acute angle on the top of the foot and swing down between the great and first toes, first encircling the great toe and then coming up, over, and across the starting point. Repeat this process, starting each series separately.
2. After the required number of half-figure-8 strips are in position, place one lock piece around the ball of the foot (4).

HAMMER, OR CLAWED, TOES

This technique is designed to reduce the pressure of the bent toes against the shoe (Figure 10-9).

MATERIALS NEEDED: One roll of ½- or 1-inch (1.25 or 2.5 cm) adhesive tape and tape adherent.

POSITION OF THE ATHLETE: The athlete sits on a table with the affected leg extended over the edge.

PROCEDURE

1. Tape one affected toe; then lace under the adjacent toe and over the next toe.
2. Tape can be attached to the next toe or can be continued and attached to the fifth toe.

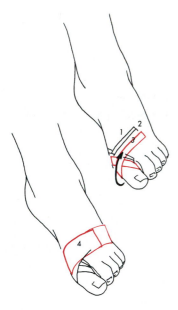

Figure 10-8

Taping for a sprained great toe.

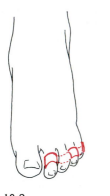

Figure 10-9

Taping for hammer or clawed toes.

FRACTURED TOES

MATERIALS NEEDED: One roll of ½- to 1-inch (1.25 to 2.5 cm) tape, ⅛-inch (0.82 cm) sponge rubber, and tape adherent.

POSITION OF THE ATHLETE: The athlete assumes a sitting position.

PROCEDURE

1. Cut a ⅛-inch sponge rubber wedge and place it between the affected toe and a healthy one.
2. Wrap two or three strips of tape around the toes (Figure 10-10). This technique splints the fractured toe with a nonfractured one.

BUNIONS

MATERIALS NEEDED: One roll of 1-inch (2.5 cm) tape, tape adherent, and ¼-inch (0.62 cm) sponge rubber or felt.

POSITION OF THE ATHLETE: The athlete assumes a sitting position.

PROCEDURE

1. Cut the ¼-inch sponge rubber to form a wedge between the great and second toes.
2. Place anchor strips to encircle the midfoot and distal aspect of the great toe (Figure 10-11, 1 and 2).
3. Place two or three strips on the medial aspect of the great toe to hold the toe in proper alignment (3 through 5).
4. Lock the ends of the strips with tape (6 and 7).

The Ankle Joint

ROUTINE NONINJURY

Ankle taping applied directly to the athlete's skin affords the greatest support; however, when applied and removed daily, skin irritation will occur. To avoid this problem apply an underwrap material. Before taping, follow these procedures:

1. Shave all the hair off the foot and ankle.
2. Apply a coating of a tape adherent to protect the skin and offer an adhering base.

    NOTE: It may be advisable to avoid the use of a tape adherent, especially if the athlete has a history of developing tape blisters. In cases of skin sensitivity the ankle surface should be thoroughly

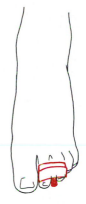

Figure 10-10

Taping for fracture of a toe.

If the athlete has sensitive skin, thoroughly clean the area to be wrapped.

Figure 10-11

Taping for a bunion.

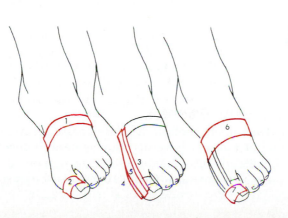

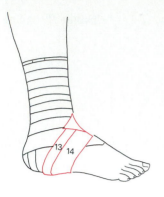

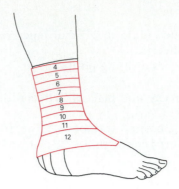

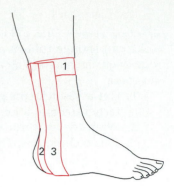

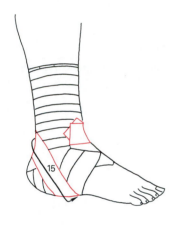

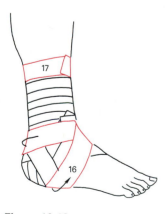

Figure 10-12

Routine noninjury ankle taping.

cleansed of dirt and oil and an underwrap material applied; or tape directly to the skin.

3. Apply a gauze pad coated with friction-proofing material such as grease over the instep and to the back of the heel.

4. If underwrap is used, apply a single layer. The tape anchors extend beyond the underwrap and adhere directly to the skin.

5. Do not apply tape if skin is cold or hot from a therapeutic treatment.

MATERIALS NEEDED: One roll of 1½-inch (3.8 cm) tape and tape adherent.

POSITION OF THE ATHLETE: The athlete sits on a table with the leg extended and the foot held at a 90-degree angle.

PROCEDURE

1. Place an anchor around the ankle approximately 5 or 6 inches (12.7 to 15.2 cm) above the malleolus (Figure 10-12, 1).

2. Apply two strips in consecutive order, starting behind the outer malleolus, with care that each one overlaps half the width of the piece of tape it adjoins (2 and 3).

3. After applying the strips, wrap seven or eight circular strips around the ankle, from the point of the anchor downward until the malleolus is completely covered (4 through 12).

4. Apply two or three arch strips from lateral to medial, giving additional support to the arch (13 through 15).

5. Additional support is given by a heel lock. Starting high on the instep, bring the tape along the ankle at a slight angle, hooking the heel, leading under the arch, then coming up on the opposite side, and finishing at the starting point. Tear the tape to complete half of the heel lock (16). Repeat on the opposite side of the ankle. Finish with a band of tape around the ankle (17).

OPEN BASKETWEAVE

This modification of the closed basketweave, or Gibney, technique is designed to give freedom of movement in dorsiflexion and plantar flexion while providing lateral and medial support and giving swelling room. Taping in this pattern (Figure 10-13) may be used immediately after an acute

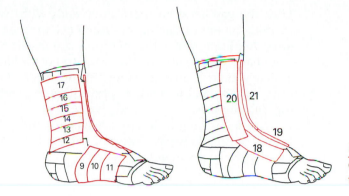

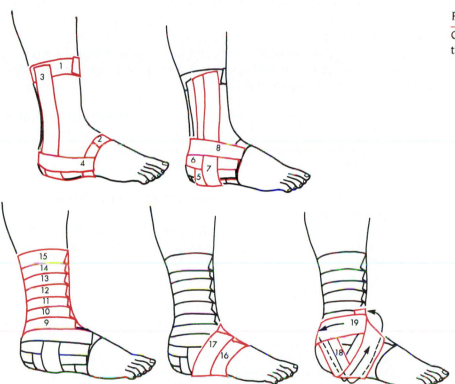

Figure 10-13

Open basketweave ankle taping.

Figure 10-14

Closed basketweave ankle taping.

sprain in conjunction with a pressure bandage and cold applications, since it allows for swelling.

MATERIALS NEEDED: One roll of 1½-inch (3.8 cm) tape and tape adherent.

POSITION OF THE ATHLETE: The athlete sits on a table with the leg extended and the foot held at a 90-degree angle.

PROCEDURE

1. The procedures are the same as for the closed basketweave (Figure 10-14) with the exception of incomplete closures of the Gibney strips.

2. Lock the gap between the Gibney ends with two pieces of tape
running on either side of the instep (11 through 21).
NOTE: Application of a 1½-inch (3.8 cm) elastic bandage over the
open basketweave affords added control of swelling; however, the
athlete should remove it before retiring. Apply the elastic bandage
distal to proximal to assist in preventing the swelling from moving into the toes.

Of the many ankle-taping techniques in vogue today, those using combinations of strips, basketweave pattern, and heel lock have been determined to offer the best support.

CLOSED BASKETWEAVE (GIBNEY)

The closed basketweave technique (Figure 10-14) offers strong tape support and is primarily used in athletic training for newly sprained or
chronically weak ankles.

MATERIALS NEEDED: One roll of 1½-inch (3.8 cm) tape and tape adherent.

POSITION OF THE ATHLETE: The athlete sits on a table with the leg extended
and the foot at a 90-degree angle.

PROCEDURE

1. Place one anchor piece around the ankle approximately 5 or 6
inches (12.7 or 15.2 cm) above the malleolus just below the belly
of the gastrocremius muscle, and a second anchor around the instep directly over the styloid process of the fifth metatarsal
(1 and 2).
2. Apply the first strips posteriorly to the malleolus and attach it to
the ankle strips (3).
NOTE: When applying strips, pull the foot into eversion for
an inversion strain and into a neutral position for an eversion
strain.
3. Start the first Gibney directly under the malleolus and attach it to
the foot anchor (4).
4. In an alternating series place three strips and three Gibneys on
the ankle with each piece of tape overlapping at least half of the
preceding strip (5 through 8).
5. After applying the basketweave series, continue the Gibney strips
up the ankle, thus giving circular support (9 through 15).
6. For arch support apply two or three circular strips lateral to medial (16 and 17).
7. After completing the conventional basketweave, apply two or
three heel locks to ensure maximum stability (18 and 19).

CONTINUOUS STRETCH TAPE TECHNIQUE

This technique provides a fast alternative to other taping methods for the
ankle (Figure 10-15).[3]

MATERIALS NEEDED: One roll of 1½-inch (3.75 cm) linen tape, one roll of
2-inch (5 cm) stretch tape, and tape adherent.

POSITION OF THE ATHLETE: The athlete sits on a table with the leg extended
and the foot at a 90-degree angle.

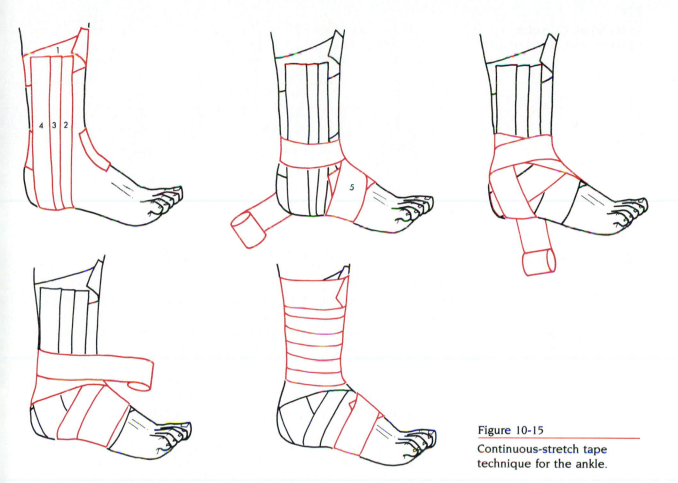

Figure 10-15

Continuous-stretch tape technique for the ankle.

PROCEDURE

1. Place one anchor strip around the ankle approximately 5 to 6 inches (12.5 to 15 cm) above the malleolus (1).
2. Apply three strips, covering the malleolli (2 through 4).
3. Start the stretch tape in a medial-to-lateral direction around the midfoot and continue it in a figure-8 pattern to above the lateral malleolus (5).
4. Continue to stretch tape across the midfoot, then across the heel.
5. Apply two heel locks, one in one direction and one in the reverse direction.
6. Next, repeat a figure-8 pattern followed by a spiral pattern, filling the space up to the anchor.
7. Use the lock technique at the top with a linen tape strip.

The Lower Leg

ACHILLES TENDON

Achilles tendon taping (Figure 10-16) is designed to prevent the Achilles tendon from overstretching.

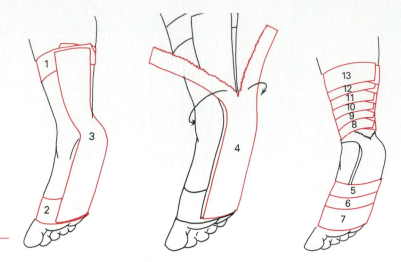

Figure 10-16

Achilles tendon taping.

MATERIALS NEEDED: One roll of 3-inch (7.5 cm) elastic tape, one roll of 1½-inch (3.8 cm) linen tape, and tape adherent.

POSITION OF THE ATHLETE: The athlete kneels or lies face down, with the affected foot hanging relaxed over the edge of the table.

PROCEDURE

1. Apply two anchors with 1½-inch (3.8 cm) tape, one circling the leg loosely approximately 7 to 9 inches (17.8 to 22.9 cm) above the malleoli, and the other encircling the ball of the foot (1 and 2).

2. Cut two strips of 3-inch (7.5 cm) elastic tape approximately 8 to 10 inches (20 to 25 cm) long. Moderately stretch the first strip from the ball of the athlete's foot along its plantar aspect up to the leg anchor (3). The second elastic strip (4) follows the course of the first, but cut it and split it down the middle lengthwise. Wrap the cut ends around the lower leg to form a lock. CAUTION: Keep the wrapped ends above the level of the strain.

3. Complete the series by placing two or three lock strips of elastic tape (5 through 7) loosely around the arch and five or six strips (8 through 13) around the athlete's lower leg.

NOTES:

1. Locking too tightly around the lower leg and foot will tend to restrict the normal action of the Achilles tendon and create more tissue irritation.

2. A variation to this method is to use three 2-inch-wide (5 cm) elastic strips in place of strips 3 and 4. Apply the first strip at the plantar surface of the first metatarsal head and end it on the lateral side of the leg anchor. Apply the second strip at the plantar surface of the fifth metatarsal head and end it on the medial side of the leg anchor. Center the third strip between the other two strips and end it at the posterior aspect of the calf. Wrap strips of 3-inch elastic tape around the forefoot and lower calf to close them off.[1]

MEDIAL SHINSPLINTS

Proper taping can afford some relief of the symptoms of shinsplints (Figure 10-17).

MATERIALS NEEDED: One roll of 1½-inch (3.75 cm) linen or elastic tape and adherent.

POSITION OF THE ATHLETE: The athlete sits on a table with the knee bent and the foot flat on the table. The purpose of this position is to fully relax the muscles of the lower leg.

PROCEDURE

1. Apply two anchor tape strips, the first to the anterolateral aspect of the ankle and lower leg and the second to the posterolateral aspect of the midcalf (1 and 2).
2. Starting at the lowest end of the first anchor, run a strip of tape to the back of the lower leg, spiraling it over the shin to attach on the lower end of the second anchor strip. Apply three strips of tape in this manner, with each progressively moving upward on the leg. As each strip comes across the previous strip, make an effort to pull the muscle toward the tibia (3 through 9).
3. After applying seven pieces of tape, lock their ends with one or two cross-strips (10 and 11).
4. After completing the procedure, you may apply an elastic wrap in a spiral fashion.

NOTE: A variation to this method is to place a ½-inch thickness of felt 1 inch wide by 6 inches long on the medial border of the tibia secured by underwrap. Beginning distally, use 6-inch strips of white tape to hold the pad in place and provide support. The strips do not encircle the leg but are completely covered by elastic tape or a 3-inch elastic bandage.[2]

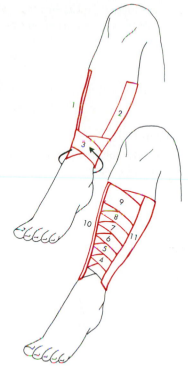

Figure 10-17

Taping for shinsplints.

The Knee

MEDIAL COLLATERAL LIGAMENT

As with ankle instabilities, the athlete with an unstable knee should never use tape and bracing as a replacement for proper exercise rehabilitation. If properly applied, taping can help protect the knee and aid in the rehabilitation process (Figure 10-18).[4]

MATERIALS NEEDED: One roll of 2-inch (5 cm) linen tape, one roll of 3-inch (7.5 cm) elastic tape, a 1-inch (2.5 cm) heel lift, and skin adherent.

POSITION OF THE ATHLETE: The athlete stands on a 3-foot (90 cm) table with the injured knee held in a moderately relaxed position by a 1-inch (2.5 cm) heel lift. The hair is completely removed from an area 6 inches (15 cm) above to 6 inches (15 cm) below the patella.

PROCEDURE

1. Lightly encircle the thigh and leg at the hairline with a 3-inch (7.5 cm) elastic anchor strip (1 and 2).
2. Precut 12 elastic tape strips, each approximately 9 inches (22.5 cm) long. Stretching them to their utmost, apply them to the knee as indicated in Figure 10-18 (3 through 14).
3. Apply a series of three strips of 2-inch (5 cm) linen tape (15

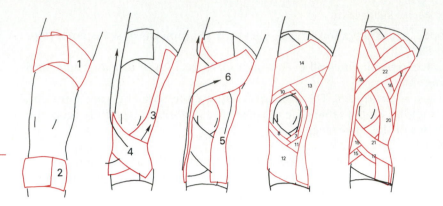

Figure 10-18

Taping for injuries to the
collateral ligament of the
knee.

through 22). Some individuals find it advantageous to complete a
knee taping by wrapping loosely with an elastic wrap, thus providing an added precaution against the tape's coming loose from
perspiration.

NOTE: Precaution—tape must not constrict patella.

ROTARY TAPING FOR INSTABILITY OF AN INJURED KNEE

The rotary taping method is designed to provide the knee with support
when it is unstable from injury to the medial collateral and anterior cruciate ligaments (Figure 10-19).

MATERIALS NEEDED: One roll of 3-inch (7.5 cm) elastic tape, skin adherent,
4-inch (10 cm) gauze pad, and scissors.

POSITION OF THE ATHLETE: The athlete sits on a table with the affected knee
flexed 15 degrees.

PROCEDURE

1. Cut a 10-inch (25 cm) piece of elastic tape with both the ends
   snipped. Place the gauze pad in the center of the 10-inch (25 cm)
   piece of elastic tape to limit skin irritation and protect the popliteal nerves and blood vessels.
2. Put the gauze with the elastic tape backing on the popliteal fossa
   of the athlete's knee. Stretch both ends of the tape to the fullest
   extent and tear them. Place the divided ends firmly around the
   patella and interlock them (1).
3. Starting at a midpoint on the gastrocremius muscle, spiral a 3-inch
   (7.5 cm) elastic tape strip to the front of the leg, then behind,
   crossing the popliteal fossa, and around the thigh, finishing anteriorly (2).
4. Repeat procedure 3 on the opposite side (3).
5. You may apply three or four spiral strips for added strength (4 and
   5).
6. Once they are in place, lock the spiral strips by the application of
   two strips around the thigh and two around the calf (6 and 7).

NOTE: Tracing the spiral pattern with linen tape yields more rigidity.

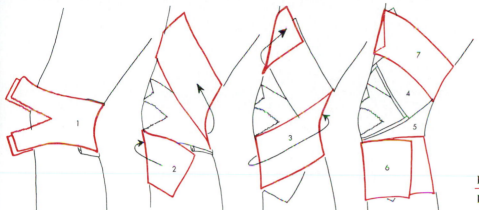

Figure 10-19

Rotary taping for instability in an injured knee.

HYPEREXTENSION

Hyperextension taping (Figure 10-20) is designed to prevent the knee from hyperextending and also may be used for strained hamstring muscles or slackened cruciate ligaments.

MATERIALS NEEDED: One roll of 2½-inch (5.5 cm) tape or 2-inch (5 cm) elastic tape, cotton or a 4-inch (10 cm) gauze pad, tape adherent, underwrap, and a 2-inch (5 cm) heel lift.

POSITION OF THE ATHLETE: The athlete's leg should be completely shaved above midthigh and below midcalf. The athlete stands on a 3-foot (90 cm) table with the injured knee flexed by a 2-inch (5 cm) heel lift.

PROCEDURE

1. Place two anchor strips at the hairlines, two around the thigh, and two around the leg (1 through 4). They should be loose enough to allow for muscle expansion during exercise.
2. Place a gauze pad at the popliteal space to protect the popliteal nerves and blood vessels from constriction by the tape.
3. Start the supporting tape strips by forming an **X** over the popliteal space (5 and 6).
4. Cross the tape again with two more strips and one up the middle of the leg (7 through 9).
5. Complete the technique by applying four or five locking strips around the thigh and calf (10 through 18).
6. Apply an additional series of strips if the athlete is heavily muscled.
7. Lock the supporting strips in place by applying two or three overlapping circles around the thigh and leg.

PATELLOFEMORAL TAPING (MCCONNELL TECHNIQUE)

Patellofemoral orientation may be corrected to some degree by using tape. The McConnell technique evaluates four components of patellar orientation: glide, tilt, rotation, and anteroposterior (AP) orientation.[6]

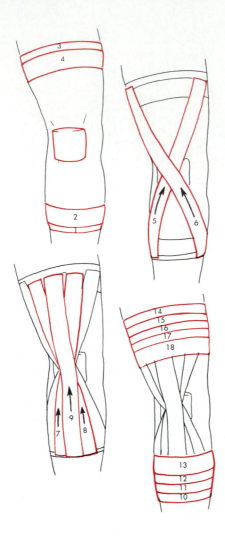

Figure 10-20

Hyperextension taping.

The glide component looks at side-to-side movement of the patella in the groove. The tile component assesses the height of the lateral patellar border relative to the medical border. Patellar rotation is determined by looking for deviation of the long axis of the patella from the long axis of the femur. Anteroposterior alignment evaluates whether the inferior pole of the patella is tilted either anteriorly or posteriorly relative to the superior pole. Correction of patellar position and tracking is accomplished by passive taping of the patella in a more biomechanically correct position. In addition to correcting the orientation of the patella, the tape provides a prolonged gentle stretch to soft-tissue structures that affect patellar movement.[6]

MATERIALS NEEDED: Two special types of extremely sticky tape are required. Fixomull and Leuko Sportape are manufactured by Biersdorf Australia, Ltd.

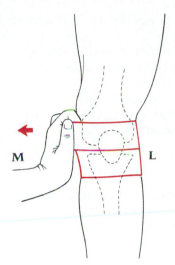

Figure 10-21

The first two strips of tape in the McConnell technique serve as the base to which additional tape is adhered.

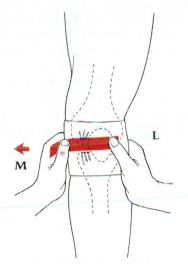

Figure 10-22

Taping technique to correct a lateral glide of the patella.

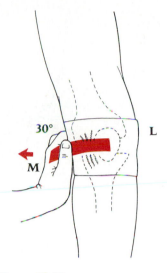

Figure 10-23

Taping technique to correct a lateral tilt of the patella.

POSITION OF THE ATHLETE: The athlete should be seated with the knee in full extension.

PROCEDURE

1. Two strips of Fixomull are extended from the lateral femoral condyle just posterior to the medial femoral condyle around the front of the knee. This tape is used as a base to which the other tape may be adhered. Leuko Sportape is used from this point on to correct patellar alignment (Figure 10-21).

2. To correct a lateral glide, attach a short strip of tape one thumb's width from the lateral patellar border, pushing the patella medially in the frontal plane. Crease the skin between the lateral patellar border and the medial femoral condyle and secure the tape on the medial side of the joint (Figure 10-22).

3. To correct a lateral tilt, flex the knee to 30 degrees, adhere a short strip of tape beginning at the middle of the patella, and pull medially to lift the lateral border. Again, crease the skin underneath and adhere it to the medial side of the knee (Figure 10-23).

4. To correct an external rotation of the inferior pole relative to the superior pole, adhere a strip of tape to the middle of the inferior pole, pulling upward and medially while internally rotating the patella with the free hand. The tape is attached to the medial side of the knee (Figure 10-24).

5. For correcting AP alignment in which there is an inferior tilt, take a 6-inch piece of tape, place the middle of the strip over the up-

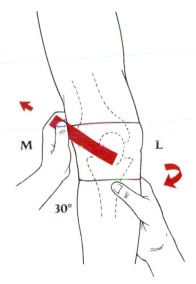

Figure 10-24

Taping technique to correct external rotation of the inferior pole of the patella.

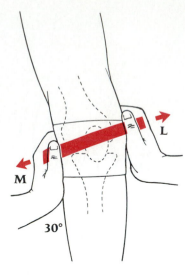

Figure 10-25

Taping technique to correct AP alignment with an inferior tilt.

per one half of the patella and attach it equally on both sides to lift the inferior pole (Figure 10-25).

6. Once patellar taping is completed, the athlete should be instructed to wear the tape all day during all activities. The athlete should periodically tighten the strips as they loosen.

NOTE: The McConnell technique for treating patellofemoral pain also stresses the importance of more symmetrical loading of the patella through reeducation and strengthening of the vastus medialis.[1]

The Thigh

QUADRICEPS SUPPORT

The taping of the quadriceps muscle group (Figure 10-26) is designed to give support against the pull of gravity. In cases of moderate or severe contusions or strains, taping may afford protection or mild support and give confidence to the athlete. Various techniques fitted to the individual needs of the athletes can be used.

MATERIALS NEEDED: One roll of 1½- or 2-inch (3.75 or 5 cm) tape, skin toughener, and a 6-inch (15 cm) elastic bandage.

POSITION OF THE ATHLETE: The athlete stands on the massage table with leg extended.

PROCEDURE

1. Place two anchor strips, each approximately 9 inches (22.5 cm) long, respectively, on the lateral and medial aspects of the thigh, half the distance between the anterior and posterior aspects (1 and 2).

2. Apply strips of tape to the thigh, crossing one another to form an X. Begin the crisscrosses 2 or 3 inches (5 or 7.5 cm) above the kneecap and carry them upward, overlapping one another. It is important to start each tape strip at the anchor piece and carry it upward and diagonally over the quadriceps, lifting against gravity. Continue this procedure until the quadriceps is completely covered (3 through 9).

3. After applying the diagonal series, place a lock strip longitudinally over the medial and lateral borders of the series (11 and 12).

4. To ensure more effective stability of the quadriceps taping, encircle the entire thigh with either a 3-inch (7.5 cm) elastic tape or a 6-inch (15 cm) elastic bandage, paying special attention to lift against gravity for additional support.

HAMSTRING SUPPORT

It is extremely difficult to relieve the injured hamstring muscles completely by any wrapping or taping technique, but some stabilization can be afforded by each. The hamstring taping technique (Figure 10-27) is designed to stabilize the moderately to severely contused or torn hamstring muscles, enabling the athlete to continue to compete.

MATERIALS NEEDED: One roll of 2- or 1½-inch (5 or 3.75 cm) tape, skin toughener, and a roll of 3-inch (7.5 cm) elastic tape or a 6-inch (15 cm) elastic wrap.

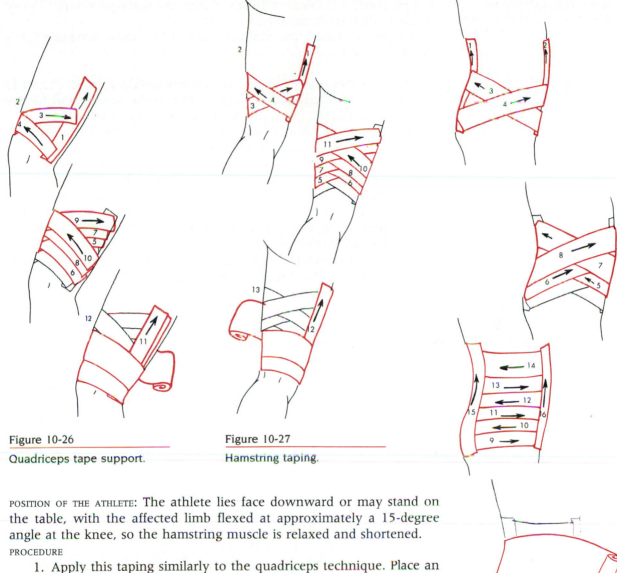

Figure 10-26

Quadriceps tape support.

Figure 10-27

Hamstring taping.

Figure 10-28

Iliac tape support.

POSITION OF THE ATHLETE: The athlete lies face downward or may stand on the table, with the affected limb flexed at approximately a 15-degree angle at the knee, so the hamstring muscle is relaxed and shortened.

PROCEDURE

1. Apply this taping similarly to the quadriceps technique. Place an anchor strip on either side of the thigh (1 and 2), and then crisscross strips, approximately 9 inches (22.5 cm) in length, diagonally upward on the posterior aspect of the thigh, forming an **X** (3 through 11).

2. After the hamstring area is covered with a series of crisscrosses, apply a longitudinal lock on either side of the thigh (12 and 13).

3. Place 3-inch (7.5 cm) elastic tape or a 6-inch (15 cm) elastic wrap around the thigh if needed to hold the crisscross taping in place.

ILIAC SUPPORT

Iliac crest adhesive taping (Figure 10-28) is designed to support, protect, and immobilize the soft tissue surrounding the iliac crest.

MATERIALS NEEDED: One roll of 2-inch (5 cm) adhesive tape, 6-inch (15 cm) bandage, skin toughener, and tape adherent.

POSITION OF THE ATHLETE: The athlete stands on the floor, bending slightly laterally toward the injured side.

PROCEDURE

1. Apply two anchor strips, each approximately 9 inches (22.5 cm) long, one longitudinally, just lateral to the sacrum and lumbar spine, and the other lateral to the umbilicus (1 and 2).
2. Commencing 2 to 3 inches (5 to 7.5 cm) below the crest of the ilium, tape crisscrosses from one anchor to the other, lifting the tissue against the pull of gravity. Carry the crisscrosses upward to a point just below the floating rib (3 through 8).
3. If additional support is desired, lay horizontal strips on alternately in posteroanterior and anteroposterior directions (9 through 14).
4. Put lock strips over approximately the same positions as the anchor strips (15 and 16).
5. Apply a 6-inch (15 cm) elastic bandage to secure the tape and to prevent perspiration from loosening the taping.

Figure 10-29

Sternoclavicular
immobilization.

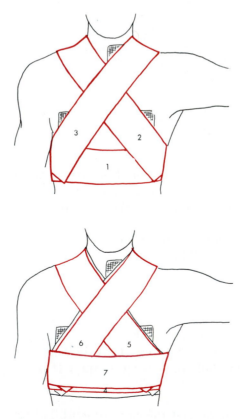

The Shoulder

STERNOCLAVICULAR IMMOBILIZATION

MATERIALS NEEDED: A felt pad ¼ inch (0.63 cm) thick, cut to a circumference of 4 inches (10 cm); 3-inch (7.5 cm) roll of elastic tape; two gauze pads; and tape adherent.

POSITION OF THE ATHLETE: Reduction of the most common sternoclavicular dislocation is performed by traction, with the athlete's arm abducted. Traction and abduction are maintained by an assistant while the immobilization taping is applied.

PROCEDURE

1. Apply an anchor strip around the chest at the level of the tenth rib while the chest is expanded (Figure 10-29, 1).
2. Lay a felt pad over the sternoclavicular joint and apply gauze pads over the athlete's nipples.
3. Depending on the direction of displacement, apply tape pressure over the felt pad. With the most common dislocation (upward, forward, and anterior), taping starts from the back and moves forward over the shoulder. The first pressure strip runs from the anchor tape on the unaffected side over the injured site to the front anchor strip (2).
4. A second strip goes from the anchor strip on the affected side over the unaffected side to finish on the front anchor strip (3).
5. Apply as many series of strips as are needed to give complete immobilization (4 through 6). Lock all series in place with a tape strip placed over the ends (7).

ACROMIOCLAVICULAR SUPPORT

Protective acromioclavicular taping (Figure 10-30) is designed to stabilize the acromioclavicular articulation in proper alignment and still allow normal movement of the shoulder complex.

MATERIALS NEEDED: One ¼-inch (0.63 cm) thick felt pad, roll of 2-inch (5 cm) adhesive tape, tape adherent, 2-inch (5 cm) gauze pad, and 3-inch (7.5 cm) elastic bandage.

Figure 10-30

Protective acromioclavicular taping.

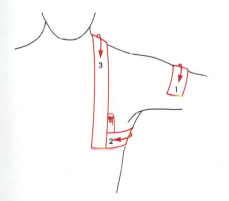
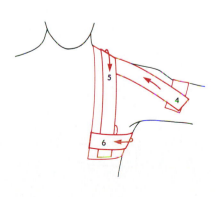
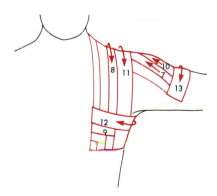

POSITION OF THE ATHLETE: The athlete sits in a chair with the affected arm resting in a position of abduction.

PROCEDURE

1. Apply three anchor strips: the first in a three-quarter circle just below the deltoid muscle (1); the second just below the nipple, encircling half the chest (2); and the third over the trapezius muscle near the neck, attaching to the second anchor in front and back (3).

2. Apply the first and second strips of tape from the front and back of the first anchor, crossing them at the acromioclavicular articulation and attaching them to the third anchor strip (4).

3. Place the third support over the ends of the first and second pieces, following the line of the third anchor strip (5).

4. Lay a fourth support strip over the second anchor strip (6).

5. Continue this basketweave pattern until the entire shoulder complex is covered. Follow it with the application of a shoulder spica with an elastic bandage (7 through 13).

SHOULDER SUPPORT AND RESTRAINT

This taping supports the soft tissues of the shoulder complex and restrains the arm from abducting more than 90 degrees (Figure 10-31).

Figure 10-31

Taping for shoulder support and restraint.

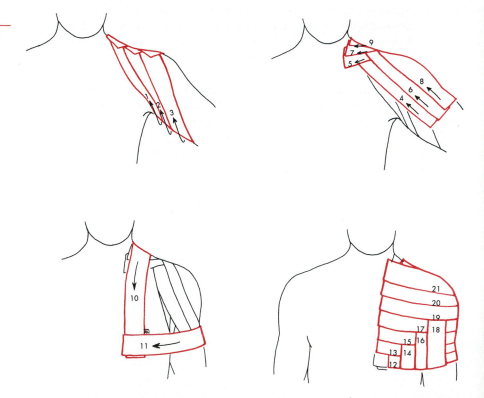

MATERIALS NEEDED: One roll of 2-inch (5 cm) tape, 2-inch (5 cm) gauze pad, cotton pad, tape adherent, and 3-inch (7.5 cm) elastic bandage.

POSITION OF THE ATHLETE: The athlete stands with the affected arm flexed at the elbow and the shoulder internally rotated and slightly abducted.

PROCEDURE

1. The first phase is designed to support the capsule of the shoulder joint. After placing a cotton pad in the axilla, run a series of three loops around the shoulder joint (1 through 3). Start the first loop at the top of the athlete's scapula, pull it forward across the acromion process, around the front of the shoulder, back underneath the axilla, and over the back of the shoulder, crossing the acromion process again. Terminate it at the clavicle. Begin each of the subsequent strips down the shoulder half the width of the preceding strip.

2. Run strips of tape upward from a point just below the insertion of the deltoid muscle and cross them over the acromion process, completely covering the outer surface of the shoulder joint (4 through 8).

3. Before the final application of a basketweave shoulder taping, place a gauze pad over the nipple area and bring the arm back to the side of the thorax. Lay a strip of tape over the shoulder near the neck and carry it to the nipple line in front and to the scapular line in back (9 and 10).

4. Take a second strip from the end of the first strip, pass it around the middle of the upper arm, and end it at the back end of the first strip (11).

5. Continue the above alternation with an overlapping of each preceding strip by at least half its width until the shoulder has been completely capped (12 throgh 21).

6. Apply a shoulder spica to keep the taping in place.

ELBOW RESTRICTION

The procedure for taping the elbow to prevent hyperextension follows (Figure 10-32).

MATERIALS NEEDED: One roll of 1½-inch (3.8 cm) tape, tape adherent, and 2-inch (5 cm) elastic bandage.

POSITION OF THE ATHLETE: The athlete stands with the affected elbow flexed at 90 degrees.

PROCEDURE

1. Apply two anchor strips loosely around the arm, approximately 2 inches (25 cm) to each side of the curve of the elbow (antecubital fossa) (1 and 2).

2. Construct a checkrein by cutting a 10-inch (25 cm) and a 4-inch (10 cm) strip of tape and laying the 4-inch (10 cm) strip against the center of the 10-inch (25 cm) strip, blanking out that portion. Next place the checkrein so that it spans the two anchor strips with the blanked-out side facing downward. Leave checkrein extended 1 to 2 inches past anchor strips on both ends. This allows

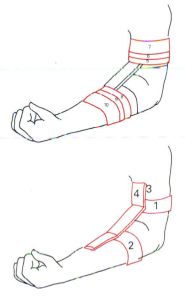

Figure 10-32

Taping to restrict elbow tension.

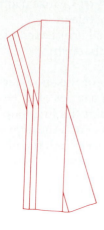

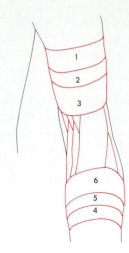

Figure 10-33

Fanned checkrein technique.

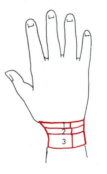

Figure 10-34

Wrist-taping technique no. 1.

anchoring of the checkreins with circular strips to secure against slippage (3 and 4).

3. Place five additional 10-inch (25 cm) strips of tape over the basic checkrein.

4. Finish the procedure by securing the checkrein with three lock strips on each end (5 through 10). A figure-8 elastic wrap applied over the taping will prevent the tape from slipping because of perspiration.

NOTE: A variation to this method is to fan the checkreins, dispersing the force over a wider area (Figure 10-33).

The Wrist and Hand

WRIST TECHNIQUE NO. 1

This wrist taping (Figure 10-34) is designed for mild wrist strains and sprains.

MATERIALS NEEDED: One roll of 1-inch (2.5 cm) tape and tape adherent.

POSITION OF THE ATHLETE: The athlete stands with the affected hand flexed toward the injured side and the fingers moderately spread to increase the breadth of the wrist for the protection of nerves and blood vessels.

PROCEDURE

1. Starting at the base of the wrist, bring a strip of 1-inch (2.5 cm) tape from the palmar side upward and around both sides of the wrist (1).

2. In the same pattern, with each strip overlapping the preceding one by at least half its width, lay two additional strips in place (2 and 3).

WRIST TECHNIQUE NO. 2

This wrist taping (Figure 10-35) stabilizes and protects badly injured wrists. The materials and positioning are the same as in technique 1.

MATERIALS NEEDED: One roll of 1-inch tape and tape adherent.

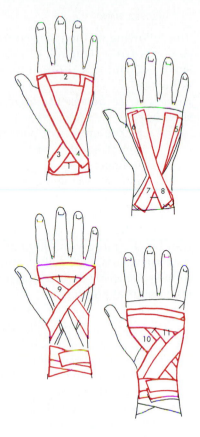

Figure 10-35

Wrist-taping technique no. 2.

POSITION OF THE ATHLETE: The athlete stands with the affected hand flexed toward the injured side and the fingers moderately spread to increase the breadth of the wrist for the protection of nerves and blood vessels.

PROCEDURE

1. Apply one anchor strip around the wrist approximately 3 inches (7.5 cm) from the hand (1); wrap another anchor strip around the spread hand (2).

2. With the wrist bent toward the side of the injury, run a strip of tape from the anchor strip near the little finger obliquely across the wrist joint to the wrist anchor strip. Run another strip from the anchor strip on the index finger side across the wrist joint to the wrist anchor. This forms a crisscross over the wrist joint (3 and 4). Apply a series of four or five crisscrosses, depending on the extent of splinting needed (5 through 8).

3. Apply two or three series of figure-8 tapings over the crisscross taping (9 through 11). Start by encircling the wrist once, carry a strip over the back of the hand obliquely, encircling the hand twice, and then carry another strip obliquely upward across the back of the hand to where the figure-8 started. Repeat this procedure to ensure a strong, stabilizing taping.

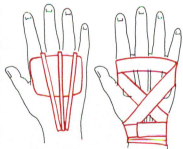

Figure 10-36

Taping for a bruised hand.

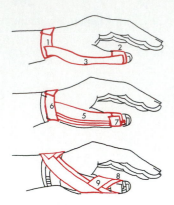

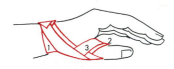

Figure 10-37

Taping for a sprained thumb.

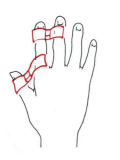

Figure 10-38

Thumb spica.

BRUISED HAND

The following method is used to tape a bruised hand (Figure 10-36).

MATERIALS NEEDED: One roll of 1-inch (2.5 cm) adhesive tape, one roll of ½-inch (1.3 cm) tape, ¼-inch (0.63 cm) thick sponge rubber pad, and tape adherent.

POSITION OF THE ATHLETE: The fingers are spread moderately.

PROCEDURE

1. Lay the protective pad over the bruise and hold it in place with three strips of ½-inch (1.3 cm) tape laced through the webbing of the fingers.
2. Apply a basic figure-8 made of 1-inch (2.5 cm) tape.

SPRAINED THUMB

Sprained thumb taping (Figure 10-37) is designed to give both protection for the muscle and joint and support to the thumb.

MATERIALS NEEDED: One roll of 1-inch (2.5 cm) tape and tape adherent.

POSITION OF THE ATHLETE: The athlete should hold the injured thumb in a relaxed neutral position.

PROCEDURE

1. Place an anchor strip loosely around the wrist and another around the distal end of the thumb (1 and 2).
2. From the anchor at the tip of the thumb to the anchor around the wrist apply four splint strips in a series on the side of greater injury (dorsal or palmar side) (3 through 5) and hold them in place with one lock strip around the wrist and one encircling the tip of the thumb (6 and 7).
3. Add three thumb spicas. Start the first spica on the radial side at the base of the thumb and carry it under the thumb, completely encircling it, and then cross the starting point. The strip should continue around the wrist and finish at the starting point. Each of the following spica strips should overlap the preceding strip by at least ⅔ inch (1.7 cm) and move downward on the thumb (8 and 9). The thumb spica with tape provides an excellent means of protection during recovery from an injury (Figure 10-38).

FINGER AND THUMB CHECKREINS

The sprained finger or thumb may require the additional protection afforded by a restraining checkrein (Figure 10-39).

MATERIALS NEEDED: One roll of 1-inch (2.5 cm) tape.

POSITION OF THE ATHLETE: The athlete spreads the injured fingers widely but within a range free of pain.

PROCEDURE

1. Bring a strip of 1-inch (2.5 cm) tape around the middle phalanx of the injured finger over to the adjacent finger and around it also. The tape left between the two fingers, which are spread apart, is called the checkrein.
2. Add strength with a lock strip around the center of the checkrein.

Figure 10-39

Finger and thumb checkreins.

SUMMARY

Historically, taping has been an important aspect of athletic training. Sports tape is used in a variety of ways—as a means of holding a wound dressing in place, as support, and as protection against musculoskeletal injuries. For supporting and protecting musculoskeletal injuries, two types of tape are currently used—linen and stretch. Sports tape must be stored in a cool place and must be stacked on the flat side of each roll.

The skin of the athlete must be carefully prepared before tape is applied. The skin should first be carefully cleaned; then all hair should be removed. An adherent may be applied, followed by an underwrap material, if need be, to help avoid skin irritation. When tape is applied, it must be done in a manner that provides the least amount of irritation and the maximum support. All tape applications require great care that the proper materials are used, that the proper position of the athlete is ensured, and that procedures are carefully followed.

REVIEW QUESTIONS AND CLASS ACTIVITIES

1. What types of tape are available? What is the purpose of each type? What qualities should you look for in selecting tape?
2. How should you prepare an area to be taped?
3. How should you tear tape?
4. How should you remove tape from an area? Demonstrate the various methods and cutters that can be used to remove tape.
5. What are some general rules for tape application and why should you follow them?
6. What are some common taping procedures?
7. Bring the different types of tape to class. Discuss their uses and the qualities to look for in purchasing tape. Have the class practice tearing tape and preparing an area for taping.
8. Take each joint or body part and demonstrate the common taping procedures used to give support to that area. Have the students pair up and practice these taping jobs on each other. Discuss the advantages and disadvantages of using tape as a supportive device.

REFERENCES

1. Ellison AE, ed: *Athletic training and sports medicine*, Chicago, 1984, American Academy of Orthopaedic Surgeons.
2. Bisek AM: Shin splint taping: something extra, *Ath Train* 22:216, 1987.
3. The continuous technique of ankle support, *Sports Med Guide* 3:14, 1984.
4. Handling KA: Taping procedure for an unstable knee, *Ath Train* 16:371, 1984.
5. Kosmahl EM et al: Painful plantar heel, plantar fascitis and calcaneal spur: etiology and treatment, *J Orthop Sports Phys Ther* 9:17, 1987.
6. McConnell J: The management of chondro-malacia patella: a long term solution, *Aust J Physiother* 32:215, 1986.
7. Zylks DR: Alternative taping for plantar fascitis, *Ath Train* 22:317, 1987.

BIBLIOGRAPHY

Athletic Training, National Athletic Training Association, Dallas.
  Each volume of the quarterly journal contains practical procedures for taping.
Beuersdorf's Medical Program: Manuals of taping and strapping technique, Agoura,
  Calif, 1988, Macmillan.
  A complete detailed guide to various taping and strapping techniques.

PART III

Sports Conditions

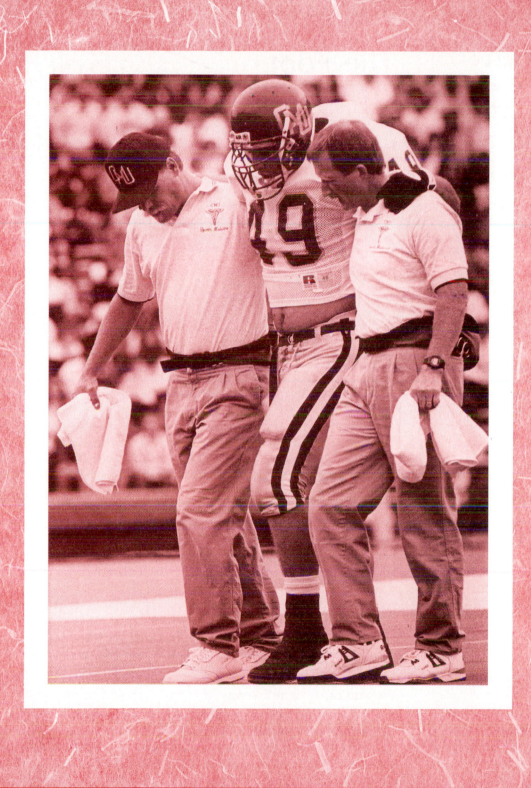

The Foot

When you finish this chapter, you will be able to:

- Explain how to recognize the most common injuries sustained by the foot
- Evaluate common foot injuries
- Explain how to apply appropriate immediate and superficial follow-up care to the foot

T he foot region has a high incidence of sports injuries. Dealing effectively with these injuries at the coach's level is a major challenge.

FOOT ANATOMY

The human foot is a marvel of strength, flexibility, and coordinated movement. It transmits the stresses throughout the body when walking, running, and jumping. It contains 26 bones that are held together by an intricate network of ligaments and fascia and moved by a complicated group of muscles (Figures 11-1 and 11-2).

SKIN TRAUMA AND INFECTION OF THE FOOT

Many sports place demands on the feet that are far beyond the normal daily requirements. The skin of the feet becomes traumatized from abnormal mechanical forces within the socks and shoes.

Prevention of Skin Trauma

Nearly all foot skin conditions are preventable.

The majority of foot skin conditions are preventable. In those sports where skin problems are common, a team meeting dedicated to prevention should be scheduled. The athlete is instructed on proper foot hygiene, which includes proper washing and drying of the feet following activity and changing to clean socks daily. The coach emphasizes the wearing of properly fitting shoes and socks. Where athletes have abnor-

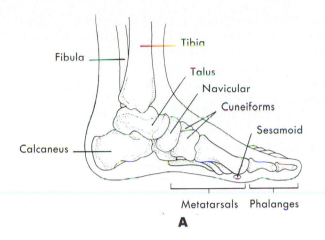

Fibula

Tibia

Talus

Navicular

Cuneiforms

Sesamoid

Calcaneus

Metatarsals   Phalanges

A

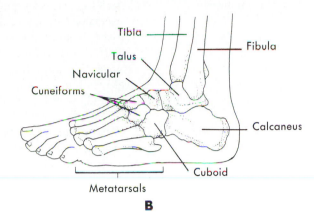

Tibia

Fibula

Talus

Navicular

Cuneiforms

Calcaneus

Metatarsals

Cuboid

B

Figure 11-1

Bony structure of the foot. **A**, Medial. **B**, Lateral.

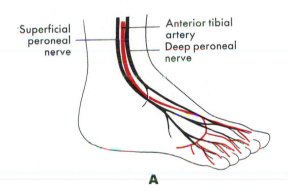

Superficial peroneal nerve

Anterior tibial artery

Deep peroneal nerve

A

Figure 11-2

The major nerves of the foot (**A** and **B**) and muscles of the plantar aspect of the foot (**C**).

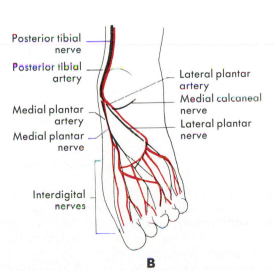

Posterior tibial nerve

Posterior tibial artery

Medial plantar artery

Medial plantar nerve

Interdigital nerves

Lateral plantar artery

Medial calcaneal nerve

Lateral plantar nerve

B

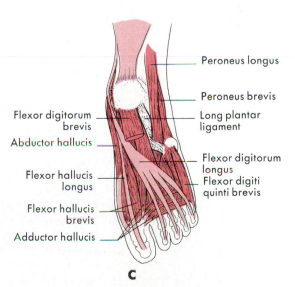

Flexor digitorum brevis

Abductor hallucis

Flexor hallucis longus

Flexor hallucis brevis

Adductor hallucis

Peroneus longus

Peroneus brevis

Long plantar ligament

Flexor digitorum longus

Flexor digiti quinti brevis

C

mal foot stresses due to faulty mechanics, referral to a podiatrist (foot specialist) is made. Some of the more common conditions such as calluses, blisters, corns, ingrown toenails, and athlete's foot should be discussed regarding prevention and possible care.

NOTE: The person caring for an athlete's skin problem should wear latex gloves for his or her own protection.

Foot Calluses

Excessive callus development must be avoided.

Foot calluses may be caused by shoes that are too narrow or too short. Calluses that develop from friction can be painful because the fatty layer loses its elasticity and cushioning effect. The excess callus moves as a gross mass, becoming highly vulnerable to tears, cracks, and, ultimately, infections.

Callus Prevention

Athletes whose shoes are properly fitted but who still develop heavy calluses commonly have foot mechanics problems that may require special orthotics. Special cushioning devices such as wedges, doughnuts, and arch supports may help to distribute the weight on the feet more evenly and thus reduce skin stress. Excessive callus accumulation can be prevented by (1) wearing two pairs of socks, a thin cotton or nylon pair next to the skin and a heavy athletic pair over the cotton pair, or a single double-knit sock; (2) wearing shoes that are the correct size and in good condition; and (3) routinely applying materials such as petroleum jelly to reduce friction.

When Excess Callosity Occurs

Athletes who are prone to excess calluses should be encouraged to use an emery callus file after each shower. Massaging small amounts of lanolin into devitalized calluses once or twice a week after practice may help maintain some tissue elasticity. The coach may have the athlete decrease

---

CARING FOR A TORN BLISTER

1. Cleanse the blister and surrounding tissue with soap and water; rinse with an antiseptic.
2. Using sterile scissors, cut the torn blister halfway around the perimeter.
3. Apply antiseptic and a mild ointment, such as zinc oxide, to the exposed tissue.
4. Lay the flap of skin back over the treated tissue; cover the area with a sterile dressing.
5. Check daily for signs of infection.
6. Zinc oxide, when applied, protects and hardens new skin.
7. Within 2 or 3 days, or when the underlying tissue has hardened sufficiently, remove the dead skin. This should be done by trimming the skin on a bevel and as close as possible to the perimeter of the blister.

the calluses' thickness and increase their smoothness by sanding or pumicing. NOTE: Great care should be taken not to remove the callus totally and the protection it affords at a given pressure point.

Blisters

Like calluses, blisters are often a major problem of sports participation, especially early in the season. As a result of shearing forces acting on the skin, fluid accumulates below the outer skin layer. This fluid may be clear, bloody, or infected. Blisters are particularly associated with rowing, pole-vaulting, basketball, football, and weight events in track and field, such as the shot put and discus.

Blister Prevention

Soft feet coupled with shearing skin stress can produce severe blisters. It has been found that a dusting of cornstarch or the application of petroleum jelly can protect the skin against abnormal friction. Wearing tubular socks or two pairs of socks can protect the athlete with sensitive skin or the one who perspires excessively. Wearing the correct-size shoe is essential. Shoes should be broken in before being used for long periods of time. If, however, a friction area (hot spot) does arise, the athlete has several options: (1) cover the irritated skin with a friction-proofing material, such as petroleum jelly, (2) place a blanked-out piece of tape (Figure 11-3) tightly over the irritated area, (3) cover the area with a piece of moleskin, or (4) apply ice massage to skin areas that have developed abnormal friction.

When Blisters Develop

When caring for a blister (see box on p. 298), be aware at all times of the possibility of severe infection from contamination. Any blister that appears to be infected requires medical attention. In sports, two approaches are generally used to care for blisters: the conservative approach and the torn blister approach. Follow the conservative approach whenever possible. Its main premise is that a blister should not be contaminated by cutting or puncturing but should be protected from further insult by a small doughnut until the initial irritation has subsided (Figure 11-4). If puncturing is necessary to prevent the blister from tearing, introduce a sterilized needle underneath the skin approximately ⅛ inch (0.3 cm) outside the diameter of the raised tissue. Open the blister wide enough that it does not become sealed. After the fluid has dispersed, place a pressure pad directly over the blister to prevent its refilling. A blister should be penetrated at a point where tearing can be avoided; for example, a ball of the foot blister should be opened closest to the heel. When the tenderness has subsided in about 5 or 6 days, cut away the loose skin. Conservative care of blisters is preferred when there is little danger of tearing or aggravation through activity. A product called Second Skin by Spenco can be sprayed on blisters where raw skin is exposed to provide a protective coating.

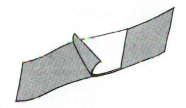

Figure 11-3

A good way to prevent a blister is to blank out a piece of tape and fit it tightly over an irritated skin area.

Blisters can be prevented by:
    Dusting shoes and socks
        with talcum powder
    Applying petroleum jelly
    Wearing tubular socks or
        two pairs of socks

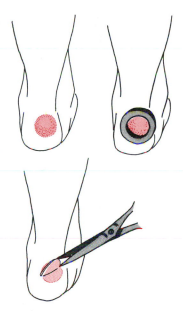

Figure 11-4

Take the conservative approach in caring for a blister whenever possible: use a protective doughnut. If the blister is torn, a flap can be formed by cutting the skin halfway around its perimeter to allow the treatment of the underlying tissue.

Corns

The *hard corn (clavis durum)* is the most serious type of corn. It is caused by the pressure of improperly fitting shoes, the same mechanism that causes calluses. Hammer toes and hard corns are usually associated; the hard corns form on the tops of the deformed toes (Figure 11-5, *A*). Symptoms are local pain and disability, with inflammation and thickening of soft tissue. Because of the chronic nature of this condition, it requires a physician's care.

The coach can aid the situation by issuing shoes that fit properly and then having athletes with such a condition soak their feet daily in warm, soapy water to soften the corn. To alleviate further irritation, the corn should be protected by a small felt or sponge rubber doughnut.

The *soft corn (clavis molle)* is the result of a combination of wearing narrow shoes and having excessive foot perspiration. Because of the pressure of the shoe coupled with the exudation of moisture, the corn usually forms between the fourth and fifth toes (Figure 11-5, *B*). A circular area of thickened, white, **macerated skin** appears between and at the base of the toes. There also appears to be a black dot in the center of the corn. Both pain and inflammation are likely to be present.

macerated skin
Skin softened by soaking

Soft Corn Care

When caring for a soft corn the best procedure is to have the athlete wear properly fitting shoes, keep the skin between the toes clean and dry, decrease pressure by keeping the toes separated with cotton or lamb's wool, and apply a **keratolytic** agent such as 40% salicylic acid in liquid or plasters.

keratolytic
Pertaining to loosening of the upper layer of the skin

Ingrown Toenails

An ingrown toenail is a condition in which the leading side edge of the toenail has grown into the soft tissue nearby, usually resulting in a severe inflammation and infection.

It is important that the athlete's shoes be of the proper length and width, since continued pressure on a toenail can lead to serious irritation or cause it to become ingrown. The length of the sports socks is also at times a factor, since they can cause pressure on the toenails. It is im-

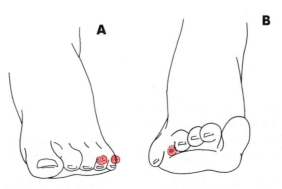

Figure 11-5

Hammer toes with hard corn, **A**, and soft corn, **B**.

portant to know how to trim the nails correctly. Two things must be taken into consideration: first, the nail must be trimmed so that its margins do not penetrate the tissue on the sides (Figure 11-6); second, the nail should be left sufficiently long that it is clear of the underlying tissue and still should be cut short enough that it is not irritated by either shoes or socks (see box below).

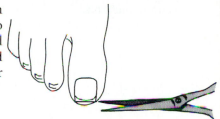

Figure 11-6

Prevention of ingrown toenails requires routine trimming so that the margins do not penetrate the skin on the side of the nail.

Direct Toenail Trauma

An athlete can sustain direct trauma, such as being stepped on by another player. Nails can also incur repetitive shearing forces to the nail apparatus as may occur in the shoe of a long distance runner. In both cases fluid can accumulate underneath the nail, producing extreme pain.[7]

The toe should be placed in ice water or an ice pack applied while being elevated to decrease the extent of bleeding. Fluid pressure and the severe pain can be eliminated by releasing it through the use of a heated paper clip.[7]

Acute Foot Injuries

Evaluation of the Foot Injury

In order to apply proper first aid measures to the athlete and to expedite healing of the foot injury, the coach must carry out a brief preliminary evaluation following the procedure outlined by the acronym HOPS—History, Observation, Palpation, Seriousness of Injury (see box on p. 302).

Contusions

Two common contusions sustained in sports are to the heel and instep.

Heel bruise Of the many contusions and bruises that an athlete may receive, there is none more disabling than the heel bruise. Sport activities that demand a sudden stop-and-go response or sudden change from a horizontal to a vertical movement, such as basketball jumping, high jumping, and long horse vaulting, are particularly likely to cause heel bruises. The heel has a thick, cornified skin layer and a heavy fat pad covering, but even this thick padding cannot protect against a sudden abnormal force directed to this area.

Heel bruises and instep bruises can be temporarily disabling.

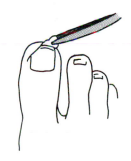

Figure 11-7

Once an ingrown toenail occurs, proper management is necessary to avoid infection. A wisp of cotton is applied under the ingrown side.

MANAGING THE INGROWN TOENAIL

1. Soak the toe in hot water (110° to 120° F) [43.3° to 48.8° C]) for approximately 20 minutes, two or three times daily.
2. When the nail is soft and pliable, use forceps to insert a wisp of cotton under the edge of the nail and lift it from the soft tissue (Figure 11-7).
3. Continue the chosen procedure until the nail has grown out sufficiently that it can be trimmed straight across. The correct trimming of nails is shown in Figure 11-6.

An ingrown toenail can easily become infected. If this occurs, it should be immediately referred to a physician for treatment.

The athlete who is prone to heel bruises should routinely wear a padded heel cup.

Care When injury occurs, the athlete complains of severe pain in the heel and is unable to withstand the stress of weight bearing.

A bruise of the heel usually develops into chronic inflammation of the bone covering (periosteum). Follow-up management of this condition by the athletic trainer should be started 2 to 3 days after insult and include a variety of superficial and deep-heat therapies. If the athlete recognizes the problem in its earliest stage, the following procedures should be adhered to:

1. Initially, cold is applied to the heel bruise and, if possible, the athlete should not step on the heel for at least 24 hours.
2. On the third and subsequent days, warm whirlpool or ultrasound can be administered by the athletic trainer.
3. If pain when walking has subsided by the third day, the athlete may resume moderate activity—with the protection of a heel cup, or protective doughnut (Figure 11-8).

The coach should be aware that an athlete who is prone to or who needs protection from a heel bruise should routinely wear a heel cup with a foam rubber pad as a preventive aid. Surrounding the heel with a firm heel cup diffuses traumatic forces.

Instep bruise The bruised instep, like the bruised heel, can cause disability. Such bruises commonly occur when the instep is stepped on

---

ON-THE-FIELD INJURY EVALUATION (HOPS PROCEDURE)

History of Injury

1. Is this a recurrent injury? When before? How bodily?
2. What events led to this injury?
3. How did this injury occur?
4. Was there something unusual felt or heard when injury first occurred?
5. Was there and/or is there pain and weakness?

Observation of Injury

1. Is there swelling and/or discoloration?
2. Is there a deformity?
3. Can athlete carry out function of that part? Move it without pain, bear weight, walk without a limp?

Palpation of Injury

1. Check for temperature difference between injured and non-injured part.
2. Check for pulse.
3. Feel for localized tenderness, swelling, deformity, abnormal noises.

Seriousness of Injury (making decisions)

1. How serious is the injury? Is there possibility of fracture or joint dislocation?
2. Should athlete be immobilized?
3. How should athlete be transported?
4. Does this injury require further evaluation by a health care professional?

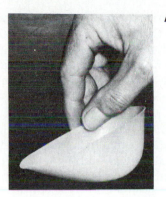
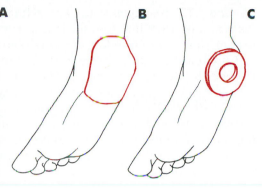

Figure 11-8

Heel protection with heel cup (**A** and **B**) and protective doughnut (**C**).

or hit with a fast-moving, hard projectile such as a baseball or hockey puck. Immediate application of cold compresses must be performed, not only to control inflammation but most importantly to avoid swelling. Irritation of the tendons on the top of the foot can make wearing a shoe difficult. If the force is of great intensity, there is a good chance of fracture. If this is likely, it requires an x-ray examination.[1] Once inflammation is reduced and the athlete returns to competition, a ⅛-inch (0.3 cm) pad should be worn directly on the skin over the bruise and a rigid instep guard should be worn over the shoe.

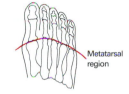

Figure 11-9

Bones of the metatarsal region.

Strains of the Foot

Insufficient conditioning of musculature, structural imbalance, and incorrect mechanics can cause the foot to become prone to strain. Common strains are to the metatarsal arch, the longitudinal arch, and the plantar fascia.

Acute Ball of Foot (Metatarsal) Arch Strain   The athlete who has a fallen metatarsal arch or who has a high arch longitudinal (pes cavus) is susceptible to an acute metatarsal arch strain. In both cases malalignment of the forefoot subjects the flexor tendons on the bottom of the foot to increased tension (Figure 11-9). Pain in this region and/or cramping is called metatarsalgia. Management of acute metatarsalgia usually consists of applying a pad to elevate the depressed metatarsal heads. The pad is placed in the center and just behind the ball of the foot (metatarsal heads) (Figure 11-10).

Longitudinal arch strain   Longitudinal arch strain is usually an early-season injury caused by subjecting the musculature of the foot to unaccustomed severe exercise and forceful contact with hard playing surfaces. In this condition there is a flattening or depressing of the longitudinal arch while the foot is in the midsupport phase, resulting in a strain to the arch. Such a strain may appear quite suddenly, or it may develop rather slowly over time.

As a rule, pain is experienced only when running is attempted and usually appears just below the inner ankle bone (medial malleolus) and the medial ankle tendons, accompanied by swelling and tenderness along the inner aspect of the foot.

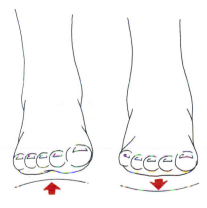

Figure 11-10

Normal and fallen metatarsal arches.

Care The management of a longitudinal arch strain involves immediate care of RICE followed by appropriate therapy, reduction of weight bearing, and exercise rehabilitation. Exercise and weight bearing must be pain free. Arch taping technique no. 1 or no. 2 may allow earlier pain-free weight bearing (see Figures 10-3 and 10-4, p. 267 and 268).

The Sprained Great Toe

Sprains of the great toe are caused most often by kicking some nonyielding object. Sprains result from a considerable force applied in such a manner as to extend the joint beyond its normal range of motion (jamming it) or to twist the toe, thereby twisting and tearing the supporting tissues.

Another major cause of the sprained great toe is forcing the toe backward (hyperextension), called "turf toe," which usually occurs on a synthetic playing surface.

Symptoms of an acute injury appear. Care involves the following considerations:

1. The injury should be handled as an acute sprain.
2. The severity of the injury should be determined through palpation and, if there are signs of a fracture, through x-ray examination.
3. When a sprain is present, the athlete should wear a stiff-soled shoe.
4. The injury should be taped (see Figure 10-8, p. 270).

Fractures and Dislocations of the Foot

Because of the foot's susceptibility to trauma in sports, fractures and dislocations can occur. After any moderate to severe contusion or twisting, fracture must be suspected. X-ray examination is routine in these situations.

Strains and Sprains

In sports like basketball, the foot is prone to numerous problems of muscles and joints. The actions of quick starts, sudden stops, changing directions, and jumping can lead to major strains and sprains.[4]

Tendons of the foot can also be specifically injured by direct trauma or by being overused, leading to pain inflammatory condition.[11]

Fractures and dislocations of the toes Fractures of the toes are usually the bone-crushing type such as may be incurred in kicking an object or stubbing a toe. Generally they are accompanied by swelling and discoloration. Any suspected fracture of the great toe should be referred to a physician immediately. If the break is in the bone shaft, an adhesive taping is applied (see Figure 10-10, p. 271). However, if more than one toe is involved, a cast may be applied for a few days. As a rule, 3 or 4 weeks of inactivity permits healing, although tenderness may persist for some time. A shoe with a wide toe box should be worn; in cases of a great toe fracture a stiff sole should be worn.

Dislocation of the toe is less common than fracture. If one occurs, it

Any suspected fracture must be referred to a physician.

is usually to the uppermost joint of the middle toe bone. The mechanism of injury is the same as for fractures. Restoring it to its normal relationship (reduction) is usually performed easily without anesthesia by the physician.

Fractures of the metatarsals Fractures of the metatarsals can be caused by direct force, such as being stepped on by another player, a severe torque of the midfoot, or by abnormal repetitive stress. [5] They are characterized by swelling and pain. The most common acute fracture, called a Jones fracture, is to the *base of the fifth metatarsal*. It is normally caused by a sharp twisting inward of the foot as in an ankle sprain. It has all the appearances of a severe sprain. Care is usually symptomatic, with RICE employed to control swelling. Once swelling has subsided, a short leg walking cast is applied for 3 to 6 weeks. Ambulation is usually possible by the second week. A shoe with a large toe box should be worn.

Note that the Jones fracture has a high rate of nonunion.

Chronic and Overuse Foot Conditions

Lower extremity stress problems in sports very often begin in the foot region.

Arch Problems

Painful arches are usually the result of improperly fitting shoes, overweight, excessive activity on hard surfaces, overuse, faulty posture, or fatigue—any of which may cause damage in the supporting tissue of the arch. The symptoms in this case are divided into three degrees, each characterized by specific symptoms. The first degree shows itself as a slight soreness in the arch. The second degree is indicated by a chronic inflammatory condition that includes soreness, redness, swelling, and a slight visible drop in the arch. In the third degree a completely fallen arch is accompanied by extreme pain, immobility, and deformity (Figure 11-10). NOTE: A number of taping techniques may be used in helping to support longitudinal arch problems (see arch taping techniques in Figures 10-3, 10-4, 10-5, 10-6, 10-7, pp. 267 to 269).

Fatigue, poor posture, overuse, excessive weight, or improperly fitting shoes may damage the supporting tissue of the arch.

Fallen metatarsal arch Activity on hard surfaces or prolonged stresses on the balls of the feet may cause weak or fallen anterior metatarsal arches (Figure 11-11). When the supporting ligaments and muscles lose their ability to hold the metatarsal heads in a domelike shape, the arch falls, placing pressure on the nerves and blood vessels in the area. The athlete first notices irritation and redness on the ball of the foot. As the condition progresses, pain, callus formation, toe cramping, and often a severe burning sensation develop. Care of a fallen anterior metatarsal arch should include hydrotherapy, light friction massage, exercise, and metatarsal pads (box on p. 307 and Figure 11-12).

Fallen Medial Longitudinal Arch (Flatfoot)

Various stresses weaken ligaments and muscles that support the arch. The athlete may complain of tiredness and tenderness in the arch and heel. Ankle sprains frequently result from weakened arches, and abnormal

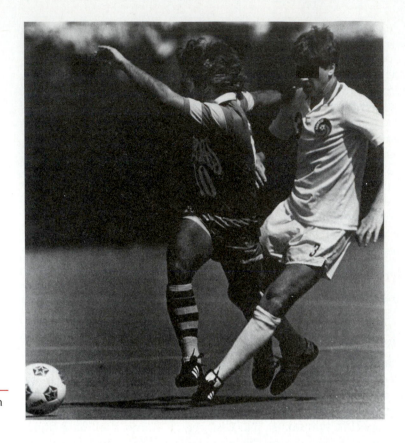

Figure 11-11

Activity on hard surfaces can weaken feet.

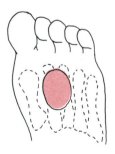

Figure 11-12

Metatarsal pad.

pes planus

Flat feet

pes cavus

Feet having an abnormally high arch

friction sites may develop within the shoe because of changes in weight distribution. This condition may be the result of several factors: shoes that cramp and deform the feet, weakened supportive tissues, overweight, postural deviations that subject the arches to unnatural strain, or overuse, which may be the result of repeatedly subjecting the arch to a severe pounding through participation on an unyielding surface. Commonly, the fallen medial longitudinal arch is associated with a foot that rolls inward, known as foot pronation (Fig. 11-13)(see also arch taping technique in Figure 10-5, p. 268).[12]

High Arch (Pes Cavus)

Pes cavus (Figure 11-14), commonly called claw foot, hollow foot, or an abnormally high arch, is not as common as flatfoot or **pes planus.** In the rigid type of pes cavus, shock absorption is poor and can lead to problems such as general foot pain, painful metatarsal arch (metatarsalgia), and clawed or hammer toes. Pes cavus also may be without symptoms.

The accentuated high medial longitudinal arch may be congenital or may indicate a neurological disorder. Commonly associated with this condition are clawed toes and abnormal shortening of the heel cord. The heel cord is directly linked with the plantar fascia. Also, because of the

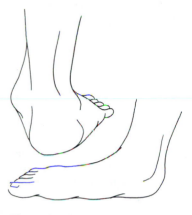

Figure 11-13

Fallen and medial longitudinal arch with pronation.

abnormal distribution of body weight, heavy calluses develop on the ball and heel of the foot.

Forefoot Problems

A number of deformities and structural deviations affect the forefoot of many athletes.

Bunion (hallux valgus)   Bunions are one of the most frequent painful deformities of the great toe.

The reasons a bunion develops are complex. Commonly, it is associated with a congenital deformity of the first metatarsal head, combined with wearing shoes that are pointed, too narrow, too short, or high-heeled. The bursa over the side of the great toe becomes inflamed and eventually thickens. The joint becomes enlarged and the great toe becomes malaligned, moving medially toward the second toe, sometimes to such an extent that it eventually overlaps it. This type of bunion is also associated with the depressed or flattened transverse arch and a **pronated foot.**

The bunionette, or tailor's bunion, is much less common. It affects the third joint of the fifth (little) toe; the little toe angulates toward the fourth toe.

In the beginning of a bunion there is tenderness, swelling, and enlargement of the joint. Poor-fitting shoes increase the irritation and pain. As the inflammation continues, angulation of the toe progresses, eventually leading to instability in the entire forefoot.

Care   Each bunion has unique characteristics. Early recognition and care can often prevent increased irritation and deformity. Management procedures include the following:

1. Wear correctly fitting shoes with a wide toe box.
2. Place a felt or sponge rubber doughnut pad or lamb's wool over the medial side of the joint.

valgus
Bent outward

foot pronation
A lowering of the inside edge of the foot or eversion and adduction of the foot

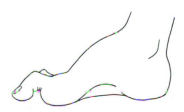

Figure 11-14

High arches (pes cavus).

3. Wear a tape splint, along with a resilient wedge placed between the great toe and the second toe (Figure 11-15).
4. Apply superficial heat therapy to reduce inflammation.
5. Engage in daily foot exercises to strengthen both the extensor and flexor muscles of the toes.

If the condition progresses, a special orthotic device may help normalize foot mechanics. Surgery may be required in the later stages of this condition.

Metatarsalgia   Although **metatarsalgia** is a general term to describe pain or cramping in the ball of the foot, it is more commonly as-

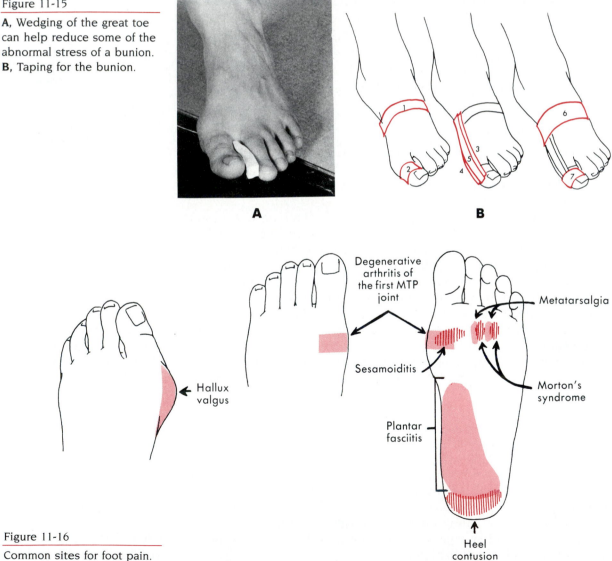

Figure 11-15

A, Wedging of the great toe can help reduce some of the abnormal stress of a bunion. **B,** Taping for the bunion.

A   **B**

Figure 11-16

Common sites for foot pain.

sociated with pain under the second and sometimes the third metatarsal head. A heavy callus often forms in the area of pain. Figure 11-16 shows some of the common pain sites in the foot.

The most prevalent cause of this condition is the fallen metatarsal arch. Normally the head of the first and fifth metatarsal bones bears slightly more weight than the second, third, and fourth: the first metatarsal head bears two sixths of the body weight, the fifth bears slightly more than one sixth, and the second, third, and fourth each bear one sixth. If the foot tends toward pronation, or if the metatarsal ligaments are weak, allowing the foot to spread abnormally (splayed foot), a fallen metatarsal arch is probable (Figure 11-17).

Care Care of metatarsalgia usually consists of applying a pad to elevate the depressed metatarsal heads (see box below). NOTE: The pad is placed behind, not under, the metatarsal heads (see Figure 11-12).

metatarsalgia
Pain in the metatarsal

METATARSAL PAD SUPPORT

The purpose of the metatarsal pad is to reestablish the normal relationships of the metatarsal bones. It can be purchased commercially or constructed out of felt or sponge rubber.

MATERIALS NEEDED: One roll of 1-inch (2.5 cm) tape, a ⅛-inch (0.3 cm) adhesive felt oval cut to a 2-inch (5 cm) circumference, and tape adherent.

POSITION OF THE ATHLETE: The athlete sits on a table or chair with the bottom surface of the affected foot turned upward.

POSITION OF THE OPERATOR: The operator stands facing the bottom of the athlete's foot.

PROCEDURE

1. The circular pad is placed just behind the metatarsal heads.
2. Two or three circular strips of tape are placed loosely around the pad and foot.

Figure 11-17

Normal weight bearing of the forefoot and abnormal spread (splayed foot).

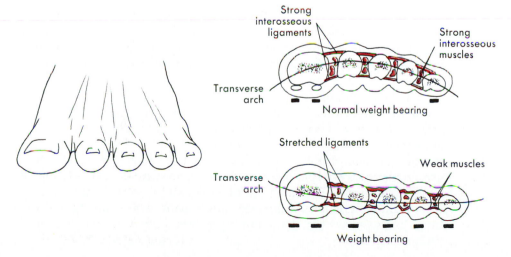

Strong interosseous ligaments

Strong interosseous muscles

Transverse arch

Normal weight bearing

Stretched ligaments

Weak muscles

Transverse arch

Weight bearing

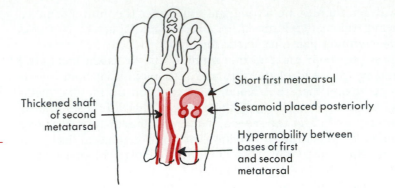

Figure 11-18

Morton's syndrome with an abnormally short first metatarsal bone.

Thickened shaft of second metatarsal

Short first metatarsal

Sesamoid placed posteriorly

Hypermobility between bases of first and second metatarsal

A daily regimen of exercise should concentrate on strengthening foot muscles and stretching the heel cord.[6]

Morton's syndrome   Another foot deformity causing major forefoot pain is Morton's syndrome. Metatarsalgia is produced by an abnormally short first metatarsal bone. Weight is borne mainly by the second metatarsal bone, and there is hypermobility between the first and second proximal metatarsal joints (Figure 11-18). The management is the same as for foot pronation.

Hammer, or clawed, toes   Hammer, or clawed, toes may be congenital, but more often the condition is caused by long-term wearing of shoes that are too short and that cramp the toes. Hammer toe usually involves the second or third toe, whereas clawed toes involve more than one toe. In both conditions the toe joints become malaligned, along with overly contracted flexor tendons and overly stretched extensor tendons. This deformity eventually results in the formation of hard corns or calluses on the exposed joints. Quite often surgery is the only cure. However, proper shoes and protective taping (see Figure 10-9, p. 270) can help prevent irritation.

Chronic and Overuse Syndromes

Because of the hard use that feet receive in many sports, they are prone to chronic and overuse syndromes. This is especially true if weight-transmission or biomechanical problems exist. Because distance running is becoming increasingly popular, musculoskeletal problems of the feet are also becoming more prevalent.

Bony outgrowths (exostoses)   **Exostoses** are benign bony outgrowths from the surface of a bone and are usually capped by cartilage. Sometimes called *spurs,* such outgrowths occur principally at the head of the first metatarsal bone on the dorsum of the foot (Figure 11-19). In certain instances what at first appears to be an exostosis actually may be a partial dislocation (subluxation) of a midfoot joint. The causes of exostoses include hereditary influences, faulty patterns of walking and running, excessive weight, joint impingements, and continual use of ill-fitting footwear.

exostoses

Benign bony outgrowths that protrude from the surface of a bone and are usually capped by cartilage

Adolescent Heel Pain

Adolescent athletes may be prone to heel pain due to a variety of causations such as stress fractures, plantar fasciitis, inflammation of the bursa at the back of the heel, irritation of the projection of **apophysis** at the back of the heel where the heel cord attaches, or heel cord tendinitis (discussed in the next chapter).

A common bursitis occurs to the bursa at the back of the heel, located under the skin just above the attachment of the heel cord (Figure 11-20). It often occurs because of pressure and rubbing of the upper edge of the sports shoe. Irritation produces an inflamed, swollen area. At the first sign of this condition a soft resilient pad should be placed over the bursa site. If necessary, larger shoes with a softer heel contour should be worn.

An inflammation of the bony outgrowth can produce a very disabling condition known as calcaneal **apophysitis.** A true apophysitis is an inflammation of the bony outgrowth's growth plate. Such a condition can cause a great deal of pain and heel cord weakness. In this case early management usually includes a ¼-inch heel left in both shoes, rest, ice massage, and a nonsteroidical antiinflammatory medication.[2]

Heel spur syndrome (plantar fasciitis)   Plantar fasciitis, or heel spur syndrome, is one of the most frequent hindfoot problems among athletes who run and/or jump.

The plantar fascia runs forward from the head bone tuberosity on the sole of the foot to insert on the heads of the metatarsal bones.[10]

Because of the stress that is placed on the heel bone tuberosity by the plantar soft tissue during repeated running or jumping, a chronic irritation and/or bone spur can occur. Tight heel cords, wearing shoes with a lose heel, a rigid high arch foot, or flat feet can predispose the athlete to plantar fasciitis.[10]

The athlete complains of a sharp pain like a stone bruise or a burning sensation. Palpation usually reveals pain on the bottom of the heel and radiating toward the sole of the foot. Often the pain intensifies when the athlete gets out of bed in the morning and first puts weight on the foot; the pain lessens after a few steps.

Care   Care of this condition follows the same procedures as for a chronic foot strain, including longitudinal arch support or LowDye arch support (see Figure 10-7, p. 269). Of major importance is a vigorous regimen of the heel cord stretching, especially if the athlete's ankle cannot dorsiflex 10 to 15 degrees from a neutral position. Stretching should be conducted at least three times a day with the foot straight ahead, toe in, and toe out. The athlete should wear a shoe that is not too stiff, with a firm heel counter, and that has a heel cushion elevated ½ to ¾ inch (1.3 to 1.9 cm) above the level of the sole.

Foot stress fractures   Over 18% of all stress fractures in the body occur in the foot.[1] The most common stress of the foot occurs to one or more of the metatarsal bone shafts (Figure 11-21).

Management of this stress fracture usually consists of 3 to 4 days of

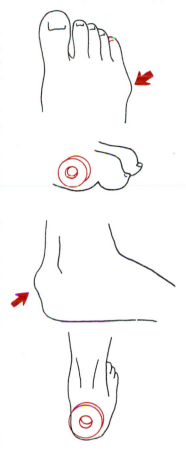

Figure 11-19

Exostoses (bony outgrowths).

apophysis
Bony outgrowth to which muscles attach

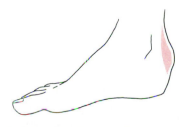

Figure 11-20

Heel bursitis.

crutch walking or a short leg walking cast for 1 to 2 weeks. Weight bearing may be resumed when pain has significantly subsided. Tape support and therapy for swelling and tenderness is given. Running should be resumed very gradually for 3 to 4 weeks.

Foot tendinitis   Because of the many muscle tendons in the foot region, tendinitis is a common occurrence (Figure 11-22). These problems are often caused by structural foot imbalances coupled with overuse. Care of these difficulties include rest, heat or cold therapy, antiinflammatory medications such as aspirin, and orthotics to alleviate structural problems.

RECONDITIONING FOOT EXERCISES

In most painful conditions of the foot, weight bearing is prohibited until pain has subsided significantly. During this period and until the athlete is ready to return to full activity, a graduated program of exercise can be instituted. Exercises are divided into two stages. Each exercise should be performed three times a day with 3 to 10 repetitions of each exercise and should progress to two or three sets.[6]

Stage 1

In Stage 1, primary exercises are employed in the non-weight–bearing or early phase of the condition. They include "writing the alphabet," picking up objects, ankle circumduction, and gripping and spreading.

1. *Writing the alphabet*—with the toes pointed, the athlete proceeds to write the complete alphabet in the air three times.
2. *Picking up objects*—the athlete picks up 10 small objects, such as marbles, with the toes and places them in a container.
3. *Ankle circumduction*—the ankle is circumducted in as extreme a range of motion as possible (10 circles in one direction and 10 circles in the other).
4. *Gripping and spreading*—of particular value to toes, the exercise of gripping and spreading is conducted up to 10 repetitions.

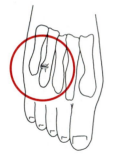

Figure 11-21

Stress fracture on the metatarsal region.

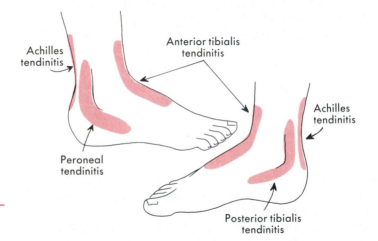

Figure 11-22

Common tendinitis of the foot and ankle region.

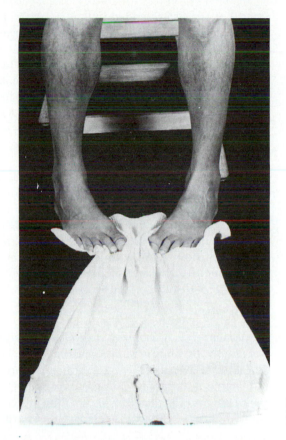

Figure 11-23
The "towel gather" exercise.

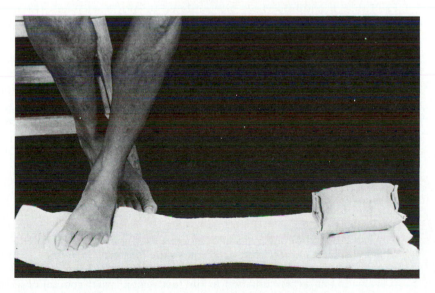

Figure 11-24
The "towel scoop" exercise.

Stage 2

Stage 2 exercises are added to Stage 1 when the athlete is just beginning to bear weight. They include the "towel gather" and "towel scoop" exercises.

1. *Towel gathering*—a towel is extended in front of the feet. The heels are firmly planted on the floor, the forefoot on the end of the towel. The athlete attempts to pull the towel with the feet without lifting the heels from the floor. As execution becomes easier, a weight can be placed at the other end of the towel for added resistance. Each exercise should be performed 10 times (Figure 11-23).

2. *Towel scoop*—a towel is folded in half and placed sideways on the floor. The athlete places the heel firmly on the floor, the forefoot on the end of the towel. To ensure the greatest stability of the exercising foot, it is backed up with the other foot. Without lifting the heel from the floor, the athlete scoops the towel forward with the forefoot. As with the towel gather, a weight resistance can be added to the end of the towel. The exercise should be repeated up to 10 times (Figure 11-24).

SUMMARY

The human foot is a highly complicated structure requiring a great deal of strength, flexibility, and coordinated movement. The foot within the shoe can sustain forces that produce abnormal calluses, blisters, corns, and ingrown toenails. Common musculoskeletal injuries are bruises, metatarsal and longitudinal arch strains, fractures, and dislocations of the toes. Fractures, primarily stress fractures, are common to the metatarsal bones.

Painful arch conditions are often related to sports activities; the most common are in the metatarsal and longitudinal arch regions. Pain is commonly related to falling arches.

Chronic and overuse foot conditions can lead to stress problems in the lower extremities. Common chronic problems occur to the arches of the foot, toes, and forefoot. The bunion, a common chronic condition, occurs when the great toe becomes deflected medially. Metatarsalgia also is a chronic conditions of the forefoot. Other problems include deformities such as hammer (clawed) toes, bony outgrowths, heel bursitis, heel spurs, tendinitis, and stress fractures.

REVIEW QUESTIONS AND CLASS ACTIVITIES

1. How can the foot be protected against skin trauma?
2. Discuss the steps in caring for a foot blister.
3. Why is the heel prone to bruising? How can heel bruises be prevented?
4. What are some common acute problems in the foot that frequently occur in athletes? How would you care for them?
5. In evaluating an acute condition in the foot region, what general observations can be made? What bony and soft tissue structures should be palpated?

6. What common chronic and overuse conditions can be seen in the foot and forefoot? How are they cared for?
7. What kinds of foot deformities can be associated with the wearing of improperly fitting shoes?
8. How are stress fractures managed?
9. Invite a podiatrist to speak to the class concerning congenital abnormalities in the foot, major sports injuries of the foot, the treatment of injuries, and the role of orthotic devices in assisting biomechanical foot problems.
10. What are some preventive and reconditioning exercises that strengthen the musculature of the foot?

REFERENCES

1. Calliet R: *Foot and ankle pain,* Philadelphia, 1986, FA Davis.
2. Crosby LA, McMullen ST: Heel pain in an active adolescent? *Phys Sports Med* 21:125, 1993.
3. Irvine WO: Feet under force, *Phys Sports Med* 20:137, 1992.
4. McDermott EP: Basketball injuries of the foot and ankle, *Clin Sports Med* 12:373, 1993.
5. Myerson M: Tarsometatarsal joint injury, *Phys Sports Med* 21:97, 1993.
6. Prentice WE: *Rehabilitation techniques in sports medicine,* St Louis, 1990, Times Mirror/Mosby College Publishing.
7. Scioli M: Managing toenail trauma, *Phys Sports Med* 20:107, 1992.
8. Singer KM, Jones DC: Ligament injuries of the ankle and foot. In Nicholas JA, Hershman EB, eds: *The lower extremity and spine in sports medicine,* vol 1, St Louis, 1986, CV Mosby.
9. Stephens MM: Heel pain. *Phys Sports Med* 20:87, 1992.
10. Tanner SM: Plantar fasciitis: healing heel pain, *Sports Med Dig* 14:2, 1992.
11. Trevino S et al: Tendon injuries of the foot and ankle, *Clin Sports Med* 11:727, 1992.
12. Waller JF: Hindfoot and midfoot problems in the runner. In Mack RP, ed: *Running sports,* St Louis, 1982, CV Mosby.
13. Warren BL, Jones CJ: Predicting Plantar fasciitis in runners, *Med Sci Sports Exerc* 19:71, 1987.

ANNOTATED BIBLIOGRAPHY

Donatelli R: *The biomechanics of the foot and ankle,* Philadelphia, 1990, FA Davis.
  A practical book on the basic mechanics of the foot and ankle.
Nigg BM: *Biomechanics of running shoes,* Champaign, Ill, 1986, Human Kinetics Publishers.
  Describes the biomechanics of running, running shoe design and construction, and how running shoes should be selected.
Yocum LA, editor: Foot and ankle injuries: *Clin Sports Med* 7: 1988.
  This book provides an overview of the major factors related to foot and ankle injuries.

Chapter

12

The Ankle and Lower Leg

When you finish this chapter, you will be able to:

- Discuss the possible procedures that can be taken to prevent ankle injuries
- Identify the most common injuries sustained by the ankle and lower leg in sports
- Generally assess common ankle and lower leg injuries
- Explain the procedures that can be taken in caring for ankle and lower leg injuries

The regions of the ankle and lower leg have a high incidence of sports injuries. Dealing effectively with these injuries at the coach's level is a major challenge.

THE ANKLE

The ankle is a hinge joint (ginglymus) formed by the articulation of two long bones, the tibia and fibula, with the talus (Figure 12-1). The ligamentous support of the ankle (Figure 12-2) further fortifies the bony arrangement. Laterally, at the most injured site, it is composed of relatively weak ligaments: the anterior and posterior tibiofibular, the anterior and posterior talofibular, the lateral talocalcaneal, and the posterior calcaneofibular. The stronger and less-injured medial side contains the large deltoid ligament. The weakest aspect of the ankle is its muscular arrangement, because the long muscle tendons that cross on all sides of the ankle afford a maximum of muscle leverage but at the same time provide poor lateral stability (Figure 12-3).

Prevention of Ankle Injuries

Many ankle injuries, especially sprains, can be reduced by heel cord (Achilles tendon) stretching, strengthening of key muscles, balance training, proper footwear, and in some cases proper taping or bracing (Figure 12-4).

Heel Cord Stretching

An ankle that can easily dorsiflex at least 15 degrees or more is essential for injury prevention. The athlete, especially one with a tight heel cord, should routinely stretch before and after practice (Figure 12-5). Stretching should be performed first with toes pointed in, second with toes pointed straight ahead, and finally with toes pointed outward. To adequately stretch the heel, cold complex stretching should be performed with the knee extended and then flexed 15 to 30 degrees.

Strength Training

Of major importance to ankle injury prevention is to achieve both static and dynamic joint stability through strength training (Figure 12-6). A normal range of motion must be maintained, along with strength of the muscles that turn the foot inward and outward and the muscles that point the foot downward and backward.

Position Sense—Proprioceptive Training

Athletes who have ankle injuries or who spend most of their time on even surfaces may develop a position sense deficiency.

It is important that the ankle and foot maintain a balance of soft tissue tension to avoid injury. This means the foot and ankle must respond quickly to any imbalancing surface situation. The ankle and foot proprioceptive sense can be enhanced by locomotion over uneven surfaces or by spending time each day on a balance board, or wobble board, Figure 12-7.

Footwear

As discussed in Chapters 5 and 11, proper footwear can be an important factor in reducing injuries to both the foot and the ankle. Shoes should not be used in activities for which they were not intended—for example, do not wear running shoes, which are designed for straight-ahead activity, to play tennis, a sport demanding a great deal of lateral movement. Cleats on a shoe should not be centered in the middle of the sole but should be placed close enough to the border to avoid ankle sprains. Ath-

Adequate ankle flexibility is important for injury prevention.

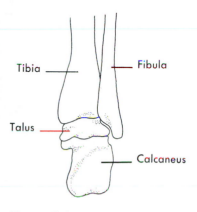

Figure 12-1

The ankle is a hinge-type joint formed by the tibia, fibula, and talus.

Figure 12-2

Major ligaments of the ankle. **A**, Lateral aspect. **B**, Medial aspect.

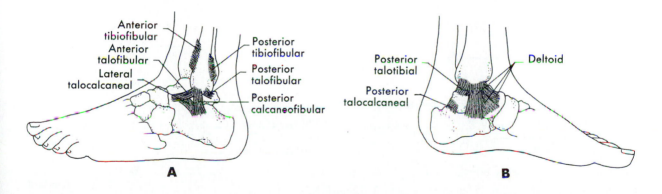

A

B

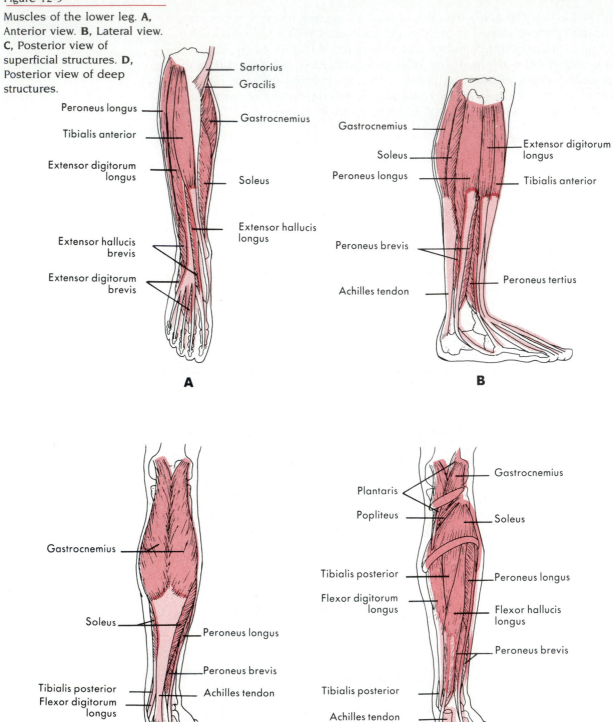

Figure 12-3

Muscles of the lower leg. **A,** Anterior view. **B,** Lateral view. **C,** Posterior view of superficial structures. **D,** Posterior view of deep structures.

Sartorius
Gracilis
Peroneus longus
Gastrocnemius
Tibialis anterior
Extensor digitorum longus
Soleus
Extensor hallucis longus
Extensor hallucis brevis
Extensor digitorum brevis

A

Gastrocnemius
Soleus
Peroneus longus
Extensor digitorum longus
Tibialis anterior
Peroneus brevis
Peroneus tertius
Achilles tendon

B

Gastrocnemius
Soleus
Peroneus longus
Peroneus brevis
Tibialis posterior
Achilles tendon
Flexor digitorum longus

C

Plantaris
Popliteus
Tibialis posterior
Flexor digitorum longus
Tibialis posterior
Achilles tendon
Gastrocnemius
Soleus
Peroneus longus
Flexor hallucis longus
Peroneus brevis

D

Continued.

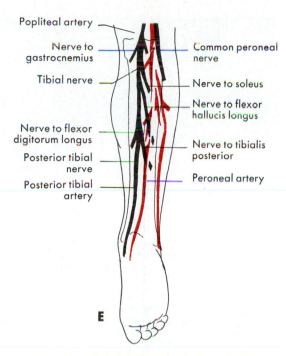

Popliteal artery

Nerve to
gastrocnemius

Tibial nerve

Nerve to flexor
digitorum longus

Posterior tibial
nerve

Posterior tibial
artery

Common peroneal
nerve

Nerve to soleus

Nerve to flexor
hallucis longus

Nerve to tibialis
posterior

Peroneal artery

E

Figure 12-3 cont'd.

E, Blood and nerve supply of
the lower leg

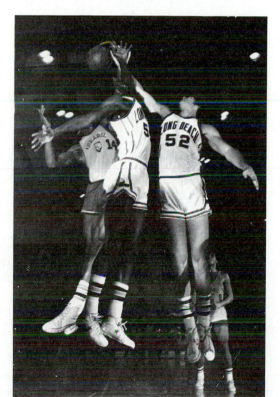

Figure 12-4

Many ankle injuries, such as
those common to basketball,
can be reduced by proper
preventive care.

A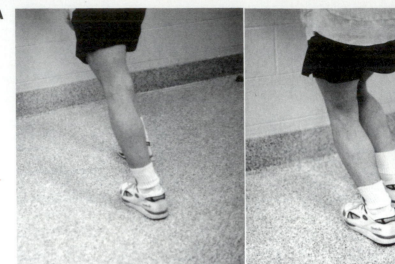

Figure 12-5

Stretching techniques for the heelcord complex. **A,** Stretching position for the gastrocnemius muscle. **B,** Stretching position for the soleus muscle.

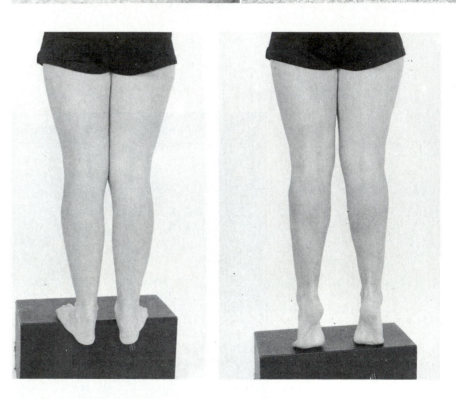

Figure 12-6

Strength training is essential for the prevention of ankle sprains.

history of ankle sprains should wear high-top shoes, which offer greater support than low-top shoes.

Preventive Ankle Wrapping, Taping, and Bracing

As discussed in Chapter 5, there is some doubt about whether it is beneficial routinely to tape ankles that have no history of sprain. There is

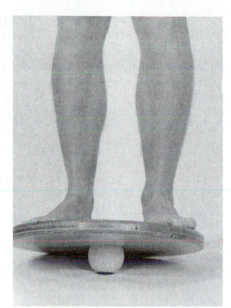

Figure 12-7

The wobble board is an
excellent device for
establishing ankle
proprioception.

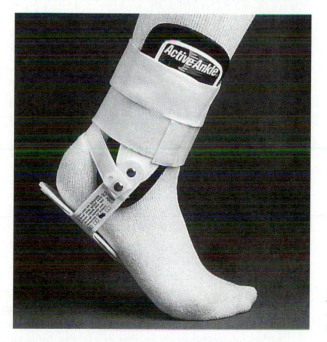

Figure 12-8

Ankle braces may be used to
support weakened ankles.

some indication that tape, properly applied, can provide some prophylactic protection. Poorly applied tape will do more harm than good. Tape
that constricts soft tissue and blood circulation or disrupts normal biomechanical function can in time create serious physical problems. Although taping is preferred, a much cheaper cloth muslin wrap may provide limited protection (see Chapter 9).

plantar flexion
When the forepart of the foot is depressed relative to the ankle.

Too often athletes are permitted to return to their sports before adequate recovery had taken place; therefore the ankle becomes chronically inflamed.

Ankle bracing, another purported means to protection, can be constructed from orthoplast or Hecelite material or it can be purchased commercially. Braces may be effective in preventing lateral and inversion movement of the foot without inhibiting **plantar flexion**; however, research is needed to verify whether ankle braces are effective (see Chapter 5).

Acute Ankle Injuries

Sprains

Because of their frequency and the disability that results, ankle sprains present a major problem for the coach, trainer, and team physician.[3] It has been said that a sprained ankle can be worse than a fracture. Fractures are usually conservatively cared for, with immobilization and activity restriction, whereas the athlete with a sprained ankle is often rushed through management and returned to activity before complete healing has occurred. Incompletely healed, the ankle becomes chronically inflamed and unstable, eventually causing a major problem for the athlete.

Injury causations   Ankle sprains are generally caused by a sudden lateral or medial twist. The inversion sprain, in which the foot turns inward from a plantar flexed position, is the most common type of ankle sprain. This is because there is more bony stability on the lateral side, which tends to force the foot into inversion rather than eversion. If the force is great enough, inversion of the foot continues until the medial malleolus loses its stability and creates a fulcrum to further invert the ankle. The peroneal or everting muscles resist the inverting force; and when they are no longer strong enough, the lateral ligaments become stretched or torn (Figure 12-9, *A*).

Usually a lateral ankle sprain involves either one or two torn ligaments (Figure 12-9, *B*). The tight heel cord forces the foot into inversion, making it more susceptible to a lateral sprain. In contrast, a foot that is pronated or hypermobile or that has a depressed medial longitudinal arch is more susceptible to an eversion sprain (Figure 12-10).

The eversion sprain occurs less frequently than the inversion sprain. The usual mechanism is that the athlete suddenly steps in a hole in the playing field, causing the foot to evert and abduct and the planted leg to rotate externally (Figure 12-11).

A sudden inversion force may be of such intensity as to produce a fracture of the lower leg. An unexpected wrenching of the lateral ligaments can avulse a portion of bone from the malleolus (Figure 12-12)

Although less common, the ankle can be seriously injured by an internal or external rotation with the foot planted. Such a mechanism can tear the supporting connective tissue between the tibia and fibula, leading to an unstable ankle.[11,12]

Evaluating the Injured and Painful Ankle

The injured or painful ankle should be carefully evaluated to determine the possibility of fracture and whether medical referral is necessary. Use

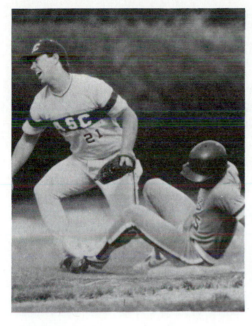

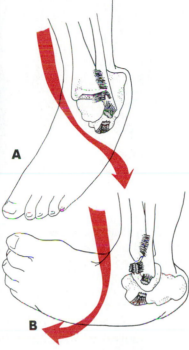

Figure 12-9

Mechanism of a serious inversion ankle sprain. **A** and **B** show tears of lateral ankle ligaments.

A

B

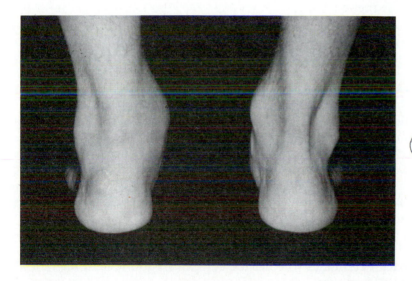

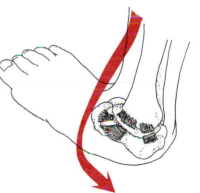

Figure 12-10

Mechanisms of an eversion ankle sprain.

of the HOPS principle may be helpful (see the box on page 302, Chapter 11).

H History

The athlete's history may vary, depending on whether the problem is the result of sudden trauma or is of long standing.

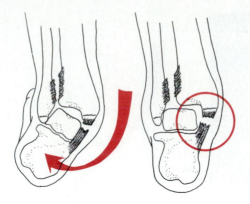

Figure 12-11

An eversion ankle sprain creates an abnormal space between the medial malleolus and the talus.

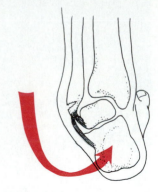

Figure 12-12

The mechanism that produces an ankle sprain can also cause an avulsion fracture.

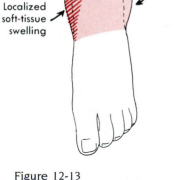

Figure 12-13

Local and diffuse ankle swelling.

Do not ask the athlete to perform any motions that will aggravate the injury.

O Observation

The first inspection should be observation of the athlete's walk. Is the injured individual walking in the usual manner or on the toes or is there an inability to bear any weight? When the athlete is seated, compare both ankles for the following:

1. Position of the foot—a sprained ankle is usually in a more inverted position if an inversion sprain.
2. Range of ankle motion—normal range is approximately 20 degrees of dorsiflexion and 45 to 50 degrees of plantar flexion.

P Palpation of Bony and Soft Tissue

Palpation in the ankle region should start with key bony sites and ligaments and progress to the musculature, especially the major tendons in the area. The purpose of palpation in this region is to detect obvious structural defects, swellings, and localized tenderness (Figure 12-13).

If there is a possibility of impeded blood flow to the ankle area, the pulse should be measured at the dorsal pedal artery and at the posterior tibial artery (Figure 12-14).

Functional Test for the Coach

The coach determines whether the athlete can do the following:

1. Walk on toes
2. Walk on heels
3. Hop on affected foot without heel touching surface
4. Start or stop the running motion
5. Change direction rapidly
6. Run Figure 8s

Functional tests should be given only if they will not aggravate an existing

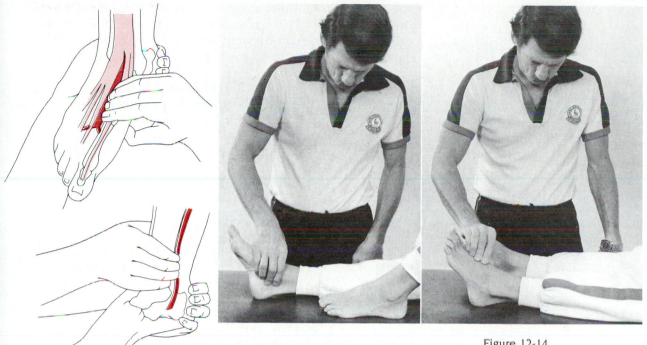

Figure 12-14

Ankle or other lower limb injuries may impede blood flow. The pulse should be taken routinely following injury.

injury. If the athlete is unable to perform any test or has pain when the test starts, the athlete should not return to activity and perhaps should be referred for further evaluation to the athletic trainer or physician.

General Immediate Care

In managing a sprained ankle, follow these first aid measures:

1. Determine the extent of the injury. The main purpose of the ankle sprain examination is to estimate the injury's severity. **NOTE:** Swelling is not an indication of the severity of the injury.

2. Employ RICE

   a. Apply crushed ice in a moist pack over the injury site with an elastic wrap providing pressure and holding the pack in place. Compression should be applied distal to proximal to relieve fluid pooling.

   An alternate procedure is to soak an elastic wrap in ice water and apply it directly to the skin. Apply an ice pack over it and hold it in place with another elastic wrap. **NOTE:** Take great care not to damage the skin by overuse of a coolant. Ice packs should be applied 30 minutes out of every 1½-hour to 2-hour period, five to six times a day. Cold should be continued until all signs of swelling have subsided. If a cold medium is not available, a horseshoe pad cut to fit around the malleolus and held in place with an elastic wrap will help confine the internal hemorrhage (Figure 12-15).

  b. Promptly elevate the injured limb, if at all practical, so that fluid pooling of the internal hemorrhage does not take place.

  c. Initially the open basketweave taping can be used in conjunction with cold application. NOTE: In most cases joint swelling can be limited if the RICE routine is carefully followed for 24 hours.

3. If there is a possibility of fracture, splint the ankle and refer the athlete to the physician for x-ray examination and immobilization.

4. For most moderate and severe ankle sprains continue cold applications through the second or even the third day.

5. Begin heat or cold therapy if hemorrhaging has stopped by the third day.

Inversion Ankle Sprains

Inversion ankle sprains are generally graded according to the ligament or ligaments involved. In each instance of injury the foot is forcibly turned inward on the leg, as when a basketball player jumps and comes down on the foot of another player. An inversion sprain can also occur while an individual is walking or running on an uneven surface or suddenly steps into a hole.

First-degree inversion ankle sprains The first-degree ankle sprain is the most common type of sprain. Most result from an inversion stress with the foot in plantar flexion. In general the first-degree ankle sprain consists of a mild stretching of specific lateral ligaments with little loss of function, range of motion, or strength.

A first-degree ankle sprain involves mild overstretching of the ligaments.

There is mild pain and disability with point tenderness and in some cases localized swelling over the anterior talofibular ligament. The anterior drawer test is negative with no discoloration and minimal loss of function.

    Care   RICE is used for 20 minutes every 1½ to 2 hours for 1 to 2

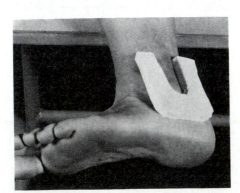

Figure 12-15

A horseshoe-shaped sponge rubber pad provides an excellent compress when held in place by an elastic wrap.

days. It may be advisable for the athlete to limit weight-bearing activities for a few days. An elastic wrap may provide comfortable pressure when weight bearing begins. When the athlete's ankle is pain free and not swollen, begin a routine of circumduction. Instruct the athlete to circle the foot 10 times in one direction, then 10 times in the other several times per day. When the athlete returns to weight bearing, taping and/or bracing may provide an extra measure of protection.

Second-degree inversion ankle sprains   Because it has a high incidence among sports participants and causes a great deal of disability with many days of lost time, the second-degree ankle sprain is a major problem for the coach and health care professionals.

A second-degree ankle sprain involves both stretching and tearing of ligaments.

The second-degree ankle sprain may completely tear some of the supporting ligaments and stretch others. There is a moderate loss of function, loss of range of motion, and loss of strength. There is a great deal of pain, with the athlete complaining of pop or snap when the ligament gave way. Even with the proper RICE procedure some swelling may occur along with some discoloration a few days after injury.

Over time, such an injury can produce a persistently unstable ankle that recurrently becomes sprained and later develops traumatic arthritis.

Care   RICE therapy should be employed intermittently for 24 to 72 hours. X-ray examination should be routine for this degree of injury. The athlete should use crutches for 5 to 10 days to avoid bearing weight. A short-leg walking cast may be applied for 2 to 3 days. The athletic trainer might begin a limited exercise program to help maintain proprioception, flexibility, and strength.

Early exercise of this type helps to maintain range of motion and normal proprioception. After 1 or 2 weeks of not bearing weight, when swelling and pain have decreased, weight bearing can be resumed.

Taping in the early inflammatory phase is of the open basketweave type (see Figure 10-13, p. 273), followed by the closed basketweave technique (see Figure 10-14, p. 273) when walking is resumed. The athlete must avoid walking and running on uneven or sloped surfaces for 2 to 3 weeks after weight bearing has begun.

Once hemorrhage has subsided, begin a therapy routine of superficial cold or heat three times per day. Two or three weeks after the injury, start circumduction exercises. Exercises can progress gradually to resistive types (see pp.337-339).

Third-degree inversion ankle sprains   The third-degree inversion ankle sprain is relatively uncommon in sports. When it does happen, it is quite disabling. Often the force partially dislocates and then spontaneously reduces the ankle (Figure 12-16). With this degree of ankle sprain there is a tearing of most supportive ligaments in the lateral side. As with the second-degree sprain, the third-degree ankle sprain is associated with a fracture.

A third-degree ankle sprain involves tearing of most of the ligaments.

The athlete complains of severe pain in the region of the lateral malleolus. Swelling is general and rapid, with tenderness over the entire lateral ankle region.

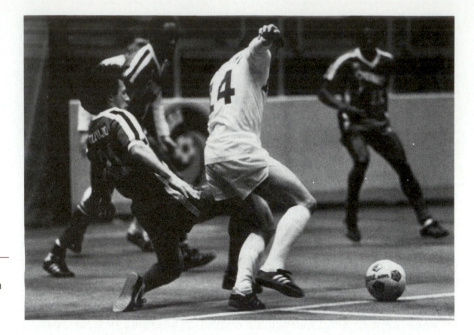

Figure 12-16

Player hitting the ground instead of the ball during an inside kick can severely injure ankle ligaments.

Care   Normally RICE is employed intermittently for 2 to 3 days. It is not uncommon for the physician to apply a short-leg walking cast, when the swelling has subsided, for 4 to 6 weeks. Crutches are usually given to the athlete when the cast is removed. Circumduction exercises begin immediately after the cast is removed and are followed by a progressive program of strengthening.

Eversion Ankle Sprains

Eversion ankle sprains are less common than inversion sprains. Athletes who have hypermobile, pronated, or flat feet have a high incidence of eversion sprains.

A second- or third-degree eversion sprain can damage the deltoid ligament and the medial longitudinal arch.

Depending on the degree of injury, the athlete complains of pain, sometimes severe, over the foot and lower leg. Usually the athlete is unable to bear weight on the foot. Most movement of the foot and ankle causes pain.

Ankle Fractures

There are two major situations in which ankle fractures occur: (1) when the foot is forcibly turned outward or inward and (2) when the foot is fixed to the ground and the lower leg is forcibly rotated either internally or externally. [5,6]

In most fracture cases, swelling and pain are extreme (Figure 12-17). There may be some or no deformity; however, if fracture is suspected, splinting is essential. RICE is employed as soon as possible to control hemorrhage and swelling. Once swelling is reduced, casting can take place, allowing the athlete to bear weight. Immobilization will usually last for at least 6 to 8 weeks. [7]

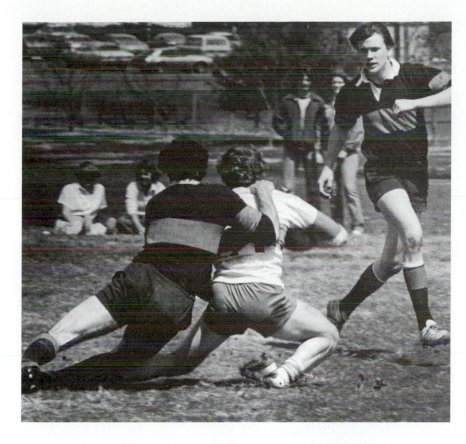

Figure 12-17

An ankle fracture or
dislocation can be a major
sports injury.

Strains About the Ankle

Heel cord strain   Heel cord strains, which are not uncommon in sports, occur from a sudden dorsiflexion of the ankle. A tight Achilles tendon is prone to strain. The resulting injury may range from mild to severe. The severe injury may result in partial or complete rupturing of the tendon.

While receiving this injury, the athlete feels acute pain and extreme weakness when pointing the foot downward.

Care   Apply the following first aid measures:

1. As with other acute injuries, apply pressure with an elastic wrap together with cold application.
2. Unless the injury is minor, hemorrhage may be extensive, requiring RICE over an extended period of time.
3. After hemorrhage has subsided, lightly apply an elastic wrap for continued pressure and send the athlete home. Follow-up care should begin the following day.

NOTE: The tendency for Achilles tendon trauma to develop into a chronic condition requires a conservative approach to therapy and immediate referral to the health care professional.

A ruptured Achilles tendon usually occurs when inflammation has been chronic.

Initiate follow-up care in the following manner:

1. Use hydromassage until soreness has subsided, beginning on the third day and continuing on subsequent days.
2. Elevate both heels, affected and unaffected, by placing a ¼-inch sponge rubber pad in the heel of each shoe. Elevation decreases the extension of the tendon and relieves some of the irritation.
3. In a few days the athlete will be able to return to activity. Restrict the Achilles tendon with a tape support and a sponge rubber heel lift placed in each sports shoe. Place heel lifts in both shoes or tape them directly on the bottoms of both heels to avoid leg length asymmetry and consequent adverse muscle and skeletal stresses (see Achilles tendon taping, Figure 10-16, p. 276)

Heel cord (Achilles) tendinitis   Achilles tendinitis usually arises from overstretching, which causes a constant inflammation (Figure 12-18). This condition may develop gradually over a long time and may require weeks or even months to heal completely. Rest and cold are the most important factors in healing. Heel lifts in shoes relieve tension on the tendon. Gentle heel cord stretching is an adjunct of cold (see p. 338).

Heel cord (Achilles tendon) rupture   A rupture of the Achilles tendon (Figure 12-19) is a possibility in sports that requires stop-and-go action. Although most common in athletes who are 30 years of age or older, rupture of the Achilles tendon can occur in athletes of any age. It usually follows chronic inflammation and gradual degeneration caused by

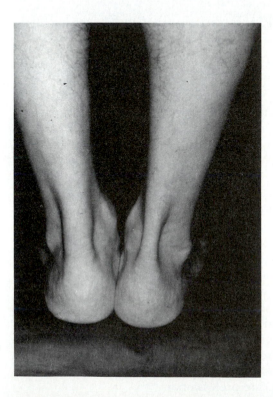

Figure 12-18

Diffuse swelling in Achilles tendinitis.

microtears. The ultimate insult normally is the result of sudden pushing-off action of the forefoot, with the knee forced into complete extension.

When the rupture occurs, the athlete complains of a sudden snap or that something hit the lower leg. Severe pain, point tenderness, swelling, discoloration, and loss of ability to point the toes are usually associated with the trauma. The major problem in the Achilles tendon rupture is accurate diagnosis. Often a partial rupture is thought to be a sprained ankle. In any acute injury to the Achilles tendon, rupture should be suspected. Signs indicative of a rupture are obvious indentation in the tendon site or a positive result to a Thompson test. The Thompson test (Fig. 12-20) is performed by simply squeezing the calf muscle while the leg is extended and the foot is hanging over the edge of the table. A positive Thompson sign is one in which squeezing the calf muscle does not cause the heel to move or pull upward or in which it moves less than the uninjured heel.

Care Usual care of a complete Achilles tendon rupture is surgical repair. On occasion, however, the physician may decide on a conservative approach.

Chronic Ankle Injuries

The second-degree sprain, with its torn and stretched ligaments, tends to have a number of serious complications. Because of laxity there is a tendency to twist and sprain the ankle repeatedly. This recurrence over time

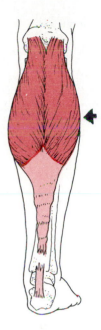

Figure 12-19

Achilles tendon rupture.

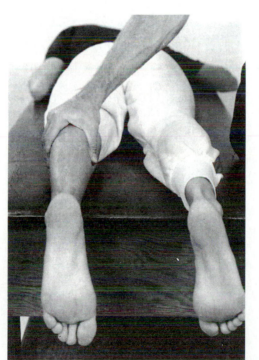

Figure 12-20

The Thompson test to determine an Achilles tendon rupture is performed by squeezing the calf muscles while the leg is extended. If the heel does not move, the tendon is damaged.

can lead to joint degeneration and traumatic arthritis. Once a second-degree sprain has occurred, there must be a concerted effort to protect the ankle against future trauma.

An eversion sprain of second or third degree can produce significant joint instability. Because the deltoid ligament supports the medial longitudinal arch, a sprain can cause weakness in this area. Repeated sprains can lead to flatfoot (pes planus).

THE LOWER LEG

The portion of the anatomy between the knee and the ankle is the lower leg. It is composed of the thicker tibia bone, the more slender fibula bone, and the soft tissues that surround them. The soft tissue of the leg is organized in four compartments bounded by fascia or bone. The compartments are named for their various locations: anterior, lateral, superficial posterior, and deep posterior (Figure 12-21).

Acute Leg Injuries

The leg is prone to a number of acute injuries, of which contusions and strains are most common. Although less common, fractures can follow

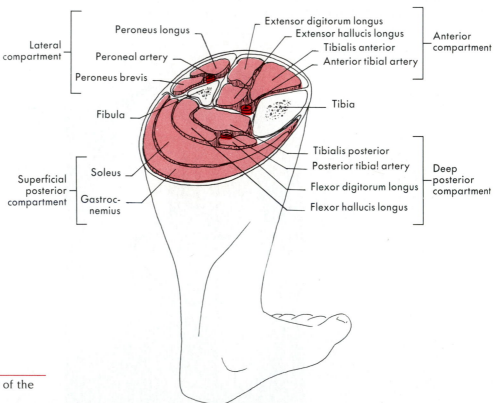

Figure 12-21

The four components of the lower leg.

direct trauma, such as occurs when being struck by a blow or through torsional forces with the foot fixed to the ground.[1]

Leg Contusions

The shin bruise   The shin, lying just under the skin, is exceedingly vulnerable and sensitive to bruising. Because of the absence of muscular or fat padding here, blows are not dissipated as they are elsewhere, and the covering of the bone, the periosteum, receives the full force of any impact delivered to the shin. Severe blows to the tibia often lead to a chronic inflammatory state. The shin is an extremely difficult area to heal, particularly the lower third, which has a considerably smaller blood supply than the upper position (Figure 12-22).

In sports in which the shin is particularly vulnerable, such as soccer and field and ice hockey, adequate padding must be provided. All injuries in this area are potentially serious and should never go untended.

Muscle contusions   Contusions of the leg, particularly in the calf muscle, are common in sports. A bruise in this area can be an extremely handicapping injury. Such a bruising blow to the leg results in pain, weakness, and some loss of function.

When this condition occurs, it is advisable to stretch the muscles in the region immediately to prevent spasm and then for approximately 1 hour to apply a compress bandage and cold packs to control internal hemorrhaging.

If cold therapy and other superficial therapy such as massage and whirlpool do not return the athlete to normal activity within 2 to 3 days, the use of ultrasound may be warranted. An elastic wrap or tape support will stabilize the part and permit the athlete to participate without aggravation of the injury.

A shin bruise is particularly difficult to heal because there is less blood supplied to the shin than other areas.

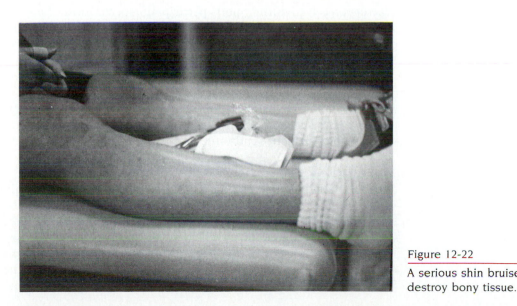

Figure 12-22

A serious shin bruise can destroy bony tissue.

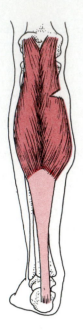

Figure 12-23

Tennis leg calf strain.

Leg Spasms and Muscle Strains

Muscle spasms Spasms are sudden, violent, involuntary contractions of one or several muscles and may be either clonic or tonic (see Chapter 6). How and why muscle spasms happen to athletes is often difficult to ascertain. Fatigue, excess loss of fluid through perspiration, and inadequate reciprocal muscle coordination are some of the factors that may predispose an individual to a contracture. The leg, particularly the gastrocnemius muscle, is prone to this condition.

Care When a muscle goes into spasm, there is severe pain and considerable apprehension on the part of the athlete. Care in such cases includes putting the athlete at ease and relaxing the contracted site. Firmly grasping the contracted muscle, together with mild gradual stretching, has been found to relieve most acute spasms. Vigorously rubbing an extremity during spasm will often increase its intensity. In cases of recurrent spasm the coach or athletic trainer should make certain that fatigue or abnormal mineral loss through perspiring is not a factor.

Calf strain (tennis leg) Sports that require quick starts and stops, such as tennis, can cause a calf strain. Usually the athlete makes a quick stop with the foot planted flatfooted and suddenly extends the knee, placing stress on the medial head of the gastrocnemius (Figure 12-23). In most cases it can be prevented by a regular routine of gradually stretching the calf region and exercising the antagonist and agonist muscles. If the pain is sustained, immediate application of RICE is necessary and should be followed by a gentle, gradual stretch routine. Follow-up care should include a regimen of cold, heat, and mild exercise, together with walking in low-heeled shoes, accentuating a heel-toe gait. A ¼-inch heel lift in each shoe will reduce muscle tension.

Leg Fractures

Fractures received during sports participation occur most often to the finger, hand, face, and leg. Of leg fractures, the fibula has the highest incidence, principally to the middle third of the leg. Fractures of the larger tibia occur predominantly to the lower third (Figure 12-24).

Chronic Leg Injuries

A number of problems of the leg can be attributed to repetitive use and overuse. Three of these conditions are medial shin stress syndrome (shinsplints), compartment syndrome, and stress fracture.

Medial Tibial Stress Syndrome (Shinsplints)

Shinsplints is a general term applied to a variety of conditions that seasonally plague many athletes. It is characterized by pain and irritation in the shin and is usually attributed to an inflammation localized primarily in the tendon of the posterior tibial muscle or long flexor muscles of the toes. It has been believed that chronic medial tibial pain was a compartment syndrome; however, recent studies have discounted this view. Speculations as to the cause include faulty posture alignment, fallen

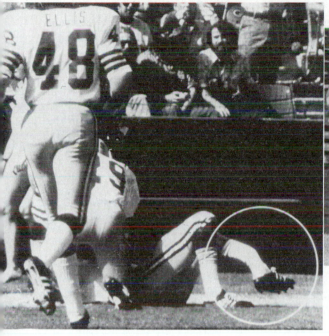

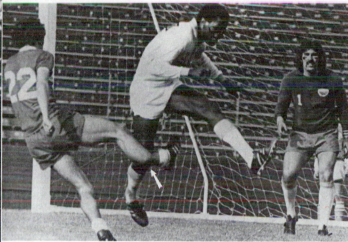

Figure 12-24

The lower leg has a high incidence of fractures in active sports.

arches, muscle fatigue, overuse stress, body chemical imbalance, and lack of proper reciprocal muscle coordination between anterior and posterior aspects of the leg. Other possible causes are tight soleus muscles, fallen longitudinal arches, and pronated ankles. All these factors, in various combinations or singly, may contribute to medial tibial stress syndrome.

This condition is regarded as a muscle or bone inflammation that occurs either acutely, as in preseason preparation, or chronically, developing slowly throughout the entire competitive season. Persistent shin irritation and incapacitation must be referred to a health care professional for further examination and monogram. Conditions such as stress fracture, muscle herniation, severe swelling within the anterior fascia chamber, muscle strain, tendinitis, fasciitis, arterial insufficiency, and nerve entrapment may be present and mistaken for a medial tibial stress syndrome.[9]

Care   Care of medial shin stress syndrome (shinsplints) can be as varied as its causes. The health care professional may opt for ice therapy, heat in the form of hot packs or whirlpool, or application of a penetrating heat modality. Supportive taping to the longitudinal arch and/or shin might be selected (see Figure 10-17, p. 277).

Ice massage to the shin region and taking two aspirins have been found to be beneficial before a workout. Apply ice massage for 10 minutes or until redness shows. Follow ice application with a gradual stretch to both the anterior and posterior aspects of the leg directly after the massage. Static stretching should be a routine procedure before and after physical activity for all athletes who have a history of shinsplints. Exercise must also accompany any therapy program, with special considerations of reconditioning the calf muscles concerned with plantar flexion.

Compartment Syndromes

As Figure 12-21 shows, there are four separate compartments of the lower leg. Injury to the lower leg that results in a fluid pressure within a compartment can compress muscles, blood vessels, and nerves. Compression of these structures, if not relieved quickly, could lead to permanent disability. Injury could stem from strain or a direct blow to the lower leg.

Acute Compartment Syndrome

syndrome
Group of typical symptoms or conditions that characterize an injury, a deficiency, or a disease

The acute compartment **syndrome** resulting from exercise is much less common than the chronic or recurrent type. It is usually caused by unaccustomed exercise such as running a long distance. This is a very serious condition and needs to be promptly referred to a physician.

In an acute condition the affected compartment continues to show signs of compression of nerves and blood vessels after the athlete stops exercising. The following signs are characteristic of anterior compartment syndrome, by far the most common form: (1) weakness of foot dorsiflexion or extension of the great toe and (2) numbness (paresthesia) or tingling of the web between the first and second toe or over the foot's entire dorsal region.

If by chance there is an acute posterior compartment syndrome there is (1) weakness in plantar flexion, (2) weakness of great toe and little toe flexion, and (3) paresthesia of the sole of the foot.

Care Because the acute compartment syndrome is a major emergency, it must be treated immediately with elevation and a cold pack. NOTE: Do not wrap the part, as it is necessary to avoid additional constriction of the lower leg. In many cases acute compartment syndrome requires immediate decompression by the surgical release of the fascia covering the area.

Exercise-Induced Compartment Syndrome

Exercise-induced compartments compression syndromes are most commonly seen in runners and soccer players.

The exercise-induced compartment compression syndrome is most frequently seen among runners and in sports such as soccer, which involve extensive running. The compartments most often affected are the anterior and deep posterior, with the anterior having by far the highest incidence. On occasion the lateral compartment may be involved.

The compartment compression syndrome occurs when the tissue's fluid pressure has increased because the confines of fascia or bone adversely compress muscles, blood vessels, and nerves. With the increase in fluid pressure, muscle blood circulation is impeded, which can lead to permanent disability.

The exercise-induced compartment compression syndrome is classified as acute or chronic (recurrent). The acute syndrome should be considered a medical emergency requiring immediate decompression to prevent permanent damage. The acute exercise-induced compartment compression syndrome resembles a fracture or a severe contusion.

The second type is chronic or recurrent. Internal pressures rise slowly during exercise and subside after discontinuance of exercise. If exercise is not stopped in time, an acute emergency may occur. In chronic exercise-induced compartment compression syndrome, constriction of blood vessels produces ischemia and pain but seldom neurological involvement.

Tibia and Fibular Stress Fractures

Stress fracture to the tibia or fibula is a common overuse stress condition, especially among distance runners.[11] As with many other overuse syndromes, athletes who have biomechanical foot problems along with improper performance skills are more prone to stress fractures in the lower leg.[11] Athletes who have hypermobile, pronated, or flat feet are more susceptible to fibular stress fracture, and those with rigid pes cavus are more prone to tibial stress fractures. Runners frequently develop a stress fracture in the lower third of the leg.

The athlete complains of pain in the leg that is more intense on activity but relieved when resting. There is usually point tenderness, but it may be difficult to discern the difference between bone pain and soft-tissue pain.

Detection of a stress fracture may be extremely difficult. X-ray examination may not determine a bone defect, which means more definitive testing by the physician is required.

Care The following regimen may be used for a stress fracture of the leg:

1. Discontinue or restrict running intensity and other stressful locomotor activities for 3 to 6 months.
2. When pain is severe, use crutches or wear a cast.
3. Weight bearing may be resumed as pain subsides.
4. Bicycling may be used before returning to running.
5. After at least 6 weeks and a pain-free period of at least 2 weeks, running can begin again.
6. Biomechanical foot correction may be necessary.

PREVENTIVE AND RECONDITIONING EXERCISE OF THE ANKLE AND LOWER LEG

Preventive and/or reconditioning exercises of the ankle and lower leg should be performed two to three times daily, progressing from one to three sets of 10 repetitions. The athlete must consider all the major muscles associated with the foot, ankle, and lower leg. The following exercises are grouped according to their level of intensity. All exercises must be performed with no pain.

Level 1

1. *Writing the alphabet*—with toes pointed, three times.

> The athlete with hypermobile and/or pronated feet is especially susceptible to fibular stress fracture. The athlete with rigid pes cavus is especially susceptible to tibial fractures.

2. *Picking up objects*—one at a time with the toes, such as 10 marbles, and placing them in a container.
3. *Gripping and spreading toes*—10 repetitions.
4. *Ankle circumduction*—10 circles in one direction and 10 circles in the other.
5. *Flatfoot Achilles tendon stretching*—with foot flat on the floor, the Achilles tendon, representing the gastrocnemius muscle, is stretched with the knee held straight followed by stretching the soleus muscle with the knee bent. The stretch occurs first with foot straight ahead, then adducted, and finally abducted. Each stretch is maintained for 20 to 30 seconds and repeated two to three times.
6. *Toe raises*—standing flat on floor, the athlete rises onto toes as far as possible, with toes pointed straight ahead, pointed in, and finally pointed out; 10 repetitions, two or three times.
7. *Walking on toes and heels*—the athlete walks 10 paces forward on toes and 10 paces backward on heels. Repeated two or three times.

Level 2

1. *Towel gather* —10 repetitions, two or three times.
2. *Towel scoop* —10 repetitions, two or three times.
3. *Achilles tendon stretching and toe raise* —the athlete stand with toes on a raised area, such as a step, with heels over the edge. The heels are raised as far as possible and then returned to stretch the Achilles tendon as much as possible. This is performed with toes pointed straight ahead, pointed in, and then pointed out; 10 repetitions, two or three times.
4. *Resistance* —exercise muscles against a resistance, such as surgical tubing or an inner-tube strip. The rubber is attached around a stationary table or chair leg. The athlete places the tubing around the foot and pulls the forefoot into dorsiflexion and eversion, then reverses position and exercises the foot in plantar flexion inversion; 10 repetitions, three or four times.
5. *Manual resistance* —manual resistance can be applied by another athlete. The exercise is performed in a complete range of motion and in all four ankle movements. Exercise is performed until fatigue or pain is felt.
6. *Proprioceptive ankle training* —the athlete spends 3 to 5 minutes daily on a balance board (wobble board) to reestablish ankle proprioception.

Level 3

1. *Rope jumping*—5 to 10 minutes daily.
2. *Heel-toe and then on-toe running*—the athlete starts with heel-toe jogging until a mile distance can be performed easily. Jogging is then shifted to jogging 50 yards and on-toe running 50 yards, graduating to all on-toe running for 1 mile.

3. *Zigzag running*—the athlete runs a zigzag pattern, graduating from slow to full speed without favoring the leg.
4. *Backward running*—a final exercise for returning full ankle and lower leg function is running backward on the toes.

SUMMARY

The ankle has a high incidence of injury in sports activities. Although the ankle has relatively strong bony arrangement, its soft tissue is very weak laterally. To offset the ankle's susceptibility to injuries, the coach and athletic trainer can use preventive procedures. Heel cord stretching, strength training, wearing of proper footwear, and the application of appropriate taping or wrapping can prevent many injuries.

A second- or third-degree sprained ankle requires immediate RICE care. Cold is applied for 20 minutes intermittently 5 to 6 times per day and lasting for 2 to 3 days. Compression is applied by an elastic wrap. The ankle is elevated above the level of the heart whenever possible. Weight bearing should be eliminated by the use of crutches.

The mechanisms that strain a heel cord also can cause rupture. The Thompson test is standard for the suspected heel-cord rupture. Repeated minor heel-cord tears can cause tissue degeneration and, subsequently, a rupture.

The lower leg is subject to bruises, acute and chronic strain, and, on occasion, fractures. Chronic strain can lead to shinsplints or the more serious exercise-induced compartment syndrome.

REVIEW QUESTIONS AND CLASS ACTIVITIES

1. How can ankle and lower leg injuries be prevented?
2. Describe the common mechanisms of injury for acute ankle sprains. What structures are damaged?
3. How can the coach rule out fractures in the lower leg and ankle?
4. How is a heel cord strain cared for? What are some indications of a heel cord rupture?
5. What acute injuries occur in the lower leg? Can any be serious enough to cause permanent damage?
6. How should you evaluate an athlete who complains of shin pain? How are shinsplints managed?
7. Contrast acute compartment syndrome with exercise-induced chronic or recurrent compartment syndrome.
8. What exercises should you include in the various levels of managing a moderate ankle sprain? What criteria should you use to determine when the athlete is ready to return to practice?

REFERENCES

1. Ekstrom M: Lower-leg pain can stop athletes in their tracks, *First Aider* 56:1, 1987.
2. Fick DS et al: Relieving painful "shinsplints," *Phys Sportmed* 20:105, 1992.
3. Franking JR et al: A comparison of ankle taping methods, *Clin J Sports Med* 3:20, 1993.
4. Glick JM, Sampson TG: Ankle and foot fractures in athletics. In Ni-

cholas JA, Hershman LB, eds: *The lower extremity and spine in sports medicine,* vol 1, St Louis, 1986, Mosby–Year Book.

5. Kimura IF et al: Effect of the air stirrup in controlling ankle inversion stress, *J Orthop Sports Phys Ther* 9:190, 1987.

6. McDermott EP: Basketball injuries of the foot and ankle, *Clin Sports Med* 12:373, 1993.

7. Mehlman CT: Ankle fractures: common mechanism, classifications, and complications, *Ath Tr* 23:110, 1988.

8. Meisterling RC: Recurrent lateral ankle sprains, *Phys Sports Med* 21:123, 1993.

9. Singer KM, Jones DC: Ligament injuries of the ankle and foot. In

Nicholas JA, Hershman EB, eds: *The lower extremity and spine in sports medicine,* vol 1, St Louis, 1986, Mosby–Year Book.

10. Schon LC et al: Chronic exercise-induced leg pain in active people, *Phys Sportsmed* 20:230, 1992.

11. Tanbe RR, Wadsworth LT: Managing tibial stress fractures, *Phys Sportsmed* 21:123, 1993.

12. Taylor DC, Bassett FH III: Syndesmosis ankle sprains, *Phys Sportsmed* 21:39, 1993.

13. Taylor DC et al: Syndesmosis sprains of the ankle, *Am J Sports Med* 20:146, 1992.

14. Weiker GG: Sprains and pseudo-sprains of the athlete's ankle, *Sports Med Dig* 9:1, 1987.

ANNOTATED BIBLIOGRAPHY

Booher JM, Thibodeau GA: *Athletic injury assessment,* St Louis, 1993, Times Mirror/Mosby College Publishing.

Chapter 15 discusses the anatomy of the ankle and lower leg; injuries to the foot, ankle, and lower leg; and the injury assessment process.

Shangold MM, Mirkin G: *Women and exercise: physiology and sports medicine,* Philadelphia, 1988, FA Davis.

Provides a brief overview of ankle impingement syndromes common to gymnasts, dancers, and divers.

Yocum LA, ed: Foot and medicine, vol 7, no 1, Philadelphia, 1988, WB Saunders.

Provides a good overview of the major factors related to foot and ankle injuries.

The Knee and Related Structures

When you finish this chapter, you will be able to:

- Describe the most common knee injuries and injuries to its related structures
- Identify the most common knee injuries
- Explain how to apply appropriate immediate and superficial follow-up care to a knee injury

Muscles and ligaments provide the main source of stability in the knee.

Major actions of the knee:
  Flexion
  Extension
  Gliding
  Rotation

anterior cruciate ligament
Stops external rotation

The knee joint is one of the most complex joints in the human body. Because so many sports place extreme stress on the knee, it is also one of the most traumatized joints in sports (Figure 13-1). The primary actions of the knee are flexion, extension, gliding, and rotation. Secondary movements consist of a slight internal (medial) and external (lateral) rotation of the tibia. The movements of flexion and extension take place above the menisci (Figure 13-2), crescent-shaped fibrocartilages, and rotation is performed below the menisci. Rotation is caused mainly by the greater length of the medial condyle of the femur, which rolls forward more than the lateral condyle does. Because the knee's bony arrangements are weak, compensation is provided through the firm support of ligaments and muscles (Figure 13-3). The knee is designed primarily for stability in weight bearing and mobility in locomotion; however, it is especially unstable laterally and medially.

Ligaments and the deeper capsular structures serve to stabilize the knee. Those that stabilize the knee medially and laterally are the tibial (medial) collateral ligament and the fibular (lateral) collateral ligament. Internal stability is also provided by the cruciate ligaments. The **anterior cruciate ligament** attaches to the front of the tibia's upper surface between the two menisci and passes to the medial aspect of the lateral condyle of the femur. In contrast, the posterior cruciate ligament attaches to the back of the tibia's upper surface and passes forward to the lateral aspect of the medial condyle of the femur. In general, the anterior cruciate ligament stops excessive external rotation, stabilizes the knee in full ex-

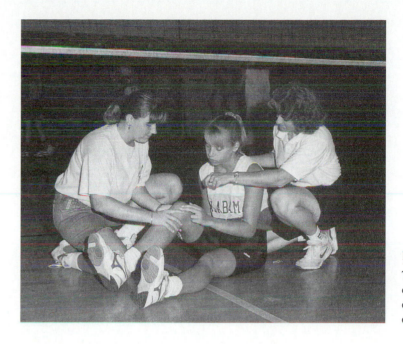

Figure 13-1

The knee is a highly
complicated joint that is
often traumatized during
competitive sports.

tension, and prevents hyperextension. The **posterior cruciate liga-**
ments prevent internal rotation, guide the knee in flexion, and act as a
drag during the initial glide phase of flexion.

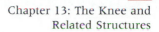

posterior cruciate
ligament
Stops internal rotation

PREVENTION OF KNEE INJURIES

Preventing knee injuries in sports is a complex problem. First in importance is physical conditioning and proper skill development followed by
the wearing of correct shoes. A questionable practice may be the routine
use of protective bracing.

Physical Conditioning

Proper conditioning of the knee plays an important role in injury prevention. Specific and total body conditioning must take place. This includes maximum strength, flexibility, stamina, agility, speed, and balance.
A balance of strength must be present. For example, in football players
the hamstring muscles should have 60% to 70% of the strength of the
quadriceps muscles. All prior knee injuries must be properly rehabilitated.[2]

Shoe Type

Over recent years, athletes in collision-type sports such as football have
been using soccer-style shoes. The change from a few long, conical cleats
to a large number of cleats that are short (no longer than ½ inch [1.3
cm]) and broad has significantly cut down on knee injuries in football.
The higher number of shorter cleats is better because the foot does not

Menisci of the knee.

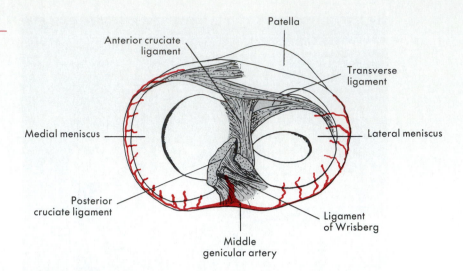

The bony and ligamentous
arrangement of the knee.

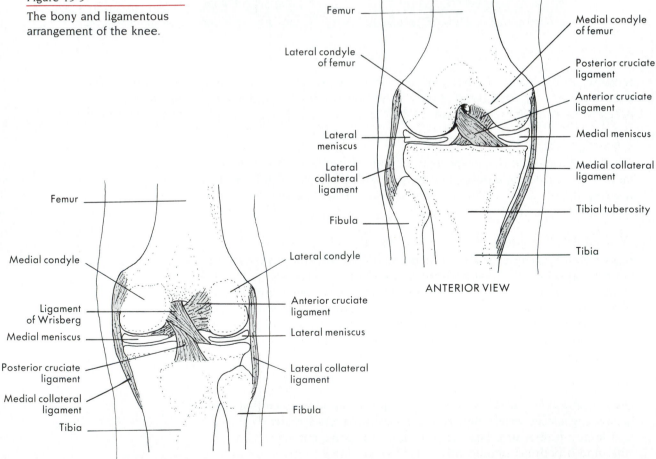

POSTERIOR VIEW

ANTERIOR VIEW

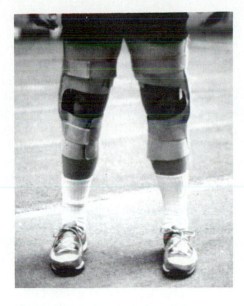

Figure 13-4

Prophylactic knee braces.

become fixed to the surface and the shoe still allows controlled running and cutting.

Protective Knee Bracing

Protective knee braces have been designed to prevent or reduce the severity of knee injuries. The effectiveness of these braces is controversial. To date there is not enough information to support the use of prophylactic bracing as a protective device[7,8] (Figure 13-4). The wearing of a prophylactic knee brace has been found to alter the knee's muscle coordination.[13]

Acute Injuries

Knee Bruise (Contusion)

A blow struck against the bony tissue and muscles crossing the knee joint can result in a severe handicap. Bruises to the inner aspect of the thigh region (vastus medialis muscle) produce all the appearances of a knee sprain, including severe pain, loss of movement, and signs of acute inflammation. Such bruising is often manifested by swelling and discoloration caused by the tearing of muscle tissue and blood vessels. If adequate first aid is given immediately, the knee will usually return to function 24 to 48 hours after the trauma (see box on p. 347).

Bruising to the region of the knee joint can penetrate to the bone. A traumatic compressive force delivered to the knee joint causes bleeding and results in profuse fluid swelling into the joint cavity and surrounding spaces. Swelling often takes place slowly. It is advisable to prevent the athlete from engaging in further activity for at least 24 hours after receipt of a joint bruise.

Care Care of a bruised knee depends on many factors. However, management principally depends on the location and severity of the contusion. The following procedures are suggested:

1. Apply compression bandages and cold along with elevation until hemorrhage has stopped.
2. Have the athlete rest for 24 hours.
3. If swelling occurs, continue cold application for 72 hours. If swelling and pain are intense, refer the athlete to the physician.
4. Once the acute stage has ended and the swelling has diminished to little or none, cold application with active range-of-motion exercises should be conducted within a pain-free range. If a gradual use of heat is elected, great caution should be taken to avoid swelling.
5. Allow the athlete to return to normal activity with protective padding when pain and the initial irritation have subsided.
6. If swelling is not resolved within a week, a chronic problem may exist, indicating the need for further rest and medical attention.

Bursitis

Where tissue such as a tendon moves in relation to a bone, a fluid cushion known as a bursa develops. A bursa has an outer coat of dense fibrous tissue with a soft lining that secretes a small amount of fluid. When this lining becomes irritated, bursitis occurs. Bursitis in the knee can be acute, chronic, or recurrent. Any one of numerous knee bursae can become inflamed.

Bursae (Figure 13-5) often become inflamed from continued kneeling or from overuse of the patellar tendon. Swelling in the knee posteriorly may indicate an irritation of one of the bursae in this region. Swelling in the back of the knee (popliteal fossa) may be a sign of *Baker's cyst* (Figure 13-6), an irritation of the bursa associated with the calf and hamstring muscles (gastrocnemius-semimembranous bursae). Baker's cyst is

Figure 13-5

Common bursae of the knee.

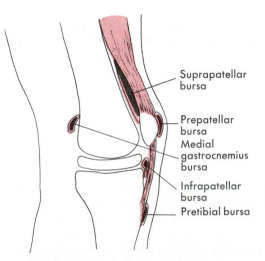

Suprapatellar bursa

Prepatellar bursa

Medial gastrocnemius bursa

Infrapatellar bursa

Pretibial bursa

EVALUATION OF THE INJURED KNEE JOINT

Although diagnosis of a specific knee injury is charged to the physician, a coach can learn to recognize key indicators of an injury. Once recognized, a coach can make a referral to the athletic trainer and/or physician. By following the acronym HOPS the coach may be able to differentiate a more serious injury from a less serious one.

History

1. What were you doing when the knee was hurt?
2. What position was your body in?
3. Did you hear a noise or feel any sensation at the time of injury, such as a pop or crunch? (A pop could indicate an anterior cruciate tear, a crunch could be a sign of a torn meniscus, and a tearing sensation might indicate a capsular tear.)
4. Could you move the knee immediately after the injury? If not, was it locked in a bent or extended position? (Locking could mean a meniscal tear.) After being locked, how did it become unlocked?
5. Did swelling occur? If yes, was it immediate, or did it occur later? (Immediate swelling could indicate a cruciate or tibial fracture, whereas later swelling could indicate a capsular, synovial, or meniscal tear.)
6. Where was the pain? Was it local, all over, or did it move from one side of the knee to the other?
7. Have you hurt the knee before?

Observation

A visual evaluation should be performed after the major complaints have been determined. The athlete should be observed in a number of situations: walking, half-squatting, and going up and down stairs. These activities should not be performed if there is any indication of a fracture. The leg also should be observed for alignment and symmetry or asymmetry.

Walking

1. Does the athlete walk with a limp, or is the walk free and easy? Is the athlete able to fully extend the knee during heel-strike?
2. Can the athlete fully bear weight on the affected leg?
3. Can the athlete go up and down stairs with ease? (If stairs are unavailable, stepping up on a box or stool will suffice.)

Leg Alignment

The athlete should be observed for leg alignment. Anteriorly, the athlete is evaluated for bowleg, knock-knees, and the position of the patella. Next, the athlete is observed from the side to ascertain conditons such as the hypeflexed or hyperextended knee.

Knee Symmetry or Asymmetry

The athletic trainer or coach must establish whether both of the athlete's knees look the same:

1. Do the knees appear symmetrical?
2. Is one knee obviously swollen?

Palpation

The knee can be palpated for sites of point tenderness and/or tissue discrepancies. Four different anatomical areas are palpated, including bone, joint supportive tissue (ligament and capsule), muscle and tendons, and areas of swelling. Bony palpation is concerned with pain and deformities that might reveal a fracture or dislocation. The supportive tissue surrounding the joint is palpated for pain and defects. Muscles and tendons are felt for their symmetry of definition, defects of continuity revealing rupture or tears. Swelling due to bleeding or edema can be determined by palpation. Blood in the knee joint feels heavy and moves like jelly, whereas edema feels light and, when pushed, runs back and forth.

Seriousness

Pain or lack of pain is not always the best indicator of a serious knee injury. One of the best indicators is a loss of function. An athlete unable to bend a knee or bear weight should be referred to the athletic trainer or physician for an in-depth evaluation.

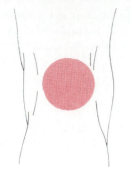

Figure 13-6

Baker's cyst in the popliteal fossa.

Figure 13-7

Various forces applied to the knee can produce serious injuries.

commonly painless, causing no discomfort or disability. Some inflamed bursae may be painful and disabling because of the swelling and should be treated accordingly.

Care Care usually follows a pattern of eliminating the cause, prescribing rest, and reducing inflammation. Contrast baths may help to reduce swelling. When the bursitis is chronic or recurrent and the synovium has thickened, aspiration and a steroid injection may be carried out by the physician.

Collateral Ligament and Capsular Joint Injuries

Ligament and capsular sprains are the most frequently reported knee injuries in sports. Many knee sprains involve the medial collateral ligament either by a direct blow from the lateral side in a medial direction or by a severe outward twist (Figure 13-7). Greater injury results from medial sprains than from lateral sprains because of their more direct relation to the articular capsule and the medial meniscus. Medial and lateral sprains appear in varying degrees, depending on knee position, previous injuries, the strength of muscles crossing the joint, the force and angle of the trauma, fixation of the foot, and conditions of the playing surface.

Any position of the knee, from full extension to full flexion, can re-

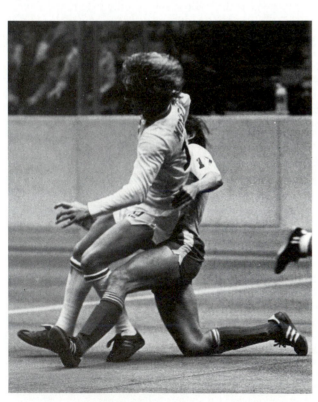

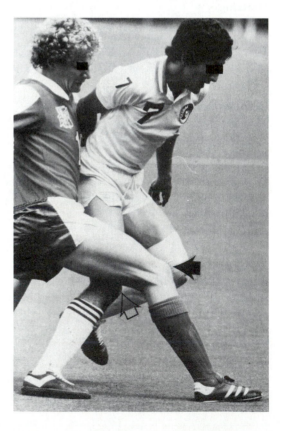

sult in injury if there is sufficient force. Full extension tightens both lateral and medial ligaments. However, flexion affords a loss of stability to the lateral ligament but maintains stability in various portions of the broad medial ligament. Medial collateral ligament sprains occur most often from a violently adducted and internally rotated knee. The most prevalent mechanism of a lateral collateral ligament or capsular sprain is one in which the foot is turned inward and the knee is forced laterally outward.

Speculation among medical authorities is that torn menisci seldom happen as the result of an initial trauma; most occur after the collateral ligaments have been stretched by repeated injury. Many mild to moderate sprains leave the knee unstable and thus vulnerable to additional internal derangements. The strength of the muscles crossing the knee joint is important for supporting the ligaments and capsules. These muscles should be conditioned to the highest possible degree for sports in which knee injuries are common (Figure 13-8).

Sprains are common when the foot is turned inward and the knee is forced outward.

Acute Medial Knee Sprains

Medial injuries to the knee can involve the medial collateral or deeper capsular ligaments (Figures 13-9 and 13-10). The major cause of this type of injury is from a direct blow from the lateral, as in a football clip, or from a severe outward twist.

First-Degree Medial Collateral Ligament Sprain

A first-degree medial collateral ligament injury of the knee has the following characteristics (Figure 13-11):

1. A few ligamentous fibers are torn and stretched.
2. The joint is stable in valgus stress tests.
3. There is little or no joint swelling.

Figure 13-8

Musculature of the knee.

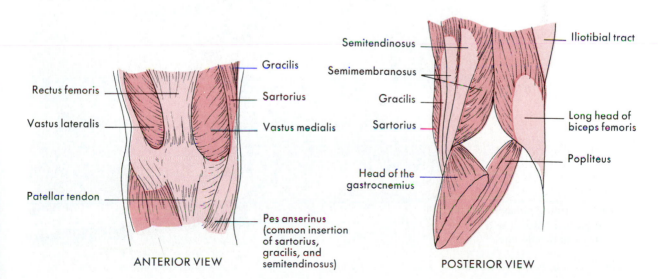

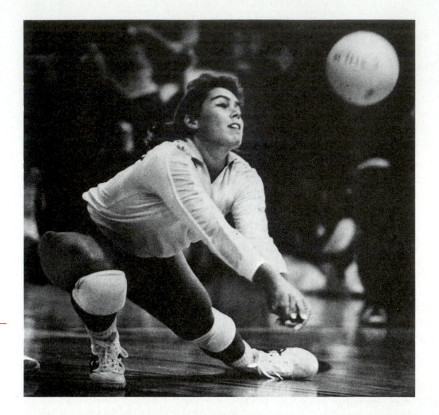

Figure 13-9

Constant stress on the medial aspect of the knee can stretch the supportive tissue, making the knee susceptible to acute sprain.

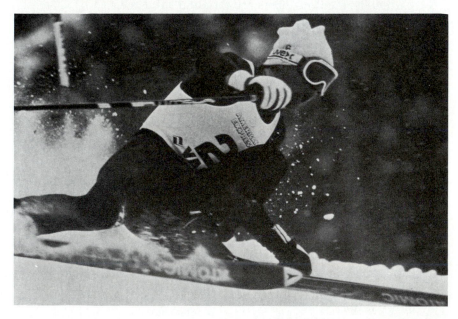

Figure 13-10

Competitive skiing places extreme medial, lateral, and rotary stresses on the knee.

4. There may be some joint stiffness and point tenderness just below the medial joint line.
5. Even with minor stiffness, there is almost full passive and active range of motion.

Care Immediate care consists of RICE for at least 24 hours. After immediate care, the following procedures should be undertaken:

1. Crutches are prescribed if the athlete is unable to walk without a limp.
2. Follow-up care may involve cryokinetics, including 5 minutes of ice-pack treatment preceding exercise or a combination of cold and compression or ultrasound.
3. Proper exercise is essential, with early movement suggested.

Isometrics and straight-leg exercises are important until the knee can be moved without pain. The athlete then graduates to stationary bicycle riding or a high-speed isokinetic program. This helps the athlete progress to knee muscle contraction near that of a particular running sport.

The athlete is allowed to return to full participation when the knee has regained normal strength, power flexibility, endurance, and coordination. Usually 1 to 3 weeks is necessary for recovery. On returning to activity the athlete may require tape support for a short period.

Second-Degree Medial Collateral Ligament Sprain

A second-degree medial collateral ligament knee sprain indicates both microscopic and gross disruption of ligamentous fibers (Figure 13-12). The only structures involved are the medial collateral ligament and the medial capsular ligament. It is characterized by the following:

1. A complete tear of the deep capsular ligament and partial tear of the superficial layer of the medial collateral ligament or a partial tear of both areas.
2. There is no general joint instability; however, there may be a minimal or slight laxity in full extension.
3. Swelling is slight or absent unless the meniscus or anterior cruciate ligament has been torn. An acutely torn or pinched synovial membrane, subluxated or dislocated patella, or an osteochondral fracture can produce extensive swelling and **hemarthrosis.**
4. Moderate to severe joint tightness with an inability to fully and actively extend the knee. The athlete is unable to place the heel flat on the ground.
5. Definite loss of passive range of motion.
6. Pain in the medial joint line, with general weakness and instability.

Care The following steps should be followed when caring for a second-degree medial collateral ligament strain:

1. RICE for 48 to 72 hours.
2. Crutches are used with a three-point gait until the acute phase of injury is over and the athlete can walk without a limp.
3. Depending on the severity and possible complications, a full-leg

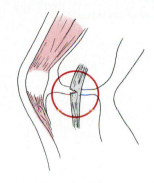

Figure 13-11

First-degree sprain of the medial collateral ligament.

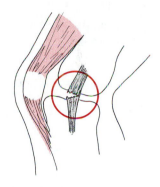

Figure 13-12

Second-degree sprain of the medial collateral ligament.

hemarthrosis
Blood in a joint cavity

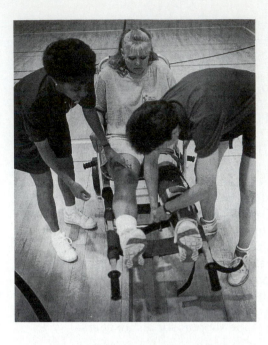

Figure 13-13

Knee immobilizer used after a ligamentous injury.

cast or postoperative knee immobilizing splint may be applied by the physician (Figure 13-13).

4. Cryokinetics or other therapeutic modalities are employed three or four times daily.
5. Isometric exercise along with exercise to all the adjacent joints is performed three or four times daily.
6. Depending on the extent of injury and swelling, the immobilizing splint is removed and gentle range of movement may be performed.
7. Although currently employed less than in the past, taping may be appropriate to provide some support and confidence to the athlete (see Figures 10-18 and 10-19, pp. 278-279).

Third-Degree Medial Collateral Ligament Sprain

Third-degree medial collateral ligament sprain is a complete tear of the supporting ligaments. The following are major signs (Figure 13-14):

1. Complete loss of medial stability
2. Minimal to moderate swelling
3. Medial pain and point tenderness
4. Loss of range of motion because of effusion and hamstring spasm
5. Some joint opening at full extension and significant opening at 30 degrees of flexion during the valgus stress test

An anterior cruciate ligament tear or medial meniscus disruption may be present and should be tested for.

Care Immediately refer the athlete to a physician. RICE for 20 minutes every 1½ to 2 hours during the waking day should be performed for at least 72 hours. In many cases such an injury is surgically repaired

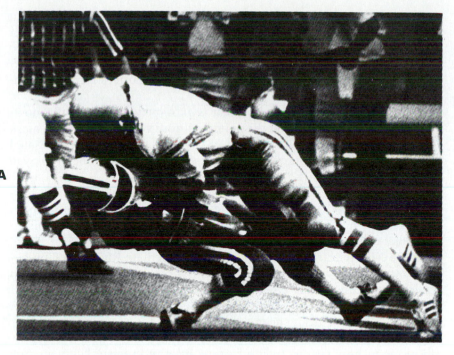

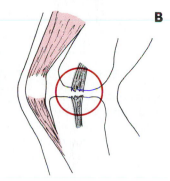

Figure 13-14

A, A knee injury that tears both medial and collateral and anterior cruciate ligaments. **B,** Third-degree sprain of the medial collateral ligament.

as soon as possible after the acute inflammatory phase of 3 or 4 days after injury.

Acute Lateral Knee Sprains

Lateral knee sprains are due to an outward force to the lateral capsule and collateral ligament. The most common situation for injury is when the lower leg is internally rotated and the knee is suddenly forced outward. If the force is great enough, fragments can be pulled from the bone.

The major signs include the following:

1. Pain and point tenderness are felt along the joint line.
2. Depending on the degree of injury, there is usually some joint instability with joint opening on the varus stress test at 30 degrees of knee flexion.
3. Swelling is usually minimal because of bleeding into joint spaces.
4. The greater the ligamentous injury, the less pain is felt on the varus stress test.

Care of the lateral collateral ligament injury should follow procedures similar to those described for medial collateral ligament injuries.

Internal Knee Joint Problems

The most common internal knee joint problems are injuries to the cruciate ligament and to the meniscus.

Acute Anterior Cruciate Ligament Tear

Until recently the medial collateral ligament tear was considered much more prevalent than the complete anterior cruciate ligament tear. Today

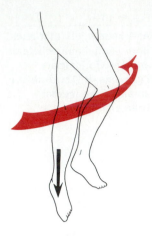

Figure 13-15

A major mechanism causing an anterior cruciate tear occurs when a running athlete suddenly decelerates and makes a sharp "cutting" motion.

the anterior cruciate is considered the most commonly disrupted ligament in the knee. The anterior cruciate ligament can be injured in a number of ways, including internal rotation of the thigh with the knee flexed while the foot is planted and forced hyperextension. Forced hyperflexion can conceivably injure both the anterior and posterior cruciate ligaments.

The anterior cruciate ligament tear is extremely difficult to diagnose. The earlier the determination the better, because swelling often will mask the full extent of injury. In addition to swelling, this injury is associated with joint instability. Therefore ligament stress tests should be employed as soon as possible by the athletic trainer or physician.

The athlete often feels or hears a pop, followed by immediate disability. The athlete complains that the knee feels like it is coming apart. Although the tear may be isolated, it can be associated with a meniscus or medial collateral ligament tear (Figure 13-15).

Care Even with proper first aid and immediate RICE, swelling begins within 1 to 2 hours and becomes a noticeable hemarthrosis within 4 to 6 hours. The athlete typically cannot walk without help.

Anterior cruciate ligament injury can lead to serious knee instability; an intact anterior cruciate ligament is necessary for a knee to function in high-performance running and jumping. Controversy exists among physicians as to how best to treat an acute anterior cruciate ligament rupture and when surgery is warranted. Before surgery an examination is commonly conducted with an arthroscope and/or magnetic resonance imaging (MRI). It is well accepted that an unsatisfactorily treated anterior cruciate ligament rupture will eventually lead to major joint degeneration.

The routine use of braces such as the Lenox Hill derotation brace, along with rotary and hyperextension taping, can provide some protection during activity (Figure 13-16) (see knee taping, Figures 10-18 and 10-19, pp. 278-279).

Posterior Cruciate

The posterior cruciate ligament has been called the most important ligament in the knee, providing a central axis for rotation. It also is the major restraint of the knee in hyperextension.

The posterior cruciate is most susceptible to injury when the knee is flexed to 90 degrees. A fall on a bent knee with the foot pointed or receiving a hard blow to the front of the knee can tear the posterior cruciate ligament.[11] A rotational force can also injure this ligament.

The major indicators of a torn posterior cruciate ligament are the following:

1. The athlete reports feeling a pop in the back of the knee.
2. There is a feeling of tenderness in the back of the knee but little swelling.
3. Testing will reveal a posterior knee sag.

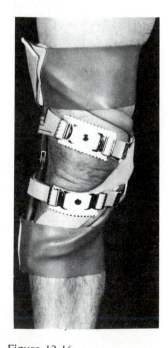

Figure 13-16

The Lenox Hill derotation knee brace.

Care

1. RICE is applied immediately.
2. Immediate referral is made to the health professional for a clinical evaluation.
3. Follow-up care might include immobilization for 6 weeks or longer, crutch walking, followed by a progressive program of exercise rehabilitation (Figure 13-17).

Meniscal Lesions

The medial meniscus has a much higher incidence of injury than the lateral meniscus. [2]

A blow from the lateral side directed inward can often tear or stretch the medial collateral ligament and pull the medial meniscus out of its bed. Repeated mild sprains reduce the strength of the knee to a state favorable for a cartilage tear through lessening of its normal ligamentous stability. A large number of medial meniscus injuries are the outcome of a sudden, strong internal rotation of the femur with a partially flexed knee while the foot is firmly planted. As a result of this action, the cartilage is pulled out of its normal bed and pinched between the femoral condyles. The higher number of medial meniscus tears is a result of the coronary ligament attaching the meniscus peripherally to the tibia and also to the capsular ligament. The lateral meniscus does not attach to the capsular ligament and is more mobile during knee movement. Because of the attachment to the medial structures, the medial meniscus is prone to disruption from inward and rotary tears (Figure 13-18). Tears within the cartilage fail to heal because of lack of adequate blood supply. However, some peripheral meniscus tears do heal when an adequate supply of blood is available.

Determination of menisci injuries should be made immediately after the injury and before muscle spasm and swelling obscure the normal shape of the knee.

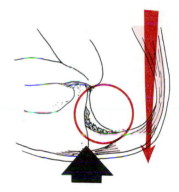

Figure 13-17

A fall or being hit on the anterior aspect of the bent knee can tear the posterior cruciate ligament.

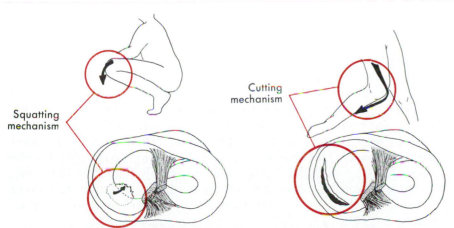

Figure 13-18

Common mechanisms of injury to the meniscus.

Squatting
mechanism

Cutting
mechanism

A knee that locks and unlocks during activity may indicate a fractured meniscus.

A meniscal tear may or may not result in the following:

1. Severe pain and loss of motion
2. A locked knee with inability to fully flex or extend
3. Pain in the area of the tear

Care   The knee that is locked by a displaced cartilage may require unlocking under anesthesia so that a detailed examination can be conducted. If discomfort, disability, and locking of the knee continue, surgery may be required. For the nonlocking acute meniscus tear, immediate care should follow a second- or third-degree sprain care routine. The knee is cared for by splinting, crutch walking, muscle setting, and isometric exercise followed by gradual range-of-movement (ROM) and progressive resistance exercises.

Chronic injuries   Once a knee cartilage has been fractured, its ruptured edges harden and may eventually atrophy. Occasionally portions of the meniscus may become detached and wedge themselves between the articulating surfaces of the tibia and femur, imposing a locking, catching, or giving way of the joint. Chronic meniscus lesions also may display recurrent swelling and obvious muscle atrophy about the knee. The athlete may complain of an inability to perform a full squat or to change direction quickly when running without pain, a sense of the knee collapsing, or a popping sensation.

Knee Plica

Knee plica stems from fetal synovial cavities that fail to fully absorb after birth. In about 20% of all individuals some of the synovial tissue does not absorb completely. The unabsorbed tissue forms into, for the most part, pliable tissue, with the exception of the mediopatellar plica. This can become thick and rigid, producing many complaints similar to a meniscus injury.[2]

Knee Fat Pads

The two most important fat pads of the knee lie between the synovial membrane and patellar ligament and between the quadricep tendon and the bursa in that region. The first fat pad is most often injured by becoming wedged between the knee cap and tibia. Usually the injury results from chronic kneeling or direct blows.

Care   Care usually involves rest, heel elevation (both heels) of ½ to 1 inch, and the therapeutic use of cold.

Loose bodies within the knee joint (joint mice)   Following repeated trauma to the knee in sports activities, loose bodies can develop within the joint cavity. Loose bodies can be fragments of the menisci, torn synovial tissue, a torn cruciate ligament, or osteochondritis dissecans. The loose body may move around in the joint space and become lodged, causing locking, popping, and giving way. When the loose body becomes wedged between articulating surfaces, irritation can occur. If not surgically removed, the loose body can lead to joint degeneration.[2]

KNEECAP (PATELLAR) AND RELATED PROBLEMS

The position and function of the patella and surrounding structures expose it to a variety of traumas and diseases related to sports activities (Figure 13-19).

Patellar Fracture

Fractures of the patella can be caused by either direct or indirect trauma. Most fractures are the result of indirect violence in which a severe pull of the patellar tendon occurs against the femur when the knee is semi-flexed. This position subjects the patella to maximal stress from the quadriceps tendon and the patellar ligament. Forcible muscle contraction may then fracture the patella at its lower half. Direct injury most often produces fragmentation with little displacement. A fall, jumping, or running may result in a fracture of the patella.

The fracture causes hemorrhage and joint effusion, resulting in a generalized swelling. Indirect fracture causes capsular tearing, separation of bone fragments, and possible tearing of the quadriceps tendon. Direct fracture involves little bone separation.

Care Diagnosis is accomplished by use of the medical history, the palpation of separated fragments, and an x-ray confirmation. As soon as the examiner suspects a patellar fracture, a cold wrap should be applied, followed by an elastic compression wrap, splinting, and crutch walking. The coach or athletic trainer should then refer the athlete to the team physician. The athlete normally will be immobilized for 2 to 3 months.

Acute Patellar Subluxation or Dislocation

When an athlete plants his or her foot, decelerates, and simultaneously cuts in an opposite direction from the weight-bearing foot, the thigh rotates internally while the lower leg rotates externally, causing a forced knee *valgus*. The quadriceps muscle attempts to pull in a straight line and as a result pulls the patella laterally—a force that may dislocate the patella. As a rule, displacement takes place outwardly with the patella resting on the lateral condyle.

An athlete who has a subluxated patella will complain that the knee catches or gives way. The knee may be swollen and painful. Pain is due to swelling but also occurs because the medial capsular tissue has been stretched and torn. Because of blood in the joint, the knee is restricted in flexion and extension.

The Dislocated Patella

An acute patellar dislocation is often associated with sudden twisting of the body while the foot or feet are planted. The athlete experiences a complete loss of knee function, pain, and swelling, with the patella resting in an abnormal position. The physician immediately puts the patella back in place (reduces the dislocation). If time has elapsed before reduction, a general anesthesia may have to be used. After removal of the blood from the joint, ice is applied and the joint is splinted. Swelling often oc-

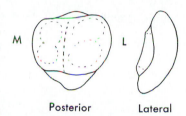

M   L

Posterior   Lateral

Figure 13-19

Patella.

The semi-flexed position subjects the patella to maximal stress from tendons and ligaments.

Knees that give way or catch may have a number of possible pathological conditions:
  Subluxating patella
  Meniscus tear
  Anterior cruciate
    ligament tear
  Hemarthrosis

curs on the medial side. A first-time patellar dislocation is always suspected of being associated with a fracture. X-ray evaluation is performed before and after reduction.

Care After reduction the knee is immobilized in extension for 4 weeks or longer, and the athlete is instructed to use crutches when walking. During immobilization, isometric exercises are performed at the knee joint. After immobilization the athlete should wear a horseshoe–shaped felt pad that is held in place around the patella by an elastic wrap or is sewn into an elastic sleeve that is worn while running or performing in sports (Figure 13-20). Commercial braces are also available. A gradual program of exercise is guided by the athletic trainer.

Pain Related to the Kneecap and Femoral Groove

The knee cap, in relation to the femoral groove, can be subject to direct trauma or disease, leading to chronic pain and disability. Of major importance among athletes are conditions that stem from abnormal patellar tracting within the femoral groove; the two most common are chondromalacia and degenerative arthritis.

Chondromalacia

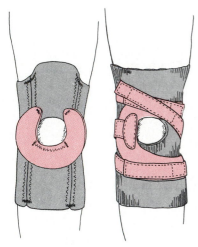

Occurring most often among teenagers and young adults, chondromalacia is a gradual degenerative process. The exact cause is unknown, but abnormal patellar tracking may be a major causative factor. Some of the more common causes are: knock-knee, abnormal rotation of the tibia, foot pronation, forward rotation of the hip, and an abnormal pull of the quadriceps muscles due to a wide hip. Chondromalacia undergoes three stages:

Stage 1—swelling and softening of the articular cartilage

Stage 2—fissuring of the softened articular cartilage

Stage 3—deformation of the surface of the articular cartilage as a result of fragmentation

The athlete may experience pain in the anterior aspect of the knee while walking, running, ascending and descending stairs, or squatting. There may be recurrent swelling around the kneecap and a grating sensation on flexing and extending the knee.

On palpation there may be pain around the borders of the patella or when the patella is compressed within the femoral groove while the knee is passively flexed and extended. The athlete may have one or more lower-limb alignment deviations (Figure 13-21).

In general, the care of chondromalacia is rest for at least 6 weeks. A physician may prescribe antiinflammatory medication and a regime of straight leg raising.

Figure 13-20

Special pads for the dislocated patella.

Other Extensor Mechanism Problems

Many other extensor mechanism problems can occur in the physically active individual. They can occur in the immature knee or through jumping and running.[12]

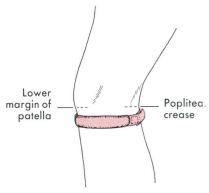

Lower margin of patella — Poplitea. crease

Figure 13-21

The chondromalacia brace.

Osgood-Schlatter Disease

Osgood-Schlatter disease is a condition of the tibial tuberosity growth region under the general classification of osteochondritis. To call this condition a *disease* is misleading because it comprises a number of conditions related to the growth center of the tibial tuberosity. The tibial tuberosity is an apophysis for the attachment of the patellar tendon.

The most commonly accepted cause is the repeated pull of the patellar tendon at the epiphysis of the tibial tubercle. Complete pulling away of the tibial tuberosity by the patellar tendon is a major complication of Osgood-Schlatter disease (see chapter 6, p. 160).

Repeated irritation causes swelling, hemorrhage, and gradual degeneration of the growth region due to impaired circulation. The athlete complains of pain on kneeling, jumping, and running. There is point tenderness over the tibial tuberosity (Figure 13-22, *B*).

Larsen-Johansson disease is similar to Osgood-Schlatter disease, but it occurs at the bottom of the kneecap. It is commonly caused by repeated muscle contraction (Figure 13-22, *A*.)

Care   Physician-directed care is usually conservative and includes the following:

1. Stressful activities should be decreased until the epiphyseal union occurs, within 6 months to 1 year.
2. Severe cases may require a cylindrical cast.
3. Ice should be applied to the knee before and after activities.
4. Quadriceps and hamstring muscles should be isometrically strengthened.
5. Only in the most severe cases should surgery be performed.

Jumper's and Kicker's Knee

Jumping, kicking, and running may place extreme tension on the knee extensor muscle complex. As a result of injury, tendinitis occurs in the patellar or quadriceps tendon. On rare occasions a patellar tendon may completely fail and rupture.

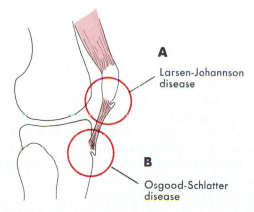

A
Larsen-Johannson
disease

B
Osgood-Schlatter
disease

Figure 13-22

Two conditions of the immature extensor mechanism. **A,** Larsen-Johansson disease. **B,** Osgood-Schlatter disease.

Patellar or Quadriceps Tendinitis

Sudden or repetitive forceful extension of the knee may begin an inflammatory process that will eventually lead to tendon degeneration.[2]

Patellar or quadriceps tendinitis can be described in three stages of pain:

Stage 1—pain after sports activity

Stage 2—pain during and after activity (the athlete is able to perform at the appropriate level)

Stage 3—pain during activity and prolonged after activity (athletic performance is hampered), which may progress to constant pain and complete rupture

Care Any pain in the extensor mechanism must preclude sudden explosive movement such as that characterized by heavy plyometric-type exercising. Athletes with first- or second-stage tendinitis should carefully warm the tendons for 5 to 10 minutes in a whirlpool at 100° to 102° F (37.7° to 38.8° C) before performing an activity. Moist heat packs can be used instead of the whirlpool. After warming, a gradual static stretch should be applied as the tendons return to normal preexercise temperature. A gradual exercise warm-up should follow. The athlete should cease all activity at once if there is pain during exercise. An ice massage or pack should follow exercise. Third-stage jumper's knee should be rested until it is symptom free.

Patellar or quadriceps tendon rupture An inflammatory condition of the knee extensor mechanism over time can cause degeneration and weakness at the tendon attachment.[2] Seldom does a rupture occur in the middle of the tendon, but usually it is torn from its attachment. The quadriceps tendon ruptures from the superior pole of the patella, whereas the patellar tendon ruptures from the inferior pole of the patella. Proper conservative care of jumper's knee is essential to avoid such a major injury.

Runner's and Cyclist's Knee

Runner's or cyclist's knee is a general description of many repetitive and overuse conditions that occur primarily to distance runners and cyclists. Many of these problems originally stem from structural asymmetrics of the foot and lower leg or from a leg-length discrepancy. Besides problems of patellar tendinitis, two common conditions are *iliotibial band tendinitis* and *pes anserinus tendinitis,* or bursitis. A chronic pain occurs on the outer or inside aspect of the runner's knee. There may be a dull ache to a sharp pain.

Care Care of runner's or cyclist's knee includes correcting foot and leg malalignments. Rest and superficial therapy such as cold packs may also be necessary. Athletes must warm up properly and avoid aggravating the problem by running on inclines. It is also necessary for both cyclists and runners to stretch the legs thoroughly. Runners should alternate sides of the road.

The Collapsing Knee

The most common causes of frequent knee collapse are a weak quadriceps muscle; chronic instability of the medial collateral ligament, anterior cruciate ligament, or posterior capsule; a torn meniscus; loose bodies within the knee; and a subluxating patella. Chondromalacia and a torn meniscus have also been known to cause the knee to give way.

RECONDITIONING EXERCISE OF THE KNEE REGION

As discussed earlier in the chapter, to avoid knee injuries the athlete must be as highly conditioned as possible; this means total body conditioning that includes strength, flexibility, cardiovascular and muscle endurance, agility, speed, and balance. Once a knee injury occurs, a gradual program of reconditioning is instituted by the athletic trainer.

The coach should be apprised that many types of knee injuries, such as cruciate tear, may require surgery and an extensive period of time for reconditioning.

The major components of knee conditioning and reconditioning are general conditioning, weight bearing, joint mobilization, flexibility, muscle strength, balance, and basic function. These components, as discussed earlier, are concerned with injury prevention, as well as reconditioning following injury.[2]

Major components of knee reconditioning:
General conditioning
Weight bearing
Joint mobilization
Flexibility
Muscle strength
Balance
Basic function

Body Conditioning

It is essential that the athlete focus on maintaining existing levels of strength, flexibility, and balance of the entire body even when there is a knee injury. A separate rehabilitation program is carried out on the injured knee.

Weight Bearing

Normally the athlete with an acute injured knee undergoes a period of time of non–weight bearing on crutches. This period allows the healing process to progress until the inflammation period has resolved. Wearing a brace may also occur when a progressive program is followed to encourage the knee to withstand normal forces and strains.

Joint Mobilization

Mobilization of the injured joint is carried out as soon as possible. The purpose of mobilization is to avoid the complications of immobilization.[5]

Flexibility

Flexibility of the knee joint is a goal following any knee injury. It often is begun on the first day.

Muscle Strength

Strengthening generally follows a progression from isometric exercise (for example, straight leg raises, quad setting) (Figure 13-23) to isotonic ex-

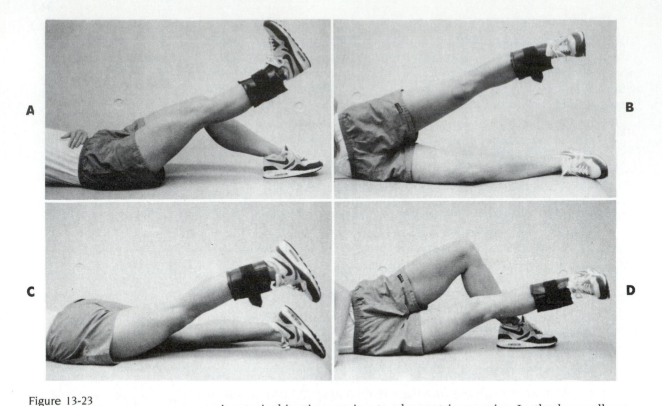

Figure 13-23

Straight leg raising. **A**, High flexion. **B**, High abduction. **C**, Hip extension. **D**, Hip adduction.

ercise, to isokinetic exercise, to plyometric exercise. In the knee all supportive muscles must be focused on.

Balance

As with the injured ankle, the knee must regain control of the balance of joint motion following injury. Injured joints lose their memory for coordinated balance and movement (Figure 13-24).

Bracing

Athletes often wear a brace that allows protective motion in a nonoperative knee. These rehabilitative knee braces are removed during rehabilitation sessions.

Functional knee braces are worn by athletes to provide some degree of support to the unstable knee when returning to activity.[9] Some braces use custom-molded thigh and calf enclosures to hold the brace in place, whereas others rely on straps for suspension (Figure 13-25).

Basic Function

Any time an athlete receives a serious injury to the lower limb, especially a knee injury, reconditioning must include a review and practice of basic locomotor skills. Skills such as walking, and jogging followed by running must be re-experienced. The return to full activity has to be

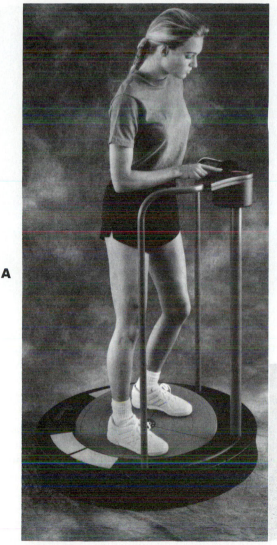

A

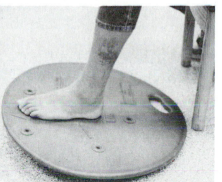

B

Figure 13-24

Proprioceptive devices. **A,**
KAT system. **B,** Seated BAPS
board.

gradual. The criteria for full knee injury recovery is full knee strength, flexibility, speed, and agility before returning to a sport.

The criteria for an athlete returning to his or her sport depend a great deal on the requirements of the specific sport. In general, the athlete's injured leg must have muscle strength equal to or greater than that of the normal leg. The muscles of greatest concern are the quadriceps, hamstrings, and gastrocnemius. The range of motion of the knee must be equal to or greater than that of the nonaffected side. It is also important that the circumference of the thigh 3 inches (7.5 cm) above the top of the patella be no less than 90% of the other thigh. A final test for a safe

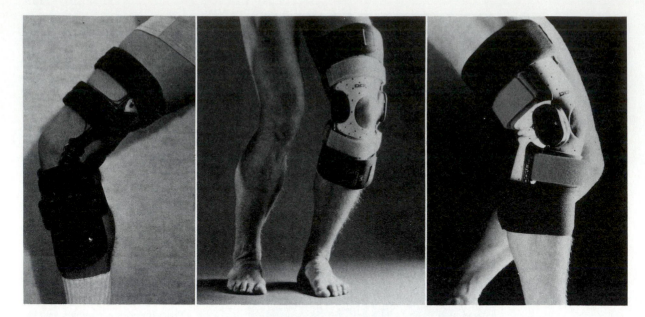

Figure 13-25

Functional knee braces.

return to a running sport should be the ability to run full-speed in a figure-8 pattern around obstacles such as goalposts—first in one direction and then in the other—placing stress equally on each side of the knee.

SUMMARY

The knee is one of the most complex joints, if not the most complex joint, in the human body. As a hinge joint that also glides and has some rotation, it is also one of the most traumatized joints in sports. Three structures are most often injured: medial and lateral collateral capsules and ligaments, the menisci, and cruciate ligaments.

Prevention of knee injuries requires maximizing muscle strength, wearing protective bracing when needed, and wearing appropriate shoes.

Acute knee troubles include superficial problems such as contusions and bursitis. Ligament and capsular sprains occur frequently to the medial aspect of the knee and less often to the lateral aspect. The most common ligament injury is to the anterior cruciate ligament.

The immediate care of a knee sprain requires ice, compression, and elevation (ICE) for 20 minutes intermittently every 1½ hours during waking periods. ICE may be extended for several days depending on the extent of the injury. Rest is also essential during this inflammatory phase.

A meniscus can be injured in a variety of ways, including a rotary force to the knee with the foot planted, a sudden valgus or varus force, and a sudden flexion or extension of the knee. There may be severe pain and loss of motion, a locking of the knee, and pain in the area of the tear.

Chronic knee joint problems can occur when the articular cartilage is disrupted. Sometimes pieces of cartilage or bone become loose bodies in the knee joint. These floating pieces can cause chronic knee inflammation, locking, catching, or a giving way of the joint.

The kneecap and surrounding area can develop a variety of injuries from sports activities. Some of these are fracture, dislocation, and chronic articular degeneration such as chondromalacia. Other conditions in the region include Osgood-Schlatter disease and Larsen-Johansson disease.

REVIEW QUESTIONS AND CLASS ACTIVITIES

1. What are the various structures that give the knee stability? What are their functions?
2. What motions occur at the knee? What muscles provide these movements?
3. How can knee injuries be prevented?
4. How are knee contusions cared for? Bursitis?
5. Contrast the characteristics of first-, second-, and third- degree medial collateral ligament sprains.
6. What signs or symptoms may present themselves that would indicate a possible acute anterior cruciate ligament injury?
7. What mechanism of injury could damage the meniscus? What signs or symptoms would be present? How are they cared for?
8. What are some acute injuries to the patella? How is a dislocated patella cared for?
9. Discuss the different stages of chondromalacia.
10. What other extensor mechanism problems can occur at the knee? How are they managed?
11. What are some goals of reconditioning? What are some exercises and activities that should be included in knee reconditioning?
12. What criteria would be used to determine when the athlete is ready to return to sports participation?
13. Invite an orthopedist to discuss evaluation techniques, treatment, rehabilitation methods, and the new diagnostic tools that are used to treat internal derangements of the knee without having to perform extensive surgery.

REFERENCES

1. Anderson K et al: A biomechanical evaluation of taping and bracing in reducing knee joint translation and rotation, *Am J Sports Med* 20:416, 1992.
2. Arnheim D, Prentice W: *Principles of athletic training*, ed 8, St Louis, 1993, Mosby-Year Book.
3. Colvile MR et al: The Lenox Hill brace: an evaluation of effectiveness in treating knee instability, *Am J Sports Med* 14:257, 1986.
4. Coughlin L et al: Knee bracing and anterolateral rotary instability, *Am J Sports Med* 15:161, 1987.
5. Davis M: Rehabilitation of the knee. In Prentice W, ed: *Rehabilitation techniques in sports medicine*, St Louis, 1990, Mosby-Year Book.
6. Doucette SA, Gable EM: The effect of exercise on patellar tracking in the lateral patellar compression syndrome, *Am J Sports Med* 20: 434, 1992.
7. Fujiwara L et al: Effect of three lateral knee braces on speed agility in experienced and non-experienced wearers, *Ath Train* 25:160, 1990.
8. Jackson RW et al: An evaluation of knee injuries in a professional football team-risk factors, type of

prophylactic knee bracing, *Clin J Sports Med* 1:1, 1991.

9. Johnson C, Back B: Use of knee braces in athletic injuries. In Scott N, ed: *Ligament and extensor mechanism injuries of the knee: diagnosis and treatment,* St Louis, 1991, Mosby-Year Book.

10. Main WK, Hershman EB: Chronic knee pain in active adolescents, *Phys Sports Med* 20:139, 1992.

11. Miller MD, Harner CD: Posterior cruciate ligament injuries, *Phys Sports Med* 21:38, 1993.

12. O'Neill DB et al: Patellofemoral stress, *Am J Sports* 20:151, 1992.

13. Osternig LR, Robertson RN: Effects of prophylactic knee bracing on lower extremity joint position and muscle activation during running, *Am J Sports Med* 21:733, 1993.

ANNOTATED BIBLIOGRAPHY

Cailliet R: *Knee pain and disability,* ed 3, Philadelphia, 1992, FA Davis.

Presents and excellent overview of the knee's structural and functional anatomy and discusses in an easy-to-read manner the conditions that produce disability pain.

Engle RP, ed: *Knee ligament rehabilitation,* New York, 1991, Churchill Livingstone.

A clear and complete treatment of knee injury management and rehabilitation.

Steingard PM, ed: Basketball injuries clinics in sports medicine, Vol 12, No 2, Apr 93 WB Saunders Co. Phil.

Four chapters address the major injuries common to basketball.

Tria AJ, Klein KS: *An illustrated guide to the knee,* New York, 1992, Churchill Livingstone.

A basic concise, easy-to-read illustrated guide to the knee.

The Thigh, Hip, Groin, and Pelvis

When you finish this chapter, you will be able to:

- Describe the major anatomical features of the thigh, hip, groin, and pelvis as they relate to sports injuries
- Identify and evaluate the major sports injuries to the thigh, hip, groin, and pelvis
- Establish a management plan for a sports injury to the thigh, hip, groin, or pelvis

Although the thigh, hip, groin, and pelvis have lower incidences of injury than the knee and lower limb, they receive considerable trauma from a variety of sports activities. Of major concern are thigh strains and contusions and chronic and overuse stresses affecting the thigh and hip.

THE THIGH REGION
Anatomy

The thigh is generally considered that part of the leg between the hip and the knee. Several important anatomical units must be considered in relationship to sports injuries: the shaft of the femur, musculature, nerves and blood vessels, and the fascia that envelops the thigh (Figures 14-1 through 14-6).

Soft-Tissue Thigh Injuries

Injuries to the thigh muscles are among the most common in sports. Contusions and strains occur most often, with the former having the higher incidence.

Quadriceps Contusions

The quadriceps group is continually exposed to traumatic blows in a variety of rigorous sports. Contusions of the quadriceps display all the classic symptoms of most muscle bruises. They usually develop as the result of a severe impact on the relaxed thigh, compressing the muscle against

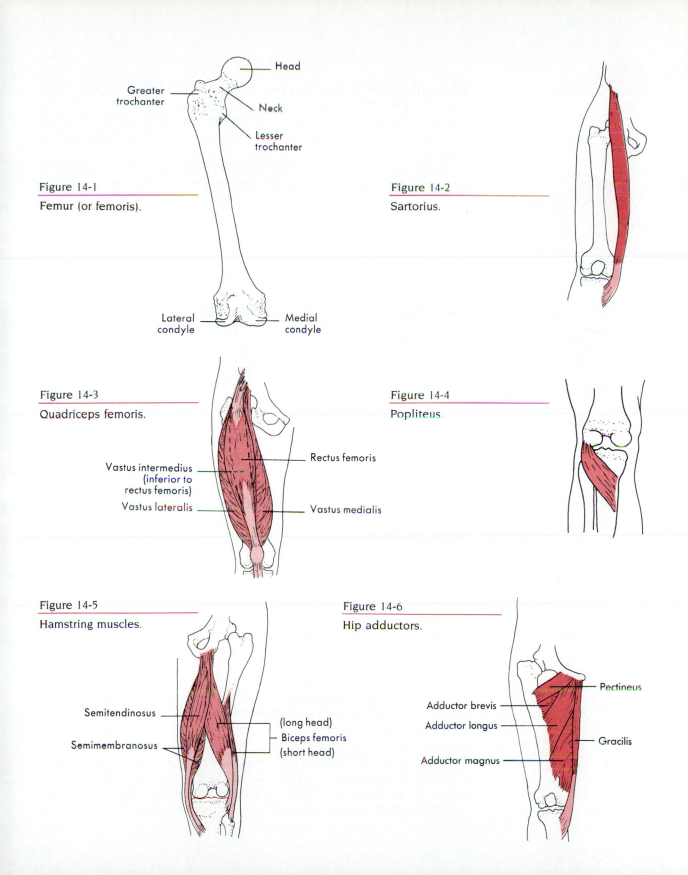

Figure 14-1

Femur (or femoris).

Head

Greater trochanter

Neck

Lesser trochanter

Lateral condyle

Medial condyle

Figure 14-2

Sartorius.

Figure 14-3

Quadriceps femoris.

Vastus intermedius (inferior to rectus femoris)

Vastus lateralis

Rectus femoris

Vastus medialis

Figure 14-4

Popliteus.

Figure 14-5

Hamstring muscles.

Semitendinosus

Semimembranosus

(long head)

Biceps femoris (short head)

Figure 14-6

Hip adductors.

Adductor brevis

Adductor longus

Adductor magnus

Pectineus

Gracilis

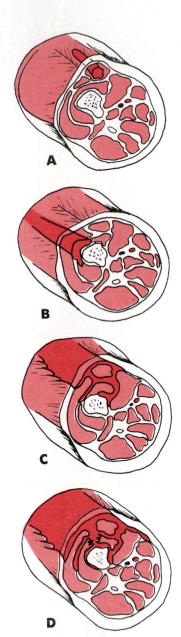

A

B

C

D

Figure 14-7

Quadriceps contusion.

the hard surface of the femur. At the instant of trauma, pain, a transitory loss of function, and immediate capillary effusion usually occur. The extent of the force and the degree of thigh relaxation determine the depth of the injury and the amount of structural and functional disruption that take place.[2]

Early detection and avoidance of profuse internal hemorrhage are vital, both in effecting a fast recovery by the athlete and in the prevention of widespread scarring. The athlete usually describes having been hit by a sharp blow to the thigh, which produced intense pain and weakness. The coach observes that the athlete is limping and holding the thigh. Palpation may reveal a circumscribed swollen area that is painful to the touch. The seriousness or extent of injury is determined by the amount of weakness and decreased range of motion.

First-degree contusions   The first-degree quadriceps contusions can have either a very superficial intramuscular bruise or a slightly deeper one. The very superficial contusion (Figure 14-7, *A*) creates a mild hemorrhage, little pain, no swelling, and a mild point tenderness with no restriction of the range of motion. In contrast, a deeper first-degree (Figure 14-7, *B*) produces pain, mild swelling, point tenderness, and a knee flexion of no more than 90 degrees.

Second-degree contusions   The second-degree or quadriceps contusion is of moderate intensity, causing pain, swelling, and a range of knee flexion that is less than 90 degrees with an obvious limp present (Figure 14-7, *C*).

Third-degree contusions   The severe quadriceps, or grade IV, contusion represents a major disability. A blow may have been so intense as to split the fasciae, allowing the muscle to protrude (muscle herniation) (Figure 14-7, *D*). A characteristic deep intramuscular hematoma with an intermuscular spread is present. Pain is severe, and swelling may lead to hematoma. Movement of the knee is severely restricted, and the athlete has a decided limp.

Care   Compression by pressure bandage and the application of a cold medium can help control superficial hemorrhage (Figure 14-8). The thigh contusion should be handled conservatively with RICE, gentle static stretch, and crutch walking when a limp is present. A variety of therapeutic modalities might be chosen, e.g., gentle passive stretch with cold application. After the hemorrhage has been completely controlled, heat application may be selected.

Generally the reconditioning of a thigh contusion should be handled conservatively. Cold pack combined with gentle stretching may be a preferred treatment. If heat therapy is used, it should not be initiated until the acute phase of the injury has clearly passed. An elastic bandage should be worn to provide constant pressure and mild support to the quadriceps area. Manual massage and hydromassage are best delayed until resolution of the injury has begun. Exercise should be graduated from mild stretching of the quadriceps area in the early stages of the injury to swim-

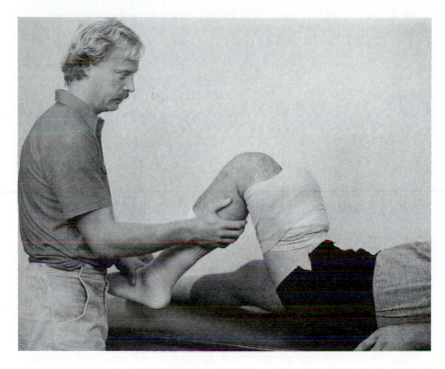

Figure 14-8

Immediate care of the thigh
contusion; applying cold pack
and pressure bandage along
with a mild stretch may
provide some relief.

ming, if possible, and then to jogging and running. Exercise should not
be conducted if it produces pain.

Once an athlete has sustained a second- or third-degree thigh contusion, great care must be taken to avoid the occurrence of another one.
The athlete should routinely wear a protective pad held in place by an
elastic wrap while engaged in sports activity.

Muscle Ossification

A severe blow or repeated blows to the thigh, usually the quadriceps
muscle, can produce **ectopic bone formation** known as myositis ossification traumatica. It commonly follows bleeding into the quadriceps
muscle and formation of a hematoma.[2] The contusion to the muscle
causes a disruption of muscle fibers, capillaries, fibrous connective tissue,
and periosteum of the femur. Acute inflammation follows resolution of
hemorrhage. The irritated tissue may produce tissue formations resembling cartilage or bone. In 2 to 4 weeks, particles of bone may be noted
under x-ray examination. If the injury is to a muscle belly, complete absorption or a decrease in size of the formation may occur. This is less likely
if calcification is at a muscle origin or insertion. Some formations are completely free of the femur, whereas another may be stalklike and yet another broadly attached (Figure 14-9).

Improper care of a thigh contusion can lead to *myositis ossificans traumatica,* bony deposits or ossification in muscle. The following can cause

ectopic bone formation
Bone formation occurring in
an abnormal place

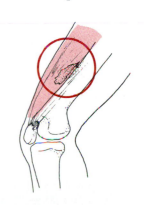

Figure 14-9

Myositis ossificans.

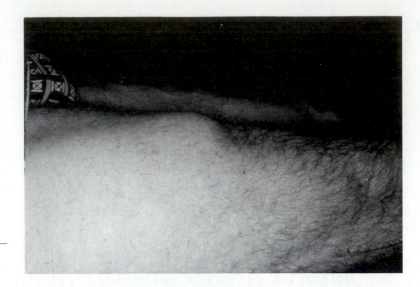

Figure 14-10

Rupture of the rectus femoris.

the condition or, once present, aggravate it, causing it to become more pronounced:

1. Attempting to run off a quadriceps contusion
2. Too vigorous treatment of a contusion—for example, massage directly over the contusion, ultrasound therapy, or superficial heat to the thigh.

Myositis ossificans traumatica can occur following:
  A single severe blow
  Many blows to a muscle area
  Improper care of a contusion

Care Once myositis ossificans traumatica is apparent, treatment should be extremely conservative. If the condition is painful and restricts motion, the formation may be surgically removed after 1 year with much less likelihood of its return. Too early removal of the formation may cause it to return. Recurrent myositis ossificans may indicate a problem with blood clotting such as hemophilia, which is a very rare condition.[2]

Thigh Strains

The two major areas for thigh strains are the quadriceps and hamstring groups.

Quadriceps muscle strain The rectus uppermost muscle of the quadriceps muscle group, femoris muscle, occasionally becomes strained by a sudden stretch (for example, falling on a bent knee) or a sudden contraction (for example, jumping in volleyball or kicking in soccer). Usually it is associated with a muscle that is weakened or overly constricted.

A tear in the region of the rectus femoris may cause partial or complete disruption of muscle fibers (Figure 14-10). The incomplete tear may be located centrally within the muscle or more peripheral to the muscle.

In order of incidence of sports injury to the thigh, quadriceps contusions rank first and hamstring strains second.

A peripheral quadriceps rectus femoris tear causes fewer symptoms than the deeper tear. In general, there is less point tenderness, and no hematoma develops. A more centrally located partial muscle tear causes more pain and discomfort than the peripheral tear. With the deep tear there is a great deal of pain, point tenderness, spasm, and loss of func-

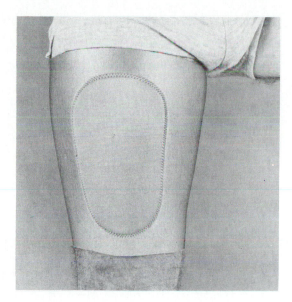

Figure 14-11

A neoprene sleeve may be worn for soft tissue support.

tion, but with little discoloration from internal bleeding. In contrast, complete muscle tear of the rectus femoris may leave the athlete with little disability and discomfort but with some deformity of the anterior thigh.

Care Immediate care employs RICE. The extent of the tear should be ascertained as soon as possible before swelling, if any, masks the degree of injury. Crutches may be warranted for the first, second, and third days. After the acute inflammatory phase has progressed to resolution and healing, a regimen of isometric muscle contraction, within pain-free limits, can be initiated along with cryotherapy. Other therapy, such as cold whirlpool and ultrasound, also may be employed. Gentle stretching should not be begun until the thigh is pain free (see Figure 10-26, p. 283 for tape support). A neoprene sleeve can be worn to provide soft-tissue support (Figure 14-11).

Hamstring strains Hamstring strains rank second in incidence of sports injuries to the thigh; of all the muscles of the thigh that are subject to strain, the hamstring group ranks the highest.

The exact cause of hamstring strain is not known. It is speculated that a quick change of the hamstring muscle from knee stabilization to extension of the hip when running may be a major cause of strain (Figure 14-12). What leads to this muscle failure and deficiency in the complementary action of opposing muscles is not clearly understood. Some possible reasons are muscle fatigue, sciatic nerve irritation, faulty posture, leg-length discrepancy, tight hamstrings, improper form, and imbalance of strength between hamstring muscle groups.

In most athletes the hamstring muscle group should have 60% to 70% of the strength of opposing the quadriceps group. Stretching after exercise is imperative to avoid muscle contraction.

Hamstring strain can involve the muscle belly or bony attachment.

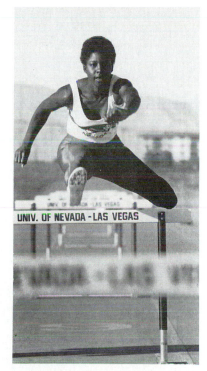

Figure 14-12

In many sports, severe stretching of the hip region can cause a groin strain.

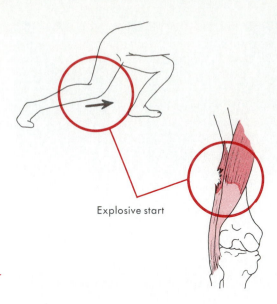

Explosive start

Figure 14-13

Hamstring tear.

The extent of injury can vary from the pulling apart of a few muscle fibers to a complete rupture or an avulsion fracture (Figure 14-13).

Capillary hemorrhage, pain, and immediate loss of function vary according to the degree of trauma. Discoloration may occur 1 or 2 days after injury.

A first-degree hamstring strain usually is evidenced by muscle soreness on movement, accompanied by point tenderness. These strains are often difficult to detect when they occur. Irritation and stiffness do not become apparent until the athlete has cooled down after activity. The soreness of the mild hamstring strain in most instances can be attributed to muscle spasm rather than to the tearing of tissue.

A second-degree strain of a hamstring muscle represents partial tearing of muscle fibers, identified by a sudden snap or tear of the muscle accompanied by severe pain and a loss of function of knee flexion.

A third-degree hamstring strain is the rupturing of tendinous or muscular tissue, involving major hemorrhage and disability.

Care Initially an ice pack with crushed ice and compression by an elastic wrap should be employed. Activity should be cut down until soreness has been completely alleviated. Ballistic stretching and explosive sprinting must be avoided.

In first-degree hamstring strain, as with the other degrees, before the athlete is allowed to resume full sports participation, complete function of the injured part must be restored.

Second- and third-degree strains should be treated very conservatively. For second-degree strains RICE should be used for 24 to 48 hours; for third-degree strains RICE should be used for 48 to 72 hours. Athletes with third-degree hamstring strains should be sent to a physician immediately. After the early inflammatory phase of injury has stabilized, a treatment regimen of isometric exercise, cryotherapy, and ultrasound may be beneficial. In later stages of healing, gentle stretching within pain limits, jogging, stationary cycling, and isokinetic exercise at high speeds may be beneficial. Following elimination of soreness, the athlete may begin isotonic knee curls. Full recovery may take from 1 month to a full season (see Figure 10-20, p. 280 for support).

Strains are always a problem to the athlete; they tend to recur because of their sometimes healing with inelastic fibrous scar tissue. The higher the incidence of strains at a particular muscle site, the greater the amount of scar tissue and the greater the likelihood of further injury. The fear of another pulled muscle becomes to some individuals almost a neurotic obsession, often more handicapping than the injury itself.

Femoral Fractures

Acute Fractures

In sports, fractures of the femur occur most often in the shaft rather than at the bone ends and are almost always caused by a great force, such as falling from a height or being hit directly by another participant. A fracture of the shaft most often takes place in the middle third of the bone because of the anatomical curve at this point, as well as the fact that the majority of direct blows are sustained in this area. Shock generally accompanies a fracture of the femur as a result of the extreme amount of pathology and pain associated with this injury. Bone displacement is usually present as a result of the great strength of the quadriceps muscle, which causes overriding of the bone fragments. Direct violence produces extensive soft-tissue injury, with lacerations of the vastus intermedius muscle, hemorrhaging, and muscle spasms.

A fractured femur is recognized by the classic signs of (1) deformity, with the thigh rotated outward; (2) a shortened thigh, caused by bone displacement; (3) loss of function; (4) pain and point tenderness; and (5) swelling of the soft tissues. To prevent danger to the athlete's life and to ensure adequate reconditioning, immediate immobilization and referral to a physician must be made.[8]

Femoral stress fracture

The popularity of jogging and the increased mileage covered by serious runners has increased the incidence of femoral stress fractures. It must be considered when the athlete complains of constant pain. It occurs most often at the neck of the femur. Rest and limited weight bearing is the treatment of choice.[3]

Femoral stress fractures are becoming more prevalent because of the increased popularity of repetitive, sustained activities such as distance running.

Thigh Reconditioning

In general, exercise rehabilitation of the thigh is primarily concerned with the quadriceps and hamstring muscles. Hip adductors and abductor muscles are discussed in the hip exercise rehabilitation section. (Because of the relationship of thigh reconditioning to the knee region, review

Chapter 13.) Normally, the progression for strength begins with muscle setting and isometric exercise until the muscle can be fully contracted, followed by active isotonic contraction and then by isotonic progressive resistance exercise or isokinetic exercise. Flexibility exercises include gently passive stretching followed by gradual static stretching. Relaxation methods and more vigorous manual stretching may also be employed. As with strengthening, flexibility exercises are performed within pain-free limits.

THE HIP AND PELVIC REGION

The pelvis is a bony ring formed by the two innominate bones (ossa coxae), the sacrum, and the coccyx (Figure 14-14). The two innominate bones are each made up of an ilium, ischium, and pubis. The functions of the pelvis are to support the spine and trunk and to transfer their weight to the lower limbs. In addition to providing skeletal support, the pelvis serves as a place of attachment for the trunk and thigh muscles and a protection for the pelvic viscera. The basin formed by the pelvis is separated into a false and a true pelvis. The false pelvis is composed of the wings of the ilium; the true pelvis is made up of the coccyx, the ischium, and the pubis.

Evaluating Hip, Groin, and Pelvic Injuries

The hip and pelvis form the body's major power source for movement. The body's center of gravity is just in front of the upper part of the sacrum. Injuries to the hip or pelvis cause the athlete major disability in the lower limb or trunk or both.

Because of the close proximity of the hip and pelvis to the low back region, many evaluative procedures overlap.

To evaluate hip, groin, and pelvic injuries follow acronym HOPS in box on p. 378.

Groin Strain

The groin is the depression between the thigh and the abdomen. The musculature of this area includes the iliopsoas, the rectus femoris. and the adductor group (the gracilis, pectineus, adductor brevis, adductor longus, and adductor magnus). Any one of these muscles can be torn in sports activity and elicit a groin strain (Figure 14-16). In addition, over-extension of the groin musculature may result in a strain. Running, jumping, and twisting with external rotation can produce such injuries.

The groin strain is one of the most difficult injuries to care for in sports. The strain can appear as a sudden twinge or feeling of tearing during a movement, or it may not be noticed until after termination of activity. As is characteristic of most tears, the groin strain also produces pain, weakness, and internal hemorrhage. If it is detected immediately after it occurs, the strain should be treated by intermittent ice, pressure, and rest for 48 to 72 hours.

Rest has been found to be the best treatment for groin strains. Daily

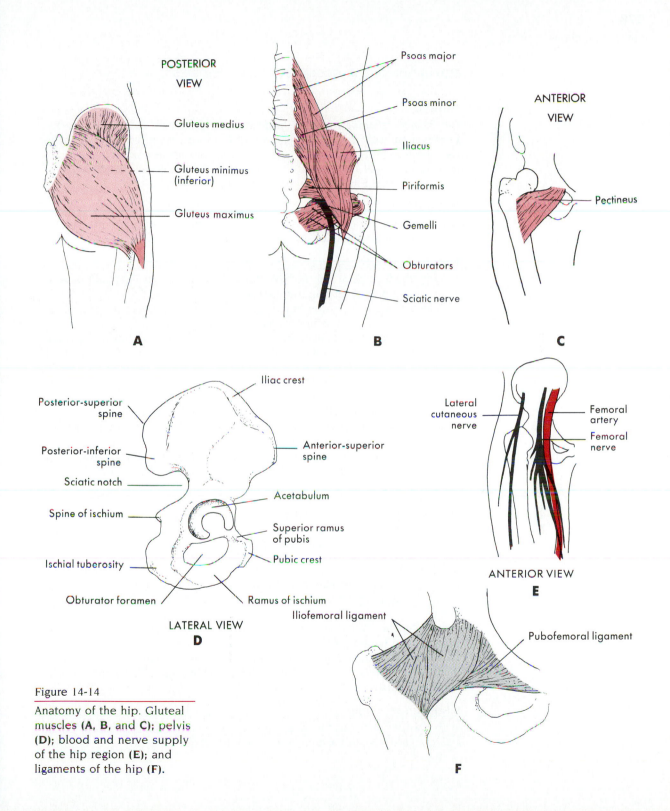

POSTERIOR VIEW

Gluteus medius

Gluteus minimus (inferior)

Gluteus maximus

A

Psoas major

Psoas minor

Iliacus

Piriformis

Gemelli

Obturators

Sciatic nerve

B

ANTERIOR VIEW

Pectineus

C

Iliac crest

Posterior-superior spine

Posterior-inferior spine

Sciatic notch

Spine of ischium

Ischial tuberosity

Obturator foramen

Anterior-superior spine

Acetabulum

Superior ramus of pubis

Pubic crest

Ramus of ischium

LATERAL VIEW

D

Lateral cutaneous nerve

Femoral artery

Femoral nerve

ANTERIOR VIEW

E

Iliofemoral ligament

Pubofemoral ligament

F

Figure 14-14

Anatomy of the hip. Gluteal muscles (**A**, **B**, and **C**); pelvis (**D**); blood and nerve supply of the hip region (**E**); and ligaments of the hip (**F**).

EVALUATION OF HIP, GROIN, AND PELVIC INJURIES

H-History

Did the athlete suddenly feel a sharp pain or did the pain develop slowly, reflecting a dull ache? A sudden pain may be from an acute strain; a dull ache may mean a chronic muscle or bone involvement such as a stress fracture. All movement should be checked if a fracture is not suspected. Specific evaluation should be conducted only by a trained professional.

O-Observation

A general observation including postural asymmetry, standing balance, and ambulation should be made by the coach or health professional.

Postural asymmetry

1. From the front view, do the hips look even? An uneven hip could mean a leg length discrepancy and/or abnormal muscle contraction.
2. Taking a side view of the hip an abnormal tilt is observed. A forward tilt indicates a swayback whereas a backward tilt indicates a flat back.
3. In lower-limb alignment facing forward—can the athlete touch the ankle malleoli and knee medial condyles together. Separation of the malleoli while touching the medial knee condyles indicates knock-knees while touching the malleoli together and not the medial knee condyles indicates bowlegs.
4. Looking at the pelvis from the rear, lateral tilting is checked for.

   It should be noted that an existing postural asymmetry can cause an injury or an injury can produce an asymmetry.

Standing on one leg—Standing on one leg may produce pain in the hip region or show a fall of the pelvis on the opposite side, indicating a muscle weakness.

Ambulation—Observe the athlete walking and sitting. Guarding against pain in the hip and pelvic region will cause the athlete to distort these movements. Exposed bony sites in thigh, hip, groin, and pelvic regions should be gently palpated for pain and deformities.

P-Palpation

Soft-Tissue Palpation—Palpation can contrast soft-tissue injuries from bony injuries. Concern areas are the groin and other muscle or fleshy regions in the area.

Groin Palpation—Palpation can reveal groin pain that stems from a strain or from swollen lymph glands, indicating a lower limb infection.

Other Muscle or Fleshy Regions—Soft-tissue areas other than the groin should be palpated for pain, swelling, and/or disruption of muscle fibers, indicating a possible rupture.

S-Seriousness of injury

With fracture ruled out, the athlete is led through all possible hip movements, actively, passively, and against some resistance (Figure 14-15).

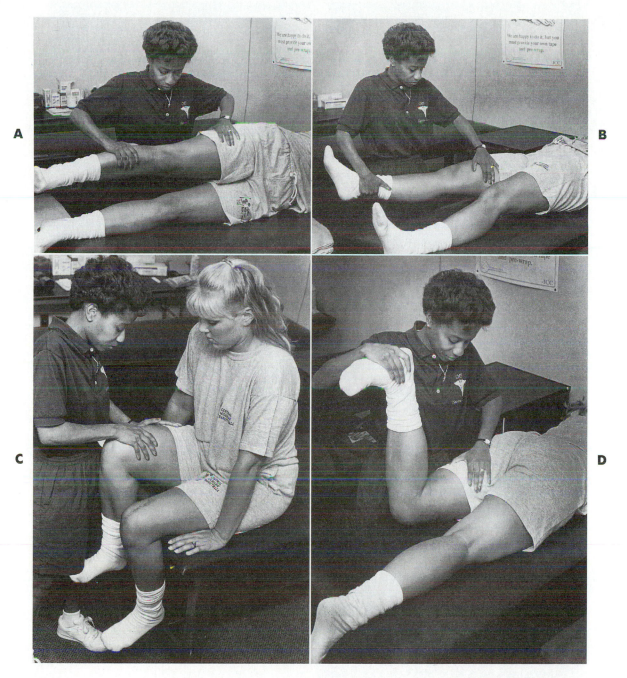

Figure 14-15

Manual muscle tests for the hip. **A**, Abduction. **B**, Adduction. **C**, Flexion (iliopsoas muscle). **D**, Extension. *Continued.*

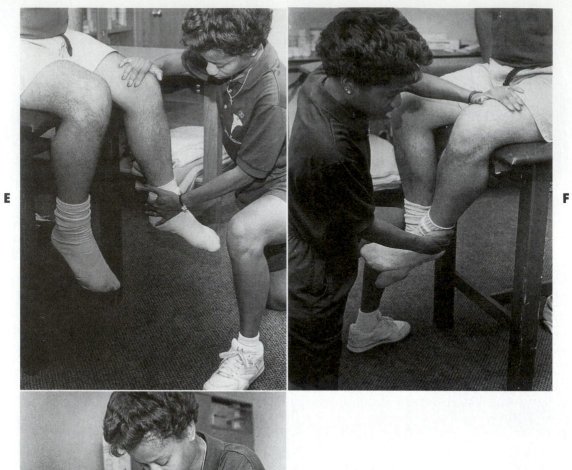

E

F

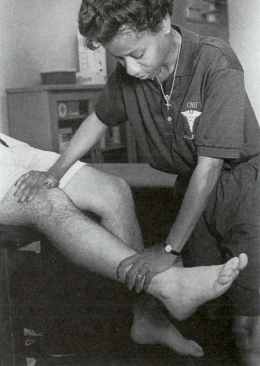

G

Figure 14-5 cont'd

E, Internal rotation. **F,** External rotation. **G,** Rectus femoris at the hip.

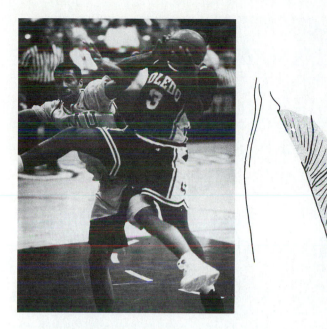

Figure 14-16

Contact and collision sports
can produce serious pelvic
injuries.

whirlpool therapy and cryotherapy are palliative; ultrasound offers a
more definite approach. Exercise should be delayed until the groin is pain
free. Exercise reconditioning should emphasize gradual stretching and restoring the normal range of motion. Until normal flexibility and strength
are developed, a protective spica bandage should be applied (see Figures
9-5 and, 9-6, p. 252). Commercial restraints are also on the market to
protect the injured groin (Figure 14-17). Note that a pelvic stress fracture may produce groin pain. Therefore distance runners particularly
should be referred to a physician for examination when they suffer severe groin pain.

Bursitis of the Trochanter

Trochanteric bursitis is a relatively common condition of the greater trochanter of the femur. Although commonly called *bursitis,* it may also be
an inflammation at a muscle insertion or at the iliotibial band as it passes
over the trochanter. It is most common among women runners. Care
should include elimination of running on inclined surfaces and correction of leg-length discrepancy and faulty running form. Cold packs or ice
massage together with gentle stretching and rest with antiinflammatory
medication may be helpful.[2]

Trochanteric bursitis is most
common among women
runners.

Problems of the Hip Joint

The hip joint, the strongest and best-protected joint in the human body,
is seldom seriously injured during sports activities.

Sprains of the hip joint   The hip joint is substantially supported by
the ligamentous tissues and muscles that surround it, so any unusual
movement that exceeds the normal range of motion may tear tissue. Such
an injury may follow a violent twist, either produced through an impact

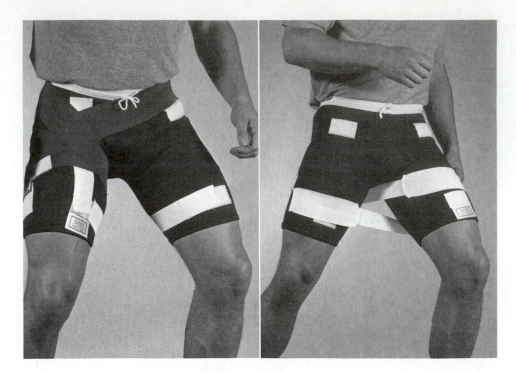

Figure 14-17

Commerical restraints such as the Sowa groin and thigh braces are increasingly being used in athletic training.

force delivered by another participant or by forceful contact with another object, or a situation in which the foot is firmly planted and the trunk forced in an opposing direction. A hip sprain displays all the signs of a major acute injury but is best revealed through the athlete's *inability to circumduct* the thigh.

Dislocated hip joint Dislocation of the hip joint rarely occurs in sports, and then usually only as the result of traumatic force along the long axis of the femur or by the athlete falling on his or her side. Such dislocations are produced when the knee is bent. The most common displacement is posterior to the acetabulum and with the femoral shaft adducted and flexed.

The luxation presents a picture of a flexed, adducted, and internally rotated thigh. Palpation will reveal that the head of the femur has moved to a position posterior to the acetabulum. A hip dislocation causes serious pathology by tearing capsular and ligamentous tissue. A fracture is often associated with this injury, accompanied by possible damage to the sciatic nerve and the nutrient artery, causing **atrophic necrosis.**

Care Medical attention must be secured immediately after displacement, or muscle contractures may complicate the reduction. Immobilization usually consists of 2 weeks of bed rest and the use of a crutch for walking for a month or longer.

Complications Complication of the posterior hip dislocation is likely. Such complications include muscle paralysis as a result of nerve injury in the area and a later development of a degeneration of the head of the femur (osteoarthritis).

Immature Hip Joint Problems

The coach or athletic trainer working with a child or adolescent should understand two major problems stemming from the immature hip joint. They are (1) Legg-Perthes avascular necrosis of the femoral head (coxa plana) and (2) a slipping of the femoral head called slipped capital femoral epiphysis.

Legg-Perthes disease (coxa plana)   Legg-Perthes disease is an avascular necrosis of the femoral head (Figure 14-18). It occurs in children ages 3 to 12 and in boys more often than in girls. The reason for this condition is not clearly understood. It is listed under the broad heading of osteochondroses. Because of a disruption of circulation at the head of the femur, articular cartilage becomes necrotic and flattens.

The young athlete commonly complains of pain in the groin that sometimes is referred to the abdomen or knee. Limping is also typical. The condition can have a rapid onset, but more often it comes on slowly over a number of months.[4] Examination may show limited hip movement and pain.

Care   Care of this condition could warrant complete bed rest to alleviate synovitis. A special brace to avoid direct weight bearing on the hip may have to be worn. If treated in time, the head of the femur will revascularize and regain its original shape.

Complications   If the condition is not treated early enough, the head of the femur will become ill shaped, producing osteoarthritis in later life.

Slipped capital femoral epiphysis   The slipped capital femoral epiphysis (Figure 14-19) is found mostly in boys between the ages of 10 and 17 who are very tall and thin or are obese. Although the cause is unknown, it may be related to the effects of a growth hormone. In one quarter of these cases both hips are affected.

As with Legg-Perthes disease, the athlete has a pain in the groin that arises suddenly as a result of trauma or over weeks or months as a result of prolonged stress. In the early stages of this condition, signs may be minimal; however, in its most advanced stage there is hip and knee pain on passive and active motion, limitations of abduction, flexion, medial rotation, and a limp. X-ray examination may show femoral head slippage backward and downward.

Care   In cases of minor slippage rest and non–weight bearing may prevent further slipping. Major displacement usually requires corrective surgery.

Complications   If the slippage goes undetected or if surgery fails to restore normal hip mechanics, severe hip problems may occur in later life.

Snapping Hip Phenomenon

The snapping hip phenomenon is common among dancers, gymnasts, and hurdlers. It stems from habitual movements that cause muscles surrounding the hip to become imbalanced in strength. It commonly occurs when the participant laterally rotates and flexes the hip joint repeatedly, causing the hip joint and associated soft tissues to become unstable. The

A young athlete who complains of pain in the groin, abdomen, or knee and who walks with a limp may display signs of Legg-Perthes disease or a slipped capital femoral epiphysis.

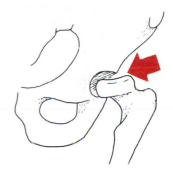

Figure 14-18

Legg-Perthes disease (coxa plana). Arrow indicates the avascular necrosis of the femoral head.

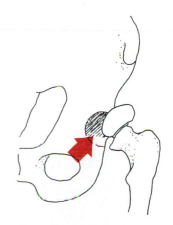

Figure 14-19

Slipped capital femoral epiphysis.

individual complains of a snapping, mainly when balancing on one leg. Care of this condition involves avoiding the action that causes snapping, stretching tight musculature, and strengthening weakened musculature. If there is pain, the athlete should be referred to a physician.

Pelvic Conditions

Athletes who perform activities involving violent jumping, running, and collisions can sustain serious acute and overuse injuries to the pelvic region (Figure 14-20).

Figure 14-20

Athletes who perform activities involving violent jumping, running, and collisions can sustain serious acute and overuse injuries to the pelvic region.

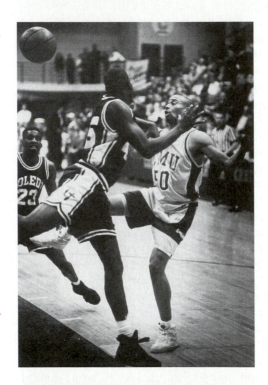

Figure 14-21

A blow to the pelvic rim can cause a bruise and hematoma known as hip pointer.

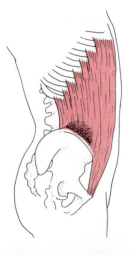

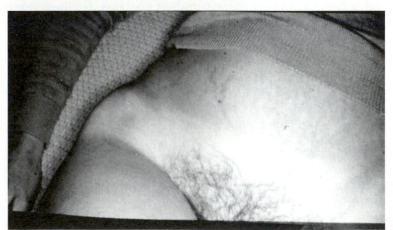

Contusion (hip pointer)   Iliac crest contusion, commonly known as *hip pointer*, occurs most often in contact sports. The hip pointer results from a blow to the inadequately protected iliac crest (Figure 14-21). The hip pointer is one of the most handicapping injuries in sports and is difficult to manage. A direct force to the unprotected iliac crest causes a severe pinching action to the soft tissue of that region.

Such an injury produces immediate pain, spasms, and transitory paralysis of the soft structures. As a result, the athlete is unable to rotate the trunk or to flex the thigh without pain.

Care   Cold and pressure should be applied immediately after injury and should be maintained intermittently for at least 48 hours. In severe cases bed rest for 1 to 2 days will speed recovery. Note that the mechanisms of the hip pointer are the same as those for an iliac crest fracture or epiphyseal separation.

Referral to a physician must be made and an x-ray examination given. A variety of treatment procedures can be employed for this injury. Ice massage and ultrasound have been found to be beneficial. Initially the injury site may be injected with a steroid. Later, oral antiinflammatory agents may be used. Recovery time usually ranges from 1 to 3 weeks. When the athlete resumes normal activity, a protective pad must be worn to prevent reinjury (see Figure 10-28, p. 283 for support).

Osteitis pubis   Since the popularity of distance running has increased, a condition known as *osteitis pubis* has become more prevalent. It is also caused by soccer, football, and wrestling. Repetitive stress on the *pubic symphysis* and adjacent bony structures by the pull of muscles in the area creates a chronic inflammatory condition (Figure 14-22). The athlete has pain in the groin region and area of the symphysis pubis. There is point tenderness on the pubic tubercle and pain when movements such as running, sit-ups, and squats are performed.

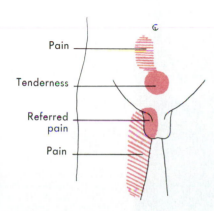

Figure 14-22

Osteitis pubis and other pain sites in the region of the pelvis.

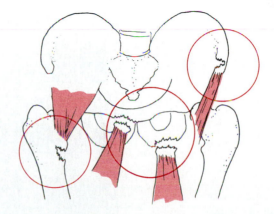

Figure 14-23

Where pelvic avulsion fractures occur.

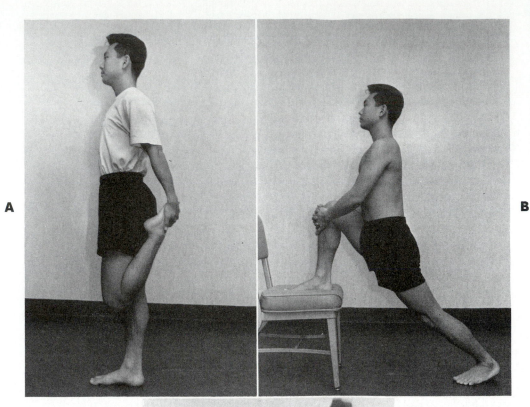

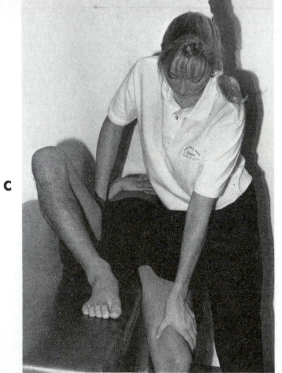

Figure 14-24

Selected basic exercises for
hip rehabilitation. **A,** Active
hip flexor standing stretch. **B,**
Active hip flexor chair stretch.
C, Manual hip flexor stretch.

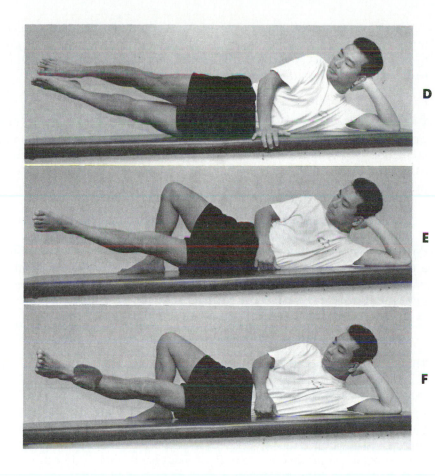

Figure 14-24 cont'd

D, Hip abduction and adduction. **E,** Hip adduction against gravity. **F,** Hip adduction against a resistance.

Care   Follow-up care usually consists of rest and an oral antiinflammatory agent. A return to activity should be gradual.

Fracture of the Pelvis

Acute fractures   The pelvis is an extremely strong structure, with fracture stemming from sports being rare. Those that do occur are usually the result of direct trauma such as a crushing blow. The athlete responds to such an injury with severe pain, loss of function, and shock.

If a pelvic fracture is suspected, the athlete should be immediately treated for shock and referred to a physician. The seriousness of this injury depends on the extent of shock and the possibility of internal injury.

Stress fractures   As with other stress fractures, repetitive abnormal overuse forces can produce pelvic stress fractures and femur fractures.

Commonly the athlete complains of groin pain, along with an aching sensation in the thigh that increases with activity and decreases with rest. Pelvic stress fractures tend to occur during intensive internal training or competitive racing.

Avulsion fractures The pelvis has a number of sites where major muscles attach. Pain at these sites could mean that a muscle has begun to pull away from its attachment (Figure 14-23). Early conditions require rest, limited activity, and graduated exercise reconditioning.

Hip Reconditioning Exercise

When considering the reconditioning of the hip and groin region, one must consider its major movements: internal rotation, external rotation, adduction, abduction, extension, flexion, and the combined movement of internal and external circumduction. Because of the wide variety of possible movements, it is essential that exercise be conducted as soon as possible after injury, without aggravating the condition.

As with all exercise designed for reconditioning, extreme caution should be taken at all times. All rehabilitation programs must be conducted by highly qualified personnel. Exercise should be practiced within a pain-free range of movement. A program should be organized to start with free movement and lead to resistive exercises. A general goal is to perform 10 to 15 repetitions of each exercise, progressing from one set to three sets two or three times daily (Figure 14-24).

SUMMARY

The thigh is composed of the femoral shaft, musculature, nerves and blood vessels, and the fascia that envelops the soft tissue. It is the part of the leg between the hip and the knee.

The quadriceps contusion and hamstring strain are the most common sports injuries to the thigh, with the quadriceps contusion having the highest incidence.

Of major importance in acute thigh contusion is early detection and the avoidance of internal bleeding. One major complication to repeated contusions is myositis ossificans.

Jumping or falling on a bent knee can strain the quadriceps muscle. A more common strain is that of the hamstring muscle. It is not clearly known why hamstring muscles become strained. Strain occurs most often to the short head of the biceps femoris.

The groin is the depression between the thigh and abdominal region. Groin strain can occur to any one of a number of muscles in this region. Running, jumping, or twisting can produce a groin strain.

A common problem of women runners is trochanteric bursitis. An irritation occurs in the region of the greater trochanter of the femur.

The hip joint, the strongest and best-protected joint in the human body, has a low incidence of acute sports injuries. More common are conditions stemming from an immature hip joint. These include Legg-Perthes disease (coxa plana) and the slipped capital femoral epiphysis.

A common problem in the pelvic region is the hip pointer. This condition results from a blow to the inadequately protected iliac crest. The contusion causes pain, spasm, and malfunction of the muscles in the area.

Major movements of the hip and groin:
Internal rotation
External rotation
Adduction
Abduction
Extension
Flexion
Internal/external
Circumduction

REVIEW QUESTIONS AND CLASS ACTIVITIES

1. What signs and symptoms are seen in each of the three degrees of quadriceps/contusions? How are they managed?
2. What complications can occur if a thigh contusion is mishandled?
3. Why do hamstring strains often become recurrent? How are they managed?
4. Where do fractures occur most often in the femur? How are they recognized? Treated?
5. What muscles are most often injured in a groin strain? How is this type of injury managed?
6. What causes trochanteric bursitis? How is it managed?
7. Contrast a hip sprain with a subluxation or dislocation.
8. What type of hip problems occur in the young athlete?
9. Describe the hip pointer. Prevention and care.

REFERENCES

1. Estwanik JJ et al: Groin strain and other possible causes of groin pain, *Phys Sports Med* 18:54, 1990.
2. Fox JM: Injuries to the thigh. In Nicholas JA, Hershman EB, eds: *The lower extremity and spine in sports medicine*, vol 2, St Louis, 1986, Mosby–Year Book.
3. Jackson DL: Stress fracture of the femur, *Phys Sports Med* 19:39, 1991.
4. Karlin LI: Injuries to the hip and pelvis in the skeletally immature athlete. In Nicholas JA, Hershman ED, eds: *The lower extremity and spine in sports medicine*, vol 2, St Louis, 1989, Mosby–Year Book .
5. Keene JS: Thigh muscle injuries in athletes, *Sports Med Dig* 14:1, 1991.
6. Klein KK: Managing hamstring pulls in runners, *First Aider* 56:15, 1987.
7. Parris HG et al: Traumatic hip dislocation, *Phys Sports Med* 21:67, 1993.
8. Strachley DJ: A life threatening femur fracture, *Phys Sports Med* 19:33, 1991.
9. Weicker GG, Munnings F: How to manage hip and pelvis injuries in adolescents, *Phys Sports Med* 21:72, 1993.

ANNOTATED BIBLIOGRAPHY

Arnheim D: *Modern principles of athletic training*, St Louis, 1993, Mosby-Year Book, Inc.
Excellent textbook that provides information on athletic injuries. Chapter 20 covers the thigh, hip, and pelvis.
Sim FH, Scott SG: *Injuries of the pelvis and hip in athletics: anatomy and function*. In Nicholas JA, Hershman EB, eds: *The lower extremity and spine in sports medicine*, vol 2, St Louis, 1986, Mosby-Year Book.
Provides a detailed discussion of hip and pelvic anatomy and sports injuries.

The Abdomen and Thorax

When you finish this chapter, you will be able to:

- Identify and care for the major abdominal injuries
- Identify and provide immediate care for a spleen rupture and kidney contusion
- Identify and care for major injuries of the thorax

This chapter deals with major sports injuries to the abdomen and thorax. Although lower in incidence of injuries than the extremities, injuries in these areas could be serious (Figure 15-1).

THE ABDOMEN
Anatomy

The abdominal cavity lies between the diaphragm and the pelvis and is bounded by the margin of the lower ribs, the abdominal muscles, and the vertebral column. Lying within this cavity are the abdominal viscera, which include the stomach and the lower intestinal tract, the urinary system, the liver, the kidneys, spleen, and genitalia (Figure 15-2).

The abdominal muscles are the rectus abdominis, the external oblique, the internal oblique, and the transverse abdominis (Figure 15-3). They are invested with both superficial and deep fasciae.

A heavy fascial sheath encloses the rectus abdominis muscle, holding it in its position but in no way restricting its motion. The inguinal ring, which serves as a passageway for the spermatic cord, is formed by the abdominal fascia.

Abdominal Injuries

Although abdominal injuries only comprise approximately 10% of sports injuries, they can require long recovery periods and can be life threatening.[4] The abdominal area is particularly vulnerable to injury in all con-

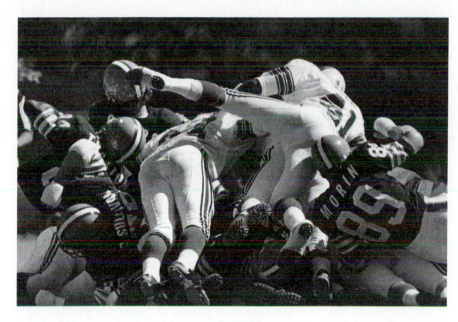

Figure 15-1

Collision sports can produce
serious trunk injuries.

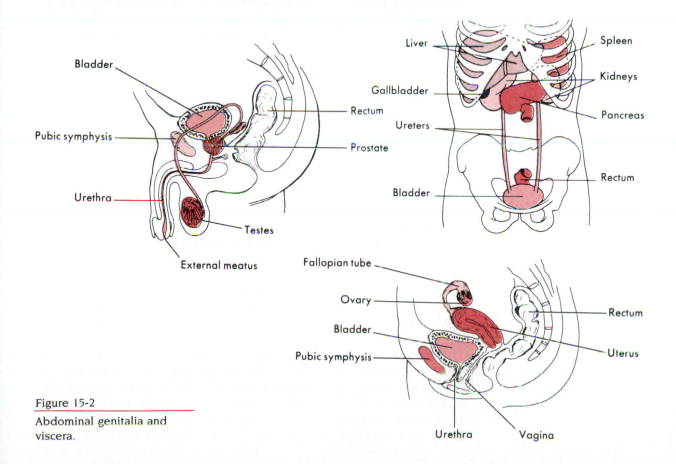

Figure 15-2

Abdominal genitalia and
viscera.

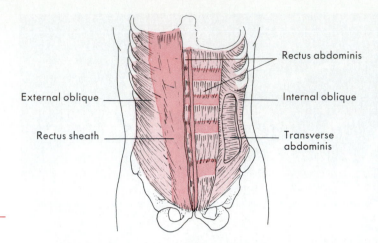

External oblique

Rectus sheath

Rectus abdominis

Internal oblique

Transverse abdominis

Figure 15-3

The abdominal musculature.

The abdominal area is particularly vulnerable to injury in all contact sports.

tact sports. A blow can produce superficial or even deep internal injuries, depending on its location and intensity. Strong abdominal muscles give good protection when they are tensed, but when relaxed, they are easily damaged. It is very important to protect the trunk region properly against the traumatic forces of collision sports. Good conditioning is essential, as is the use of proper protective equipment and the application of safety rules. Any athlete with a suspected internal injury must be referred immediately to a physician.

Injuries to the Abdominal Wall

Contusions Compressive forces that injure the abdominal wall are not common in sports. When they do happen, they are more likely to occur in collision sports such as football or ice hockey; however, any sports implements or high-velocity projectiles can injure. Hockey goalies and baseball catchers would be very vulnerable to injury without their protective torso pads. Contusion may occur superficially to the abdominal skin or subcutaneous tissue or much deeper to the musculature. The extent and type of injury vary, depending on whether the force is blunt or penetrating.

A contusion of the rectus abdominis muscle can be very disabling. A severe blow may cause a hematoma that develops under the fascial tissue surrounding this muscle. The pressure that results from hemorrhage causes pain and tightness in the region of the injury. A cold pack and a compression elastic wrap should be applied immediately after injury. Signs of possible internal injury must also be looked for in this type of injury.

Abdominal muscle strains Sudden twisting of the trunk or reaching overhead can tear an abdominal muscle. Potentially these types of injuries can be very incapacitating, with severe pain and hematoma formation. Initially ice and an elastic wrap compress should be used. Treatment should be conservative, with exercise staying within pain-free limits.

Hernia   The term *hernia* refers to the protrusion of abdominal viscera through a portion of the abdominal wall. Hernias may be congenital or acquired. A congenital hernial sac is developed before birth and an acquired hernia after birth. Structurally a hernia has a mouth, a neck, and a body. The mouth, or hernial ring, is the opening from the abdominal cavity into the hernial protrusion; the neck is the portion of the sac that joins the hernial ring and the body. The body is the sac that protrudes outside the abdominal cavity and contains portions of the abdominal organs.

The acquired hernia occurs when a natural weakness is further aggravated by either a strain or a direct blow. Athletes may develop this condition as the result of violent activity. An acquired hernia may be recognized by the following:

1. Previous history of a blow or strain to the groin area that has produced pain and prolonged discomfort
2. Superficial protrusion in the groin area that is increased by coughing
3. Reported feeling of weakness and pulling sensation in the groin area

The danger of a hernia in an athlete is the possibility that it may become irritated by falls or blows. Besides the aggravations caused by trauma, a strangulated hernia may arise in which the inguinal ring constricts the protruding sac and occludes normal blood circulation. If the strangulated hernia is not surgically repaired immediately, gangrene and death may ensue.

Hernias resulting from sports most often occur in the groin area; inguinal hernias, which occur in men (over 75%), and femoral hernias, most often occurring in women, are the most prevalent types (Figure 15-4). Externally the inguinal and femoral hernias appear similar because of the groin protrusion, but a considerable difference is indicated internally. The inguinal hernia results from an abnormal enlargement of the opening of the inguinal canal through which the vessels and nerves of the male reproductive system pass. In contrast to this, the femoral hernia arises in the canal that transports the vessels and nerves that go to the thigh and lower limb.

Under normal circumstances the inguinal and femoral canals are protected against abnormal opening by muscle control. When intra-abdominal tension is produced in these areas, muscles produce contraction around these canal openings. If the muscles fail to react or if they prove inadequate in their shutter action, abdominal contents may be pushed through the opening. Repeated protrusions serve to stretch and increase the size of the opening. Most physicians think that any athlete who has a hernia should be prohibited from engaging in hard physical activity until surgical repair has been made.

The treatment preferred by most physicians is surgery. Mechanical devices, which prevent hernial protrusion, are for the most part unsuitable in sports because of the friction and irritation they produce. Exer-

Femoral hernias occur most often in women.

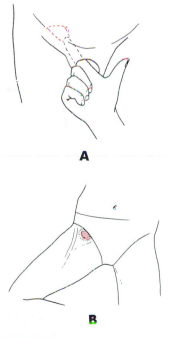

A

B

Figure 15-4

A, Inguinal hernia. **B,** Femoral hernia.

cise has been thought by many to be beneficial to a mild hernia, but such is not the case. Exercise will not affect the stretched inguinal or femoral canals.

Intra-abdominal Conditions

idiopathic

Of unknown cause

Stitch in the side   A "stitch in the side" is the name given an **idiopathic** condition that occurs in some athletes. It is best described as a cramplike pain that develops on either the left or right costal angle during hard physical activity. Sports that involve running apparently produce this condition.

The cause is obscure, although several hypotheses have been advanced. Among these causes are the following:

1. Constipation
2. Intestinal gas
3. Overeating
4. Diaphragmatic spasm as a result of poor conditioning
5. Lack of visceral support because of weak abdominal muscles
6. Distended spleen
7. Faulty breathing techniques leading to a lack of oxygen in the diaphragm
8. Decreased circulation of either the diaphragm or the intercostal muscles

Immediate care of a stitch in the side demands relaxation of the spasm, for which two methods have proved beneficial. First, the athlete is instructed to stretch the arm on the affected side as high as possible. If this is inadequate, flexing the trunk forward on the thighs may prove of some benefit.

Athletes with recurrent abdominal spasms may need special study. The identification of poor eating habits, poor elimination habits, or an inadequate athletic training program may explain the athlete's particular problem. It should be noted that a stitch in the side, although not considered serious, may require further evaluation by a physician if abdominal pains persist.

Appendicitis can be mistaken for a stomach virus.

Appendicitis   Appendicitis is discussed because of the importance of its early detection in the athlete and the fact that it can be mistaken for a common gastric complaint.

Inflammation of the vermiform appendix can be chronic or acute; it is caused by a bacterial infection from a variety of causes such as a fecal obstruction, parasites, lymph swelling, or even a carcinous tumor. Its highest incidence is between the ages of 15 and 24. In its early stages, the appendix becomes red and swollen; in later stages it may become gangrenous, rupturing into the bowels or peritoneal cavity (the membrane that coats the abdominal cavity and viscera) and causing peritonitis.

The athlete may complain of a mild-to-severe cramp in the lower abdomen, associated with nausea, vomiting, and a low-grade fever ranging from 99° to 100° F (37° to 38° C). Later, the cramps may localize into a pain in the right side, and palpation may reveal tenderness at a point between the anterior superior spine of the ilium and the navel (McBurney's point), about 2.5 to 5.1 cm above the latter.

Another indicator that strongly suggests appendicitis is the psoas pain sign elevated in the lower right abdominal quadrant when the thigh is passively hyperextended.

Care   If appendicitis is suspected, the athlete must be referred immediately to a physician for diagnostic tests. Surgery is the usual treatment.

Blow to the solar plexus   A blow to the sympathetic celiac plexus (solar plexus) produces a transitory paralysis of the diaphragm ("wind knocked out"). Paralysis of the diaphragm stops respiration and leads to **anoxia.** When the athlete is unable to inhale, hysteria because of fear may result. It is necessary to allay such fears and instill confidence in the athlete. On occasion, the sudden lack of oxygen to the brain may cause an anoxic seizure. These symptoms are usually transitory.

Care   In dealing with an athlete who has had the wind knocked out of him or her, the coach or athletic trainer should adhere to the following procedures:

1. Help the athlete overcome apprehension by talking in a confident manner.
2. Loosen the athlete's belt and the clothing around the abdomen; have the athlete bend the knees.
3. Encourage the athlete to relax by initiating short inspirations and long expirations.

Because of the fear of not being able to breathe, the athlete may hyperventilate, which means to breathe at an abnormal rate. Hyperventilation results in the delivery of too much oxygen to the circulatory system and causes a variety of physical reactions such as dizziness, a lump in the throat, pounding heart, and fainting to occur.[3]

There should always be some concern that a blow hard enough to knock out the wind could also cause internal organ injury.

Spleen injury   Every year there are reports of athletes who suddenly die—hours, days, or even weeks after a severe blow received in a sports event. These deaths are often attributed to delayed hemorrhage of the spleen, the organ most often injured by blunt trauma.

The spleen is a spongelike organ consisting of lymphatic tissue and enclosed by a dense capsule. The spleen stores blood and filters various bacteria and other matter.

Injuries to the spleen usually result from a fall that jars or a direct blow to the left upper quadrant of the abdomen (Figure 15-5).

Infectious mononucleosis commonly enlarges and weakens the spleen, predisposing it to injury from a blunt external blow to the trunk. An athlete with mononucleosis must not engage in jarring sports activities.

The gross indications of a ruptured spleen must be recognized so that an immediate medical referral can be made. Indications include a history of a severe blow to the abdomen and possibly signs of shock, abdominal

A blow to the solar plexus can lead to transitory paralysis of the diaphragm and unconsciousness.

anoxia
Lack of oxygen

An athlete with mononucleosis must not engage in any jarring activities.

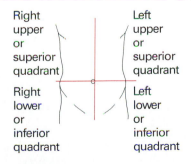

Figure 15-5

Abdominal quadrants for the purpose of diagnostic description.

rigidity, nausea, and vomiting. There may be a reflex pain occurring about 30 minutes after injury, called *Kehr's sign*, which radiates to the left shoulder and one third of the way down the left arm or upper left quadrant. Pain is often constant and worsens with movement and deep breathing.

Complications   The great danger in a ruptured spleen lies in its ability to splint itself and then produce a delayed hemorrhage. Splint of the spleen is formed by a loose hematoma and the constriction of the supporting and surrounding structures. Any slight strain may disrupt the splinting effect and allow the spleen to hemorrhage profusely into the abdominal cavity, causing the athlete to die of internal bleeding days or weeks after the injury. A ruptured spleen must be surgically removed.

Liver contusion   Compared with other organ injuries from blunt trauma, injuries to the liver rank second. [4] In sports activities, however, liver injury is relatively infrequent. A hard blow to the right side of the rib cage can tear or seriously contuse the liver, especially if it has been enlarged as a result of some disease such as hepatitis. Such an injury can cause hemorrhage and shock, requiring immediate surgical intervention. Liver injury commonly produces a referred pain that is just below the right scapula, right shoulder, and substernal area and, on occasion, the anterior left side of the chest.

Hollow visceral organ injuries   When compared to hollow organs, the solid organs are more often injured in sports; however, on rare occasions a severe blunt blow to the abdomen may cause rupture or laceration of the duodenum or other structures of the small intestine.[2]

Injuries to the Genitourinary System

Kidney contusion   A kidney is one of a pair of organs positioned at the back of the abdominal cavity, one on each side of the spinal column. Their purpose is to excrete urine and to help in the regulation of water, electrolyte, and acid-base content of the blood. The kidneys are seemingly well protected within the abdominal cavity. However, on occasion, contusions and even ruptures of these organs occur. The kidney may be susceptible to injury because of its normal distention by blood. A severe outside force, usually to the back of the athlete, will cause abnormal extension of an engorged kidney, which results in injury. The degree of renal injury depends on the extent of the distention and the angle and force of the blow. An athlete who has received a contusion of the kidney may display signs of shock, nausea, vomiting, rigidity of the back muscles, and blood in the urine (hematuria). As with other internal organs, kidney injury may cause referred pain to the outside of the body. Pain may be felt high on the back and may radiate forward around the trunk into the lower abdominal region. Any athlete who reports having received a severe blow to the abdomen or back region should be instructed to urinate two or three times and to look for blood in the urine. If there is any sign of blood in the urine, immediate referral to a physician must be made.

Medical care of the contused kidney usually consists of a 24-hour hospital observation, with a gradual increase of fluid intake. If the hem-

Athletes who complain of external pain in the shoulders, trunk, or pelvis after a severe blow to the abdomen or back may be describing referred pain from an injury to an internal organ.

orrhage fails to stop, surgery may be indicated. Controllable contusions usually require 2 weeks of bed rest and close surveillance after activity is resumed. In questionable cases complete withdrawal from one active playing season may be required.

Injuries of the ureters, bladder, and urethra   On rare occasions a blunt force to the lower abdominal region may avulse a ureter or contuse or rupture the urinary bladder. Injury to the urinary bladder only arises if it is distended by urine.

After a severe blow to the pelvic region, the athlete may display the following recognizable signs:

1. Pain and discomfort in the lower abdomen, with the desire but inability to urinate
2. Abdominal rigidity
3. Nausea, vomiting, and signs of shock
4. Blood dripping from the urethra
5. Passing a great quantity of bloody urine, which indicates possible rupture of the kidney

With any contusion to the abdominal region, the possibility of internal damage must be considered, and after such trauma the athlete should be instructed to check periodically for blood in the urine. To lessen the possibility of rupture, the athlete must always empty the bladder before practice or game time. The bladder can also be irritated by intra-abdominal pressures during long-distance running. In this situation repeated impacts to the bladder's base are produced by the jarring of the abdominal contents, resulting in hemorrhage and blood in the urine. Bladder injury commonly causes referred pain to the lower trunk, including the upper thigh anteriorly and above the pubis.

> The athlete should look for blood in the urine after any blow to the abdominal region.

Injury to the urethra is more common in men, because the male's urethra is longer and more exposed than the female's. Injury may produce severe perineal pain and swelling.

Blow to the testicles   A severe blow to the testicles can produce an accumulation of fluid. After trauma the athlete complains of pain, swelling in the lower abdomen, and nausea (Figure 15-6). Cold packs should be applied to the scrotum, and referral to the physician should be made. A contusion to the scrotal region causes testicular spasms that add to the athlete's discomfort. A good technique to relieve such spasms is to have the athlete lie on his back and instruct him to flex his thighs to his chest. This position helps to relieve pain and relax the muscle spasms (Figure 15-7).

Gynecologic injuries   In general, the female reproductive organs have a lower incidence of injury in sports; however, a woman water skier may injure her vulva when water is forced into the vagina and fallopian tubes, later causing infection. On occasion the external genital organs (vulva) of the female may become contused, resulting in hematoma.

Other reasons for abdominal pain   A number of other abdominal pain sites can be disabling to the athlete. The coach or athletic trainer should be able to discern the potentially more serious pain sites and re-

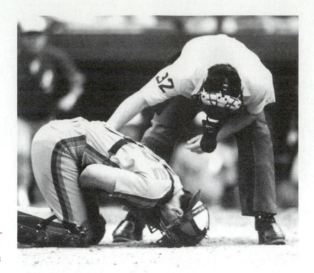

Figure 15-6

A blow to the testicles region can produce excruciating pain and spasm.

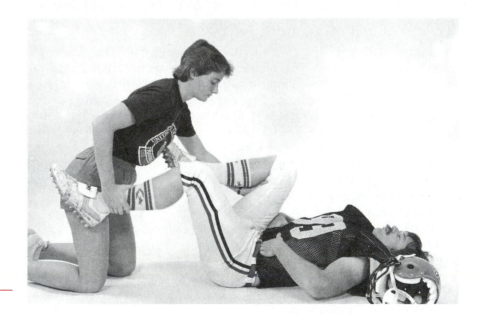

Figure 15-7

Reducing testicular spasm.

fer the athlete accordingly (Figure 15-8). Indigestion or dyspepsia commonly causes pain just below the sternum. NOTE: Appendicitis is often mistaken for indigestion and/or an upset stomach.

THE THORAX
Anatomy

The thorax is that portion of the body commonly known as the chest, which lies between the base of the neck and the diaphragm. It is contained within the thoracic vertebrae and the 12 pairs of ribs that give it

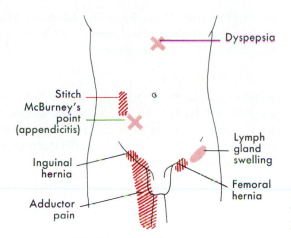

Dyspepsia

Stitch
McBurney's
point
(appendicitis)

Inguinal
hernia

Adductor
pain

Lymph
gland
swelling

Femoral
hernia

Figure 15-8

Common sites of abdominal
pain.

conformation (Figure 15-9). Its main functions are to protect the vital respiratory and circulatory organs and to assist the lungs in inspiration and expiration during the breathing process. The ribs are flat bones that are attached to the thoracic vertebrae in the back and to the sternum in the front. The upper seven ribs are called *sternal* or *true ribs,* and each rib is joined to the sternum by a separate costal cartilage. The eighth, ninth, and tenth ribs *(false ribs)* have cartilages that join each other and the seventh rib before uniting with the sternum. The eleventh and twelfth ribs *(floating ribs)* remain unattached to the sternum but do have muscle attachments. The individual rib articulation produces a slight gliding action.

Thoracic Injuries

The chest is vulnerable to a variety of soft-tissue injuries, depending on the nature of the sport.

Breast Problems

It has been suggested that many women athletes can have breast problems in connection with their sports participation. Violent up-and-down and lateral movements of the breasts, such as are encountered in running and jumping, can bruise and strain the breast, especially in large-breasted women. Constant uncontrolled movements of the breast over a period of time can stretch the Cooper's ligament, which supports the breast at the chest wall, leading to premature ptosis of the breasts.

Another condition occurring to the breasts is *runner's nipples,* in which the shirt rubs the nipples, causing an abrasion that can be prevented by placing a Band-Aid over each nipple before participation. *Bicyclist's nipples* can also occur as the result of a combination of cold and evaporation of sweat, causing the nipples to become painful. Wearing a windbreaker can prevent this problem.[4]

Wearing a well-designed bra that allows little vertical or horizontal breast movement is most desirable. Breast injuries usually occur during

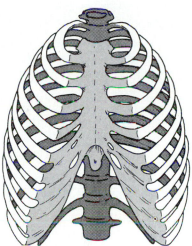

Figure 15-9

The thorax.

physical contact with either an opponent or equipment. In sports such as fencing or field hockey, women athletes should be protected by wearing plastic cup-type brassieres.

Rib Contusions

A blow to the rib cage can contuse intercostal muscles or, if severe enough, produce a fracture. Because the intercostal muscles are essential for the breathing mechanism, when they are bruised, both expiration and inspiration become very painful. Characteristically the pain is sharp during breathing, there is point tenderness, and pain is elicited when the rib cage is compressed. X-ray examination should be routine in such an injury. RICE and antiinflammatory agents are commonly used. As with most rib injuries, contusions to the thorax are self-limiting, responding best to rest and cessation of sports activities.

Rib Fractures

Rib fractures are not uncommon in sports. They have their highest incidence in contact sports, particularly in wrestling and football (Figure 15-10).

Fractures can be caused by either direct or indirect traumas and can infrequently be the result of violent muscular contractions. A direct injury is the type caused by a kick or a well-placed block, with the fracture developing at the site of forced application. An indirect fracture is produced by a general compression of the rib cage, such as may occur in football or wrestling.

The structural and functional disruption sustained in rib fractures var-

Figure 15-10

Rib fractures have their highest incidence in contact sports, particularly wrestling and football.

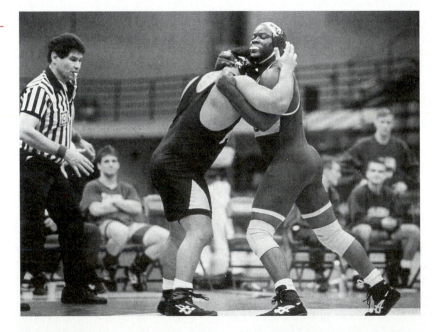

ies according to the type of injury. The direct fracture causes the most serious damage, since the external force fractures and displaces the ribs inwardly. Such a mechanism may completely displace the bone and cause an overriding of fragments. The jagged edges of the fragments may cut, tear, or perforate the delicate tissue surrounding the lung (pleura), causing hemothorax, or they may collapse one lung (pneumothorax). Contrary to the pattern with direct violence, the indirect type usually causes the rib to spring and fracture outward, which produces an oblique or transverse fissure.

The rib fracture is usually quite easily detected. The medical history informs the coach or athletic trainer of the type and degree of force to which the rib cage has been subjected. After trauma, the athlete complains of having a severe pain on breathing in and has point tenderness. A fracture of the rib will be readily evidenced by a severe sharp pain and possibly crepitus on palpation.

Care The athlete should be referred to the team physician for x-ray examination if there is any indication of fracture.

An uncomplicated rib fracture is often difficult to identify on x-ray film. Therefore the physician plans the treatment according to the symptoms presented. The rib fracture is usually managed with support and rest. A simple transverse or oblique fracture heals within 3 to 4 weeks. A rib brace can offer the athlete some rib cage stabilization and comfort (Figure 15-11).

Sternal Fracture

Fracture of the sternum occurs infrequently in sports. It can result from a direct blow to the sternum, from a violent compression force applied

A rib fracture is usually indicated by a severe, sharp pain on breathing.

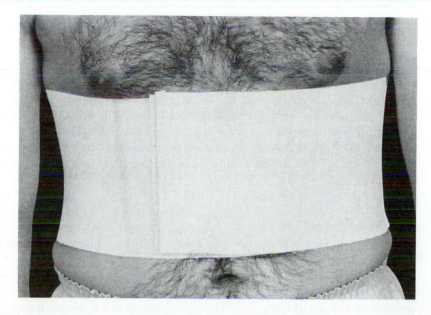

Figure 15-11

A commercial rib brace can provide moderate support to the thorax.

posteriorly, or from hyperflexion of the trunk. The most frequently affected area of the sternum is the *manubrium*. This fracture produces sharp chest pain that occurs particularly on inhalation and is localized over the sternum; as a result of this injury the athlete assumes a position in which the head and shoulders drop forward.

Palpation indicates mild swelling and possibly displaced fragments. An x-ray film must be taken by a physician to determine the extent of displacement.

The treatment may require bed rest for 2 to 3 weeks along with immobilization or the use of a sand weight over the fracture site. After activity is resumed, a posterior figure-8 bandage is applied to maintain the shoulders in an erect position (see Figure 10-29, p. 284).

Costochondral Separation and Dislocation

The rib is connected to the sternum, or breastbone, by cartilage. This cartilage connection can be separated or even be dislocated from its attachment by traumas. In sports activities the costochondral separation or dislocation has a higher incidence than fractures. This injury can occur from a direct blow to the athlete's chest or indirectly from a sudden twist or a fall on a ball, compressing the rib cage. The costochondral injury displays many signs similar to those of the rib fracture, with the exception being that pain is localized in the junction of the rib cartilage and rib (Figure 15-12).

The athlete complains of sharp pain on sudden movement of the trunk, with difficulty in breathing deeply. There is point tenderness with swelling. In some cases there is a rib deformity and a complaint that the rib makes a crepitus noise as it moves in and out of place.

Care   As with a rib fracture, the costochondral separation is managed best by rest and immobilization. Healing takes anywhere from 1 to 2 months, precluding any sports activities until the athlete is symptom free.

Muscle Injuries of the Thorax

The muscles of the thorax are the intercostals and the erector spinae, latissimus dorsi, trapezius, serratus anterior, serratus posterior, and pectoralis major, all of which are subject to contusions and strains in sports. The intercostal muscles are especially susceptible. Traumatic injuries occur most often from a direct blow or sudden torsion of the athlete's trunk. Care of such injuries requires immediate pressure and applications of cold for approximately 1 hour; after hemorrhaging has been controlled, immobilization should be employed.

Internal Complications

Internal complications in the thorax resulting from sports trauma are rare. They pertain principally to injuries of the lungs, pleurae, and/or intercostal arteries. Because of the seriousness of internal injuries, the coach or athletic trainer should be able to recognize their basic signs. The most serious of the conditions are (1) pneumothorax, (2) hemothorax, (3)

Costochonral separation or rib fracture can take 1 to 2 months to heal.

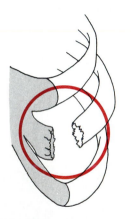

Figure 15-12

Costochondral separation.

hemorrhaging into the lungs, (4) traumatic asphyxia, and (5) heart contusion.

Pneumothorax   Pneumothorax is air in the pleural cavity. It may enter through an opening in the chest or through some tissue imperfection of the pleural sac. As the negatively pressured pleural cavity fills with air, the lung on that side collapses. The loss of one lung may produce pain, difficulty in breathing, and anoxia.

Hemothorax   Hemothorax is the presence of blood within the pleural cavity. It results from the tearing or puncturing of the lung or pleural tissue involving the blood vessels in the area.

Hemorrhaging into the lungs   A violent blow or compression of the chest without an accompanying rib fracture may cause a *lung hemorrhage.* This condition results in severe pain on breathing, difficult breathing (dyspnea), the coughing up of frothy blood, and signs of shock and cyanosis. If these signs are observed, the athlete should be treated for shock and immediately referred to a physician.

Traumatic asphyxia   Traumatic asphyxia occurs as the result of a violent blow to or a compression of the rib cage, causing a cessation of breathing. Signs include a purple discoloration of the upper trunk and head, with the mucous membrane that lines the eye (conjunctiva) displaying a bright red color. A condition of this type demands immediate mouth-to-mouth resuscitation and medical attention.

Heart contusion   A heart contusion may occur when the heart is compressed between the sternum and the spine by a strong outside force, such as being hit by a pitched ball or bouncing a barbell off the chest in a bench press. This injury produces severe shock and heart pain. Death may ensue if emergency attention is not given immediately.

Sudden death syndrome   The most common cause of exercise-induced deaths is congenital cardiovascular abnormalities. The three most prevalent conditions are hypertrophic cardiomyopathy, anomalous origin of the left coronary artery, and Marfan's syndrome (see Chapter 20).

SUMMARY

The abdominal region can sustain a superficial or deep internal injury from a blow. Good conditioning that strengthens the abdominal muscles is essential to prevent contusions and strains.

Of the two common hernias, inguinal and femoral, the most prevalent is the inguinal hernia. These conditions can be congenital or acquired. The major danger in each occurs when the protruding sac becomes constricted and circulation is impeded.

Three additional abdominal problems are the "stitch in the side," appendicitis, and a blow to the solar plexus. The causes of the cramplike stitch in the side are obscure, although poor eating habits, poor elimination habits, or inadequate training habits are possibilities. Because appendicitis can be mistaken for another gastric complaint, early detection with immediate referral to a physician is important. A blow to the solar plexus produces transitory paralysis of the diaphragm, which stops breathing for a short while.

The two major internal organs that can be injured in sports are the spleen and the kidney. A direct blow to the abdomen or a jarring fall can rupture the spleen. Shock, abdominal rigidity, nausea, and vomiting are signs of spleen injury. Although well-protected, the kidney can be contused by a severe blow to the athlete's back. Signs of contusion are shock, nausea, vomiting, and rigidity of the back muscles.

The thoracic region can sustain a number of different sports injuries such as rib contusions, fractures, separations, and dislocations. Internal thoracic complications include pneumothorax, hemothorax, traumatic asphyxia, and even heart contusions.

REVIEW QUESTIONS AND SUGGESTED ACTIVITIES

1. What muscles protect the abdominal viscera?
2. How is an abdominal contusion recognized and managed?
3. What conditions produce pain in the abdominal region?
4. Distinguish an inguinal hernia or a femoral hernia from a groin strain.
5. Describe the signs of a "stitch in the side."
6. How do you manage an athlete who has had his or her wind knocked out?
7. Contrast the signs of a ruptured spleen with signs of a severely contused kidney.
8. What are the most common sports injuries to the genitourinary system?
9. Describe the anatomy of the thorax. Contrast a rib fracture with a costochondral separation.
10. Differentiate among rib contusions, rib fractures, and costochondral separations.
11. Compare the signs of pneumothorax, hemothorax, and traumatic asphyxia.
12. List the possible causes of sudden death syndrome among athletes.

REFERENCES

1. Barret GR: First rib fractures in football players, *Am J Sports Med* 16:674, 1988.
2. Freitas JE: Renal imaging following blunt trauma, *Phys Sports Med* 17:59, 1989.
3. Hafen GQ: *First aid in health emergencies,* ed 4, New York, 1987, West Publishing.
4. Haycook CE: How I manage abdominal injuries, *Phys Sports Med* 14:86, 1986.
5. Haycock CE: How I manage breast problem in athletes, *Phys Sports Med* 15:89, 1987.
6. Janda DH et al: An analysis of preventative methods for baseball-induced chest impact injuries, *J Sports Med* 2, 1992.
7. Morden RS et al: Spleen injury in sports, *Phys Sports Med* 20:126, 1992.
8. Viano DC et al: Mechanism of fatal chest injury by baseball impact: development of an experimental model, *J Sports Med* 2, 1992.

ANNOTATED BIBLIOGRAPHY

American Academy of Orthopaedic Surgeons: *Athletic training and sports medicine,* ed 2, Park Ridge, Ill, 1991, The Academy.
Part *D* provides an in-depth discussion of the gastrointestinal and genitourinary systems.
Kulund DN: *The injured athlete,* ed 2, Philadelphia, 1988, JB Lippincott.
Chapter 11 provides a complete discussion of torso injuries.

The Spine

When you finish this chapter, you will be able to:
- Understand the causes of spinal conditions
- Establish procedures for injury prevention
- Recognize major sports injuries to the spine

ANATOMY

This chapter deals with major sports injuries to the spinal region. The spine is a complex region of the body, with the potential of receiving injuries that could cause major disability or be life threatening.

Cervical Spine

Because of the vulnerability of the cervical spine to sports injuries, coaches should have a general knowledge of the cervical spine anatomy and its susceptibility to sports injuries. The cervical spine consists of seven vertebrae, with the first two differing from the other true vertebrae (Figure 16-1). These first two are called the atlas and the axis, respectively, and they function together to support the head on the spinal column and to permit cervical rotation.

The *spinal cord* is that portion of the central nervous system that is contained within the vertebral canal of the spinal column. It extends from the foramen magnum of the cranium to the filum terminale in the vicinity of the first or second lumbar vertebra. The lumbar roots and the sacral nerves form a horselike tail (Figure 16-2) called the *cauda equina*.

Thoracic Spine

The thoracic spine consists of 12 vertebrae. The first through the tenth thoracic vertebrae articulate with ribs through articular facets. Attached to all thoracic spinous processes is the trapezius muscle; the rhomboid muscle is attached to the upper spinous processes; and the latissimus dorsi

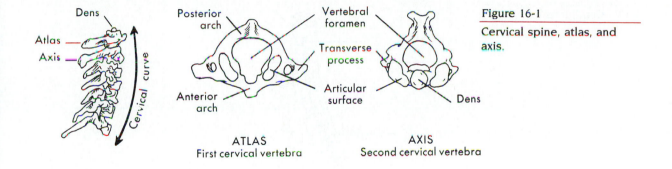

Figure 16-1

Cervical spine, atlas, and axis.

ATLAS
First cervical vertebra

AXIS
Second cervical vertebra

muscle is attached to the lower spinous processes. Deeper muscles of the back also attach to spinous and transverse processes (Figure 16-3).

Lumbar, Sacral, and Coccygeal Spine

The lumbar, sacral, and coccygeal spine is generally considered the low back region and must be thought of in terms of the entire spine.

Bony Structure

The spine or vertebral column is composed of 33 individual bones called *vertebrae*. Twenty-four are classified as *movable*, or *true*, and nine are classified as *immovable*, or *false*. The false vertebrae, which are fixed by fusion, form the sacrum and the coccyx. The design of the spine allows a high degree of flexibility forward and laterally and limited mobility backward. Rotation around a central axis in the areas of the neck and the lower back is also permitted.

Vertebrae can be movable (true) or immovable (false).

Intervertebral Articulations

Intervertebral articulations are between vertebral bodies and vertebral arches. There is an intervertebral disk composed of two components, the *annulus fibrosus* and the *nucleus pulposus*. The annulus fibrosus forms the periphery of the intervertebral disk and is composed of strong, fibrous tissue, with its fibers running in several different directions for strength. In the center is the semi-fluid nucleus pulposus compressed under pressure. The disks act as important shock absorbers for the spine.

Major Ligamentous Structures

The major ligaments that join the various vertebral parts are the anterior longitudinal, the posterior longitudinal, and the supraspinous (Figure 16-4). The anterior longitudinal ligament is a wide, strong band that extends the full length of the anterior surface of the vertebral bodies.

The Lumbar Vertebrae

The lumbar spine is usually composed of five vertebrae (Figure 16-5). They are the major support of the low back and are the strongest and most massive of the vertebrae. Movement occurs in all of the lumbar ver-

All of the lumbar vertebrae are capable of movement, particularly extension.

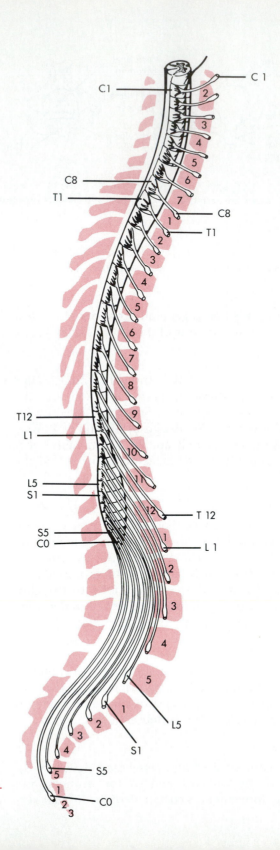

Figure 16-2

Spinal cord and the
peripheral nerves.

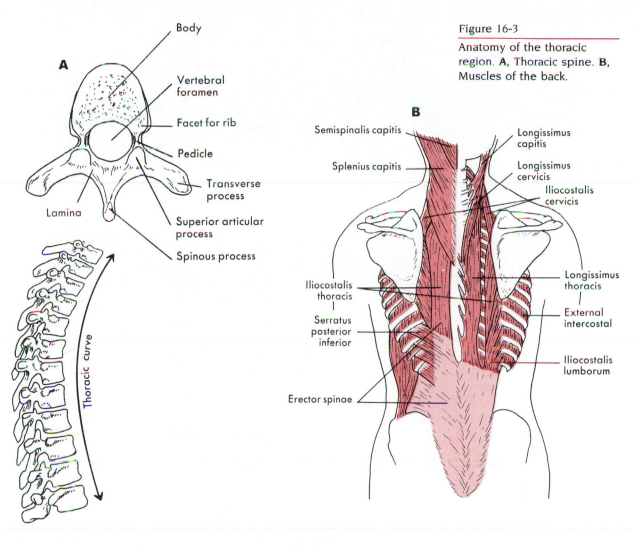

A

Body

Vertebral foramen

Facet for rib

Pedicle

Transverse process

Lamina

Superior articular process

Spinous process

Thoracic curve

Figure 16-3

Anatomy of the thoracic region. **A**, Thoracic spine. **B**, Muscles of the back.

B

Semispinalis capitis

Splenius capitis

Iliocostalis thoracis

Serratus posterior inferior

Erector spinae

Longissimus capitis

Longissimus cervicis

Iliocostalis cervicis

Longissimus thoracis

External intercostal

Iliocostalis lumborum

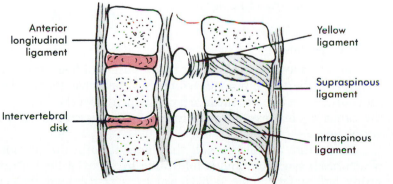

Anterior longitudinal ligament

Intervertebral disk

Yellow ligament

Supraspinous ligament

Intraspinous ligament

Figure 16-4

Major ligaments of the lumbar spine.

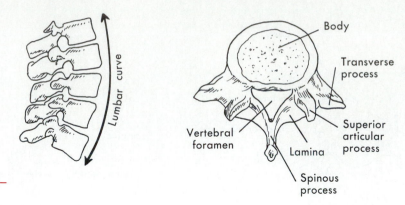

Figure 16-5

The lumbar vertebrae.

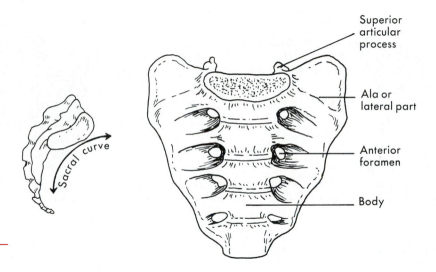

Figure 16-6

Anterior view of the sacrum.

tebrae; however, there is much less flexion than extension. Seventy-five percent of flexion occurs at the lumbosacral junction (L5-S1), whereas 15% to 70% occurs between L4 and L5; the rest of the lumbar vertebrae execute 5% to 10% of flexion.[5]

The Sacrum and Coccyx
The Sacrum

The sacrum is formed in the adult by the fusion of five vertebrae and, in addition to the two hip bones, comprises the pelvis (Figure 16-6). The roots of the lumbar and sacral nerves, which form the lower portion of the cauda equina, pass through four foramina lateral to the five fused vertebrae.

As a child grows up, the bottom five vertebrae fuse and form the sacrum.

The sacrum articulates with the ileum to form the sacroiliac joint, which has a synovium and is lubricated by synovial fluid. During both sitting and standing, the body's weight is transmitted through these joints. A complex of numerous ligaments serves to make these joints very stable.

The Coccyx

In the child the coccyx has four or five separate vertebrae, of which the lower three fuse in adulthood. The gluteus maximus muscle attaches to the coccyx posteriorly and to the levator ani muscles anteriorly.

CERVICAL SPINE CONDITIONS

Because the neck is so mobile, it is extremely vulnerable to a wide range of sports injuries. Although relatively uncommon, severe sports injury to the neck can produce catastrophic impairment of the spinal cord (Figure 16-7).

On-Site Emergency Evaluation

Unconscious athletes should be treated as if they have a cervical fracture. Every sports program should have an emergency system for caring for the severely injured athlete, especially when a neck injury is suspected The ABCs (airway, breathing, and circulation) of life support should be considered when the person is unconscious (Figure 16-8).

An athlete who has sustained a neck injury, when fracture has been ruled out, should be carefully evaluated by a health care professional. Any one or more of the following signs should preclude the athlete from further sports participation:

1. Tingling or burning sensation in the neck, shoulder, or arm
2. Neck motion that causes an abnormal sensation such as numbness or burning sensation
3. Muscle weakness in the upper or lower limbs

NOTE: Serious injury of the neck must be ruled out before motion is allowed.

Off-Site Evaluation

Even when an athlete comes into the training room from an evaluation of neck discomfort, fracture should always be considered as a possibility until it is ruled out. If there is doubt about a fracture, immediate referral to a physician for x-ray examination should be made.

History   The following factors should be considered:

1. How did the pain begin (for example, with a sudden twist or a hit to the head or neck)?
2. Does the athlete have faulty posture?
3. Does the athlete complain of radiating pain or tingling or prickling sensations?
4. Is there numbness in the arm or hand?
5. Is there a crackling or creaking sensation during movement?
6. What precipitates pain (for example, tension stress, sitting for long periods, sudden head movements)?
7. What activities relieve the neck pain?

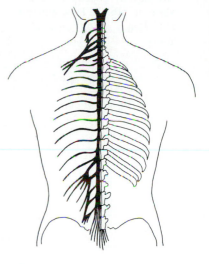

Figure 16-7

Relationship of cord and spinal nerves to the vertebral column.

The very mobile neck supporting the relatively heavy head can incur a wide range of sports injuries.

Figure 16-8

Life support measures taken
when an athlete is suspected
of having a serious cervical
injury.

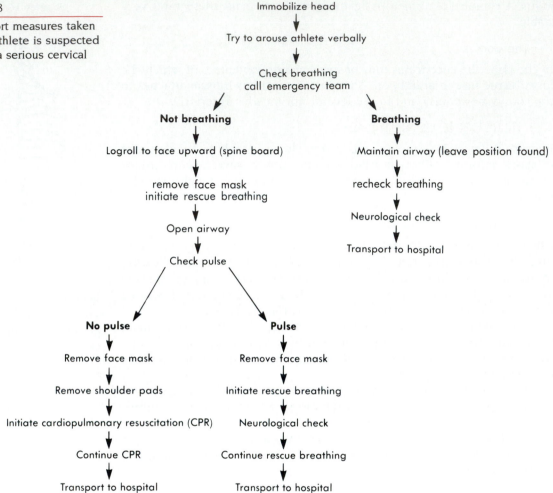

8. Does the athlete have a history of neck problems or injuries? If so, what actions were taken (for example, x-ray films, physical therapy, traction, manipulation)?

Observations   The athlete is observed for the following:

1. Postural alignment
2. How the head is carried
3. Favoring the neck by holding it in a restricted position

Bony palpation   Cervical skeletal sites are felt for pain and possible deformity.

Soft tissue palpation   Muscles in the region of the neck are palpated from their origin to their insertion. Trigger points and tonus asymmetries are also noted.

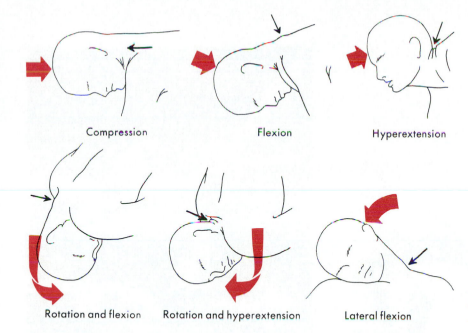

Compression   Flexion   Hyperextension

Rotation and flexion   Rotation and hyperextension   Lateral flexion

Figure 16-9

Mechanisms of cervical injuries.

Functional evaluation   Both active and passive movements, including flexion, extension, rotation, and lateral flexion, are observed for range of motion. Strength of the major neck muscles is next determined, followed by testing of the shoulders and arms.

Mechanisms of serious neck injuries   The neck can be seriously injured by the following events (Figure 16-9):

1. An **axial load** force to the top of the head
2. A flexion force
3. A hyperextension force
4. A flexion-rotation force
5. A hyperextension-rotation force
6. A lateral flexion force

The neck is also prone to subtle injuries stemming from stress, tension, and postural malalignments (Figure 16-10).

Sports and neck injuries   A number of sports can place the cervical spine at risk. Among those activities in the highest risk category are diving, tackle football, and wrestling. Diving into shallow water causes many catastrophic neck injuries. The diver usually dives into water that is less than 5 feet deep, failing to keep the arms extended in front of the face; the head strikes the bottom, producing a cervical fracture at the C5 level.

Football helmets do not protect players against neck injury. In illegal spearing, the athlete uses the helmet as a weapon, striking the opponent with its top. Most serious cervical injuries in football result from purposeful axial loading while spearing.[10] In other sports such as diving, wrestling, and bouncing on a trampoline, the athlete's neck can be flexed at

axial loading
A blow to the top of the athlete's head while in 30-degree flexion.

Figure 16-10

Many sports place a great deal of stress on the upper spine.

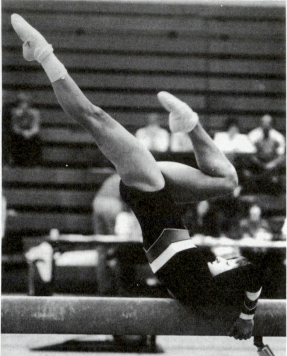

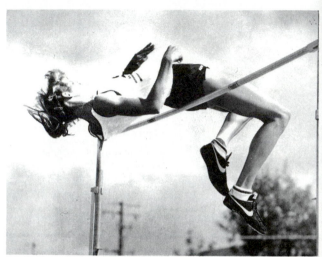

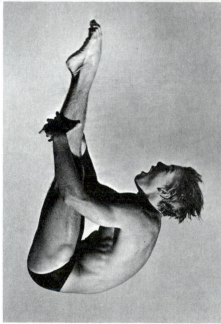

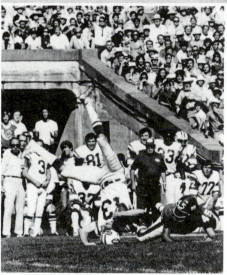

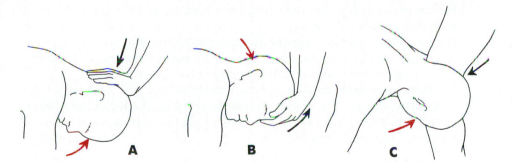

Figure 16-11

Manual resistance can provide an excellent means for helping to prevent neck injuries. **A,** Extension. **B,** Flexion. **C,** Lateral flexion.

the time of contact, energy of the forward-moving body mass cannot be fully absorbed, and fracture or dislocation or both can occur. Many of the same forces can be applied in wrestling. In such trauma, **paraplegia, quadriplegia,** or death can result.

Prevention of Neck Injuries

Prevention of neck injuries depends on flexibility of the neck, muscle strength, the state of readiness of the athlete, a knowledge of proper technique, and the use of proper protective equipment. A normal range of neck movement is necessary. Therefore neck flexibility exercises, coupled with neck-strengthening exercises, should be performed daily by the athlete.

During participation the athlete should constantly be in a state of readiness, and when making contact with an opponent should bull the neck. This is accomplished by elevating both shoulders and isometrically contracting the muscles surrounding the neck.

Strength Athletes with long, weak necks are especially at risk. Tackle football players and wrestlers must have highly stable necks. Specific strengthening exercises are essential for the development of this stability; a variety of different exercises that incorporate isotonic, isometric, or isokinetic contractions can be used. One of the best methods is manual resistance by the athlete or by a partner who selectively uses isometric and isokinetic resistance exercises.

Manual neck resistance
Manual resistance should *not* be performed just before an individual engages in a collison-type sport such as football or ice hockey because of the danger of participating in these activities with fatigued neck muscles.
1. Extension, flexion, lateral flexion, and rotation are performed (Figure 16-11).
2. Each exercise is repeated four to six times in sets of three.
3. The resisting partner accommodates to the varied strength of the mover through a full range of motion.
4. Weaker spots in the range of motion can be strengthened with isometric resistance that is held for 6 seconds .

Flexibility In addition to strong muscles, the athlete's neck should have a full range of motion. Ideally the athlete should be able to place the chin on the chest and to extend the head back until the face is par-

paraplegia
Paralysis of both legs

quadriplegia
Paralysis of all four limbs

Long-necked football players and wrestlers are at risk and need to establish neck stability through strengthening exercises.

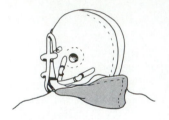

Figure 16-12

A collar for neck protection in football.

A throat contusion may ultimately lead to brain damage.

cyanosis
Slightly bluish, grayish, slatelike, or dark purple discoloration of the skin caused by a reduced amount of blood hemoglobin

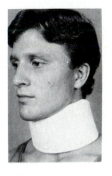

Figure 16-13

Wearing a soft cervical collar helps reduce pain and spasm in an athlete with an injured neck.

allel with the ceiling. There should be at least 40 to 45 degrees of lateral flexion and enough rotation to allow the chin to reach a level even with the tip of the shoulder. Flexibility is increased through stretching exercises and strength exercises that are in full range of motion. Where flexibility is restricted, manual static stretching can be beneficial.

Protective neck devices   The commercial neck roll attached to the shoulder pads has been found effective in reducing the incidence of neck muscle strains (Figure 16-12). The coach is cautioned against using a restrictive strap to prevent injuries.

Neck Injuries

Contusions to the throat and neck   Blows to the neck do not occur frequently in sports, but occasionally an athlete may receive a kick or blow to the throat. Recently the wearing of throat protectors in sports such as baseball, softball, hockey, and lacrosse has reduced throat injuries in those sports. In one type of trauma, known as clotheslining, the athlete strikes or is struck in the throat region. Such a force can conceivably injure the carotid artery, causing a clot to form that occludes the blood flow to the brain. This clot may become dislodged and migrate to the brain. In either case, serious brain damage may result. Immediately after throat trauma the athlete may experience severe pain and spasmodic coughing, speak with a hoarse voice, and complain of difficulty in swallowing.[2]

Fracture of throat cartilage is rare, but it is possible and may be indicated by inability to breathe and expectoration of frothy blood. **Cyanosis** may be present. Throat contusions are extremely uncomfortable and are often frightening to the athlete.

If the more severe signs appear, a physician should be called. In most situations cold may be applied intermittently to control superficial hemorrhage and swelling, and after a 24-hour rest period, moist hot packs may be applied. For the most severe neck contusions, stabilization with a well-padded collar is beneficial.

Acute torticollis (wryneck)   Acute torticollis is a very common condition, more frequently called wryneck or stiff neck. The athlete usually complains of pain on one side of the neck when awakening. This problem typically follows exposure to a cold draft of air or holding the head in an unusual position over time.

Inspection reveals palpable point tenderness and muscle spasm. Head movement is restricted to the side opposite the irritation. X-ray examination will rule out a more serious injury. Management usually involves wearing a cervical collar for the several days to relieve muscle stress and daily therapy with superficial heat (Figure 16-13).

Acute strains of the neck and upper back   In a strain of the neck or upper back the athlete has usually turned the head suddenly or has forced flexion or extension. Muscles involved are typically the upper trapezius or sternocleidomastoid. Localized pain, point tenderness, and restricted motion are present. Care usually includes using RICE immediately after the strain occurs and wearing a soft cervical collar. Follow-up management may include cryotherapy or superficial heat and analgesic medications as prescribed by the physician.

Cervical sprain (whiplash)   A cervical sprain can result from the same mechanism as the strain but usually from a more violent motion. More commonly the head snaps suddenly, as when the athlete is tackled or blocked while unprepared (Figure 16-14).

The sprain displays all the signs of the strained neck but to a much greater degree. Besides injury to the musculature, the neck sprain produces tears in the major supporting tissue of the cervical spine. Along with a sprain of the neck, an intervertebral disk may be ruptured.

Pain is not experienced initially but appears the day after the trauma. Pain stems from tissue tear and a protective muscle spasm that restricts motion.

Care   As soon as possible the athlete should have an x-ray examination to rule out the possibility of fracture, dislocation, or disk injury. Neurological examination is performed by the physician to ascertain spinal cord or nerve root injury. A soft cervical collar is applied to reduce muscle spasm. RICE is used for 48 to 72 hours while the injury is in the acute stage of healing. In an athlete with a severe injury the physician may prescribe 2 to 3 days of bed rest, along with analgesics and antiinflammation agents. Therapy may include cryotherapy or heat and massage. Mechanical traction may also be prescribed to relieve pain and muscle spasm.

Cervical fractures   The cervical vertebrae can be fractured in a number of ways. The common cause of cervical fracture and dislocation leading to very serious consequences is through axial loading. A blow to the top of the athlete's head while in 30 degrees of flexion transmits a force through a straightened cervical spine. Spinal fractures and dislocation leading to quadriplegia occur at a relatively low impact. A compression fracture is created by a sudden forced flexion of the neck, such as striking the head when diving into shallow water. If the head is also rotated when making contact, a dislocation may occur along with the fracture. Fractures can also occur during a sudden forced hyperextension of the neck.

The athlete may have one or more of the following signs of cervical fracture:

1. Cervical pain and pain in the chest and extremities
2. Numbness in trunk and/or limbs
3. Weakness or paralysis in limbs and/or trunk
4. A loss of bladder and/or bowel control
5. Neck point tenderness and restricted movement
6. Cervical muscle spasm

Care   An unconscious athlete should be treated as if a serious neck injury is present until this possibility is ruled out by the physician. Extreme caution must be used in moving the athlete. The coach must always be thinking of the possibility of the athlete's sustain-

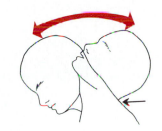

Figure 16-14

Whiplash.

ing a catastrophic spinal injury from improper handling and transportation.

Cervical dislocations Cervical dislocations are not common, but they occur much more frequently in sports than do fractures. They usually result from violent flexion and rotation of the head. Most injuries of this type happen in pool diving accidents. The mechanism is analogous to the situation that occurs in football when blocks and tackles are poorly executed. The cervical vertebrae are more easily dislocated than are the vertebrae in other spinal regions, principally because of their nearness to the horizontally facing articular facets. The superior articular facet moves beyond its normal range of motion and either completely passes the inferior facet (luxation) or catches on its edge (subluxation). The latter is far more common, and as in the case of the complete luxation, most often affects the fourth, fifth, or sixth vertebra.

For the most part a cervical dislocation produces many of the same signs as a fracture. Both can result in considerable pain, numbness, and muscle weakness or paralysis. The most easily discernible difference is the position of the neck in a dislocation: a unilateral dislocation causes the neck to be tilted toward the dislocated side with extreme muscle tightness on the elongated side and a relaxed muscle state on the tilted side.

A unilateral cervical dislocation can cause the neck to tilt toward the dislocated side, with tight muscles on the elongated side and relaxed muscles on the tilted side.

Cervical cord and peripheral nerve injuries Neck and back injuries should always be treated with caution, since they may cause paralysis. Because the spinal cord is well protected by a connective tissue sheath, fat, and fluid cushioning, vertebral dislocations and fractures seldom result in paralysis.

The spinal cord and nerve roots may be injured in five basic ways: laceration by bony fragments, hemorrhage (hematomyelia), contusion, shock, and stretching. These ways may be combined in a single trauma or may act as separate conditions. It should also be noted that often an athlete having a narrower than normal spinal canal is at higher risk for spinal cord or nerve root injury.

Laceration Laceration of the cord is usually produced by the combined dislocation and fracture of a cervical vertebra. The jagged edges of the fragmented vertebral body cut and tear nerve roots or the spinal cord and cause varying degrees of paralysis below the point of injury.

Hemorrhage Hemorrhage develops from all vertebral fractures and from most dislocations, as well as from sprains and strains. It seldom causes harm in the musculature or extradurally. However, hemorrhage within the cord itself causes irreparable damage.

Contusion Contusion in the cord or nerve roots can arise from any force applied to the neck violently but without causing a cervical dislocation or fracture. Such an injury may result from sudden displacement of a vertebra that compresses the cord and then returns to its normal position. This compression causes edematous swelling within the cord, resulting in various degrees of temporary or permanent damage.

Spinal cord shock Occasionally an athlete, after receiving a severe twist or snap of the neck, presents all the signs of a spinal cord injury.

The athlete is unable to move certain parts of the body and complains of numbness and a tingling sensation in his or her arms. After a short while all these signs leave; the athlete is then able to move his limbs quite freely and has no other symptoms other than a sore neck. This condition, a spinal cord shock, is caused by a mild contusion of the spinal cord. In such cases athletes should be cared for as with any severe neck injury.

Cervical nerve stretch syndrome Stretching (cervical nerve stretch syndrome), or cervical nerve pinch, has received increased recognition in recent years. Other terms for this condition are *cervical radiculitis, hot spots, pinched nerve,* and *burner.* The mechanism of injury is that an athlete receives a violent lateral wrench of the neck from a head or shoulder block. The player complains of a burning sensation and pain extending from the neck down the arm to the base of the thumb, with some numbness and loss of function of the arm and hand that lasts 10 to 20 seconds. It is speculated that overriding of the articular facet has caused the electric-shock-like sensation. However, it also may be an indication of a slipped cervical disk or a congenital vertebral defect. Repeated nerve stretch may result in neuritis, muscular atrophy, and permanent damage. This condition requires immediate medical evaluation. After cervical nerve stretch, medical clearance is required before the athlete can return to sports activity. In some cases functional damage is such that an athlete must not participate in certain sports. Conditions for returning to the sport include above-average neck strength, wearing of protective neckwear, and not using the head and neck in a sports activity in such a way as to cause reinjury. A similar condition can be produced by a nerve compression.

NOTE: With any indication of nerve involvement a thorough neurological evaluation by a specialist must be performed before an athlete is allowed to return to participation.

> Cervical nerve stretch syndrome is also known as stretching, cervical pinch, cervical radiculitis, hot spots, pinched nerve, and burner.

Neck Reconditioning

The first consideration in neck reconditioning should be restoration of the neck's normal range of motion. If the athlete had a prior restricted range of motion, increasing it to a more normal range is desirable. A second goal is to strengthen the neck as much as possible. NOTE: Neck exercises related to injury must be supervised by the athletic trainer and/or physician.

Increasing Neck Mobility

All mobility exercises should be performed pain free. Stretching exercises include passive and active movement.

Passive and active stretching The athlete sits in a straight-backed chair while the athletic trainer applies a gentle passive stretch through a pain-free range. Extension, flexion, lateral flexion, and rotation in each direction is sustained for a count of six and repeated three times. Passive stretching should be conducted daily.

The athlete is also instructed to actively stretch the neck two to three times daily. Each exercise is performed for five to 10 repetitions, with each end point held for a count of six. All exercises are performed without force. Figure 16-15 shows forward flexion, extension, lateral flexion, and rotation.

Stretching can progress gradually to a more vigorous procedure such as the Billig procedure. In this exercise the athlete sits on a chair with one hand firmly grasping the seat of the chair and the other hand over the top of the head and placed on the ear on the side of the support hand. Keeping that hand in place, the athlete gently pulls the opposite side of the neck (Figure 16-16). Stretch should be held for 6 seconds. A rotary stretch in each direction can also be applied in the same manner by the athlete.

Manual Neck-strengthening Exercises

When the athlete has gained near-normal range of motion, a strength program should be instituted. All exercises should be conducted pain free. In the beginning, each exercise is performed with the head in an upright position facing straight forward. Exercises are performed isometrically, with each resistance held for a count of six, starting with five repetitions and progressing to 10 repetitions (Figure 16-17).

1. Flexion—press forehead against palm of hand.
2. Extension—place fingers behind head and press head back against hands.

Figure 16-15

Active neck stretching is important for increasing neck mobility after injury. **A,** Forward flexion. **B,** Extension. **C,** Lateral flexion. **D,** Rotation.

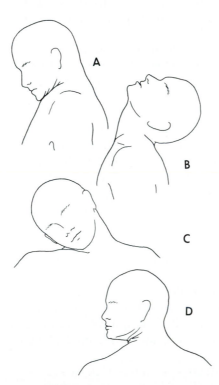

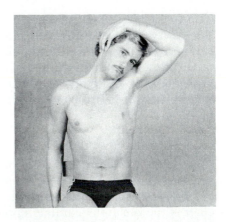

Figure 16-16

Stretching the lateral neck flexors by the Billig procedure.

3. Lateral flexion—place palm on side of head and press head into palm.
4. Rotation—put one palm on side of forehead and the other at back of the head. Push with each hand, attempting to rotate head. Change hands and reverse direction.

Strengthening progresses to isotonic exercises through a full range of motion using manual resistance, special equipment such as a towel, or weighted devices (Figure 16-18). Each exercise is performed for 10 repetitions and two to three sets. NOTE: The athlete must be cautioned against overstressing the neck and must be encouraged to increase resistance gradually.

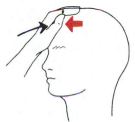
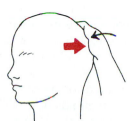
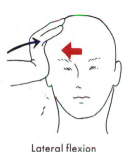

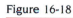

Flexion   Extension   Lateral flexion

Figure 16-17

Manual neck strengthening.

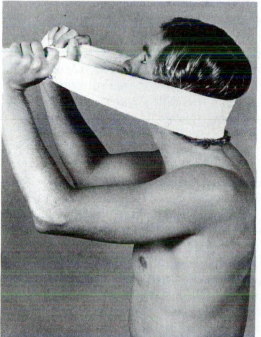

A

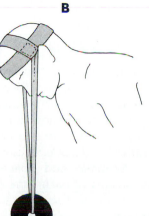

B

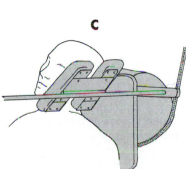

C

Figure 16-18

Neck strengthening through the use of resistive devices. **A,** Towel. **B,** Weight. **C,** Nautilus.

THORACIC SPINE CONDITIONS

Pain in the upper back can be caused by a variety of conditions, including musculoskeletal disabilities, an internal organ disorder, or nerve root irritation.

Evaluation of Thoracic Spine Conditions

History

Having the athlete respond to the following questions should provide important information:

1. What kind of pain do you feel? Describe it.
2. What is the duration, location, and intensity of the pain? (For example, is it constant? intermittent?)
3. What makes the pain more or less intense?
4. Did the pain come on gradually or suddenly?
5. Do you feel numbness or tingling anywhere?
6. Have you had this problem before?

Observation

scoliosis
A lateral deviation curve of the spine

The athlete's back is observed for obvious postural deviation, such as a round back, flat back, or **scoliosis.** An obvious muscle spasm is noted that limits motion. In a young athlete **Scheuermann's disease** is of concern.

Scheuermann's disease (osteochondrosis)
A degeneration of the vertebral epiphyseal endplates

Bony and soft-tissue palpation The back is felt for areas of point tenderness. Bony and muscle pain is differentiated by touch.

Seriousness of injury To determine whether the thoracic condition is joint or muscular active, passive and resistive movement is performed. The athlete first actively flexes the trunk forward, extends the trunk and laterally flexes the trunk, and finally rotates the trunk in each direction. Pain may indicate a muscle condition. Following active movement the athlete sits in a chair with hips and legs stabilized and is passively moved in the same directions as the active. Pain on passive movement could indicate a vertebral condition. Finally the athlete moves the trunk in all directions against a resistance. Pain on resistance indicates a muscle problem.

The Immature Athlete

spondylolisthesis
Forward slipping of a vertebral body, usually a lumbar vertebra

Because young athletes are much less likely to sustain back strains and nerve root irritation, back pain could indicate a vertebral growth disturbance. Two such conditions that could have serious disabling consequences are scoliosis and Scheuermann's disease. **Spondylolisthesis** is another condition occurring in the immature athlete. It is discussed fully under low back conditions on p. 431.

Scoliosis and Schuermann's disease Any time a young athlete complains of back pain, scoliosis should be considered. A lateral-rotary condition of the spine can be progressively disabling if not promptly treated. Scheuermann's disease (osteochondrosis of the spine) is a degeneration of vertebral epiphyseal endplates. This degeneration allows the disk's nucleus pulposus to collapse into a vertebral body. Characteristically there is an accentuation of the kyphotic curve and backache in the young athlete. Adolescents engaging in sports such as gymnastics and swimming—the butterfly stroke particularly—are prone to this condition.

The cause of Scheuermann's disease is unknown, but the occurrence of multiple minor injuries to the vertebral growth region seems to be a major factor.

In the initial stages, the young athlete will have kyphosis of the thoracic spine and lumbar lordosis without back pain. In later stages, there is point tenderness over the spinous processes, and the young athlete may complain of backache at the end of a very physically active day. Hamstring muscles are characteristically very light.

Care The major goal of management is to prevent progressive curvature of the spine **(kyphosis).** In the early stages of the disease, extension exercises and postural education are beneficial. Bracing, rest, and antiinflammatory medication may also be helpful. The athlete may stay active but should avoid aggravating movements.

kyphosis
Exaggeration of the normal thoracic spine

LOW BACK CONDITIONS

As is true of the general population, low back disability adversely affects a large number of athletes. Coaches and health care personnel must thoroughly understand the relationships of sports to low back problems.

Evaluation of the Low Back

Evaluating the low back for injuries, as for the cervical and thoracic spine, involves a great deal of skill and experience. Normally this is left to the health care professional. However, the coach should be able to recognize key signs of injury and make an appropriate referral.

History

To determine the basis for the back pain, the following questions should be answered by the athlete:

1. Where does it hurt, and how long does the pain last?
2. What events precipitated the pain? Was there sudden, direct trauma such as being hit in the back, or was there a strain from a twist or lifting a heavy object? Did the pain come on slowly?
3. Does pain radiate into legs?
4. Is there a feeling of weakness, numbness, or tingling in the legs or feet?
5. What activities or movement cause pain or make the existing pain worse?
6. Is this a new injury or one that has worsened?

Observation

1. Does the athlete move carefully to avoid pain?
2. Does posture appear altered due to a muscle spasm?
3. Can certain movement not be accomplished?

Palpation

Muscle palpation of spasm areas can be painful.

Seriousness of Injury

An athlete should be referred to a health professional when:
1. There is an acute injury that causes severe loss of function and/or the possibility of paralysis.
2. A chronic problem produces:
   a. constant pain
   b. loss of function/muscle weakness
   c. asymmetrical posture
   d. an alteration of sensation that is reflected in numbness or tingling sensation

Mechanisms of Low Back Pain in the Athlete

Back afflictions, particularly those of the lower back, are second only to foot problems in order of incidence to humans throughout their lives. In sports, back problems are relatively common and are most often the result of congenital, mechanical, or traumatic factors. Congenital back disorders are present at birth. Many authorities think that the human back is still undergoing structural changes to adapt to upright position and therefore humans are prone to slight spinal defects at birth, which later in life may cause improper body mechanics.

Congenital Anomalies

Anomalies of bony development are the underlying cause of many back problems in sports. Such conditions would have remained undiscovered had it not been for a blow or sudden twist that created an abnormal stress in the area of the anomaly. The most common of these anomalies are excessive length of the transverse process of the fifth lumbar vertebra, incomplete closure of the neural arch *(spina bifida, occulta),* nonconformities of the spinous processes, atypical lumbosacral angles or articular facets, and incomplete closures of the vertebral laminae. All these anomalies may produce mechanical weaknesses that make the back prone to injury when it is subjected to excessive postural strains.

An example of a congenital defect that may develop into a more serious condition when aggravated by a blow or a sudden twist in sports is the condition of spondylolisthesis. Spondylolisthesis is a forward subluxation of the body of a vertebra, usually the fifth lumbar.

Mechanical Defects of the Spine

Mechanical back defects are caused mainly by faulty posture, obesity, or faulty body mechanics—all of which may affect the athlete's performance in sports. Traumatic forces produced in sports, either directly or indirectly, can result in contusions, sprains, strains, and/or fractures. Sometimes even minor injuries can develop into chronic and recurrent conditions, which may have serious complications for the athlete (Figure 16-19). To

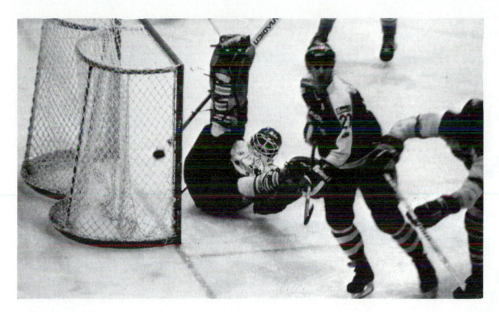

Figure 16-19

Minor injuries of the back can develop into serious chronic conditions.

aid fully in understanding a back complaint, a logical investigation should be made into the history and the site of any injury, the type of pain produced, and the extent of impairment of normal function.

Maintaining proper segmental alignment of the body during standing, sitting, lying, running, jumping, and throwing is of utmost importance for keeping the body in good condition. Habitual violations of the principles of good body mechanics occur in many sports and produce anatomical deficiencies that subject the body to constant abnormal muscular and ligamentous strain.[16] In all cases of postural deformity the athletic trainer should determine the cause and attempt to rectify the condition through proper strength and mobilization exercises.

Back Trauma

It is imperative that the coach be able to recognize and evaluate the extent of a back injury. Every football season there are stories of an athlete who has become paralyzed because of the mishandling of a fractured spine. Such episodes could be greatly reduced if field officials, coaches, and athletic trainers would use discretion, exercise good judgment, and be able to identify certain gross indications of serious spine involvement.[5]

Preventing Initial Low Back Injuries in Sports

All conditioning programs in sports should include work for the prevention of back injuries. Prevention involves the following:
1. Correction, amelioration, or compensation of functional postural deviations
2. Maintenance or increase of trunk and general body flexibility
3. Increase of trunk and general body strength

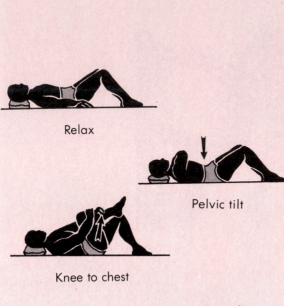

Relax

Pelvic tilt

Knee to chest

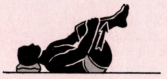

Both knees to chest

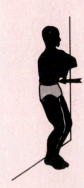

Erect pelvic tilt

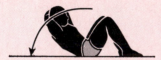

Leg raise

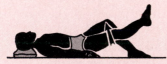

Uncurling the trunk

The Williams flexion series is an example of progressive exercises designed to stretch and strengthen the low back region.[8]

The following exercises should be avoided if the back is hurting. Start with three repetitions and increase by one every 3 days. Repeat twice daily.

Relax

While lying on a firm surface (back flat and knees bent, feet flat, hands behind head), breathe in and out slowly, relaxing as much as possible.

Pelvic Tilt

Tighten the abdomen and buttocks and press the low back against the floor. Hold for 5 seconds, then relax.

Knee to Chest

Grab behind the knee of one leg and gently pull it toward the chest. Stretch for 10 seconds; slowly release and return leg to its original position. Repeat with the other leg.

Both Knees to Chest

While lying on your back, grasp both hands behind both knees and pull toward the chest. Stretch for 10 seconds; slowly release and return to the original position.

Leg Raise

Flatten the back and grasp behind one knee. Bring it to the chest, then point the leg upward as much as possible. Hold for 10 seconds before lowering. Repeat with the other leg. NOTE: This exercise must be avoided if the athlete has numbness or weakness in the muscles of the leg.

Erect Pelvic Tilt

Stand 6 to 12 inches away from a wall facing outward. Press and flatten the low back against the wall. Hold for 10 seconds and relax.

Uncurling the Trunk

From a full trunk curl, lean back slightly from a flexed knee position until tension is felt in the abdominal muscles. Return to the full curled position. Repeat 3 to 10 times.

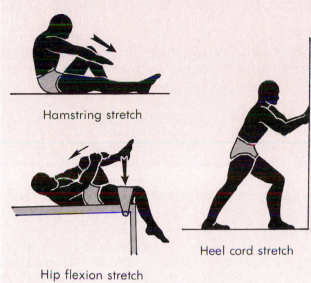

Hamstring stretch

Hip flexion stretch

Heel cord stretch

Hamstring Stretch

If hamstrings are tight, they should be stretched one at a time. Extend the leg to be stretched straight ahead; flex the other leg. As the extended leg is gradually stretched, rotate the flexed leg outward and reach forward with both arms. Hold for 30 seconds.

Heel Cord Stretch

Stand erect and lean toward the wall with one foot forward. Keep the back leg extended with the foot flat against the floor. As the body leans toward the wall, the heel cord is stretched. Keep the back straight at all times. Repeat with the other leg.

Hip Flexion Stretch

Lie supine on a table or bench with both legs dangling over the end. With the low back flat, grasp behind the knee of one leg and pull the thigh to the chest, keeping the opposite thigh flat on the table. Stretch the opposite leg. Hold for 30 seconds.

One should be aware of any postural anomalies that the athletes possess; with this knowledge, one should establish individual corrective programs. Basic conditioning should include an emphasis on trunk flexibility. Every effort should be made to produce maximum range of motion in rotation and both lateral and forward flexion. Strength should be developed to the ultimate, with stress placed on developing the spinal extensors (erector spinae) and on developing abdominal strength to ensure proper postural alignment.

Considerations in preventing low back injuries:

Postural deviations must be corrected or compensated for.

A balance of strength and flexibility in the trunk and pelvis must be maintained.

Conditions Causing Low Back Pain

Soft-Tissue Injuries

Soft-tissue injuries of the back most often occur to the lower back. Those that occur in sports are produced by acute twists, direct blows, or chronic strains resulting from faulty posture or from the use of poor body mechanics in the sport. Tearing or stretching of the supporting ligamentous tissue with secondary involvement of the musculature occurs. Repeated strains or sprains cause the stabilizing tissues to lose their supporting power, thus producing tissue laxity in the lower back area.

Back contusions   Back contusions rank second to strains and sprains in incidence. Because of its surface area the back is quite liable to bruises in sports; football produces the greatest number of these injuries. A history indicating a violent blow to the back could indicate an extremely serious condition. Contusion of the back must be distinguished from a vertebral fracture; in some instances this is possible only through an x-ray examination. The bruise causes local pain, muscle spasm, and point tenderness. A swollen area may be visible also. Cold and pressure should be applied immediately for approximately 48 hours or longer, followed by rest and a gradual introduction of various forms of superficial heat. If the bruise handicaps the movement of the athlete, deep heat in the form of ultrasound or microwave diathermy may hasten recovery. Ice massage combined with gradual stretching benefits soft-tissue injuries in the region of the lower back. The time of incapacitation usually ranges from 2 days to 2 weeks.

Lower back strain and sprain　The mechanism of the typical lower back strain or sprain in sports activities usually occurs in two ways.[1] The first happens from a sudden, abrupt, violent extension contraction on an overloaded, unprepared, or underdeveloped spine, primarily in combination with trunk rotation. The second is the chronic strain commonly associated with faulty posture, usually excessive lumbar lordosis; however, conditions such as flat lower back or scoliosis can also predispose one to strain or sprain.

Evaluation must be performed by the athletic trainer or physician immediately after injury. The possibility of fracture must first be ruled out. Discomfort in the low back may be diffused or localized in one area. There is no radiating pain farther than the buttocks or thigh and no neurological involvement causing muscle weakness, sensation impairment, or reflex impairments.

Care　In the acute phase of this injury, it is essential that cold packs and/or ice massage be used intermittently throughout the day to decrease muscle spasm. Injuries of moderate-to-severe intensity may require complete bed rest to help break the pain-muscle spasm cycle. The physician may prescribe oral analgesic medication.

Cryotherapy, ultrasound, and an abdominal support (Figure 16-20) are often beneficial following the acute phase. Exercise must not cause pain.

Recurrent and chronic low back pain　Once an athlete has a moderate to severe episode of acute back strain or sprain, there is high probability that it will occur again. With each subsequent episode the stage is set for the common problem of chronic low back pain. Recurrent and chronic low back pain have many causes. Many episodes of strain or sprain can produce vertebral malalignment or eventually produce a disk disease that later causes nerve compression and pain. Gradually this problem can lead to muscular weakness and impairments in sensation. The older the athlete, the more prone he or she is to lower back injury. Incidence of this injury at the high school level is relatively low but becomes progressively greater at college and professional levels.[8] In most cases, because of postural anomalies and numerous small injuries, a so-called acute back condition is the culmination of a progressive degeneration of long duration that is aggravated or accentuated by a blow or sudden twist. The injury is produced by an existing anatomical vulnerability.

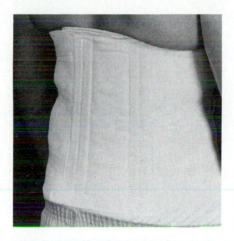

Figure 16-20

An abdominal brace must both support the abdomen and flatten the lumbar curve.

Sciatica **Sciatica** is an inflammatory condition of the sciatic nerve that can accompany recurrent or chronic low back pain. It produces pain that follows the nerve pathway, posterior and medial to the thigh. The term *sciatica* has been incorrectly used as a general term to describe all lower back pain, without reference to exact causes. It is commonly associated with peripheral nerve root compression from intervertebral disk protrusion or structural irregularities within the intervertebral foramen. This nerve is particularly vulnerable to torsion or direct blows that tend to impose abnormal stretching and pressure on it as it emerges from the spine, thus effecting a traumatic condition. The sciatic nerve is also subject to trauma at the point at which it crosses over the ischial spine. Such a contusion can cause muscular spasm, placing direct pressure on the nerve.

sciatica
Inflammatory condition of the sciatic nerve; commonly associated with peripheral nerve root compression

Lumbar disk disease (intervertebral disk syndrome) The lumbar disk is subjected to constant abnormal stresses stemming from faulty body mechanics, trauma, or both, which over a period of time can cause degeneration, that is, tears and cracks in the anulus fibrosus.

The area most often injured is the lumbar spine, particularly the disk lying between the fourth and fifth lumbar vertebrae. In sports, the mechanism of a disk injury is the same as for the lumbosacral sprain—a sudden twist that places abnormal strain on the lumbar region. Besides injuring soft tissues, such a strain may herniate an already degenerated disk by increasing the size of the crack and allowing the nucleus pulposus to spill out (Figure 16-21). This protrusion of the nucleus pulposus may place pressure on the cord of spinal nerves, thus causing radiating pains similar to those of sciatica.

The movement that produces a herniation or bulging of the nucleus pulposus may be excessive, and pain may be minimal or even absent. Initially the athlete may feel a snap or pop. After this episode the athlete complains of pain radiating down the leg. However, even without severe

Individuals with lumbar disk disease should avoid forward-bending activities.

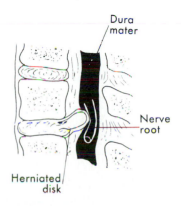

Figure 16-21

Intervertebral disk syndrome.

EDUCATING FOR THE PROPER CARE OF THE BACK

Bed Rest

1. Do not stay in one position too long.
2. The bed should be flat and firm.
3. Do not sleep on the abdomen.
4. Do not sleep on the back with legs fully extended.
5. If sleeping on the back, a pillow should be placed under the knees.
6. Ideally, sleep on the side with the knees drawn up.
7. Arms should never be extended overhead.

Sitting

1. Do not sit for long periods.
2. Avoid sitting forward on a chair with back arched.
3. Sit on a firm, straight-backed chair.
4. The low back should be slightly rounded or positioned firmly against the back of the chair.
5. The feet should be flat on the floor, with knees above the level of the hips (if unable to adequately raise the knees, the feet should be placed on a stool).
6. Avoid sitting with legs straight and raised on a stool.

Driving

1. Move seat so that knees are higher than the hips (pedals must be reached without stretching).
2. Avoid leaning forward.
3. Wear seat and shoulder harnesses.
4. Adjust headrest to appropriate height.

Standing

1. If standing in one spot for a long period of time:
   a. Shift position from one foot to the other.
   b. Place one foot on a stool.
2. Stand tall, flatten low back, and relax knees.
3. Avoid arching back.

Lifting and Carrying

1. To pick up an object:
   a. Bend at knees and not the waist.
   b. Do not twist to pick up an object—face it squarely.
   c. Tuck in buttocks and tighten abdomen.
2. To carry an object:
   a. Hold object close to body.
   b. Hold object at waist level.
   c. Do not carry object on one side of the body—if it must be carried unbalanced, change from one side to the other.

pain the athlete may complain of numbness along the nerve root and muscle weakness in the lower extremity.

Care Treatment of disk disease as directed by a physician usually includes the following:

1. Strict bed rest as required
2. Progressive ambulation
3. Antiinflammatory agent and, on occasion, muscle relaxants
4. Analgesics and cryotherapy to break the pain—muscle spasm cycle (heat may be of value for its ability to relax muscles)

A condition that leads to a progressive bladder or bowel malfunction or severe paresis is a medical emergency. When symptom free, the athlete begins a daily program of exercise rehabilitation and postural education.

Spondylolysis **Spondylolysis** refers to a degeneration of the vertebrae and, more commonly, a defect in the pars intermedia of the articular processes of the vertebrae (Figure 16-22). It is attributed to a congenital predisposition and/or repeated stress to this area. It is more common among boys.[6] Spondylolysis may produce no symptoms unless a disk herniation occurs or there is sudden trauma such as hyperextension. Sports movements that characteristically hyperextend the spine, such as the back arch in gymnastics, lifting weights, blocking in football, serving in tennis, spiking in volleyball, and the butterfly stroke in swimming, are most likely to cause this condition. Commonly spondylolysis begins unilaterally and then extends to the other side of the vertebrae.

Management usually involves restricted activity and complete bed rest; bracing may also be required.

Rehabilitative exercise usually involves resolution of hyperlordosis.

Spondylolisthesis *Spondylolisthesis* is a forward slippage of a vertebra onto the one below, stemming from a degeneration of an articular process. It has the highest incidence in the lumbar region (Figure 16-23). The athlete with this condition will usually have a swayback postural impairment. A direct blow or sudden twist or chronic low back strain may cause the defective vertebra to displace itself forward on the sacrum. When this happens, the athlete complains of localized pain or a pain that radiates into both buttocks, stiffness in the lower back, and increased irritation after physical activity.[8] The athlete with serious spondylolisthesis displays a short torso, heart-shaped buttocks, low rib cage, high iliac crest, and vertical sacrum; tight hamstring muscles and restricted hip extension may also be present. For the most part, symptoms are the same for the majority of lower back problems; therefore an x-ray film should be made to enable the physician to diagnose accurately. Discovery of a defective vertebra may be grounds for medical exclusion from collision and contact-type sports.[3]

Conservative care of acute problems usually consists of bed rest and flexion of the lumbar spine.[8] Casting to reduce hyperlordosis may also be employed. A slippage of 50% or more may cause a medical emergency, requiring surgical fusion of the spine.

spondylolysis
A degeneration of the vertebrae and a defect in the pars intermedia of the articular processes of the vertebrae

A defective vertebra may preclude an athlete from joining in full contact sports.

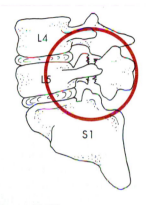

Figure 16-22

Spondylolysis.

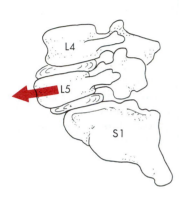

Figure 16-23

Spondylolisthesis.

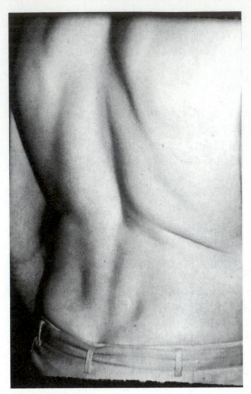

An athlete could sustain a compression fracture through violent hyperextension or jackknifing of the trunk or by falling from a height and landing on the feet or buttocks.

Sacroiliac joint

The sacroiliac is the junction formed by the ilium and the sacrum, and it is fortified by ligamentous tissue that allows little motion to take place. When the pelvis is abnormally rotated downward anteriorly, the majority of the weight of the upper trunk is carried back of the pelvis, producing stress at the sacroiliac joint. This abnormal postural alignment can cause pain and disability.

Lumbar vertebral fracture and dislocation Fractures of the vertebral column, in terms of bone injury, are not serious in themselves, but they pose dangers when related to spinal cord damage. Imprudent movement of a person with a fractured spine can cause irreparable damage to the spinal cord. All sports injuries involving the back should be considered fractures until proved otherwise by the physician. Lifting and moving the athlete should be executed in such a manner as to preclude twisting, and each body segment (neck, trunk, hips, and lower limbs) should be firmly supported. Vertebral fractures of the greatest concern in sports are compression fractures and fractures of the transverse and spinous processes.

The *compression fracture* may occur as a result of violent hyperflexion or jackknifing of the trunk. Falling from a height and landing on the feet or buttocks may also produce a compression fracture. The vertebrae that are most often compressed are those in the dorsolumbar curves. The vertebrae usually are crushed anteriorly by the traumatic force of the body above the site of injury. The crushed body may spread out fragments and protrude into the spinal canal, compressing and possibly even cutting the cord.

Recognition of the compression fracture is difficult without an x-ray examination. A basic evaluation may be made with a knowledge of the history and point tenderness over the affected vertebrae.

Fractures of the transverse and spinous processes result most often from kicks or other direct blows to the back. Because these processes are surrounded by large muscles, fracture produces extensive soft-tissue injury. As fractures they present little danger and will usually permit the athlete considerable activity within the range of pain tolerance. Most care and treatment will be oriented toward therapy of the soft-tissue pathology.

Coccyx Injuries

Coccygeal injuries in sports are prevalent and occur primarily from such direct blows as those received in forcibly sitting down, falling, or being kicked by an opponent. Most injuries to the coccyx are the result of contusions.

Athletes with persistent coccyalgia should be referred to a physician for x-ray and rectal examinations. Pain in the coccygeal region is often prolonged and at times chronic. Such conditions are identified by the term *coccygodynia* and occur as a result of an irritation to the coccygeal plexus.

Treatment consists of analgesics and a ring seat to relieve the pressure on the coccyx while sitting. Palliative measures such as sitz baths or whirlpool in warm water might alleviate some of the pain. It should be noted that pain from a fractured coccyx may last for many months. Once a coccygeal injury has healed, the athlete should be protected against reinjury by appropriately applied padding.

Care of Low Back Pain

The following treatment procedures are used to a greater or lesser degree, depending on the type and extent of the pathological condition:

1. Limitation of activity
2. Antiinflammatory and muscle relaxant medications
3. Cold and/or heat application and ultrasound
4. Passive exercise
5. Active progressive exercise
6. Relaxation training
7. Transcutaneous electrical nerve stimulation (TENS) application
8. Mobilization
9. Traction
10. Education for proper back usage (See box on p. 430.)

Limitation of Activity

Limiting physical activity is essential during acute episodes of low back pain. It can also be a positive influence in chronic pain. The least strain on the back is in the fully recombinant position with the hips and knees at angles of 90 degrees. In the case of a chronic or a subacute lower back condition, a *firm mattress will afford better rest and relaxation of the lower back.* Placing a ¾-inch plywood board over the entire area of the bed underneath the athlete's mattress prevents the mattress from sagging in the wrong places and gives a firm, stable surface for the injured back. The athlete lies supine with hips flexed by elevating the legs with pillows. It is also interesting to note that sleeping on a water bed will often relieve the symptoms of a low back problem if the athlete lies on his or her back. However, in some cases, the firm mattress or water bed may create more pain and discomfort. The value of a water bed is that it supports the body curves equally, decreasing abnormal pressures to any one body area.

Medications

Analgesics and oral antiinflammatory agents are commonly given to inhibit pain. If a highly active athlete becomes severely depressed over suddenly being severely physically restricted, an antidepressant may be given. On occasion, muscle relaxants are also given.

Cold or Heat Application

Local ice application reduces the pain–muscle spasm cycle. Superficial heat can also provide relaxation and reduction of spasm. Ultrasound and mild muscle stimulation can be used to relieve spasm and discomfort.

Exercise and Low Back Disorders

Exercise is a common approach to managing athletes with low back disorders. Many exercise approaches such as flexion and extension, passive and active exercises, postural programs, and exercise that may be predominantly isometric, isometric, isokinetic, or aerobic are available to the athletic trainer. Selecting the correct program may be difficult because research data supporting a specific approach are very sparse. (See box on p. 426.)

Exactly how exercise relieves symptoms is not known. Pain is known to be relieved by a program of gradual stretching and strengthening. Biomechanically, functional improvement occurs through a program of gradual progressive loading, along with stretching. Passive or active range of motion is necessary for stretching contracted muscles. Many exercises are designed to regain the normal lumbar curve.

The Williams flexion exercises, for many years, have been popular for reducing low back pain. However, in recent years they have waned in popularity, with extension exercise becoming increasingly popular. Flexion exercise is based on empirical knowledge acquired from clinical observation. Its basic premise is that much of lumbosacral pain is caused by overextension that can be relieved through lumbar flexion. It is also theorized that lumbar flexion relieves pain produced by the impingement of the facet joints and the intervertebral foramen. Like flexion exercises, the use of extension exercises has an empirical base acquired by observing patients with low back pain. Those individuals who seem to expand most have decreased lumbar lordosis.[2] Through extension exercises the normal lumbar lordosis is regained. It is thought that regaining lumbosacral motion during extension improves the biomechanics of the spine and, as a result, relieves pain. Extension exercise is thought to shift posteriorly displaced nucleus pulposa within the disk anteriorly.

Passive Exercise

If the condition is muscular and discogenic disease has been ruled out, a mild passive stretch can help reduce muscle spasm. Passive stretching of the hamstrings and the iliopsoas muscle may allow a more coordinated lumbar pelvic rhythm to take place without pain and discomfort. Lumbar vertebral mobilization techniques may also be of some benefit if performed gently.

Active Progressive Exercise

Active exercise is a major aspect of low back rehabilitation. Once the pain and spasm caused by a low back injury have subsided, active exercise should begin. The major goals of exercise are to establish normal flexibility and strength and to develop good postural habits in all aspects of daily activities.

Exercise should not be engaged in too vigorously before pain has diminished significantly.

Relaxation and Low Back Pain

An important aspect of treating athletes with low back pain is progressive relaxation. With constant pain comes anxiety and increased muscular tension that compounds the low back problem. By systematically contracting and completely "letting go" of the body's major muscles, the athlete learns to recognize abnormal tension and to relax the muscles consciously. The most popular method of progressive relaxation is the Jacobson[6] method, which can be found in modified form in a number of different texts.

Transcutaneous Electrical Nerve Stimulation (TENS)

Application of a TENS device has been beneficial in a high percentage of cases of low back pain.[1] However, not every machine is equally effective in all cases of low back pain. There must be experimentation as to type of machine, wave form, and sites of application.

Manual Therapeutic Procedures

Manual therapeutic procedures have been used extensively over the years to treat low back pain. The four manual therapeutic procedures currently being used for the management of low back pain include proprioceptive neuromuscular facilitation (PNF), mobilization, traction, and stretching.

PNF There is a high success rate in using PNF principles to increase range of motion and strength. Besides increasing flexibility and strength, muscles are reeducated to reestablish lost pelvic lumbar rhythm and proprioception.

Mobilization

Joint mobilization of the lumbar spine may be used to improve joint mobility or to decrease joint pain by restoring accessory movements to the joint to achieve a full nonrestricted, pain-free range of motion. Vertebral joints in the lumbar region are capable of both anterior and posterior gliding and rotation, or some combination of the two; mobilization techniques should address all restricted joint motions. Grade 1 and 2 mobilizations may be incorporated early in the rehabilitation program for managing pain. Mobilization may progress to grades 3 and 4 once pain and muscle guarding are decreased. For best results mobilization should be combined with manual traction techniques.

Traction Traction is the treatment of choice when there is a small protrusion of the nucleus pulposus. Through traction, the lumbar vertebrae are distracted, a subatmospheric pressure is created, tending to pull the protrusion to its original position, and there is tightening of the longitudinal ligament, tending to push the protrusion toward its original position within the disk. Traction may be done manually or using a traction machine. Sustained traction for at least 30 minutes with a force commensurate with body weight is preferred.

SUMMARY

Because of its mobility, the cervical spine is vulnerable to a wide range of sports injuries. The catastrophic neck injury is one that produces varying degrees of quadriplegia, so the unconscious athlete should be treated as if he or she has a serious neck injury. A major means for prevention of neck injury is maximizing its strength and flexibility.

The neck and upper back are subject to a number of acute injuries, the most common of which are wryneck, muscle strains, sprains, and contusions.

The posture defect scoliosis can be progressively disabling. Spondylolysis, spondylolisthesis, and Scheuermann's disease can cause pain in the lumbar region.

The low back can sustain a number of different injuries from sports activities. Prevention of low back injuries includes correcting or compensating for postural deviations, maintaining or increasing trunk and general body flexibility, and increasing trunk and general body strength.

Many low back problems stem from congenital defects such as spina bifida occulta or spondylolisthesis. Faulty posture is commonly the cause of mechanical defects in the spine. Faulty mechanics of the low back can eventually lead to the serious condition called lumbar disk disease. As with any musculoskeletal region, the low back can sustain traumatic sports injuries such as contusions, strains, and sprains.

REVIEW QUESTIONS AND CLASS ACTIVITIES

1. How does the cervical spine differ from the lumbar and thoracic regions in terms of functions?
2. What congenital and mechanical defects may be present in the spine?
3. Describe on-site emergency spinal evaluation.
4. Describe common neck, thoracic, and lumbar injuries.
5. Describe the mechanism of spinal injuries.
6. What steps can be taken to prevent spinal injuries?
7. Describe some reconditioning and therapeutic approaches that are taken in the care of a spinal injury.
8. Invite an athletic trainer/physical therapist/orthopedic physician to discuss his or her approach to caring for a spinal injury.

REFERENCES

1. Anderson C: Neck injuries, *Phys Sports Med* 1:23, 1993.
2. Bechman SM: Laryngeal fracture in a high school football player, *J Ath Train* 28:217, 1973.
3. Cailliet R: *Low back pain*, ed 3, Philadelphia, 1988, FA Davis.
4. Cantu RC: Cervical spinal stenosis, *Phys Sports Med* 21:57, 1993.
5. Fourre M: On-site management of cervical spine injuries, *Phy Sports Med* 19:4, 1991.
6. Jacobson E: *Progressive relaxation*, ed 2, Chicago, 1938, University of Chicago Press.
7. Lord MJ, Carson WG: Management of herniated lumbar discs in the athlete, *Sports Med Digest* 16:1, 1994.
8. Rovere GD: Low back pain in athletes, *Sports Med* 15:105, 1987.
9. Wilkerson JE, Maroon JC: Cervical spine injuries in athletes, *Phys Sports Med* 18:57, 1990.
10. Vegso JJ, Lehman RC: Field evaluation and management of head and neck injuries, In Torg JS, ed, *Clin Sports Med* 6:1987.

ANNOTATED BIBLIOGRAPHY

Cailliet R: *Low back pain syndrome*, ed 3, Philadelphia, 1988, FA Davis.
  Presents the subject of low back pain in a clear, concise, and interesting manner.
de Grout J et al: Correlative neuroanatomy, ed 12,1 Norwalk, Conn, 1991 Appleton & Lange.
  This text provides "Basic Principles," "Spinal Cord and Spine," "Anatomy of the brain," "Functional Systems," "Diagnostic Aids," and "Case Discussions."
Ishmael NK, Shorbe HB: *Care of the back*, ed 3, Philadelphia, 1985, JB Lippincott.
  A booklet with basic information about caring for back pain.
McCullough J: *Backache*, ed 2, Baltimore, 1990, Williams & Wilkins.
  In-depth text about the evaluation and treatment of back conditions.
Russell GS, Highland TR: *Care of the low back: a patient guide*, Philadelphia, 1990, FA Davis.
  A book for the individual with acute or chronic back pain.
Torg JS, ed: Head and neck injuries, *Clin Sports Med* 6:1987.
  In-depth coverage of head–neck injuries stemming from sports activities.

The Head and Face

When you finish this chapter, you should be able to

- Recognize major sports injuries to the head and face
- Provide emergency care and appropriate referral for head and face injuries

Sports injuries to the head could be life threatening.

S ports injuries to the head could be life threatening whereas facial injuries could lead to disfigurement.

THE CEREBRUM
Anatomy

The *brain*, or encephalon, is the part of the central nervous system that is contained within the bony cavity of the cranium and is divided into four sections: the cerebrum, the cerebellum, the pons, and the medulla oblongata.

Investing the spinal cord and the brain are the **meninges,** which are the three membranes that protect the brain and the spinal cord. Outermost is the dura mater, consisting of a dense, fibrous, and inelastic sheath that encloses the brain and cord. In some places it is attached directly to the vertebral canal, but for the most part a layer of fat that contains the vital arteries and veins separates this membrane from the bony wall and forms the epidural space. The arachnoid, an extremely delicate sheath, lines the dura mater and is attached directly to the spinal cord by many silklike tissue strands. The space between the arachnoid and the pia mater, the membrane that helps contain the spinal fluid, is called the *subarachnoid space*. The subarachnoid cavity projects upward and, running the full length of the spinal cord, connects with the ventricles of the brain. The pia mater is a thin, delicate, and highly vascularized membrane that

meninges
The three membranes that protect the brain and the spinal cord

adheres closely to the spinal cord and to the brain—the large extension of the cord that is housed within the skull (Figure 17-1).

Cerebrospinal fluid is contained between the arachnoid and the pia mater membrane and completely surrounds and suspends the brain. Its main function is to act as a cushion, helping to diminish the transmission of shocking forces.

Cerebral Injuries

Despite its considerable protection, the brain is subject to traumatic injury, and a great many of the head injuries incurred in sports have serious consequences (Figure 17-2). For this reason it is necessary to give special consideration to this part of the body. A constant supply of oxygen and blood to the brain is vital and critical to its survival. In the United States 7.5 million head injuries occur annually.

There are many ways to grade cerebral injuries; the following repre-

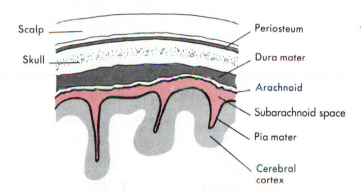

Figure 17-1

The meninges covering the brain.

Scalp

Skull

Periosteum

Dura mater

Arachnoid

Subarachnoid space

Pia mater

Cerebral cortex

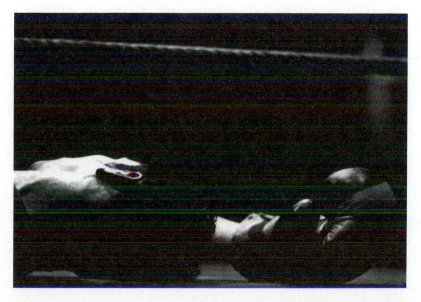

Figure 17-2

Many head injuries incurred in sports have serious consequences.

sents one procedure. Concussions are described as mild, moderate, or severe and are graded from I through VI (Table 17-1).

Grade I Concussion

Grade I concussions are minimum in intensity and represent the most common type in sports. In general the athlete becomes dazed and disoriented but does not lose memory (amenesia) or have other signs associated with a more serious condition. There may also be a mild unsteadiness in gait. The athlete is completely lucid in 5 to 15 minutes.

Grade II Concussion

A grade II concussion is characterized by minor confusion that is caused by post-traumatic amnesia. Posttraumatic amnesia is reflected by the inability of the athlete to recall events that have occurred since the time of injury. There are also unsteadiness, ringing in the ears (tinnitus), and perhaps minor dizziness. A dull headache may also follow. The athlete may also develop postconcussion syndrome, which is characterized by difficulty in concentrating, recurring headaches, and irritability. Athletes with postconcussion amnesia should not be permitted to return to play that day.[18] This amnesia may last for several weeks after the trauma, precluding sport participation until symptoms are completely gone.

Grade III Concussion

Grade III concussion includes all of the symptoms of grade II together with retrograde amnesia. Retrograde amnesia has occurred when the athlete is unable to recall recent events that occurred before the injury. There is also moderate tinnitus, mental confusion, balance disturbance, and headache. With a grade III concussion the athlete must not be allowed

TABLE 17-1 Cerebral Concussion Related to Consciousness and Amnesia

Grade	Symptoms
I	No amnesia and normal consciousness
II	Confusion and amnesia → Normal consciousness with posttraumatic amnesia
III	Confusion and amnesia → Normal consciousness with posttraumatic amnesia and retrograde amnesia
IV	Coma (paralytic) → Confusion and amnesia
V	Coma → Coma vigil
VI	Death

to return to activity until a thorough physical examination has been performed. An intracranial lesion that causes a gradual increase in intracranial pressure may be present (see box at the bottom of this page).

Grade IV Concussion

A grade IV concussion involves the athlete who is "knocked out." This state is considered a paralytic coma, from which the athlete usually recovers in a few seconds or minutes.[18] While recovering, the athlete returns to consciousness through states of being lethargic and confused, to a semilucid state with **automatism,** and finally to full alertness. There almost always are **posttraumatic amnesia** and **retrograde amnesia,** along with postconcussion syndrome.

An emergency situation is present whenever there is a loss of consciousness for more than several minutes and/or when there is a deteriorating neurological state. This situation demands immediate transportation to a hospital, with the athlete carried off the field on a spine board.

Grade V Concussion

A grade V concussion has occurred when the athlete is in a paralytic coma that is associated with secondary cardiorespiratory collapse.

Grade VI Death

The grade V concussion and coma may lead to a grade VI concussion and death.

Intracranial Hemorrhage

A blow to the head can cause intracranial bleeding. It may arise from rupture of a blood vessel's aneurysm or from tearing of a sinus separating the two brain hemispheres (Figure 17-3). Venous bleeding may be slow and insidious, whereas arterial hemorrhage may be evident in a few hours. In the beginning the athlete may be quite alert and lucid, with few or none of the symptoms of serious head injury, and then gradually display severe head pains, dizziness, nausea, inequality of pupil size, or sleepiness. Later stages of cerebral hemorrhage are characterized by de-

automatism
Automatic actions without conscious knowledge of those actions

posttraumatic amnesia
Inability of athlete to recall events since injury

retrograde amnesia
Memory loss for events occurring immediately before trauma

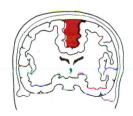

Figure 17-3
Intracranial hemorrhage.

**CONDITIONS INDICATING THE POSSIBILITY
OF INCREASING INTRACRANIAL PRESSURE**

Headache
Nausea and vomiting
Unequal pupils
Disorientation
Progressive or sudden impairment of consciousness
Gradual increase in blood pressure
Decrease in pulse rate

teriorating consciousness, neck rigidity, depression of pulse and respiration, and convulsions— a life-and-death situation.

Skull fracture   Any time an athlete sustains a severe blow to the unprotected head, a skull fracture should be suspected. Skull fractures can be difficult to ascertain. Swelling of the scalp may mask a skull depression or deformity. Until the more obvious signs caused by intracranial bleeding are present, the skull fracture, even during x-ray examination, can be missed.

Epidural, subdural, and intracerebral hemorrhage   There are three major types of intracranial hemorrhage: epidural, subdural, and intracerebral.

The three major types of intracranial hemorrhage are
epidural
subdural
intracerebral

Epidural bleeding

A blow to the head can cause a tear in one of the arteries in the dural membrane that covers the brain (Figure 17-4). It can result from a skull fracture or sudden shift of the brain. Because of arterial blood pressure, blood accumulation and the creation of a hematoma are extremely fast.[13] Often in only 10 to 20 minutes the athlete goes from appearing all right to having major signs of serious head injury. The pressure of the hematoma must be surgically relieved as soon as possible.

Subdural bleeding

In subdural bleeding, veins are torn that bridge the dura mater to the brain. A common mechanism of injury is one of contrecoup, in which the skull decelerates suddenly and the brain keeps moving, tearing blood vessels (Figure 17-5). Because of lower pressure, veins are the primary type of blood vessels injured. Hemorrhage is slow. Signs of brain injury may not appear for many hours after injury. Thus athletes who have sustained a hard blow to the head must be carefully observed for a 24-hour period for signs of pressure buildup within the skull.

Intracerebral bleeding

Intracerebral hemorrhage is bleeding within the brain itself. Most commonly it results from a compressive force to the brain[12] (Figure 17-6). Deterioration of neurological function occurs rapidly, requiring immediate hospitalization. The coach must be aware that even a mild head concussion could result in delayed problems including bleeding that may not reveal itself for several months.

Assessment of Cerebral Injuries

Cases of serious head injury almost always represent a life-threatening situation that requires that the athlete be admitted to a hospital within a crucial 30-minute period.

On-the-Field Evaluation

One must be adept at recognizing and interpreting the signs that an unconscious athlete presents. Priority first aid for any head injury must always deal with any life-threatening condition such as impaired airway or hemorrhage. When an athlete is unconscious, a neck injury is also assumed. Without moving the athlete, evaluation includes the following:

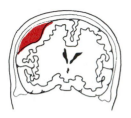

Figure 17-4

Epidural bleeding.

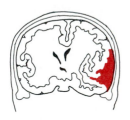

Figure 17-5

Subdural bleeding.

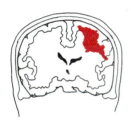

Figure 17-6

Intracerebral bleeding.

1. Looking for the possibility of airway obstruction. If breathing is obstructed, perform the following:
   a. Remove face mask by cutting it away from the helmet but leave helmet in place.
   b. Stabilize head and neck.
   c. Bring jaw forward to clear air passage (do not hyperextend neck).
   d. Take pulse: if absent, cardiopulmonary resuscitation (CPR) is given; if present, oxygen may be given.
2. A quick observation of the following physical signs of concussion and/or skull fracture:
   a. Face color may be red or pale.
   b. Skin may be cool or moist.
   c. Pulse, if present, may be strong and slow or rapid and weak.
   d. Breathing, if present, may be deep or shallow.
   e. Pupils may be dilated and/or unequal.
   f. Head may show swelling or deformity over area of injury.
3. The athlete is removed carefully from the playing site on a spine board as per Chapter 7 instructions, pp. 194 and 195.

Continued Evaluation

History   Athletes with grade III or IV concussions having distinct clinical signs should automatically be sent to the hospital for medical care. In grade I and II concussions it is often difficult to determine exactly how serious the problem is. Also, grade I and II conditions can slowly—or even quickly—deteriorate to a higher grade. This possibility makes certain evaluative procedures imperative even in so-called very minor cases (Table 17-2).

Table 17-2 Symptoms of Cerebral Concussion

Symptoms	First Degree		Second Degree	Third Degree
	Grade I	Grade II	Grade III	Grade IV
Disorientation	+	+	++	+++
Dizziness		+	++	+++
Amnesia		+	++	+++
Headache			+/++	+++
Loss of consciousness			+/++	+++
Problems in concentrating		+	++	+++
Tinnitus		+	++	+++
Balance problems		+	++	+++
Automatism			+/++	+++
Pupillary discrepancies			+/++	+++

+ Mild.
++ Moderate.
+++ Severe.

When the athlete regains awareness, testing for mental orientation and memory should be done. Questions might include the following:

- What is your name?
- How old are you?
- Where are you?
- What game are you playing?
- What period is it?
- What is the score?
- What is your assignment on the 23 trap play?

After 5 or 10 minutes, repeat the questions that were previously asked.

Testing eye signs Because of the direct connection between the eye and the brain, pupillary discrepancies provide important information. The athlete should be observed and tested for the following:

1. Dilated and/or irregular pupils. Checking pupil sizes may be particularly difficult at night and under artificial lights. To ensure accuracy, the athlete's pupil size should be compared with that of an official or another player present. It should be remembered, however, that some individuals normally have pupils that differ in size.
2. Blurred vision determined by difficulty or inability to read a game program or the score board.
3. Inability of the pupils to accommodate rapidly to light variance. Eye accommodation should be tested by covering one eye with a hand. The covered eye normally will dilate, whereas the uncovered pupil will remain the same. When the hand is removed, the previously covered pupil normally will accommodate readily to the light. A slow accommodating pupil may be an indicator of cerebral injury.
4. Inability of eyes to track smoothly. The athlete is asked to hold the head in a neutral position, eyes looking straight ahead. The athlete is then asked to follow the top of a pen or pencil, first up as far as possible, then down as far as possible. The eyes are observed for smooth movement and any signs of pain. Next, the tip of the pen or pencil is slowly moved from left to right to determine whether the eyes follow the tip smoothly across the midline of the face or whether they make involuntary movements. A constant involuntary back and forth, up and down, or rotary movement of the eyeball indicates possible cerebral involvement.

Testing balance If the athlete can stand, the degree of unsteadiness must be noted. A cerebral concussion of grade II or more can produce balance difficulties (positive Romberg's sign). To test Romberg's sign the athlete is told to stand tall with the feet together, arms at sides, eyes closed. A positive sign is one in which the athlete begins to sway, cannot keep eyes closed, or obviously loses balance. Having the athlete attempt to stand on one foot is also a good indicator of balance.

Finger-to-nose test The athlete stands tall with eyes closed and arms out to the side. The athlete is then asked to touch the index finger of one hand to the nose and then to touch the index finger of the other hand to the nose. Inability to perform this task with one or both fingers is an indication of physical disorientation and precludes reentry to the game.

An athlete with any degree of concussion should be sent immediately to the sports physician for treatment and observation. Brain injury may not be apparent until hours after the trauma occurs. The athlete may have to be observed closely throughout the night and be awakened approximately every 1 to 2 hours to check the level of consciousness and orientation.

Although the incidence of serious head injuries from football has decreased in past years when compared with catastrophic neck injuries, the occurrence of football injuries is of major concern. Every coach and athletic trainer must be able to recognize the signs of serious head injury to act appropriately.

Most traumas of the head result from direct or indirect blows and may be classified as concussion injuries. Literally, "concussion" means an agitation or a shaking from being hit, and "cerebral concussion" refers to the agitation of the brain by either a direct or an indirect blow (Figure 17-7). The indirect concussion most often comes from either a violent fall, in which sitting down transmits a jarring effect through the vertebral column to the brain, or a blow to the chin. In most cases of cerebral concussion there is a short period of unconsciousness, having mild to severe results.

Most authorities agree that unconsciousness results from a lack of oxygen to the brain that is caused by constriction of the blood vessels. Depending on the force of the blow and the athlete's ability to withstand such a blow, varying degrees of cerebral hemorrhage, edema, and tissue

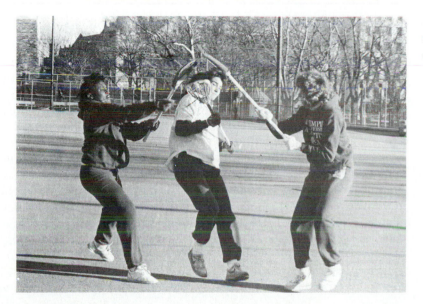

Figure 17-7

Sports using implements can cause serious head injuries.

laceration may occur that, in turn, will cause tissue changes. Because of the fluid suspension of the brain, a blow to the head can effect an injury to the brain either at the point of contact or on the opposite side. After the head is struck, the brain continues to move in the fluid and may be contused against the opposite side. This causes a contrecoup brain injury. An athlete who is knocked unconscious by a blow to the head may be presumed to have received some degree of concussion.

In determining the extent of head injury one must be aware of basic gross signs by which concussions may be evaluated. For the coach when the athlete is knocked out, the following questions must be answered: 1. the athlete breathing? 2. Does the athlete have a heart beat? 3. Has the athlete sustained a spinal fracture?

Returning to Competition After Cerebral Injury

Following a cerebral injury, an athlete must be free of symptoms and signs before returning to competition.

There is always the question of whether an athlete who has been "knocked out" several times should continue in the sport. The team physician must be the final authority on whether an athlete continues to participate in a collision sport after head injury. Each athlete must be evaluated individually.[1] One serious concussion may warrant exclusion from the sport; on the other hand, a number of minor episodes may not. In making this decision, the physician must make sure that the athlete is as follows:

1. Normal neurologically
2. Normal in all vasomotor functions
3. Free of headaches
4. Free of seizure and has a normal electroencephalogram
5. Free of lightheadedness when suddenly changing body positions[12]

NOTE: Athlete must have a written documentation for the return to competition.[17]

Secondary Conditions Associated with Cerebral Injury

Secondary brain injury conditions include the following:
  Cerebral hyperemia
  Cerebal edema
  Cerebral seizure
  Migraine headache

In addition to the initial injury to the brain, many secondary conditions can also arise following head trauma. Some of the prevalent ones are cerebral hyperemia (primarily in children), cerebral edema, postinjury epilepsy and seizures, and posttraumatic headaches.

Cerebral hyperemia   A condition common to children with head injuries is cerebral hyperemia, resulting from cerebral blood vessel dilation and a rise in intracranial blood pressure. As a result, children develop headache, vomiting, and lethargy. Cerebral hyperemia can occur within a few minutes of injury and can subside in 12 hours.

Cerebral edema   Cerebral edema is a localized swelling at the injury site. Within a 12-hour period the athlete may begin to develop edema, which causes headache and, on occasion, seizures.[12] Cerebral edema may last as long as 2 weeks and is not related to the intensity of trauma.

Seizures   Seizures can occur immediately after head trauma, indicating the possibility of brain injury. They have a higher incidence when the brain has been actually contused or there is intracranial bleeding. A small number of individuals who have sustained a severe cerebral injury will in time develop epilepsy.[12]

For athletes having a grand mal seizure, the following measures should be taken:

1. Maintain airway.
2. Make sure athlete is safe from injury.
3. Avoid sticking fingers into the athlete's mouth in an effort to withdraw the tongue.
4. Turn athlete's head to the side so that saliva and blood can drain out of the mouth once the seizure has ended.

The seizure will normally last only a couple of minutes.

Headaches   Headaches, which may range from mild to severe, may follow a single or repeated head injury (Figure 17-8). Headaches stem from physical effort. Following a head injury an athlete may experience tension, migraine, and/or cluster type headaches.

A tension headache is associated with abnormal contraction of the muscles in the neck and scalp. A migraine headache is a disorder characterized by recurrent attacks of severe headache with sudden onset, with or without visual or gastrointestinal problems. The athlete who has a history of repeated minor blows to the head such as those that may occur in soccer or who has sustained a major cerebral injury may, over a period of time, develop migraine headaches. The exact cause is unknown, but it is believed by many to be a vascular disorder. Flashes of light, blindness in half the field of vision, and numbness are thought to be caused by vessel constriction. Headache is believed to be caused by dilation of scalp arteries. The athlete complains of a severe headache that is diffused throughout the head and often accompanied by nausea and vomiting.

Cluster headaches are similar to migraines, recurring as often as two or three times per day. The athlete then becomes symptom free for weeks or months. A cluster headache comes on abruptly and is characterized by an intense throbbing pain behind a nostril and one eye. Eyes and nose water, skin over pain area becomes red with the pupil of the eye becoming constricted. Attacks last less than 2 hours.

THE FACE
Anatomy

The facial skin covers primarily subcutaneous bone with very little protective muscle, fascia, or fat. The supraorbital ridges house the frontal sinuses. In general the facial skeleton is composed of dense bony buttresses combined with thin sheets of bone (Figure 17-9). The middle third of the face consists of the maxillary bone, which supports the nose and nasal passages. The lower aspect of the face consists of the lower jaw or mandible. Besides supporting teeth, the mandible also supports the larynx, trachea, upper airway, and upper digestive tract.

Figure 17-8

Repeated blows to the head may predispose athletes to headaches.

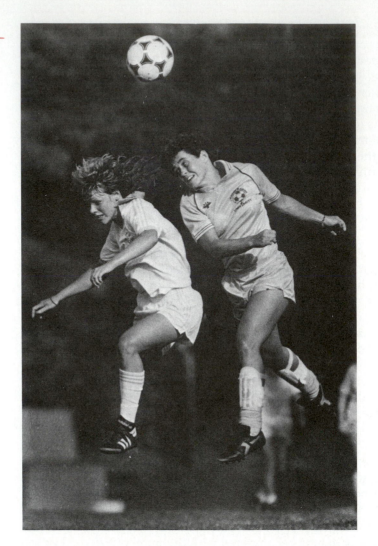

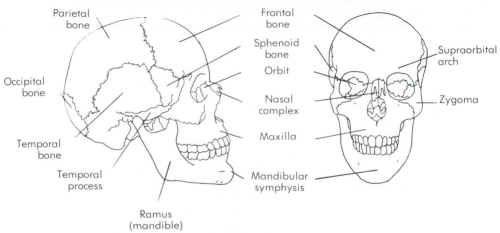

Parietal bone

Occipital bone

Temporal bone

Temporal process

Ramus (mandible)

Frontal bone

Sphenoid bone

Orbit

Nasal complex

Maxilla

Mandibular symphysis

Supraorbital arch

Zygoma

Figure 17-9

Bones of the face.

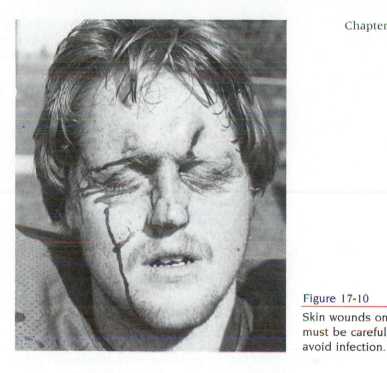

Figure 17-10

Skin wounds on the face
must be carefully managed to
avoid infection.

Facial Injuries

Serious injuries to the face have been reduced significantly from the past
by requiring athletes to wear proper protection in high-risk sports (Figure 17-10). The most prevalent cause of facial injury is a direct blow that
injures soft and bony tissue. Very common are skin abrasions, lacerations,
and contusions; less common are fractures.

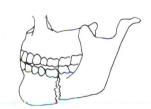

Figure 17-11

Lower jaw fracture.

Injuries of the Lower Jaw

Jaw fracture   Fractures of the lower jaw (Figure 17-11) occur most
often in collision sports. They are second in incidence of all facial fractures. Because it has relatively little padding and sharp contours, the
lower jaw is prone to injury from a direct blow. The most frequently fractured area is near the jaw's frontal angle.

The main indications of a fractured lower jaw are deformity, loss of
normal **occlusion** of the teeth, pain when biting down, bleeding around
teeth, and lower lip numbness.[10]

Care   Management usually includes cold packs to the side of the face,
immobilization by a four-tailed bandage, and immediate referral to a physician.

Occlusion
The way the teeth line up.
Malocclusion means that the
upper and lower teeth do
not line up.

Jaw Dislocations

A dislocation of the jaw, or *lower jaw luxation,* involves the temporomandibular joint. This area has all the features of a hinge and gliding articulation. Because of its wide range of movement and the inequity of size between the two pieces the jaw is somewhat prone to dislocation. The mechanism of injury in dislocations is usually initiated by a side blow to the open mouth of the athlete, forcing the mandibular condyle forward out of the temporal fossa.

The major signs of the dislocated jaw are a locked-open position, with jaw movement being almost impossible, and/or an overriding malocclusion of the teeth.

Care In cases of first-time jaw dislocation the initial treatment includes immediately applying a cold compress to control hemorrhage, splinting the jaw through the use of a four-tailed bandage, and referring the athlete to a physician for reduction.

Cheekbone fracture A fracture of the cheekbone represents the third most common facial fracture.[10] Because of its nearness to the eye orbit, visual problems may also occur.

An obvious deformity occurs in the cheek region or a bony discrepancy can be felt during palpation. There is usually a nosebleed and the athlete commonly complains of seeing double.

Care Care usually involves cold application for the control of edema and immediate referral to a physician.

Upper jaw fracture A severe blow to the upper jaw such as would be incurred by being struck by a hockey puck or stick can fracture this bone. This ranks fourth in incidence of facial fracture.[10]

After being struck a severe blow to the upper jaw, the athlete complains of pain while chewing, malocclusion, nosebleed, double vision, and numbness in the lip and cheek region.

Care Because bleeding is usually profuse, airway passages must be maintained. A brain injury may also be associated with this condition as with all injuries to the face and must be evaluated and managed accordingly. The athlete must be referred immediately for medical attention.

Dental Injuries

The tooth is a composite of mineral salts of which calcium and phosphorus are most abundant. That portion protruding from the gum, called the *crown*, is covered by the hardest substance within the body, the enamel. The portion that extends into the alveolar bone of the mouth is called the *root* and is covered by a thin, bony substance known as *cementum*. Underneath the enamel and cementum lies the bulk of the tooth, a hard material known as *dentin*. Within the dentin is a central canal and chamber containing the *pulp*, a substance composed of nerves, lymphatics, and blood vessels that supply the entire tooth (Figure 17-12).

With the use of face guards and properly fitting mouth guards most dental injuries can be prevented. Mouth protectors need to be mandated in all sports that produce mouth injuries (for example, wrestling, rugby, soccer, basketball, gymnastics, racquetball, lacrosse, field hockey, martial arts, and skiing). Any blow to the upper or lower jaw can potentially injure the teeth. Injuries to the tooth below the gum line may repair themselves because of the abundant blood supply. However, fractures of

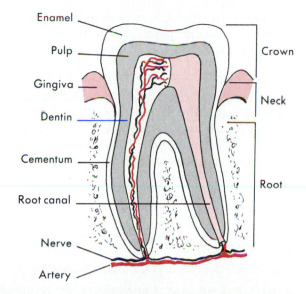

Figure 17-12

Normal tooth anatomy.

Enamel

Pulp

Gingiva

Dentin

Cementum

Root canal

Nerve

Artery

Crown

Neck

Root

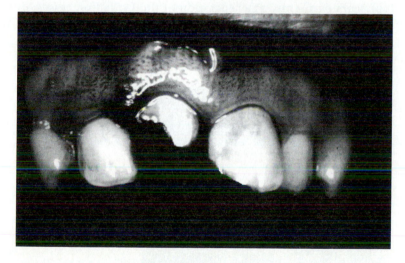

Figure 17-13

Tooth fractures exposing the pulp can predispose the tooth to infection and perhaps death.

the tooth below the gum line may not heal if there is an injury to the tooth pulp. A tooth could sustain a mild blow, which may not be obvious, that disrupts its blood and nerve supply.[13]

The Fractured Tooth

Fracture of the crown of the tooth is an enamel fracture and can usually be repaired by smoothing, capping, or even removing the entire tooth. In contrast, fractures that involve the dentin, which expose the pulp, may predispose the tooth to infection and tooth death (Figure 17-13).

Teeth in which the enamel or dentin is chipped fail to rejuvenate because they lack a direct blood supply. They can be capped for the sake of appearance. A tooth that is fractured or loosened may be extremely painful because of the damaged or exposed nerve. In such cases a small amount of calcium hydroxide (Dycol) applied to the exposed nerve area will inhibit the pain until the athlete is seen by a dentist.

Partially or Completely Dislocated Tooth

A tooth that has been knocked crooked should be manually realigned to a normal position as soon as possible. One that has been totally knocked out should be cleaned with water and replaced in the tooth socket, if possible. If repositioning the dislocated tooth is difficult, the athlete should keep it under the tongue until the dentist can replace it. If this is inconvenient, a dislodged tooth can also be kept in a glass of water. If a completely dislodged tooth is out of the mouth for more than 30 minutes, the chances of saving it are very tenuous; therefore the athlete should immediately be sent to the dentist for splinting.

A tooth that has been completely dislocated intact should be rinsed off with water and replaced in the socket.

Nasal Injuries

Nasal Fractures and Cartilage Separation

A fracture of the nose is one of the most common fractures of the face.[10] It appears frequently as a separation of the frontal processes of the maxilla, a separation of the lateral cartilages, or a combination of the two (Figure 17-14).

Figure 17-14

Nasal fracture.

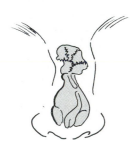

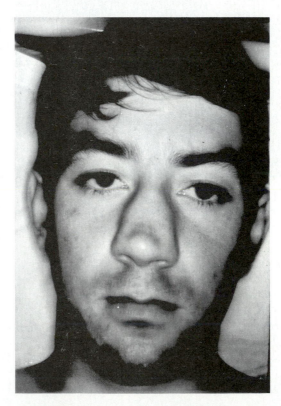

The force of the blow to the nose may either come from the side or from a straight frontal force. A lateral force causes greater deformity than a "straight-on" blow. In nasal fractures hemorrhage is profuse because of laceration of the mucous lining. Swelling is immediate. Deformity is usually present if the nose has received a lateral blow. Gentle palpation may reveal abnormal mobility and emit a grating sound (crepitus).

Care   One should control the bleeding and then refer the athlete to a physician for x-ray examination and reduction of the fracture. Simple and uncomplicated fractures of the nose will not hinder or be unsafe for the athlete, and he or she will be able to return to competition within a few days. Adequate protection can be provided through splinting (see box below and Figure 17-15).

Nasal Septal Injuries

A major nasal injury can occur to the septum. As with fracture, the mechanisms are caused by compression or lateral trauma.[14]

A careful evaluation of the nose must be made by the athletic trainer or physician after the trauma. Injury commonly produces bleeding and, in some cases, a hematoma. The athlete complains of nasal pain.

Care   At the site where a hematoma may occur, compression is applied. When a hematoma is present, it must be drained immediately through a surgical incision through the mucous lining. After surgical drainage, a small wick is inserted for continued drainage, and the nose is firmly packed to prevent reformation of the hematoma. If a hematoma is neglected, an abscess will form, causing bone and cartilage loss and, ultimately, a difficult-to-correct deformity.[11]

Nosebleed

Nosebleeds in sports are usually the result of direct blows that cause varying degrees of contusion to the septum (Figure 17-16).

Hemorrhages arise most often from the highly vascular anterior aspect of the nasal septum. In most situations the nosebleed presents only a minor problem and stops spontaneously after a short period of time.

NOSE SPLINTING

The following procedure is used for nose splinting.
MATERIALS NEEDED: Two pieces of gauze, each 2 inches (5 cm) long and rolled to the size of a pencil, three strips of 1½-inch (3.75 cm) tape, cut approximately 4 inches (10 cm) long; and clear tape adherent.
POSITION OF THE ATHLETE: The athlete lies supine on the athletic training table.
PROCEDURE:
1. The rolled pieces of gauze are placed on either side of the athlete's nose.
2. Gently but firmly, 4-inch (10 cm) lengths of tape are laid over the gauze rolls.

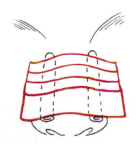

Figure 17-15

Splinting the fractured nose.

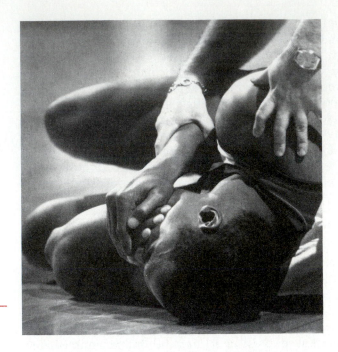

Figure 17-16

Nosebleeds are common in contact and collision sports.

cauterization

Destruction of tissue by means of a caustic, an electric current, or by freezing

However, there are persistent types that require medical attention and, possibly, **cauterization.**

Care   The care of the athlete with an acute nosebleed is as follows:
1. The athlete sits upright.
2. A cold compress is placed over the nose and the ipsilateral carotid artery.
3. The athlete applies finger pressure to the affected nostril for 5 minutes.

If the above method fails to stop the bleeding within 5 minutes, more extensive measures should be taken. After bleeding has ceased, the athlete may resume activity but should be reminded not to blow the nose under any circumstances for at least 2 hours after the initial insult.

Foreign Body in the Nose

During participation the athlete may have insects or debris lodge in one of his or her nostrils; if the object is large enough, the mucous lining of the nose will react by becoming inflamed and swollen. In most cases the foreign body will become dislodged if the nose is gently blown while the unaffected side in pinched shunt. Probing and blowing the nose violently will only cause additional irritation.

Ear Injuries

The ear (Figure 17-17) is responsible for the sense of hearing and equilibrium. It is composed of three parts: the external ear; the middle ear (tympanic membrane) lying just inside the skull; and the internal ear (labyrinth), which is formed, in part, by the temporal bone of the skull.

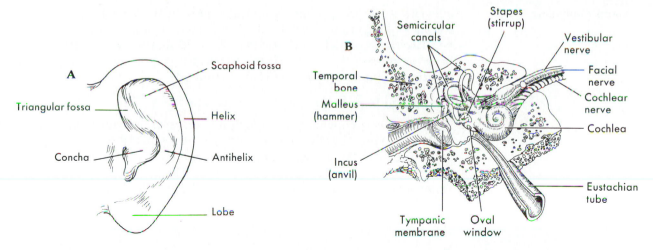

A
Triangular fossa
Scaphoid fossa
Helix
Concha
Antihelix
Lobe

B
Semicircular canals
Stapes (stirrup)
Temporal bone
Vestibular nerve
Malleus (hammer)
Facial nerve
Cochlear nerve
Incus (anvil)
Cochlea
Tympanic membrane
Oval window
Eustachian tube

Figure 17-17

Ear anatomy. **A,** Normal external ear. **B,** Inner ear.

The middle ear and internal ear are structured to transport auditory impulses to the brain. Aiding the organs of hearing and equalizing pressure between the middle and the internal ear is the eustachian tube, a canal that joins the nose and the middle ear.[15]

Sports injuries to the ear occur most often to the external portion. The external ear is separated into the auricle (pinna) and the external auditory canal (meatus). The auricle, which is shaped like a shell, collects and directs waves of sound into the auditory canal. It is composed of flexible yellow cartilage, muscles, and fat padding and is covered by a closely adhering, thin layer of skin. Most of the blood vessels and nerves of the auricle turn around its borders, with just a few penetrating the cartilage proper.

Cauliflower Ear

Contusions, wrenching, or extreme friction of the ear can lead to hematoma auris, commonly known as a "cauliflower ear"[11] (Figure 17-18).

This condition usually occurs from repeated injury to the ear and is seen most frequently in boxers and wrestlers. However, recently, it has been held to a minimum because of the protective measures that have been initiated.

Trauma may tear the overlying tissue away from the cartilaginous plate, resulting in hemorrhage and fluid accumulation. A hematoma usually forms before the limited circulation can absorb the fluid. If the hematoma goes unattended, a sequence of coagulation, organization, and fibrosis results in a **keloid** that appears elevated, rounded, white, nodular, and firm, resembling a cauliflower. Once developed, the keloid can be removed only through surgery. To prevent this disfiguring condition from arising, some friction-proofing agent such as petroleum jelly should be applied to the ears of athletes susceptible to this condition. They should also routinely wear ear guards in practice and in competition.

Care If an ear becomes "hot" because of excessive rubbing or twisting, the immediate application of a cold pack to the affected spot will

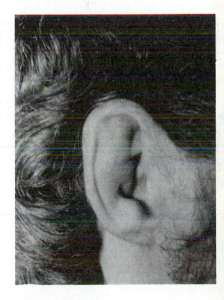

Figure 17-18

Cauliflower ear.

keloid
a raised, firm, thickened red scar progressively developing after injury or surgery

alleviate hemorrhage. Once swelling is present in the ear, special care should be taken to prevent the fluid from solidifying; a cold pack should be placed immediately over the ear and held tightly by an elastic bandage for at least 20 minutes. If the swelling is still present at the end of this time, aspiration by a physician is required.

Foreign Body in the Ear

The ears offer an opening, as do the nose and eyes, in which objects can become caught. Usually these objects are pieces of debris or flying insects. They can be dislodged by having the athlete tilt the head to one side. If removal is difficult, syringing the ear with a solution of lukewarm water may remove the object. Care should be exercised to avoid striking the eardrum with the direct stream of water.

Eye Injuries

Eye injuries account for approximately 1% of all sports injuries.[14] In the United States, baseball has the highest incidence of eye injuries.

Eye Anatomy

The eye has many anatomical protective devices. It is firmly retained within an oval socket formed by the bones of the head. A cushion of soft fatty tissue surrounds it, and a thin skin flap (the eyelid), which functions by reflex action, covers the eye for protection. Foreign particles are prevented from entering the eye by the lashes and eyebrows, which act as a filtering system. A soft mucous lining that covers the inner conjunctiva transports and spreads tears, which are secreted by many accessory lacrimal glands. A larger lubricating organ is located above the eye and secretes heavy quantities of fluid through the lacrimal duct to help wash away foreign particles. The eye proper is well protected by the sclera, a tough white outer layer possessing a transparent center portion called the *cornea* (Figure 17-19).

Figure 17-19

Eye anatomy.

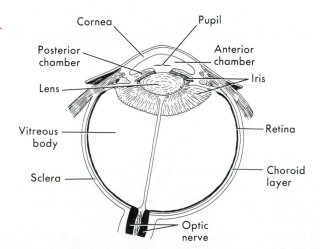

Eye Protection

The eye can be injured in a number of different ways. Shattered eyeglass or goggle lenses can lacerate; ski pole tips can penetrate; and fingers, racquetballs, and larger projectiles can seriously compress and injure the eye.[20] High-injury sports such as ice hockey, football, and lacrosse require full-face and helmet protection, whereas low-energy sports such as racquetball and tennis require eye guards that rest on the face. Protective devices must provide protection from front and lateral blows.

Sport goggles can be made with highly impact-resistant polycarbonate lenses for refraction. The major problems with sports goggles are distortion of peripheral vision and the tendency to become fogged under certain weather conditions.

Evaluation of Eye Injuries

It is essential that any eye injury be evaluated immediately. The first concern is to understand the mechanism of injury and to ascertain whether there is a related condition to the head, face, or neck.

Initial Management of Eye Injuries

Proper care of eye injuries is essential. The athletic trainer must use extreme caution in handling eye injuries. If there appears to be retinal detachment, perforation of the globe, foreign object embedded in the cornea, blood in the anterior chamber, decreased vision, loss of the visual field, poor pupillary adaptation, double vision, laceration, or impaired lid function, the athlete should be immediately referred to a hospital or an ophthalmologist. Ideally, the athlete with a serious eye injury should be transported to the hospital by ambulance in a recumbent position (see box below). Both eyes must be covered during transport. At no time should pressure be applied to the eye. In case of surrounding soft-tissue injury, a cold compress can be applied for 30 to 60 minutes to control hemorrhage (Figure 17-20).

*Extreme care must be taken with any eye injury:
Transport the athlete in a recumbent position.
Cover both eyes but put no pressure on the eye.*

Black Eye

Although well protected, the eye may be bruised during sports activity. The severity of eye injuries varies from a mild bruise to an extremely serious condition affecting vision to the fracturing of the orbital cavity. Fortunately, most of the eye injuries sustained in sports are mild. A blow to the eye may initially injure the surrounding tissue and produce capil-

---

SYMPTOMS INDICATING THE POSSIBILITY OF SERIOUS EYE INJURY

Blurred vision not clearing with blinking
Loss of all or part of the visual field
Pain that is sharp, stabbing, or throbbing
Double vision after injury

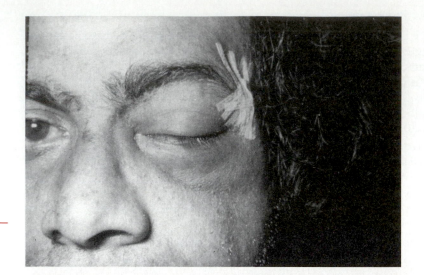

Figure 17-20

A serious eye injury should be treated as a major medical emergency.

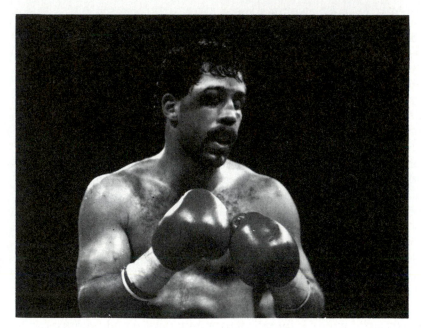

Figure 17-21

A blow to the eye region may produce capillary bleeding and later the classic black eye.

lary bleeding into the tissue spaces. If the hemorrhage goes unchecked, the result may be a classic "black eye." The signs of a more serious contusion may be displayed as a subconjunctival hemorrhage or as faulty vision (Figure 17-21).

Care of an eye contusion requires cold application for at least half an hour, plus a 24-hour rest period if the athlete has distorted vision. Under no circumstances should an athlete blow the nose following an acute eye injury. To do so might increase hemorrhaging.

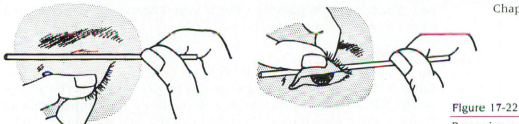

Figure 17-22

Removing a foreign body
from the eye.

REMOVING A FOREIGN BODY FROM THE EYE

MATERIALS NEEDED: One applicator stick, sterile cotton-tipped applicator, eyecup, and eyewash (solution of boric acid).

POSITION OF THE ATHLETE: The athlete lies supine on a table.

PROCEDURE:

1. Gently pull the eyelid down and place an applicator stick crosswise at its base.
2. Have the athlete look down; then grasp the lashes and turn the lid back over the stick.
3. Holding the lid and the stick in place with one hand, use the sterile cotton swab to lift out the foreign body.

Foreign Body in the Eye

Foreign bodies in the eye are a frequent occurrence in sports and are potentially dangerous. A foreign object produces considerable pain and disability. No attempt should be made to rub out the body or to remove it with the fingers. Have the athlete close the eye until the initial pain has subsided and then attempt to determine if the object is in the vicinity of the upper or lower lid. Foreign bodies in the lower lid are relatively easy to remove by depressing the tissue and then wiping it with a sterile cotton applicator. Foreign bodies in the area of the upper lid are usually much more difficult to localize. Two methods may be used. The first technique, which is quite simple, is performed as follows: gently pull the upper eyelid over the lower lid, as the subject looks downward. This causes tears to be produced, which may flush the object down on to the lower lid. If this method is unsuccessful, the second technique (see box above) should be used (Figure 17-22).

After the foreign particle is removed, the affected eye should be washed with a boric acid solution or with a commercial eyewash. Quite often there is a residual soreness, which may be alleviated by the application of petroleum jelly or some other mild ointment. If there is extreme difficulty in removing the foreign body or if it has become embedded in the eye itself, the eye should be closed and "patched" with a gauze

Rubbing an eye with a foreign object in it will often scratch the cornea.

photophobia
An intense intolerance of light

pad, which is held in place by strips of tape. The athlete is referred to a physician as soon as possible.

Corneal Abrasions

An athlete who gets a foreign object in his or her eye will usually try to rub it away. In doing so, the cornea can become abraded. The athlete will complain of severe pain and watering of the eye, **photophobia,** and spasm of the eyelid. The eye should be patched, and the athlete should be sent to a physician. Corneal abrasion is diagnosed through application of a fluorescein strip to the abraded area, staining it a bright green.

Hyphema

A blunt blow to the anterior aspect of the eye can produce a hyphema, which is a collection of blood within the anterior chamber. The blood settles inferiorly or may fill the entire chamber. Vision is partially or completely blocked. The coach must be aware that a hyphema is a major eye injury that can lead to serious problems of the lens, choroid, or retina.

Rupture of the Globe

A blow to the eye by an object smaller than the eye orbit produces extreme pressure that can rupture the globe. A golf ball or racquetball fits this category; however, larger objects such as a tennis ball or a fist will often fracture the bony orbit before the eye is overly compressed. Even if it does not cause rupture, such a force can cause internal injury that may ultimately lead to blindness.

Blowout Fracture

A blow to the face that strikes the eye and orbital ridge can cause what is commonly called a *blowout fracture of the orbit.* Because of the sudden increase in internal pressure of the eye, the very thin bone located in the inferior aspect of the orbit can fracture. Hemorrhage occurs around the inferior margins of the eye. The athlete commonly complains of double vision and pain when moving the eye. With such symptoms and signs, immediate referral to a physician is necessary.

Retinal Detachment

A blow to the athlete's eye can partially or completely separate the retina from its underlying retinal pigment epithelium. Retinal detachment is more common among athletes who have myopia (nearsightedness). Detachment is painless; however, early signs include seeing specks floating before the eye, flashes of light, or blurred vision. As the detachment progresses, the athlete complains of a "curtain" falling over the field of vision. Any athlete with symptoms of detachment must be immediately referred to an ophthalmologist.

SUMMARY

Brain injuries, which can be life-threatening, often result from blows that can be classified as concussion injuries. Depending on the severity of the concussion, the athlete may display signs of disorientation, dizziness, amnesia, headache, loss of consciousness, problems in concentrating, tinnitus, balance problems, automatism, or pupillary discrepancies.

Brain concussion is categorized into six grades. In grade I the athlete becomes dazed and disoriented. In grade II the athlete displays minor confusion caused by a posttraumatic amnesia. There may also be minor dizziness, ringing in the ears, and a dull headache. Grade III concussion includes all of the symptoms of grade II, plus retrograde amnesia. Grade IV is of the "knocked out" athlete. There are posttraumatic amnesia and retrograde amnesia, along with postconcussion syndrome. The grade V concussion includes a paralytic coma, associated with a secondary cardiorespiratory collapse. A grade VI concussion is one in which coma leads to death.

The face is subject to many different types of traumatic sports injuries. The most common are facial wounds, with lacerations ranking at the top. Less common, but usually more serious, are injuries such as jaw fractures and dislocations, dental injuries, and nasal injuries. A potentially disfiguring ear injury is hematoma auris, or cauliflower ear. The eye is also at risk; therefore it is essential that the eye be protected against fast-moving projectiles.

REVIEW QUESTIONS AND SUGGESTED ACTIVITIES

1. Pair off with another student, with one acting as the coach or athletic trainer and the other as the injured athlete. The athlete simulates concussions of various grades. The coach or athletic trainer assesses the student, attempting to determine the grade of concussion.
2. List the on-site assessment steps that should be taken when cerebral injuries occur.
3. Demonstrate the following procedures in evaluating a cerebral injury—questioning the athlete, testing eye signs, testing balance, and the finger-to-nose test.
4. Contrast a grade II with a grade III concussion.
5. What immediate care procedures should be performed for athletes with facial lacerations?
6. Describe the immediate care procedures that should be performed when a tooth is fractured and when it is dislocated.
7. Describe the procedures that should be performed for an athlete with a nose bleed.
8. How can cauliflower ear be prevented?
9. The eye can sustain an extremely serious injury during some sports activities. What are the major indicators of a possibly serious eye injury?

REFERENCES

1. Cantu RC: Guidelines for return to contact sports after a cerebral concussion, *Phys Sportsmed* 14:75, 1986.
2. Diamond S: Treating athletes who have post traumatic headaches, *Phys Sportsmed* 20:167, 1992.
3. Douglas LG: Facial injuries. In Welsh PR, Shephard RJ, eds: *Current therapy in sports medicine 1985-1986*, Philadelphia, 1985, BC Decker.
4. Dimeff RJ: Activity related headache, *Clin Sports Med* 11:339, 1992.

5. Forrest LA: Management of orbital blow-out fractures, *Am J Sports Med* 17:217, 1989.
6. Gieck JH: Evaluation and correction of common postural dysfunctions, *Ath Train* 24:310, 1989.
7. Lubell AL: Chronic brain injury in boxers: is it avoidable? *Phys Sportsmed* 17:126, 1989.
8. Mac Afee II KA: Immediate care of facial trauma, *Phys Sportsmed* 20:331, 1992.
9. Maroon JC et al: Assessing closed head injuries, *Phys Sportsmed* 4:37, 1992.
10. Matthews B: Maxillofacial trauma from athletic endeavors, *Ath Tr* 25:132, 1990.
11. McGrail JS: Ear, nose, and throat injuries. In Welsh PR, Shephard RJ, eds: *Current therapy in sports medicine 1985-1986*, Philadelphia, 1985, BC Decker.
12. McWhorter JM: Concussions and intracranial injuries in athletics, *Ath Tr* 25:129, 1990.
13. Morrow RM: Reports of a survey of oral injuries in male college and university athletes, *Ath Tr* 25:338, 1991.
14. Pashby RC, Pashby TJ: Ocular injuries. In Welsh PR, Shephard RJ, eds: *Current therapy in sports medicine 1985-1986*, Philadelphia, 1985, BC Decker.
15. Podolsky ML: Common ear problems due to trauma and temperature, *Sports Med Dig* 8:1, 1986.
16. Roob JD et al: Delayed presentation of subdural hematoma, *Phys Sportsmed* 21:61, 1993.
17. Shell D et al: Can subdural hematoma result from repeated minor head injury? *Phys Sportsmed* 21:75, 1993.
18. Sitler M: Nasal septal injuries, *Ath Train* 21:10, 1986.
19. Vegso JJ, Lehman RC: Field evaluation and management of head and neck injuries, *Clin Sports Med* 6:474, 1987.
20. Zagelbaum BM: Sports-related eye trauma, *Phy Sportsmed*, 21:25, 1993.

ANNOTATED BIBLIOGRAPHY

Lehman LB, Ravich SJ: Close head injuries in athletes *Clin Sports Med* 9:485, 1990
  A concise description of cerebral injuries common in sports.
Torg JS, ed: *Head and neck injuries, Clin Sports Med* 6:720, 1987.
  In-depth coverage of head and neck injuries stemming from sports activities. The mechanisms of these injuries are discussed, as well as their prevention, initial treatment, and rehabilitation.

The Shoulder Complex and Upper Arm

When you finish this chapter, you will be able to:

- Identify major shoulder injuries
- Provide immediate care for major shoulder injuries
- Provide follow-up care for major shoulder injuries

The shoulder complex, as the name implies, is an extremely complicated region of the human body. Sports using the shoulder in repetitive activities such as throwing, blocking, tackling, and rolling over as in tumbling may produce a serious injury (Figure 18-1).

The shoulder complex and shoulder joint comprise the clavicle, scapula, and humerus bones (Figure 18-2). The major joints of this region are the sternoclavicular joint, acromioclavicular joint, coracoclavicular joint, and glenohumeral joint, more commonly called the shoulder joint (Figure 18-3). A highly complex system of muscles, bursae, joint capsules, and ligaments is also a part of the shoulder complex (Figures 18-2 through 18-6). Movements of the shoulder include abduction, adduction, internal and external rotation, circumduction, flexion, and extension (Figure 18-7).

EVALUATION OF THE SHOULDER COMPLEX

The shoulder complex is one of the most difficult regions of the body to evaluate. The athlete who complains of pain in the shoulder region may be injured in another area of the body. Pain may be referred from a neck nerve root irritation or from an intrathoracic problem emanating from the heart, lungs, gallbladder, or other internal organ.

Pain in the shoulder region may be referred from injury to an internal organ.

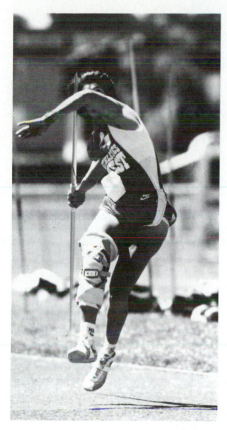

Figure 18-1

Repeated throwing often
results in shoulder injury.

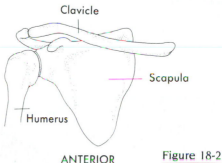

ANTERIOR

Figure 18-2

Bones of the shoulder
complex.

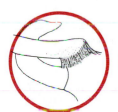

Sternoclavicular

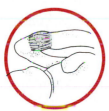

Acromioclavicular

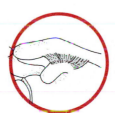

Coracoclavicular

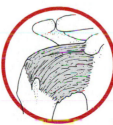

Glenohumeral

Figure 18-3

Shoulder complex
articulations.

History

It is essential that the coach or health professional understand the
athlete's major complaints and possible mechanism of the injury. It is also
necessary to know whether the condition was produced by a sudden
trauma or was of slow onset. The following questions in regard to the
athlete's complaints can help the evaluator determine the nature of the
injury and make the proper decisions:

1. If the onset was gradual, what appeared to be the cause?
2. What are the duration and intensity of the pain? Where is the
   pain located?

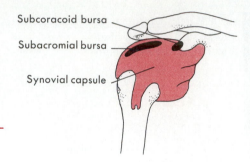

Figure 18-4

Synovial capsule and bursae of the shoulder.

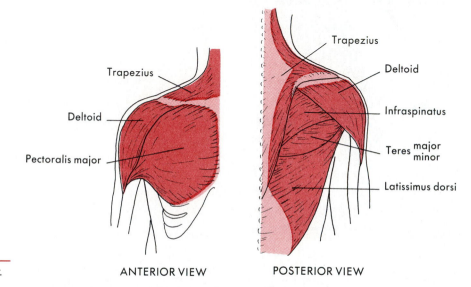

Figure 18-5

Musculature of the shoulder.

ANTERIOR VIEW   POSTERIOR VIEW

3. Is there a noise during movement, numbness, or distortion in temperature such as a cold or warm feeling?
4. Is there a feeling of weakness or fatigue?
5. What movement or body positions seem to aggravate or relieve the pain?
6. If therapy has been given before, what, if anything, offered pain relief (e.g., cold, heat, massage, or analgesic medication)?

General Observations

The athlete should be generally observed while walking and standing. Observation during walking can reveal asymmetry of arm swing or leaning toward the painful shoulder.

The athlete is next observed from the front, side, and back while standing. The evaluator looks for any postural asymmetries, bony or joint deformities, or muscle contractions and laxities. If there are no indications of fracture or dislocation, the athlete is asked to move the shoulder in all directions. The shoulder's range of motion is noted and compared to the noninjured shoulder. Painful or pain-free movement is also noted.

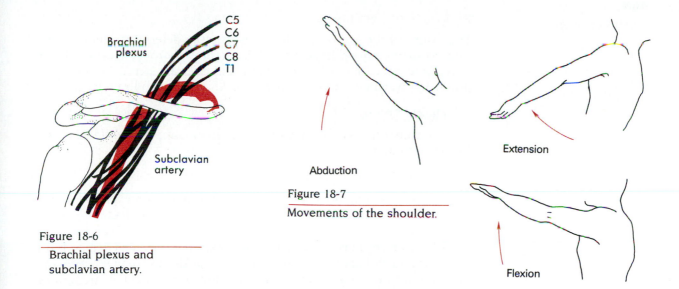

Figure 18-6

Brachial plexus and subclavian artery.

Figure 18-7

Movements of the shoulder.

PALPATION
Bony Palpation

The evaluator stands behind the athlete and palpates the shoulder anteriorly, laterally, and posteriorly. Both shoulders are palpated at the same time for pain sites and deformities.

Soft-Tissue Palpation

Palpation of the soft tissue of the shoulder detects pain sites, abnormal swelling or lumps, overly contracted muscle tissue, and trigger points. Trigger points are commonly found in shoulder muscles.

TEMPERATURE AND ARTERIAL PULSES
Temperature

Skin temperature is subjectively assessed by comparing the back of the athlete's hands. A cold temperature can be an indication of blood vessel constriction, whereas an overly warm temperature may indicate an inflammatory condition.[21]

Arterial Pulses

It is essential that athletes with shoulder complaints be evaluated for impaired circulation. In cases of shoulder complaints, pulse rates are routinely obtained over the axillary, brachial, and radial arteries (Figure 18-8). The axillary artery is found in the axilla against the shaft of the humerus. The brachial artery is a continuation of the axillary artery and follows the medial border of the biceps brachii muscle toward the elbow. The radial pulse is found at the anterior lateral aspect of the wrist over the radius. Taking the radial pulse provides an indication of the total circulation of the shoulder and arm.

trigger points
Small hyperirritable areas within a muscle

Injury to the shoulder complex can adversely affect skin sensation and the temperature of the arm and the leg.

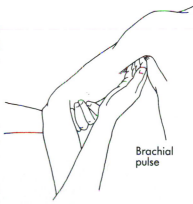

Figure 18-8

Arterial pulses related to the shoulder.

Immediate mobilization and physician referral is the proper care for a suspected fracture.

Seriousness of Injury

The extent of the loss of function is usually the determinant of the seriousness of the injury. Indication of dislocation and/or fractures calls for immediate immobilization and physician referral. Nerve involvement producing numbness and/or muscle weakness also require referral.

Muscle Strength

All major muscles associated with the shoulder complex should be tested for strength and pain.

PREVENTING SHOULDER INJURIES

Proper physical conditioning is of major importance in preventing shoulder injuries. As with all preventive conditioning, a program should be directed to general body development and development of specific body areas for a given sport.[17] If a sport places extreme sustained demands on the arms and shoulders, or if the shoulder is at risk for sudden traumatic injury, extensive conditioning must be employed. Maximal strength of muscles must be gained, along with a full range of motion in all directions.[17]

Proper warm-up must be performed gradually before explosive arm movements are attempted. This includes a general increase in body temperature followed by sport-specific stretching of selected muscles.

One of the most important things an athlete can learn is how to fall properly.

All athletes in collision and contact sports should be instructed and drilled on how to fall properly. They must be taught to avoid trying to catch themselves with an outstretched arm. Performing a shoulder roll is a safer way to absorb the shock of the fall. Specialized protective equipment, such as shoulder pads, must be properly fitted to avoid some shoulder injuries in tackle football.

To avoid shoulder injuries from overuse, it is essential that athletes be correctly taught in the appropriate techniques of throwing, spiking, overhead smashing, overhand serving, proper crawl and butterfly swimming strokes, and tackling and blocking.

SHOULDER COMPLEX INJURIES
Contusions and Strains

Injuries to the soft tissue in the area of the shoulder complex are common in sports.

Contusions

Blows about the shoulder that produce injury are most prevalent in collision and contact sports. The muscles with the highest incidence are those in the upper arm and shoulder. Characteristically, bruises of this region result in pain and restricted arm movement. The subcutaneous areas of the shoulder complex are subject to bruising in contact sports.

The shoulder pointer The most vulnerable part of the clavicle is the enlarged lateral end (acromial end), which forms a projection just before it joins the acromion process. Contusions of this type are often called *shoulder pointers,* and they may cause the athlete severe discomfort. Contusion to the lateral end of the clavicle causes a bone bruise and subsequent irritation to the bony surface. On initial inspection this injury may be mistaken for a first degree acromioclavicular separation. Management requires proper immediate first aid and follow-up therapy. In most cases these conditions are self-limiting; when the athlete can freely move the shoulder, he or she may return to sports activities.

Throwing Motion and Injuries

Overuse syndromes of the shoulder complex occur mainly in athletes who use repetitive throwing-type motions in activities such as baseball pitching, tennis serving, and overhead smashing (Figure 18-9), and swimming the crawl or butterfly. Quarterbacking and volleyball spiking also can cause microtraumas, which can lead to an overuse syndrome. In general, these sports actions have three phases in common: cocking, acceleration, and follow-through and deceleration.

Three phases of sports actions:
    Cocking
    Acceleration
    Follow-through and Deceleration

Cocking Phase

The cocking phase of throwing, where the arm is brought back while abducted and externally rotated, can produce major muscle strains. This aspect of throwing can strain the greater pectoralis muscle and the anterior deltoid muscle, the long head of the biceps, and/or the internal shoulder rotators.

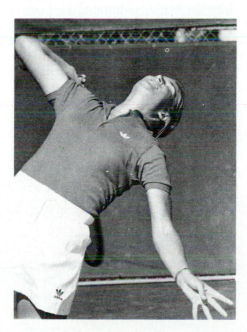

Figure 18-9

The tennis serve is a major cause of overuse syndromes of the shoulder.

Acceleration Phase

The acceleration phase, where the arm is brought forward, can cause a shoulder impingement syndrome or a bursitis resulting in the following conditions:

1. Tendinitis of the greater pectoral major muscle insertion
2. Tendinitis of the coracobrachial muscle and short head of the biceps where it joints the coracoid process
3. Synovitis of the sternoclavicular or acromioclavicular joint
4. "Little League shoulder," or osteochondrosis of the upper growth region of the humerus
5. Spontaneous throwing fractures of the proximal humerus stemming from a stress fracture

Follow-through and Deceleration Phase

In the follow-through of the throw strain can occur to the middle and inferior posterior capsule and to key ligaments supporting the glenohumeral joint.

Rotator Cuff Strains

The rotator cuff consists of the supraspinatus, infraspinatus, teres minor, and subscapular muscles.

The principal rotator cuff tendon injured is that of the supraspinatus muscle (Figure 18-10). The mechanism of shoulder strains occurs mainly as the result of a violent pull to the arm, an abnormal rotation, or a fall on the outstretched arm, tearing or even rupturing tendinous tissue. The throwing mechanism can produce a variety of abnormal stresses to the soft tissues of the shoulder—for example, impingement, overstretching, torsion, subluxation, and entrapment of nerves and blood vessels. Besides throwing, swimming in freestyle and butterfly events also place great stress on the shoulders' rotating mechanisms and can lead to an acute or chronic injury. A tear or complete rupture of one of the rotator

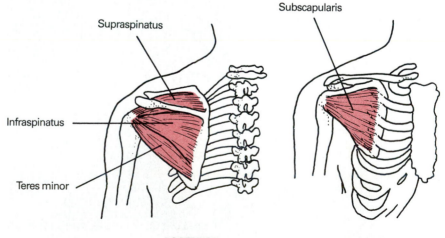

Figure 18-10

Rotator cuff muscles.

POSTERIOR   ANTERIOR

cuff tendons produces an extremely disabling condition in which pain, loss of function, swelling, and point tenderness are symptoms.

Care Care of the rotator cuff injury ranges from surgical intervention for complete ruptures to conservative care.

Rotator cuff impingement injury The continual use of the arm or arms above the horizontal plane in an athletic endeavor has been known to lead to an impingement syndrome (Figure 18-11). The major reason for impingement is the reduction of space through which the supraspinatus muscle can pass.[13]

The athlete with a rotator cuff injury may complain of the shoulder joint aching during or after activity.[8] There also may be some restriction of shoulder motion.

Care If the rotator cuff impingement injury is diagnosed in its early stages, conservative care is usually enough. This may include rest, coaching for proper arm usage, and superficial therapy such as cold or heat. Exercise rehabilitation should be concerned with full range of joint motion and strengthening of weak shoulder-complex musculature. If this condition is allowed to progress beyond its early stages, however, surgery may be necessary.

Proper coaching to prevent shoulder injuries must be undertaken for sports that involve throwing or throwinglike motions. Gradual warm-up should emphasize slow stretching and maximizing the extensibility of all major shoulder muscles. Strengthening of shoulder muscles should be general at first and then emphasize the external and internal rotator muscles for good shoulder joint control.

Athletes displaying early symptoms of shoulder impingement must modify their arm movements. A swimmer may have to decrease his or her distance or change to a different stroke. Athletes who throw or who perform throwinglike motions may have to decrease their force or develop a different technique.[5]

Athletes experiencing shoulder pain and inflammation may benefit from cold application after workouts. This can be in the form of ice massage using of an ice chip pack.

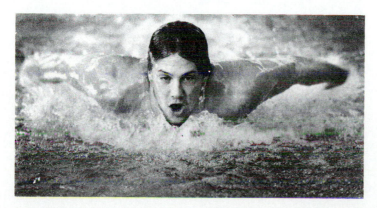

Figure 18-11

The butterfly stroke is a major cause of the rotator cuff syndrome impingement syndrome.

Rest from 1 to 2 days, along with ice applied 10 to 20 minutes several times per day, is a major factor in managing a rotator cuff injury. Under the direction of a physician, the athletic trainer may use both ultrasound to relieve inflammation and transcutaneous electrical nerve stimulation (TENS) to relieve pain from the shoulder impingement. Besides this, the physician may prescribe an oral antiinflammatory drug for a short period.

Sprains

Sternoclavicular Sprain

Sprains can occur in the three major joints of the shoulder complex:
Sternoclavicular joint
Acromioclavicular joint
Glenohumeral joint

Sternoclavicular sprain (Figure 18-12) is a relatively uncommon occurrence in sports, but occasionally one may result from one of the various traumas affecting the shoulder complex.

The mechanism of the injury can be an indirect force transmitted through the upper arm to the shoulder joint by a direct force, such as from a blow that strikes the poorly padded clavicle or by twisting or torsion of a backward elevated arm. Depending on the direction of force, the medial end of the clavicle can be displaced upward and forward, either posteriorly or anteriorly. Generally, the clavicle is displaced upward and forward.

Trauma resulting in a sprain to the sternoclavicular joint can be described in three degrees. The *first-degree sprain* is characterized by little pain and disability with some point tenderness but with no joint deformity. A *second-degree* sprain displays subluxation of the sternoclavicular joint with visible deformity, pain, swelling, point tenderness, and an inability to abduct the shoulder in full range or to bring the arm across the chest, indicating disruption of stabilizing ligaments. The *third-degree sprain*,

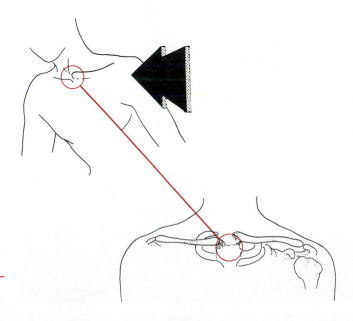

Figure 18-12

Sternoclavicular sprain and dislocation.

which is the most severe, presents a picture of complete dislocation with gross displacement of the clavicle at its sternal junction, swelling, and disability, indicating complete rupture of the supporting ligaments. If the clavicle is displaced backward, pressure may be placed on the blood vessels, esophagus, or trachea and threaten life.

Care Care of this condition is based on returning the displaced clavicle to its original position, which is done by a physician, and immobilizing it at that point so that healing may take place. Immobilization is usually maintained for 3 to 5 weeks, followed by graded reconditioning exercises. There is a high incidence of recurrence of sternoclavicular sprains.

Acromioclavicular Sprain

The acromioclavicular joint is extremely vulnerable to sprains among active sports participants, especially in collision sports. A program of prevention should entail proper fitting of protective equipment, conditioning to provide a balance of strength and flexibility to the entire shoulder complex, and teaching proper techniques of falling and the use of the arm in sports.

An acromioclavicular sprain can occur in three ways: a fall on the tip of the shoulder that drives the acromion process down, a blow from behind the shoulder driving the acromion process forward, or a fall on the outstretched hand or elbow pushing the acromion process upward (Figure 18-13).

The *first-degree* acromioclavicular sprain reflects point tenderness and discomfort on movement at the junction between the acromion process and the other end of the clavicle. There is no deformity, only a mild stretching of the supportive ligaments.

A *second-degree* sprain produces a rupture of the ligaments holding the clavicle to the acromion process. There is a definite displacement and prominence of the lateral end of the clavicle when compared with the unaffected side. In this moderate sprain there is point tenderness on palpation of the injury site, and the athlete is unable to fully abduct through a full range of motion or to bring the arm completely across the chest. NOTE: The second-degree sprain may or may not require surgery to restore stability.

Although occurring infrequently, the *third-degree* injury is considered a dislocation, involving a rupture of the supporting ligaments and major bony displacement. The mechanics of the third-degree subluxation or dislocation is a downward and outward force on the acromion process away from the clavicle. In such an injury there is gross deformity and prominence of the outer clavicular head, severe pain, loss of movement, and instability of the shoulder complex.

Care Immediate care of the acromioclavicular sprain involves three basic procedures: (1) cold and pressure to control local hemorrhage, (2) stabilization of the joint by a sling and swathe bandage, and (3) referral to a physician for definitive diagnosis and treatment. Complete severance

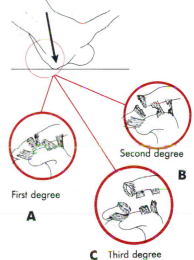

First degree

A

Second degree

B

C Third degree

Figure 18-13

Mechanism of an acromioclavicular sprain. **A,** Tear of the acromioclavicular ligament. **B,** Tear of the acromioclavicular ligament and partial tear of coracoclavicular ligaments. **C,** Complete tear of acromioclavicular and coracoclavicular ligaments.

of the major supportive ligament may demand corrective surgery. Most second-degree sprains require 4 to 6 weeks for fibrous healing to take place, and an extended period is needed for the restoration of general shoulder strength and mobility. A regimen of superficial moist heat will aid in resolving soreness. Movement in the pain-free range will be restored after the use of ice packs.

Rehabilitative exercise is concerned with reconditioning the shoulder complex to its state before the injury. Full strength, flexibility, endurance, and function must be redeveloped.

Glenohumeral Joint Sprain

Sprains of the shoulder joint involve injury to ligaments and the joint capsule. The pathological process of the sprain is comparable with that of an internal strain and along with ligament and capsule injury often affects the rotator cuff muscles.

The cause of this injury is the same as that which produces dislocation. Anterior capsular sprains occur when the arm is forced upward and sideward, such as when making an arm tackle in football. Sprain also can arise from external rotation of the arm.

The athlete complains of pain on arm movement, especially when the sprain mechanism is reproduced. There also may be decreased range of motion and pain when the shoulder joint is palpated.

Care Care after acute trauma to the shoulder joint requires the use of a cold pack for 24 to 48 hours, elastic or adhesive compression, rest, and immobilization by means of a sling. After hemorrhage has subsided, a program of gentle mobilization following cold application is performed. Ultrasound and massage may also be applied by the trainer. Once the shoulder can execute a full range of movement without signs of pain, a resistance exercise program should be initiated. Any traumatic injury to the shoulder joint can lead to a chronic inflammation, which is encouraged when there is absence of shoulder movement.

Subluxations and Dislocations

Dislocation of the humeral head is second only to finger dislocation in order of incidence in sports. When the shoulder joint is placed in an extreme range of motion, it is highly susceptible to dislocation. The most common kind of displacement is that occurring anteriorly (Figure 18-14). Of those dislocations caused by direct trauma, 85% to 90% recur.[7]

Anterior Glenohumeral Dislocation

The anterior glenohumeral dislocation occurs when an arm is in a sideward or forced abducted position and is externally rotated. An arm tackle or an abnormal force to an arm that is executing a throw can cause a dislocation. Less often a fall or inward rotation and abduction of an arm may result in a dislocation.

The athlete with an anterior dislocation outwardly displays a flattened deltoid contour. Feeling the armpit of the affected arm will reveal

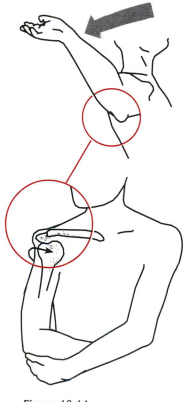

Figure 18-14

Anterior shoulder subluxation and dislocation.

an obvious prominence of the humeral head.[4] The athlete carries the affected arm in slight abduction and external rotation and is unable to touch the opposite shoulder with the hand of the affected arm. There is often severe pain and disability.

In an anterior glenohumeral dislocation, the head of the humerus is forced forward out of the joint capsule and then upward to rest under the coracoid process. There also may be torn muscles and profuse bleeding. A tear or detachment of the fibrocartilage labrum may also occur. Additional complications may arise if the head of the humerus comes into contact with and injures the major complex, the brachial nerves and blood vessels (see Figure 18-6 p. 467).

Care Care of the shoulder dislocation requires immediate reduction by a physician, control of the hemorrhage by cold packs, immobilization, and the start of muscle reconditioning as soon as possible. The question often arises as to whether a first-time dislocation should be reduced or should receive medical attention. *Physicians generally agree that a dislocation may be associated with a fracture and nerve injury, and therefore it is beyond the scope of a coach's or athletic trainer's responsibilities.* Recurrent dislocations do not present the same complications or attendant dangers as the acute type; however, risk is always involved.

After the dislocation has been reduced, immobilization and muscle rehabilitation are carried out. Immobilization takes place for about 3 weeks after reduction, with the arm maintained in a relaxed position of adduction and internal rotation. While immobilized, the athlete is instructed to perform isometric exercises for strengthening the internal and external rotator muscles (see page 466). After immobilization, the strengthening program progresses from isometrics to resisting rubber tubing and then to dumbbells and other resistance devices. A major criterion for the athlete's return to sports competition is that there must be internal and external rotation strength equal to 20% of the athlete's body weight. Once a shoulder has been dislocated, it must be protected against further injury (Figure 18-15).

> An athlete must have internal and external rotation strength equal to 20% of body weight in order to return to competition after a dislocation.

The Unstable Shoulder: Recurrent Subluxation and Dislocation

Chronic recurrent instabilities of the shoulder Increasingly shoulder instabilities are being recognized among athletes. The causes of shoulder instabilities consist of macrotraumatic, atraumatic, microtraumatic (repetitive use), congenital, and neuromuscular. These conditions could be acute, recurrent, or chronic and occur as full dislocations, subluxations, or small-joint displacements.

Macrotraumatic As discussed earlier these instabilities occur from one or more traumatic situations that cause a complete or partial joint displacement.

Atraumatic This refers to an athlete who, because of a history of injury or inherent ligamentous laxity, voluntarily displaces the shoulder joint.

Microtraumatic This term refers to instabilities created by repetitive

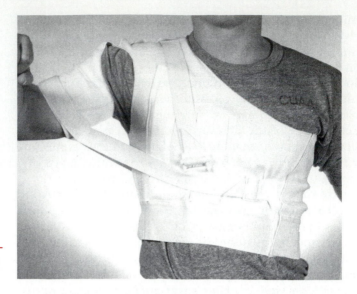

Figure 18-15

Shoulder dislocation must be protected against recurrence.

use of the shoulder, leading to soft-tissue laxity. The chances of this situation occurring are increased when faulty biomechanics is carried out. Sports activities such as baseball pitching, tennis serving, and crawl swimming may produce anterior shoulder instabilities; swimming the back stroke or backhand stroking in tennis can produce problems in posterior instability. As the supporting tissue becomes increasingly loose, more mobility of the glenohumeral head is allowed, eventually damaging the glenoid cartilage. With increased laxity of the supportive capsule and tendinous structures, instability becomes evident, eventually leading to the possibility of recurrent subluxations and/or dislocations.

The throwing athlete may complain of pain or clicking or experience a dead arm syndrome in the cocking phase of the throw. Pain is often posterior and may last for several minutes, followed by extreme weakness of the entire arm. Anterior instability may allow for repetitive traction and compressions of the rotator cuff, consequently causing an added impingement syndrome.

Care Management of the recurrent anterior dislocation falls under the heading of conservative and surgical treatment. Complete rest by immobilization lasts for a period of 5 weeks. Conservative management of the traumatic recurrent anterior instability consists of the return of range of motion and strength.

A return of external rotation is essential before the athlete can be permitted to compete. Exercise must include normal movement patterns performed manually and with specialized equipment. Surgical treatment is considered when the athlete's shoulder is resistant to conservative treatment.

Recurrent shoulder subluxation and dislocation reduction With the permission of the team physician, the coach or athletic trainer can assist the athlete in reducing a recurrent shoulder subluxation or dislocation. The safest method is the *weight on the wrist technique*. In this method the athlete lies between two tables, with the head resting on one table and the body on the other. The affected arm extends between the two tables with a 5- to 10-pound weight tied to the wrist. As the muscles of the shoulder relax, a spontaneous reduction occurs.

Shoulder protection Every protection should be given to the athlete who may be prone to recurrent dislocations. Restraint by means of a harness appliance should be used during any sports activity. Repeated dislocations continue to stretch the supporting structures and damage the articulating hyaline cartilage, eventually producing arthritis.

Shoulder Synovitis and Bursitis

The shoulder joint is subject to subacute chronic inflammatory conditions resulting from trauma or from overuse in an abnormal fashion. An injury of this type may develop from a direct blow, a fall on the outstretched hand, or the stress incurred in throwing an object (Figure 18-16). Inflammation can occur in the shoulder, extensively affecting the soft tissues surrounding it or specifically affecting various bursae. The bursa that is most often injured is the subacromial bursa, which lies underneath the deltoid muscle and the articular capsule and extends under the acromion process.[3] The apparent pathological process in these conditions is fibrous buildup and fluid accumulation developing from a constant inflammatory state.

Recognition of these conditions follows the same course as in other shoulder afflictions. The athlete is unable to move the shoulder, especially in abduction; rotation and muscle atrophy also may ensue because of disuse.

Care Care of low-grade inflammatory conditions must be initiated somewhat empirically. In some instances both the superficial heat from moist pads or infrared rays and the deep heat of diathermy or ultrasound are beneficial. In other instances heat may be aggravating, so cold packs may be more useful. Whatever the mode of treatment, the athlete must maintain a consistent program of exercise, with the emphasis placed on regaining a full range of motion, so that muscle contractures and adhesions do not immobilize the joint.

The *"frozen shoulder"* is a condition more characteristic of an older person, but occasionally it does occur in the athlete. It results from a chronically irritated shoulder joint that has had improper care. Constant, generalized inflammation causes degeneration of the soft tissues in the vicinity of the shoulder joint, resulting in an extreme limitation of movement. The main care of the frozen shoulder is a combination of deep heat therapy and mobilization exercise.

Thoracic Outlet Compression Syndrome

A number of nerve and blood vessel problems that involve compression of the brachial plexus and subclavian artery can occur in the neck and

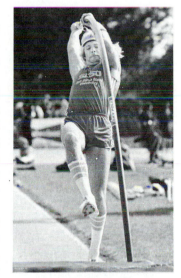

Figure 18-16

Sports such as pole vaulting place extreme stress on the arm and shoulder complex; such overuse can lead to bursitis or inflammation of the synovium.

shoulder. These are usually associated with throwing activities. Possible causes are the following:

1. Compression over a cervical rib
2. Spasm of the anterior scalene muscle
3. Compression of major nerves and blood vessels between the first rib and clavicle
4. Compression of the smaller pectoral muscle over major blood vessels and nerves as they pass beneath the coracoid process or between the clavicle and first rib

Abnormal pressure on the subclavian artery, subclavian vein, and brachial plexus produces a variety of symptoms:

1. Numbness and pain
2. Sensation of cold
3. Impaired circulation that could lead to gangrene of the fingers
4. Muscle weakness
5. Muscle atrophy
6. Radial nerve palsy

Care A conservative approach should be taken with early and mild cases of thoracic outlet syndromes. Conservative treatment is favorable in 50% to 80% of cases.

The following measures might be taken:

1. Sling support and tension reduction
2. Antiinflammatory medication
3. Exercises to strengthen the trapezius, serratus anterior, and erector muscles of the spine
4. Postural correction, especially in cases of drooped shoulders.

Peripheral Nerve Injuries

Sports injuries around the shoulder can produce and cause serious nerve injuries. The nerves that can be affected are the suprascapular, axillary, long thoracic, musculocutaneous, and spinal accessory nerves. Injuries to shoulder nerves commonly stem from blunt trauma or a stretch type of injury. Nerve injury must be considered when there is constant pain, muscle weakness, paralysis, and/or muscle atrophy.

Clavicular Fractures

Fractures in the shoulder complex can be caused by a direct blow on the bone or indirectly by a fall on either an outstretched arm or the point of the shoulder. The clavicular fracture (Figure 18-17) is one of the most frequent fractures in sports. More than 80% occur in the middle third of the clavicle, which lacks ligamentous support.

Clavicular fracture is caused by either a direct blow or a transmitted force resulting from a fall on the outstretched arm. In junior and senior high school athletes these fractures are usually the greenstick type.

The athlete with a fractured clavicle usually supports the arm on the injured side and tilts his or her head toward that side, with the chin

Nerve injury should be suspected when there is constant pain, muscle weakness, paralysis, and/or muscle atrophy.

More than 80% of all fractures to the clavicle occur in the middle third.

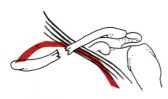

Figure 18-17

Clavicular fracture and associated brachial blood vessels and nerves.

turned to the opposite side. On inspection the injured clavicle appears a little lower than the one on the unaffected side. Palpation may also reveal swelling and mild deformity.

Care The clavicular fracture is cared for immediately by applying a sling and swathe bandage and by treating the athlete for shock, if necessary. The athlete is then referred to a physician, who in most instances will perform an x-ray examination of the area and then apply a shoulder figure-8 wrapping that will stabilize the shoulder in an upward and backward position.

INJURIES TO THE UPPER ARM

The upper arm can sustain varied stresses and traumas, depending on the nature of the sport. Crushing blows may be directed to the area by collision and contact sports; severe strain can be imposed by the throwing sports and sports that afford muscle resistance, such as gymnastics.

Contusions

Contusions of the upper arm are frequent in contact sports. Although any muscle of the upper arm is subject to bruising, the area most often affected is the lateral aspect, primarily the brachial muscle and portions of the triceps and biceps muscles.

Bruises to the upper arm area can be particularly handicapping, especially if the radial nerve is contused through forceful contact with the humerus, producing transitory paralysis and consequently inability to use the extensor muscles of the forearm.

Care Cold and pressure should be applied for 1 to 24 hours after injury, followed by cryotherapy or superficial heat therapy and massage. In most cases this condition responds rapidly to treatment, usually within a few days. If swelling and irritation last more than 2 or 3 weeks, *myositis ossificans* may have been stimulated, and massage must be stopped and protection afforded the athlete during sports participation.

Strains

Acute and chronic strains in the arm are common. The muscles most commonly affected are the biceps, triceps, and pectoral muscles. Two conditions that are unique to the arm are bicipital tenosynovitis and biceps brachii rupture.

Bicipital Tenosynovitis

Tenosynovitis of the long head of the biceps muscle is common among athletes who execute a throwing movement as part of their event. It is more prevalent among pitchers, tennis players, and javelin throwers, for whom the repeated forced internal rotations of the upper arm may produce chronic inflammation in the vicinity of the synovial sheath of the long head of the biceps muscle. A complete rupture of the transverse ligament, which holds the biceps in its groove, may take place, or a constant

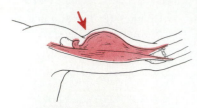

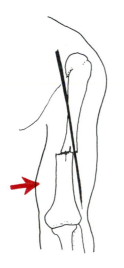

Figure 18-18

Performing the iron cross on the rings can rupture the biceps brachii.

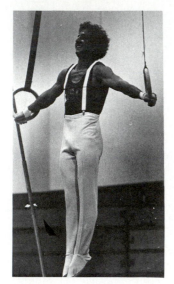

Figure 18-19

Fracture of the humeral shaft.

inflammation may result in degenerative scarring or a subluxated tendon.

The athlete may complain of an ache in the front or the side of the shoulder; deep palpation reveals point tenderness in the region of the bicipital tendon.

Care Such conditions are best cared for by complete rest for 1 to 2 weeks, with daily applications of cryotherapy or ultrasound. After the initial aching is gone, a gradual program of reconditioning can begin.

Biceps Brachii Ruptures

Ruptures of the biceps brachii occur mainly in gymnasts who are engaged in power moves (Figure 18-18). The rupture commonly takes place near the origin of the muscle. The athlete usually hears a resounding snap and feels a sudden, intense pain at the point of injury. A protruding bulge may appear near the middle of the biceps. When asked to flex the elbow joint of the injured arm, the gymnast displays a definite weakness. Care should include immediately applying a cold pack to control hemorrhage, placing the arm in a sling, and referring the athlete to the physician. Surgical repair is usually indicated.

Fractures

Fractures of the humeral shaft (Figure 18-19) happen occasionally in sports, usually as the result of a direct blow or a fall on the arm.

The pathological process is characteristic of most uncomplicated fractures, except that there may be a tendency for the radial nerve, which encircles the humeral shaft, to be severed by jagged bone edges, resulting in radial nerve paralysis and causing wrist drop and inability to perform forearm supination.

Recognition of this injury requires immediate application of a splint, treatment for shock, and referral to a physician. The athlete will be out of competition for approximately 3 to 4 months.

Fracture of the Upper Humerus

Fractures of the upper humerus (Figure 18-20) pose considerable danger to nerves and vessels of that area. They result from a direct blow, a dislocation, or the impact received when falling on the outstretched arm. Various parts of the end of the humerus may be involved. Such a fracture may be mistaken for a shoulder dislocation.

It may be difficult to recognize a fracture of the upper humerus by visual inspection alone; therefore, x-ray examination gives the only positive proof. Some of the more prevalent signs are pain, inability to move the arm, swelling, point tenderness, and discoloration of the superficial tissue. Because of the proximity of the axillary blood vessels and the brachial plexus, a fracture to the upper end of the humerus may result in severe hemorrhaging or paralysis.

Care A suspected fracture of this type warrants immediate support with a sling and swathe bandage and referral to a physician. Incapacitation may range from 2 to 6 months.

Epiphyseal Fracture

Epiphyseal fracture of the head of the humerus (Figure 18-21) is much more common in the young athlete than is a bone fracture. Epiphyseal injury in the shoulder occurs most frequently in individuals 10 years of age and younger. It is caused by a direct blow or by an indirect force traveling the long axis of the humerus. This condition causes shortening of the arm, disability, swelling, point tenderness, and pain. There also may be a false joint. This type of injury should be suspected when such signs appear in young athletes. Initial treatment should include splinting and immediate referral to a physician. Healing is initiated rapidly; immobilization is necessary for only about 3 weeks. The main danger of such an injury is the possibility of damage to the epiphyseal growth centers of the humerus.

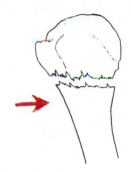

Figure 18-20

Fracture of the upper humerus.

RECONDITIONING OF THE SHOULDER COMPLEX

The shoulder complex and especially the glenohumeral joint have a tendency to become highly restricted in motion after injury or immobilization. In some cases a serious injury and immobilization lead to contractures and a tendency to develop fibrosis of the articular capsule. To prevent these problems, pain-free mobility is started as soon as possible by the athletic trainer.

Shoulder rehabilitation is highly complicated and depends on the nature of the injury and whether surgery has been performed. In general, rehabilitation progresses through early, intermediate, and advanced exercise stages.[4] Types of exercise can be isometrics, isotonics, isokinetics, stretching, and manual resistance. The following exercises may be employed, depending upon the nature of injury.

Immobilization following injury The length of the immobilization period will vary depending on the structures injured, the severity of the injury, and whether the injury is treated conservatively or surgically by the physician. Depending on the type of injury, the athlete may be required to wear a sling for all or part of the recovery. Progression in range of motion and strengthening techniques should be dictated by an understanding of the physiological process of healing and is generally determined by a lack of pain and swelling associated with increased activity.

General body conditioning It is essential for the athlete to maintain a high level of cardiorespiratory endurance throughout the rehabilitation process. In the case of the shoulder joint, activities such as running, speed walking, or riding an exercise bike could be used to maintain cardiorespiratory endurance. Because many athletic activities involve some running, recommending such training would be more useful than recommending swimming for the rehabilitation of an ankle sprain. In sports that require upper-extremity endurance, such as swimming and throwing, the athlete should be progressed to these activities as soon as they can be tolerated. The athlete must also continue to maintain strength, flexibility, and neuromuscular control throughout the rest of the body during the period of shoulder rehabilitation.

Reconditioning and rehabilitation Although not a therapist, the

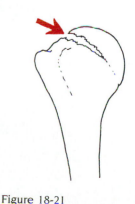

Figure 18-21

Epiphyseal fracture.

coach should have some appreciation and understanding of the complexities inherent in restoring the injured shoulder. Reconditioning and rehabilitation involve an intricate program of shoulder joint mobilization and manual exercise by the health professional and a progressional program of active exercise.

Flexibility   Regaining a full, nonrestricted, pain-free range of motion is certainly one of the most important aspects of shoulder rehabilitation. Gentle range-of-motion exercises should begin immediately using Codman's pendulum exercises (Figure 18-22) and a "sawing" motion (Figure 18-23). Exercises can be progressed to a series of active-assistive range-of-motion exercises using a T-bar, done in a pain-free arc for all the cardinal plane movements (Figure 18-24). Wall-climbing exercises (Figure 18-25) are particularly effective in regaining flexion and abduction.

Muscular strength   Strengthening exercises in the shoulder generally follow a progression from positional isometrics, full-range isotonics concentrating on both eccentric and concentric contractions, isokinetics, to plyometrics. Gentle isometrics should begin immediately after injury or following surgery while the arm is still immobilized at the side.

Isotonic exercise may be incorporated using different types of resistance including dumbbells and barbells (Figure 18-26) surgical tubing or Theraband (Figure 18-27), or manual resistance techniques including PNF strengthening techniques (Figure 18-28). Resistance exercises

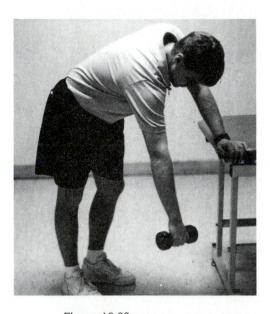

Figure 18-22

Codman's pendulum exercise may begin immediately following injury.

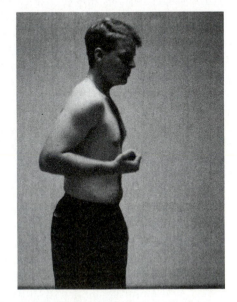

Figure 18-23

"Sawing" exercises are used as a gentle ROM activity for the glenohumeral joint.

should include all cardinal plane movements. Particular attention should be given to strengthening the scapular stabilizers by incorporating exercises to resist scapular abduction, adduction, elevation, depression, upward rotation, downward rotation, protraction, and retraction (Figure 18-29). Strengthening the muscles that control the stability of the scapula helps to provide a base for the function of the highly mobile glenohumeral joint.

Isokinetic exercises are used to exercise the muscles of the shoulder girdle at varying speeds (Figure 18-30). Plyometric exercises incorporated in the later stages of a rehabilitation program use a quick eccentric stretch of a muscle to facilitate a concentric contraction. Plyometric exercises for the upper extremity can be done using a weighted ball (Figure 18-31).

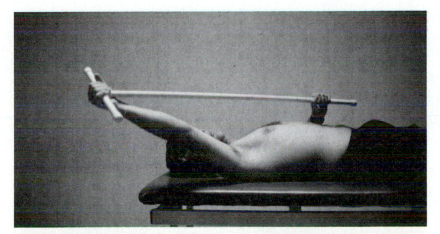

Figure 18-24

T-bar exercises are active-assistive ROM exercises that should be done for each of the cardinal plane movements.

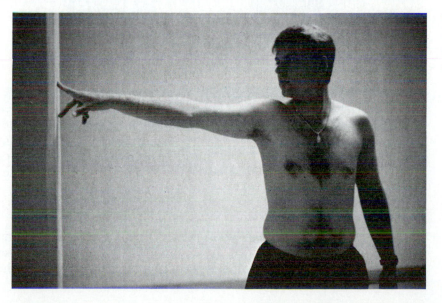

Figure 18-25

Wall-climbing exercises are useful in regaining abduction and flexion.

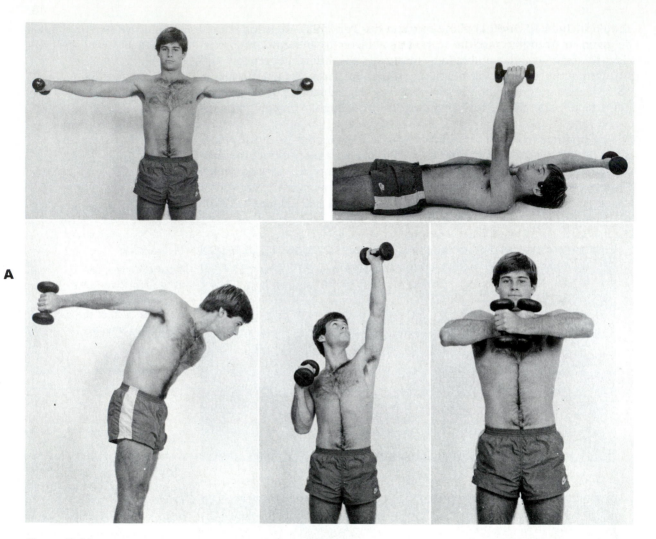

A

Figure 18-26

Isotonic exercises using **A,** Dumbbells. **B,** Barbells for strengthening in all cardinal planes.

Regaining neuromuscular control Following injury and some period of immobilization, the athlete must "relearn" how to use the injured extremity. Coordinated, highly skilled movement about the shoulder joint is essential for successful return to activity. The athlete must not only regain strength and ROM but must also develop a firing sequence for the specific muscles that are necessary to perform a highly skilled movement.

SUMMARY

The shoulder complex is a highly complicated anatomical region that can sustain numerous sports injuries. Preventing shoulder-complex injuries requires general body conditioning as well as specific conditioning for the

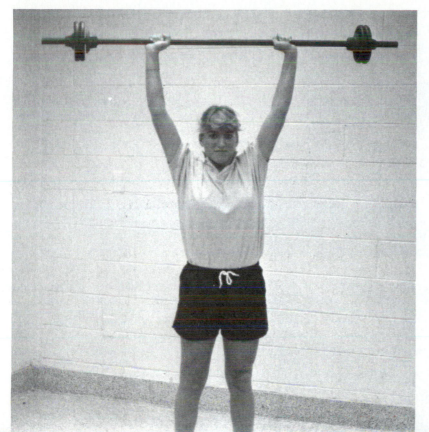

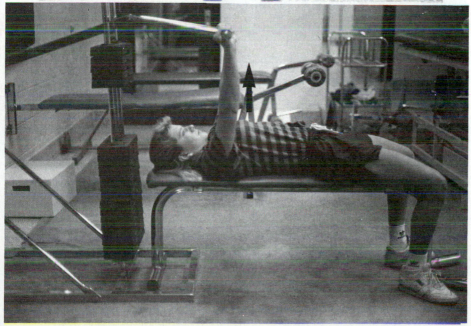

B

Figure 18-26 cont'd.

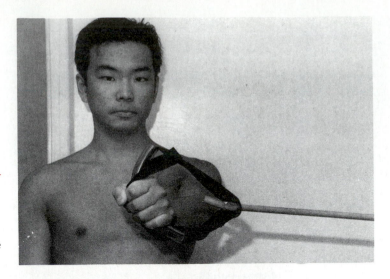

Figure 18-27

Exercises using surgical tubing are used to emphasize both eccentric and concentric strengthening contractions and can be done in all cardinal planes.

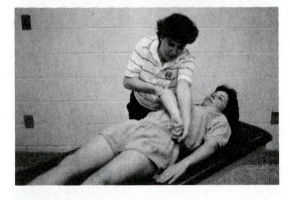

Figure 18-28

Manual resistance techniques such as a D2 upper-extremity PNF pattern are useful for strengthening.

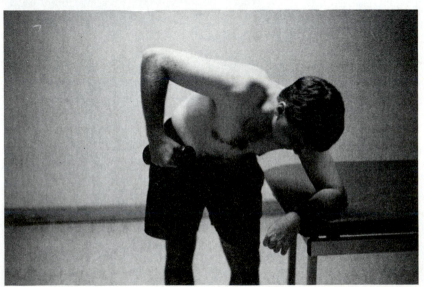

Figure 18-29

Strengthening exercises for the scapular stabilizers may provide the key for return of normal shoulder function.

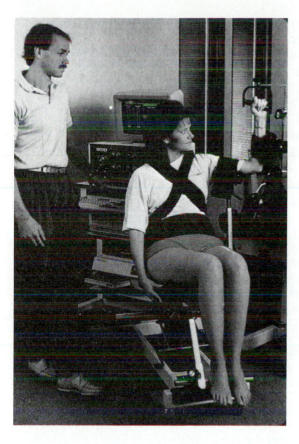

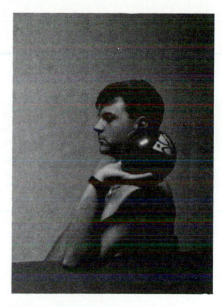

Figure 18-30

Isokinetic exercises may be incorporated in the later stages of a rehabilitation program.

Figure 18-31

Plyometric exercise for shoulder strengthening using a weighted ball.

demands of an individual sport. Proper warm-up and learning how to fall can also help to prevent shoulder complex injuries.

Overuse injuries to the shoulder commonly stem from faulty form in pitching, tennis serving, overhead smashing, and swimming the crawl or butterfly stroke.

Contusions commonly occur to the soft tissue surrounding the shoulder complex as well as to the clavicle region. Strains and impingements are common in sports that use the arms to overcome resistance or to propel objects. The rotator cuff muscles are common sites for strains and impingements. Sprains of the shoulder complex can occur at the sternoclavicular, acromioclavicular, and shoulder joints.

Shoulder joint dislocation is second only to finger dislocation in order of incidence in sports. The most common shoulder dislocation is the anterior glenohumeral dislocation. The athlete displays a flattened deltoid contour and carries the arm in slight abduction and external rotation.

The shoulder joint is also subject to chronic bursitis. Bursitis can stem from overuse or a sudden strain. The most often injured is the subacromial bursa that lies underneath the deltoid muscle and articular capsule and extends under the acromion process.

Fractures of the shoulder complex can be caused directly by a blow to the bone or indirectly by a fall on either an outstretched arm or the point of a shoulder. The most prevalent fracture occurs to the clavicle. The scapula is fractured less often.

Injuries to the upper arm include contusions, strains, and fractures. A relatively common chronic strain site is the long head of the biceps. This strain is called bicipital tenosynovitis. This tendon also can rupture. Fracture of the upper humeral shaft occurs only occasionally in sports, usually from a direct blow or a fall on the outstretched arm. A more common fracture site is the epiphysis of the humeral head in young athletes.

REVIEW QUESTIONS AND CLASS ACTIVITIES

1. What are the bony and soft-tissue structures associated with the shoulder complex?
2. What four major joints make up the shoulder complex?
3. How can shoulder injuries be prevented?
4. What are some common injuries of the shoulder? What mechanisms cause them?
5. Discuss the throwing motion and the injuries that can occur in each phase.
6. Contrast a sternoclavicular, an acromioclavicular, and a glenohumeral sprain.
7. What is the common cause of an anterior glenohumeral dislocation? How is it cared for? What types of exercises should be included in a rehabilitation program for this injury?
8. Discuss the unstable shoulder and the reduction of a recurrent shoulder subluxation and dislocation.
9. What causes clavicular fractures? How are they cared for?
10. What are some injuries of the upper arm? How are they managed?
11. What are some exercises in a rehabilitation program for the shoulder complex?
12. Invite an orthopedic surgeon to discuss injuries associated with the shoulder complex and the various surgical procedures used to repair the different joints.

REFERENCES

1. Back BR et al: Acromioclavicular injuries, *Phy Sports Med* 20:87, 1992.
2. Baker CL, Liu SH: Neurovascular injuries to the shoulder, JOSPT 18:360, 1993.
3. Botte MJ, Abrams RA: Recognition and treatment of shoulder bursitis, *Sports Med Dig* 14:81, 1992.
4. Cain TA et al: Anterior stability of the glenohumeral joint, *Am Sports Med* 15:144, 1987.
5. Ciullo JV: Swimmer's shoulder, *Clin Sports Med* 5:115, 1986.
6. Di Giovine NM, Pink M: Pitching injuries, *Sports Med Dig* 14:1, 1992.
7. Grana WA et al: How I manage acute anterior shoulder dislocations, *Phys Sportsmed* 15:88, 1987.
8. Gross ML et al: Overworked shoulders, *Phy Sportsmed* 22:81, 1994.
9. Hill JA: Overuse syndromes of the shoulders in athletes, *Sports Med Dig* 8:1, 1986.
10. Lutz Jr FR, Gieck JH: Thoracic outlet compression syndrome, *Ath Train* 21:302, 1986.
11. Mendoza FX, Main K: Peripheral

nerve injuries of the shoulder in the athlete, *Clin Sports Med* 9:331, 1990.

12. Schenkman M, Riego de Cortoya V: 1 Kinesiology of the shoulder complex, *J Orthop Sports Phys Ther* 8:438, 1987.

13. Scovaggo ML et al: The painful shoulder during freestyle swimming, *Am J Sports Med* 19:577 1991.

14. Skyhar MJ et al: Instability of the shoulder. In Nicholas JA, Hershman EB, eds: *The upper extremity in sports medicine*, St Louis, 1990, Mosby-Year Book.

15. Terry GC et al: The function of passive shoulder restraints, *Am J Sports Med* 19:26, 1991.

16. Warner JJP et al: Patterns of flexibility, laxity, and strength in normal shoulders and shoulders with instability and impingement, *Am J Sports Med* 18:366, 1990.

17. Wichiewicz TL: The impingement syndrome. In *Postgraduate advances in sports medicine*, vols I-V, Pennington, NJ, 1986, Forum Medicus.

ANNOTATED BIBLIOGRAPHY

Cailliet R: *Shoulder pain*, ed 2, Philadelphia, 1991, FA Davis.
Detailed coverage of the major causes of shoulder pain includes functional anatomy, pain caused by trauma, referred pain, and rotator cuff tears.

Hawkins RJ, ed: Basic science and clinical application in the athlete's shoulder, *Clin Sports Med* 10: 692, 1991.
A detailed monograph dedicated to all aspects of the shoulder in sports.

The Elbow, Forearm, Wrist, and Hand

When you finish this chapter, you will be able to:

- Identify common elbow, forearm, wrist, and hand injuries
- Provide immediate care of elbow, forearm, wrist, and hand injuries

The portion of the upper limb consisting of the elbow, forearm, wrist, and hand is second to the lower limb in the number of sports injuries incurred. Because of the way it is used and its relative exposure, the upper limb is highly prone to numerous acute and overuse conditions.

THE ELBOW JOINT

Although not as complicated as the knee or shoulder, the elbow still ranks as one of the more complex joints in the human body. It is the junction of three bones: the humerus, the radius, and the ulna (Figures 19-1 through 19-3). The elbow joint allows for flexion and extension. The radioulnar joint, which allows for forearm pronation and supination, is formed by the annular ligament and the head of the radius resting close to the rounded end of the humerus (capitulum). An intricate network of muscles, nerves and blood vessels serves to allow for very complicated movement patterns (Figures 19-4 and 19-5).

Evaluation of the Elbow
History

As with all sports injuries, the evaluator must first understand the mechanism of injury. The following questions will aid in evaluation of the elbow:

1. Is the pain or discomfort caused by a direct trauma such as falling on an outstretched arm or landing on the tip of a bent elbow?

2. Can the problem be attributed to sudden overextension of the elbow or to repeated overuse of a throwing-type motion?

The location and duration should be ascertained. As with shoulder pain, elbow pain or discomfort may be from internal organ dysfunction or referred from a nerve root irritation or nerve impingement.

1. Are there movements or positions of the arm that increase or decrease the pain?
2. Has a previous elbow injury been diagnosed or treated?
3. Is there a feeling of locking or crepitation during movement?

NOTE: Elbow pain may not be directly associated with an elbow injury but rather referred pain from the neck or shoulder.

Pain in the elbow could be referred pain from the neck or shoulder.

isosceles triangle
Triangle with two sides equal in length

Observation

The athlete's elbow should be observed for obvious deformities and swelling. If permissible, the carrying angle, flexion, and extensibility of the elbow should be observed. If the carrying angle is abnormally increased, a cubitus valgus is present; if it is abnormally decreased, a cubitus varus is present. Too great or too little of an angle may be indication of a bony or epiphyseal fracture. The athlete is next observed for the extent of elbow flexion and extension. The elbows are compared (Figure 19-6). A decrease in normal flexion (Figure 19-7), inability to extend fully, or extending beyond normal extension (cubitus recurvatus) may precipitate joint problems (Figure 19-8). Next, the elbow is bent to a 45-degree angle and observed from the rear to determine whether or not the two epicondyles and olecranon process form an **isosceles triangle** (Figure 19-9).

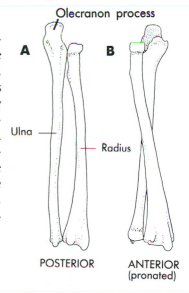

Figure 19-1

Bones of the elbow. **A,** Anterior. **B,** Posterior.

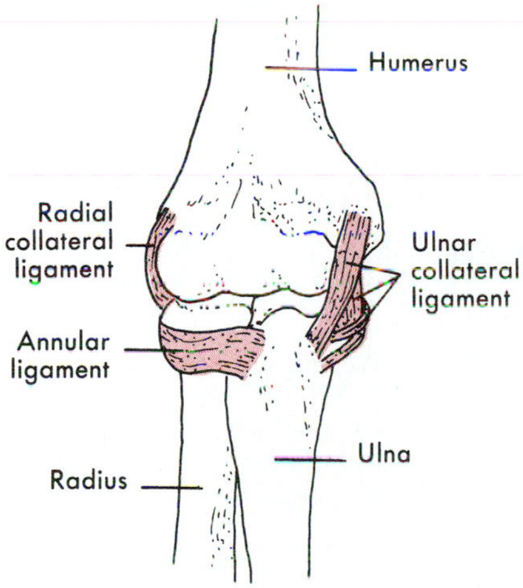

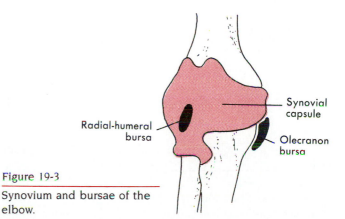

Figure 19-2

Bones and ligaments of the elbow.

Figure 19-3

Synovium and bursae of the elbow.

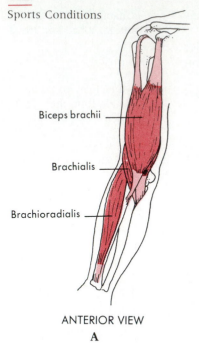

Biceps brachii

Brachialis

Brachioradialis

ANTERIOR VIEW

A

Triceps brachii

Supinator

POSTERIOR VIEW

B

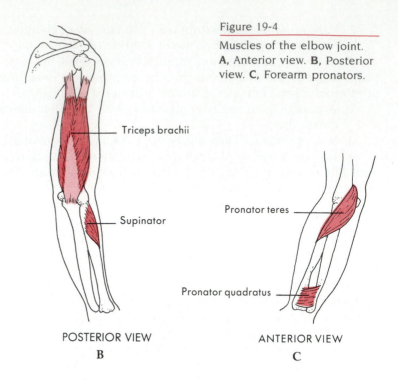

Figure 19-4

Muscles of the elbow joint.
A, Anterior view. **B**, Posterior
view. **C**, Forearm pronators.

Pronator teres

Pronator quadratus

ANTERIOR VIEW

C

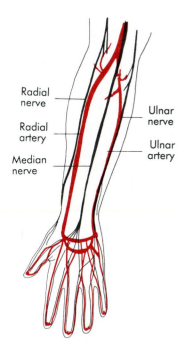

Radial
nerve

Radial
artery

Median
nerve

Ulnar
nerve

Ulnar
artery

Figure 19-5

Arteries and nerves
supplying the elbow joint,
wrist, and hand.

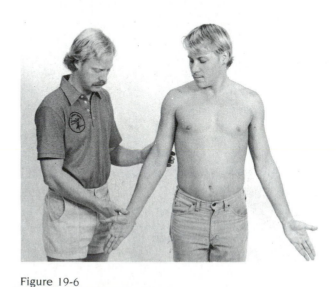

Figure 19-6

Testing for elbow carrying
angle and the extent of
cubitus valgus and cubitus
varus.

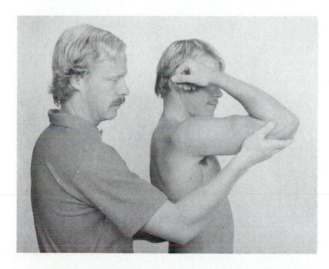

Figure 19-7

Testing for elbow flexion and
elbow extension.

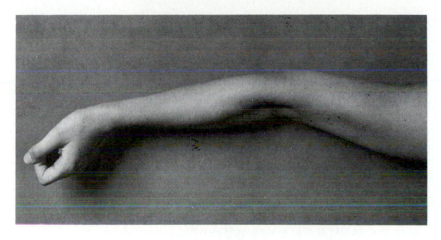

Figure 19-8

Testing for elbow
hyperextension (cubitus
recurvatus).

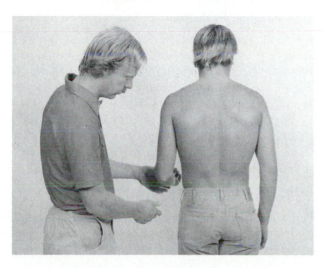

Figure 19-9

Determining whether the
lateral and medial
epicondyles, along with the
olecranon process, form an
isosceles triangle.

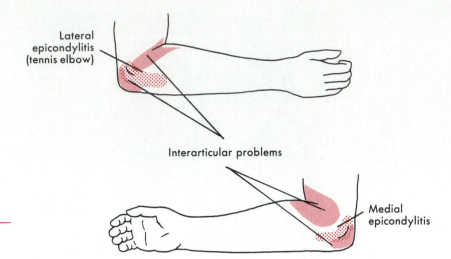

Figure 19-10

Typical pain sites in the elbow region.

Palpation
Bony Palpation

Pain sites and deformities are determined through careful palpation of the epicondyles, olecranon process, distal aspect of the humerus, and proximal aspect of the ulna (Figure 19-10).

Soft-Tissue Palpation

Soft tissue includes the muscles and muscle tendons, joint capsule, and ligaments surrounding the joint.

Circulatory Evaluation

With an elbow injury a pulse routinely should be taken at the brachial artery and at the radial artery at the wrist.

Functional Evaluation

The joint and the muscles are evaluated for pain sites and weakness through passive, active, and resistive motions, consisting of elbow flexion and extension (Figure 19-11) and forearm pronation and supination (Figure 19-12). Range of motion is particularly noted in passive and active pronation and supination (Figure 19-13).

Symptoms and signs The athlete complains of severe pain on the medial aspect of the elbow that can be relieved by flexing the elbow. There is point tenderness on the medial epicondyle, distal aspect of the ulna, or lateral collateral ligament.

Tennis Elbow Test

Resistance is applied to the athlete's extended hand with the elbow flexed 45 degrees. A positive tennis elbow test produces moderate to severe pain at the lateral epicondyle (Figure 19-14).

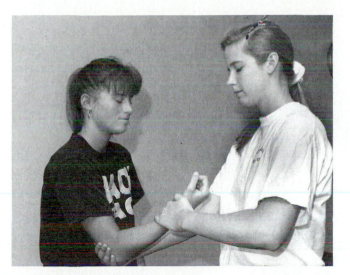

Figure 19-11

Functional evaluation
includes performing passive
resistance flexion and
extension to determine joint
restrictions and pain sites.

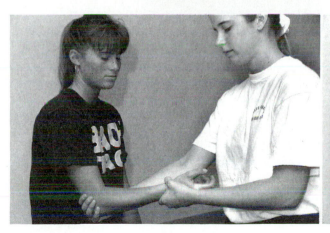 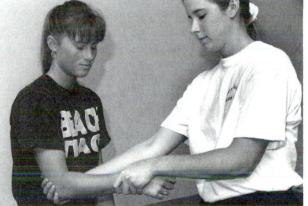

Figure 19-12

Elbow evaluation includes
performing passive, active,
and resistive forearm
pronation and supination.

Prevention of Elbow Injuries

As with other areas of the body, elbow injury prevention requires year-round conditioning consisting of strength, endurance, and flexibility activities. Because of the elbow's sensitivity to overuse problems, it is essential that sport specific techniques be carefully carried out.

Mechanism of Elbow Injuries

As discussed earlier, elbow injuries can occur from a variety of causes. The most common causes of injury are overuse throwing and falling on the outstretched hand.

Injuries to the Elbow Region

The elbow is subject to injury in sports because of its broad range of motion, weak lateral bone arrangement, and relative exposure to soft tissue

The two most common
mechanisms of elbow injury
    Throwing
    Falling on the outstretched
        hand

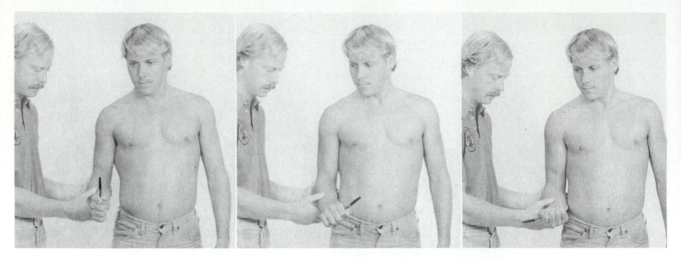

Figure 19-13

The range of motion of the forearm pronation and supination is routinely observed in athletes with elbow problems.

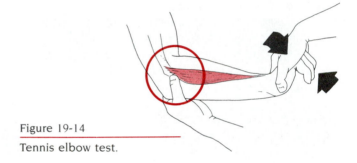

Figure 19-14

Tennis elbow test.

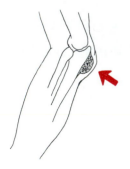

Figure 19-15

Olecranon bursitis.

damage in the vicinity of the joint.[16] Many sports place excessive stress on the elbow joint. Extreme locking of the elbow in gymnastics or using implements such as racquets, golf clubs, and javelins can cause injuries. The throwing mechanism in baseball pitching can injure the elbow during both the acceleration and follow-through phases.[3]

Soft Tissue Injuries Around Elbow

Contusions   Because of its lack of padding and its general vulnerability, the elbow often becomes contused in collision and contact sports. Bone bruises arise from a deep penetration or a succession of blows to the sharp projections of the elbow. A contusion of the elbow may swell rapidly after an irritation of the olecranon bursa or the synovial membrane and should be treated immediately with cold and pressure for at least 24 hours. If the injury is severe, the athlete should be referred to a physician for x-ray examination to determine if a fracture exists.

Olecranon bursitis   The olecranon bursa (Figure 19-15), lying between the end of the olecranon process and the skin, is the most frequently injured bursa in the elbow. Its superficial location makes it prone to acute or chronic injury, particularly as the result of direct blows. The inflamed bursa produces pain, marked swelling, and point tenderness. Occasionally, swelling will appear almost spontaneously and without the usual pain and heat. If the condition is acute, a cold compress should be applied for at least 1 hour. Chronic olecranon bursitis requires a program of superficial therapy. In some cases aspiration by a physician will hasten healing. Although seldom serious, olecranon bursitis can be annoying and should be well protected by padding while the athlete is engaged in competition.[16]

Strains The acute mechanisms of muscle strain associated with the elbow joint are usually excessive resistive motion, such as a fall on the outstretched hand with the elbow in extension that forces the joint into hyperextension. Repeated microtears causing chronic injury will be discussed under *epicondylitis*.

Care Immediate care includes RICE and sling support for the more severe cases. Follow-up care may include cryotherapy, ultrasound, and rehabilitative exercises. Conditions that cause moderate to severe loss of elbow function should routinely be referred for x-ray examination. It is important to rule out the possibility of an avulsion or epiphyseal fracture.

Sprains Sprains to the elbow are usually caused by hyperextension or a force that bends or twists the lower arm outward.

Care Immediate care for elbow sprain consists of cold and a pressure bandage for at least 24 hours with sling support fixed at 90 degrees of flexion. After hemorrhage has been controlled, superficial heat treatments in the whirlpool may be started and combined with massage above and below the injury. Like fractures and dislocations, sprains also may result in abnormal bone proliferation if the area is massaged directly and too vigorously or exercised too soon. The main concern should be to gently aid the elbow in regaining a full range of motion and then, when the time is right, to commence active exercises until full mobility and strength have returned. Taping can help and should restrain the elbow from further injury, or it may be used while the athlete is participating in sports.

Epicondylitis Epicondylitis is a chronic condition that may affect athletes who execute repeated forearm flexion and extension movements such as are performed in tennis, pitching, golf, javelin throwing, and fencing. The elbow is particularly predisposed to mechanical trauma in the activities of throwing and striking. It is also called tennis elbow, pitcher's elbow, or golfer's elbow.

Epicondylitis is an inflammation of the muscular attachments of either the long extensor muscles of the wrist and fingers at the lateral epicondyle of the humerus, or of the long flexor muscles of the wrist and fingers at the medial epicondyle of the humerus. Epicondylitis occurs from small microtears at these sites of muscle attachment; these microtears result from repeated forceful wrist flexion or extension.[10]

Regardless of the sport or exact location of the injury, the symptoms and signs of epicondylitis are similar. Pain around the epicondyles of the humerus is produced during forceful wrist flexion or extension. The pain

Common sports injuries that are forms of epicondylitis:
  Pitcher's elbow
  Tennis elbow
  Javelin thrower's elbow
  Golfer's elbow

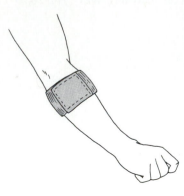

Figure 19-16

Counterforce brace for treatment of elbow and epicondylitis.

Athletes with a pronounced cubitus valgus are prone to injuring the ulnar nerve.

may be centered at the epicondyle, or it may radiate down the arm. There is usually point tenderness and, in some cases, mild swelling. Passive movement of the wrist into extension or flexion seldom elicits pain, although active movement does.[12]

Care   Conservative management of moderate-to-severe epicondylitis usually includes use of a sling, rest, cryotherapy, and/or heat through the application of ultrasound. Analgesic and/or antiinflammatory agents may be prescribed and a counterforce brace may be worn (Figure 19-16). It should be noted that the counterforce should only be used by individuals who have been diagnosed with epicondylitis. It should never be used by children or adolescents who have been diagnosed with a growth plate problem or by an individual with an elbow instability.

Elbow Osteochondritis Dissecans

Although osteochondritis dissecans is more common in knees, it also occurs in elbows. Its cause is unknown; however, impairment of the blood supply to the anterior surfaces leads to fragmentation and separation of a portion of the articular cartilage and bone, creating a loose body within the joint.[16,17]

The adolescent athlete usually complains of sudden pain and locking of the elbow joint. Range of motion returns slowly over a few days. Swelling, pain, and crepitation also may occur.

Care   If there are repeated episodes of locking, surgical removal of the loose bodies may be warranted. If they are not removed, traumatic arthritis can eventually occur.

Ulnar Nerve Injuries

Because of the exposed position of the medial humeral condyle, the ulnar nerve is subject to a variety of problems. The athlete with a pronounced cubitus valgus may develop a friction problem. The ulnar nerve can also become recurrently dislocated because of a structural deformity or impinged by a ligament during flexion-type activities.

Rather than being painful, ulnar nerve injuries usually respond with a paresthesia to the fourth and fifth fingers. The athlete complains of burning and tingling in the fourth and fifth fingers.

Care   The management of ulnar nerve injuries is conservative; aggravation of the nerve, such as placing direct pressure on it, is avoided. When stress on the nerve cannot be avoided, surgery may be performed to transpose it anteriorly to the elbow.

Dislocation of the Elbow

Dislocation of the elbow has a high incidence in sports activity and most often is caused either by a fall on the outstretched hand with the elbow in a position of hyperextension or by a severe twist while the elbow is in a flexed position. The bones of the forearm (ulna and radius) may be displaced backward, forward, or laterally. The appearance of the most common dislocation is a deformity of the olecranon process wherein it extends backward, well beyond its normal alignment with the upper arm.

Elbow dislocations involve rupturing and tearing of most of the stabilizing ligamentous tissue, accompanied by profuse internal bleeding and subsequent swelling. There is severe pain and disability. The complications of such a trauma may include injury to the major nerves and blood vessels.

Care   The primary responsibility is to provide the athlete with a sling and immediately to refer the athlete to a physician for reduction. Reduction must be performed as soon as possible to prevent spasmodic constriction and prolonged derangement of soft tissue. In most cases the physician will administer an anesthetic before reduction to relax spasmed muscles. After reduction, the physician often will immobilize the elbow in a position of flexion and apply a sling suspension, which should be used for approximately 3 weeks. While the arm is maintained in flexion, the athlete should execute hand gripping and shoulder exercises. When initial healing has taken place, gentle, passive exercise and heat may be applied to help regain a full range of motion. Above all, therapy that is too strenuous should be avoided before complete healing has occurred because of the high probability of encouraging calcification of tendons and the joint capsule. Both range of movement and a strength program should be initiated by the athlete, but forced stretching must be avoided. When an elbow is dislocated as with a fracture, neurovascular problems must be considered as a possibility.

Neurovascular problems are a possibility when an elbow is dislocated or fractured.

Fractures of the Elbow

An elbow fracture can occur in almost any sports event and is usually caused by a fall on the outstretched hand or the flexed elbow or by a direct blow to the elbow. Children and young athletes have a much higher rate of this injury than do adults. A fracture can take place in any one or more of the bones that compose the elbow. A fall on the outstretched hand quite often fractures the humerus above the condyles. The bones of the forearm or wrist also may be the recipients of trauma that produces a fracture. An elbow fracture may or may not result in visible deformity. There usually will be hemorrhage, swelling, and muscle spasm in the injured area.

Volkmann's Contracture

It is essential that athletes sustaining a serious elbow injury have their brachial or radial pulse monitored often. Swelling, muscle spasm, or pressure from a bone displacement can put pressure on the brachial artery and inhibit blood circulation to the forearm, wrist, and hand. Such inhibition of circulation can lead to muscle contracture and permanent paralysis.

Volkmann's contracture is a major complication of a serious elbow injury.

The first indication of this problem is pain in the forearm that becomes progressively greater when the fingers of the affected arm are passively extended. Volkmann's contracture is a major problem requiring immediate referral for emergency treatment.

Reconditioning of the Elbow

While the elbow is immobilized after an acute injury, the athlete should perform general body exercises as well as exercises specific to the shoulder and wrist joint. Strengthening wrist flexors and extensors are important to elbow reconditioning. In some cases isometric exercise is appropriate while the elbow is immobilized.[1] Maintaining the strength of these articulations will speed the recovery of the elbow. After the elbow has healed and free movement is permitted by the physician, the first consideration should be restoration of the normal range of movement. Lengthening the contracted tendons and supporting tissue around the elbow requires daily gentle, active exercises. NOTE: Passive stretching may be detrimental to the athlete striving to regain full range of movement. *Forced stretching must be avoided at all times.*[3] When the full range of motion has been regained, a graded, progressive resistance exercise program should be initiated, including elbow flexion and extension as well as forearm pronation and supination (Figure 19-17). Protective taping must be continued until full strength and flexibility have been restored. Long-standing chronic conditions of the elbow usually cause gradual debilitation of the surrounding soft tissue. Elbows with conditions of this type should be restored to the maximal state of conditioning without encouraging postinjury aggravation. Pitching or other throwing elbow injuries require a gradual program of reconditioning.

Figure 19-17

A very gradual program of progressive resistance exercise is important to elbow rehabilitation.

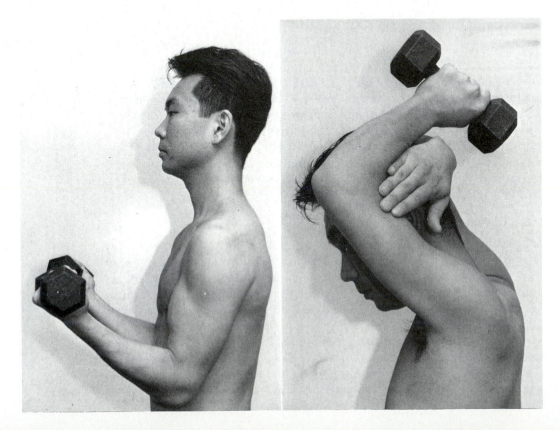

THE FOREARM

The bones of the forearm are the ulna and the radius (Figure 19-1, p. 490). The ulna, which may be thought of as a direct extension of the humerus, is long, straight, and larger at its upper end than at its lower end. The radius, considered an extension of the hand, is thicker at its lower end than at its upper end. The forearm has three articulations: the superior, middle, and distal radioulnar joints.

The forearm muscles consist of flexors and pronators, positioned anteriorly and attached to the medial elbow, and of extensors and supinators, which lie posteriorly and are attached to the lateral elbow (Figure 19-18). The flexors of the wrist and fingers are separated into superficial muscles and deep muscles.

The major blood supply stems from the brachial artery, which divides into the radial and ulnar artery in the forearm.

Except for the flexor carpi ulnaris and half of the flexor digitorum profundus, most of the flexor muscles of the forearm are supplied by the median nerve. The majority of the extensor muscles are controlled by the radial nerve.

Evaluating Forearm Injuries

Sports injuries for the forearm are easily detectable because of the amount of exposure of both the ulna and the radius. Recognition of an injury is accomplished mainly through observation of the range of motion present and visible deviations and through the use of palpation. The

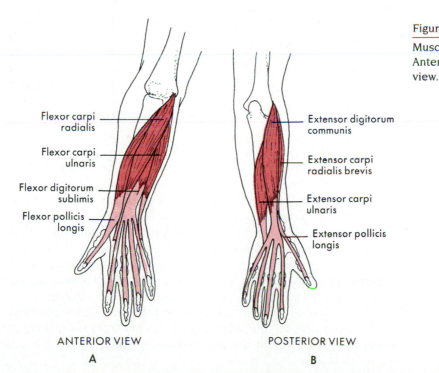

Figure 19-18

Muscles of the forearm. **A,** Anterior view. **B,** Posterior view.

Flexor carpi radialis

Flexor carpi ulnaris

Flexor digitorum sublimis

Flexor pollicis longis

Extensor digitorum communis

Extensor carpi radialis brevis

Extensor carpi ulnaris

Extensor pollicis longis

ANTERIOR VIEW

A

POSTERIOR VIEW

B

forearm is first tested for the amount of pronation and supination possible, 150 degrees being considered average. Next it is tested for wrist flexion and extension, with 150 degrees again considered normal. Injury may be reflected in the visible indications of deformity or paralysis. Palpation can reveal a false joint, bone fragments, or a lack of continuity between bones.[14]

Injuries to the Forearm

Lying between the elbow joint and the wrist and hand, the forearm is indirectly influenced by injuries to these area; however, direct injuries can also occur.

Contusions

The forearm is constantly exposed to bruising in contact sports such as football. The ulnar side receives the majority of blows in arm blocks and consequently the greater amount of bruising. Bruises to this area may be classified as acute or chronic. The acute contusion can result in a fracture, but this happens only rarely. Most often muscles or bones develop varying degrees of pain, swelling, and accumulation of blood (hematoma). The chronic contusion develops from repeated blows to the forearm with attendant multiple irritations. Extensive scar tissue may replace the hematoma and in some cases a bony callus replaces the scar tissue.

Care   Care of the contused forearm requires proper attention in the acute stages by application of RICE for 20 minutes every 1½ waking hours, followed the next day by cold and exercise. Protection of the forearm is important for athletes who are prone to this condition. The best protection consists of a full-length sponge rubber pad for the forearm early in the season.

Strains

Forearm strain occurs in a variety of sports; most such injuries come from repeated static contractions.

Forearm splints   Forearm splints, like shinsplints, are difficult to manage. They occur most often in gymnastics, particularly to those who perform on the side horse.

The main symptom is a dull ache of the extensor muscles, crossing the back of the forearm. Muscle weakness may accompany the dull ache. Palpation reveals an irritation of the deep tissue between the muscles. The cause of this condition is uncertain; like shinsplints, forearm splints usually appear either early or late in the season, indicating poor conditioning or a factor of chronic fatigue. It is speculated that the reason for this problem is static muscle contractions of the forearm, as occurs when performing on the side horse. Constant static muscle contraction causes minute tears in the deep connective tissues of the forearm.

Care   Care of forearm splints is symptomatic. If the problem occurs in the early season, the athlete should concentrate on increasing the strength of the forearm through resistance exercises, but if it arises late

Forearm splints, like shinsplints, commonly occur early and late in the sports season.

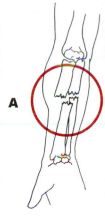

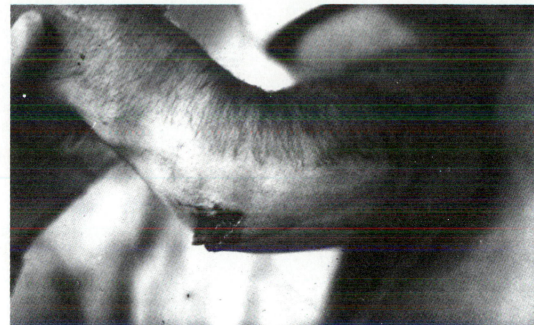

A

B

in the season, emphasis should be placed on rest, cryotherapy or heat, and use of a supportive wrap during activity.

Fractures Fractures of the forearm (Figure 19-19) are particularly common among active children and youths. They occur as the result of a blow or a fall on the outstretched hand. Fractures to the ulna or the radius singly are much rarer than simultaneous fractures to both. The break usually presents all the features of a long-bone fracture: pain, swelling, deformity, and a false joint.[4] The older the athlete, the greater the danger is of extensive damage to soft tissue and the greater the possibility of paralysis from Volkmann's contractures.

To prevent complications a cold pack must be applied immediately to the fracture site, the arm splinted and put in a sling, and the athlete referred to a physician. The athlete will usually be incapacitated for about 8 weeks.

Colles' fracture Colles' fracture (Figure 19-20), among the most common forearm fractures, involves the lower (distal) end of the radius. This mechanism of injury is usually a fall on the outstretched hand, forcing the forearm backward and upward into hyperextension.

In most cases there is a visible deformity to the wrist. Sometimes no deformity is present, and the injury may be passed off as a bad sprain—to the detriment of the athlete. Bleeding is quite profuse in this area with the accumulated fluids causing extensive swelling in the wrist and, if unchecked, in the fingers and forearm. Ligamentous tissue is usually unharmed, but tendons may be torn away from their attachment, and there may possibly be median nerve damage.

Figure 19-19

A, Fracture of the radius and ulna. **B,** Compound fracture of the ulna.

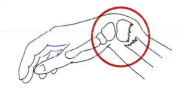

Figure 19-20

Common appearance of the forearm in Colles' fracture.

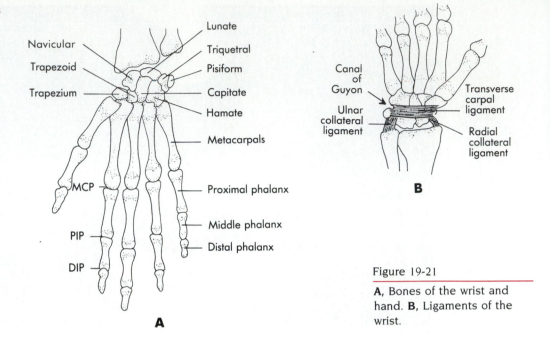

Figure 19-21

A, Bones of the wrist and hand. **B,** Ligaments of the wrist.

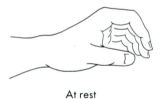

At rest

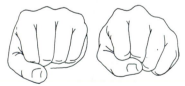

Normal fist   Clenched fist

Figure 19-22

General normal attitudes of the hand.

Care   The main responsibility is to apply a cold compress, splint the wrist, put the limb in a sling, and then refer the athlete to a physician for x-ray examination and immobilization. Lacking complications, Colles' fracture will keep an athlete out of sports for 1 to 2 months. What appears to be Colles' fracture in children and youths is often a lower epiphyseal separation. NOTE: Forearm exercise rehabilitation is discussed later in this chapter.

THE WRIST AND HAND

The wrist is formed by the union of the distal aspect of the radius and the articular disk of the ulna with three of the four proximal (of the eight diversely shaped) carpal bones (Figure 19-21).

Evaluation of the Wrist and Hand
History

As with other conditions, the evaluator asks about the location and type of pain:

1. What increases or decreases the pain?
2. Has there been a history of trauma or overuse?
3. What therapy or medications, if any, have been given?

Observations

As the athlete is observed, arm and hand asymmetries are noted. Hand usage such as writing or unbuttoning a shirt is also noted. The general attitude of the hand is observed (Figure 19-22). When the athlete is asked to open and close the hand, the evaluator notes whether this movement can be performed fully and rhythmically. Another general functional activity is to have the athlete touch the tip of the thumb to each fingertip several times. The last factor to be observed is the color of the fingernails. Nails that are very pale instead of pink may indicate a problem with blood circulation.

Palpation

Bony Palpation

Wrist region   The bones of the wrist region are palpated for pain and defects.

Soft-Tissue Palpation

Wrist region   Each tendon is palpated for pain as it crosses the wrist region.
Hand region   The soft tissue of the hand is then palpated.

Circulatory and Neurological Evaluation

The hands should be inspected to determine whether circulation is impeded. The hands should be felt for their temperature. A cold hand or portion of a hand is a sign of decreased circulation. Pinching the fingernails can also help to indicate circulatory problems. Pinching will blanch the nail, and on release there should be rapid return of a pink color.

Functional Evaluation

Range of motion is noted in all movements of the wrist and fingers. Active and resistive movements are then compared with those of the uninjured wrist and hand.

Passive, active, and resistive movements are performed in the wrist and hand.

Injuries to the Wrist

Injuries to the wrist usually occur from a fall on the outstretched hand or repeated flexion, extension, or rotary movements (Figure 19-23).[5]

Strains and Sprains

It is often very difficult to distinguish between injury to the muscle tendons crossing the wrist joint and to the supporting structure of the carpal region. Therefore, emphasis will be placed on the condition of wrist sprains, whereas strains will be considered in the discussion of the hand.

A sprain is by far the most common wrist injury and in most cases is the most poorly managed injury in sports. It can arise from any abnormal forced movement of the wrist. Falling on the hyperextended wrist is the most common cause, but violent flexion or torsion can also tear supporting tissue. Since the main support of the wrist is derived from posterior and anterior ligaments that carry the major nutrient vessels to the

Sprains are the most common wrist injury in sports and often the worst managed.

Figure 19-23

Wrist injuries commonly occur from falls on the outstretched hand or from repeated flexion, extension, lateral, or rotary movements.

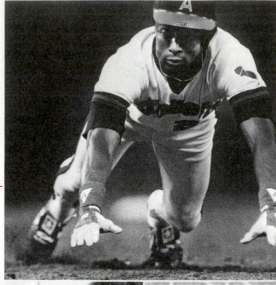

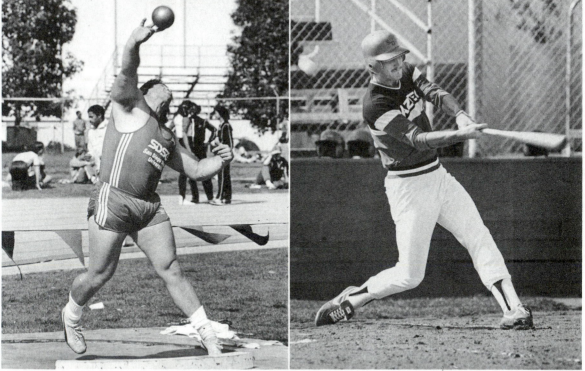

carpal bones, repeated sprains may disrupt the blood supply and consequently the nutrition to the carpal bones.

The sprained wrist may be differentiated from the carpal navicular fracture by recognition of the generalized swelling, tenderness, inability to flex the wrist, and absence of appreciable pain or irritation over the navicular bone. All athletes having severe sprains should be referred to a physician for x-ray examination to determine possible fractures.

Care Mild and moderate sprains should be given cold therapy and compression for at least 24 to 48 hours, after which cryotherapy is carried out or heat therapy is gradually increased. It is desirable to have the athlete start hand-strengthening exercises almost immediately after the injury has occurred.

Nerve Compression in the Wrist Region

Because of the narrow spaces that some nerves must travel through the wrist to the hand, compression neuropathy or **entrapment** can occur. The two most common entrapments are of the median nerve, which travels through the carpal tunnel, and the ulnar nerve, which is compressed in the tunnel of Guyon between the pisiform bone and the hook of the hamate bone (Fig. 19-21).

entrapment
Organ becomes compressed by nearby tissue

Such compression causes a sharp or burning pain that is associated with an increase or decrease in skin sensitivity or **paresthesia.** When chronic entrapment may cause irreversible nerve damage, unsuccessful conservative treatment can lead to surgical decompression.[19]

paresthesia
Abnormal or morbid sensation such as itching or prickling

Carpal tunnel syndrome The carpal tunnel is located on the anterior aspect of the wrist. The floor of the carpal tunnel is formed by the carpal bones and the roof by the transverse carpal ligament. A number of anatomical structures course through this limited space (Fig. 19-21). Carpal tunnel syndrome results from an inflammation of the tendons and synovial sheaths within this space, which ultimately leads to compression of the median nerve.

Carpal tunnel syndrome most often occurs in athletes who engage in activities that require repeated wrist flexion, although it can also result from direct trauma to the anterior aspect of the wrist.

Compression of the median nerve will usually result in both sensory and motor deficits. Sensory changes could result in tingling, numbness, and parasthesia over the thumb, index and middle fingers, and the palm of the hand. Weakness in thumb movement is associated with carpal tunnel syndrome.

Care Initially, conservative treatment involving rest, immobilization, and nonsteroidal antiinflammatory medication is recommended. If the syndrome persists, injection with a corticosteroid, and possible surgical decompression of the transverse carpal ligament may be necessary.

de Quervain's disease De Quervain's disease is due to a narrow tendon passage in the thumb causing a tenosynovitis. The first tunnel of the wrist becomes contracted and narrowed as a result of inflammation of the synovial lining. The tendons that go through the first tunnel move through the same synovial sheath. Because the tendons move through a groove, constant wrist movement can be a source of irritation.

Athletes who use a great deal of wrist motion in their sport are prone to de Quervain's disease. Its symptom is aching, which may radiate into the hand or forearm. Movements of the wrist tend to increase the pain, and there is a positive de Quervain's test. There is point tenderness and weakness during thumb extension and abduction, and there may be a painful snapping and catching of the tendons during movement.

Care Management of de Quervain's disease involves immobilization, rest, cryotherapy, and antiinflammatory medication. Ultrasound and ice massage are also beneficial.

Dislocations

Dislocations of the wrist are relatively infrequent in sports activity. Most occur from a forceful hyperextension of the wrist as a result of a fall on the outstretched hand. Of those dislocations that do happen, the bones that could be involved are the distal ends of the radius and ulna (Figure 19-24) and a carpal bone, the lunate being the most commonly affected.

The primary signs of this condition are pain, swelling, and difficulty in executing wrist and finger flexion. There also may be numbness or even paralysis of the flexor muscles because of lunate pressure on the median nerve.

Care This condition should be treated as acute, and the athlete sent to a physician. If it is not recognized early enough, bone deterioration may occur, requiring surgical removal.

Fractures

Fractures of the wrist commonly occur to the distal ends of the radius and ulna and to the carpal bones; the carpal navicular bone is most commonly affected; the hamate bone is affected less often.

Scaphoid fracture The scaphoid bone is the most frequently fractured of the carpal bones. The injury is usually caused by a force on the outstretched hand, which compresses the navicular bone between the radius and the second row of carpal bones (Figure 19-25). This condition is often mistaken for a severe sprain, and as a result the required complete immobilization is not carried out. Without proper splinting, the navicular fracture often fails to heal because of an inadequate supply of

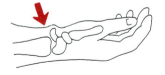

Figure 19-24

Dislocation of the wrist.

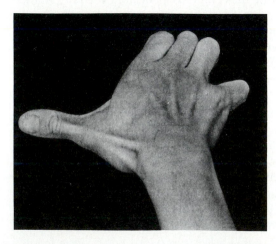

Figure 19-25

Anatomical "snuffbox" formed by extensor tendons of the thumb.

blood; thus, degeneration and **necrosis** (bone death) occur. Even after proper splinting the navicular fractures may not heal and may have to be surgically repaired. This condition is often called *aseptic necrosis* of the navicular bone. It is necessary to try in every way possible to distinguish between a wrist sprain and a fracture of the navicular bone because a fracture necessitates immediate referral to a physician.

necrosis
Death of tissue

The signs of a recent navicular fracture include swelling in the area of the carpal bones, severe point tenderness of the navicular bone in the anatomical snuffbox, and navicular pain that is elicited by upward pressure exerted on the long axis of the thumb and by radial flexion.

Care With these signs present, cold should be applied, the area splinted, and the athlete referred to a physician for x-ray study and casting. In most cases cast immobilization lasts for about 8 weeks and is followed by strengthening exercises coupled with protective taping. Following a so-called wrist sprain, x-ray examination should be conducted every two weeks to determine whether there are indications of a fracture.

Hamate fracture A fracture of the hamate bone can result from a fall but more commonly occurs after a blow from an implement such as the handle of a tennis racquet, a baseball bat, or a golf club.[20] Wrist pain and weakness are experienced. Pull of the muscular attachments can cause nonunion; therefore casting is usually the treatment of choice. Taping support should be maintained until the athlete has regained full strength and mobility.

Wrist Ganglion of the Tendon Sheath

The wrist ganglion (Figure 19-26) is often seen in sports. It is considered by many to be a herniation of the joint capsule or of the synovial sheath of a tendon; other authorities believe it to be a cystic structure. It usually appears slowly after a wrist strain and contains a clear, mucous fluid. The ganglion most often appears on the back of the wrist but can appear at any tendinous point in the wrist or hand. As it increases in size, it may be accompanied by a mild pressure discomfort. An old method of treatment was to break down the swelling by means of finger pressure and then apply a felt pressure pad for a period to encourage healing. A newer approach is the combination of drawing the fluid off using a hypodermic needle and chemical cauterization, with subsequent application of a pressure pad. Neither of these methods prevents the ganglion from recurring. Surgical removal is the best method available.

Injuries to the Hand

Injuries to the hand occur frequently in sports, yet the injured hand is probably the most poorly managed of all body areas.

Contusions and Pressure Injuries of the Hand and Phalanges

The hand and phalanges, having irregular bony structure and little protective fat and muscle padding, are prone to bruising in sports. This condition is easily identified from the history of trauma and the pain and

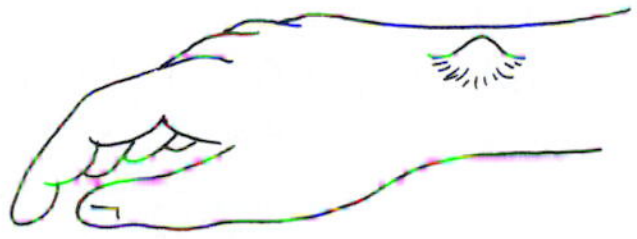

Figure 19-26

Wrist ganglion.

RELEASING BLOOD FROM BENEATH THE FINGERNAIL

The following is one common methods for releasing the pressure of the subungual hematoma:

MATERIALS NEEDED: paper clip and antiseptic.

POSITION OF THE ATHLETE: The athlete sits with the injured hand palm down on the table.

POSITION OF THE OPERATOR: The operator sits facing the athlete's affected finger and stabilizes it with one hand.

Technique:
1. A paper clip is heated to red-hot.
2. The red-hot paper clip is laid on the surface of the nail with moderate pressure. The clip melts through the nail to the site of the bleeding.

It is important to elevate the hand for the first 48 hours after injury to prevent swelling in the fingers.

swelling of soft tissues. Cold, compression, and elevation should be applied immediately for 48 hours to avoid swelling. This should be followed by gradual warming of the part in a whirlpool or immersion bath. Although soreness is still present, protection should be given by a sponge rubber pad.

A particularly common contusion of the finger is bruising of the distal phalanx, or fingertip, which results in a *subungual hematoma* (contusion of the fingernail). This is an extremely painful condition because of the accumulation of blood underneath the fingernail. The athlete should place the finger in ice water until the hemorrhage ceases, and the pressure of blood should then be released.

Bowler's thumb   Bowler's thumb can occur from the pressure of a bowling ball thumbhole. With the development of fibrotic tissue around the ulnar nerve, the athlete senses pain, tingling during pressure to the irritated area, and numbness.

Early management includes decreasing the amount of bowling and padding of the thumbhole. If the condition continues, however, surgery may be warranted.

Tendon Conditions

Tendon injuries are common among athletes. As with many other hand injuries occurring in sports, they are characteristically neglected.

Tenosynovitis   The tendons of the wrist and hand can sustain irritation from repeated movement that results in tenosynovitis. An inflammation of the tendon sheath results in swelling, crepitation, and painful movement. Most commonly affected are the extensor tendons of the wrist.

Two important forms of tenosynovitis
  deQuervain's disease
  Trigger finger or thumb

Trigger finger or thumb   The trigger finger or thumb is another example of stenosing tenosynovitis. It most commonly occurs in a flexor tendon that runs through a common sheath with other tendons. Thickening of the sheath or tendon can occur, thus constricting the sliding ten-

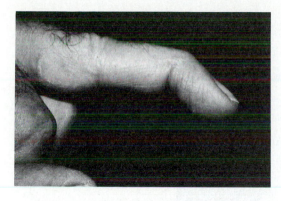
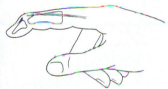

Figure 19-27
Mallet finger.

don. A nodule in the synovium of the sheath adds to the difficulty of gliding.[11]

The athlete complains that when the finger or thumb is flexed, there is resistance to re-extension, producing a snapping that is both palpable and audible. During palpation, tenderness is produced, and a lump can be felt at the base of the flexor tendon sheath.

Care   Treatment initially is the same as for de Quervain's disease (p. 508); however, if it is unsuccessful, steroid injections may produce relief. If steroid injections do not provide relief, splinting the tendon sheath is the last option.

Jamming Fingers

The jamming of a finger or thumb can lead to a variety of injuries that should never be trivialized. Mallet finger, boutonnière deformities, sprains, dislocations, and fractures represent this mechanism of injury.

Mallet Finger

The mallet finger is common in sports, particularly in baseball and basketball. It is caused by a blow from a thrown ball that strikes the tip of the finger, completely tearing the extensor tendon from its insertion along with a piece of bone.

The athlete, unable to extend the finger, carries it at about a 30-degree angle. There is also point tenderness at the site of the injury, and the pulled-away bone chip often can be felt (Figure 19-27).

Care   Pain, swelling, and discoloration from internal hemorrhage are present. The distal phalanx should be splinted in a position of extension immediately, cold should be applied to the area, and the athlete should be referred to a physician. Most physicians will splint the mallet finger into extension or hyperextension and the proximal phalanx into flexion for 6 to 8 weeks (Figure 19-28).

Boutonnière deformity   The boutonnière, or buttonhole, deformity is caused by a rupture of the extensor tendon of the middle phalanx. Trauma forces the upper joint of the middle phalanx into excessive flexion.

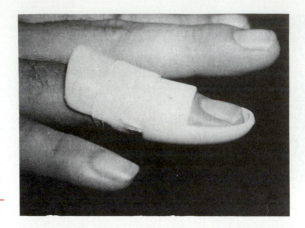

Figure 19-28

Splinting of the mallet finger.

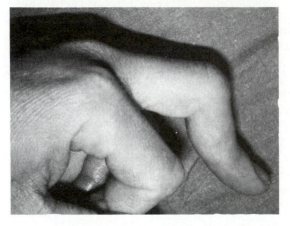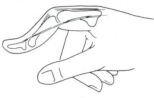

Figure 19-29

Boutonnière deformity.

The athlete complains of severe pain and inability to extend the finger. There is swelling, point tenderness, and an obvious deformity (Figure 19-29).

Care   Care of the boutonnière deformity includes cold application followed by splinting of the joint in extension. NOTE: If this condition is inadequately splinted, the classic boutonnière deformity will develop. Splinting is continued for 5 to 8 weeks.[13]

Sprains, Dislocations, and Fractures

The phalanges, particularly the thumbs, are prone to sprains caused by a blow delivered to the tip or by violent twisting. The mechanism of injury is similar to that of fractures and dislocations. The sprain, however, mainly affects the capsular, ligamentous, and tendinous tissues. Recognition is accomplished primarily through the history and the sprain symptoms: pain, marked swelling, and bleeding.

Gamekeeper's thumb   A sprain of the ulnar collateral ligament of the thumb is common among athletes, especially skiers and tackle foot-

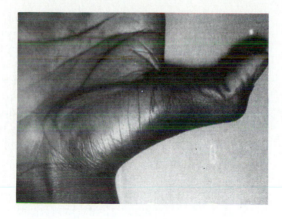

Figure 19-30

Gamekeeper's thumb.

ball players. The cause of injury is usually a forceful abduction of the thumb's uppermost phalanx, which is occasionally combined with hyperextension (Figure 19-30).

Care   Since the stability of pinching can be severely deterred by this sprain, proper immediate and follow-up care must be carried out.[13] If there is instability in the joints, the athlete should be immediately referred to an orthopedist. If the joint is stable, x-ray examination should routinely be performed to rule out fracture. Splinting of the thumb should be applied for protection over a 3-week period or until it is pain free. The splint is applied with the thumb in a neutral position extending from the end of the thumb to above the wrist.[13] After splinting, a thumb spica taping should be worn during sports participation.

Collateral ligament sprain   A collateral ligament sprain of a finger is very common in sports such as basketball, volleyball, and football. A common mechanism is an axial force producing the jammed finger.[6,9]

There is severe point tenderness at the joint site, especially in the region of the collateral ligaments. There may be a lateral or medial instability when the joint is in 150 degrees of flexion.

Care   Care includes ice packs for the acute stage, x-ray examinations, and splinting. Splinting of the joint is usually at 30 to 40 degrees of flexion for 10 days. If the sprain is to the first phalanx joint, splinting for a few days in full extension assists in the healing process. If the sprains are minor, taping the injured finger to a noninjured one will provide protective support. Later, a protective checkrein can be applied for either thumb or finger protection. (See Fig. 10-37 for special thumb strapping.)

Dislocations of the phalanges   Dislocations of the phalanges (Figure 19-31) occur frequently in sports and are caused mainly by a blow to the tip of the finger by a ball (Figure 19-32). The force of injury is usually directed upward from the palmar side, displacing either the first or second joint dorsally. The resultant problem is primarily a tearing of the supporting capsular tissue, accompanied by hemorrhaging. However, there may be a rupture of the flexor or extensor tendon and chip fractures in and around the dislocated joint. Reduction of the thumb dislocation should be performed by a physician. It is advisable to splint the dislocation as it is and refer to the team physician for reduction.

To ensure the most complete healing of the dislocated finger joints, splinting should be maintained for about 3 weeks in 30 degrees of flexion because an inadequate immobilization can cause an unstable joint and/or excessive scar tissue and possibly a permanent deformity.

Special consideration must be given to dislocations of the thumb and second or third joints of the fingers. A properly functioning thumb is necessary for hand dexterity; consequently, any injury to the thumb should be considered serious. Thumb dislocations occur frequently at the second joint, resulting from a sharp blow to its tip, with the trauma forcing the thumb into hyperextension and dislocating the second joint down-

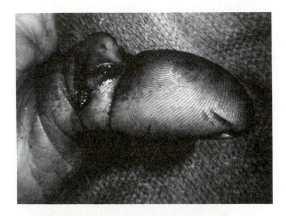

Figure 19-31

Compound dislocation of the thumb.

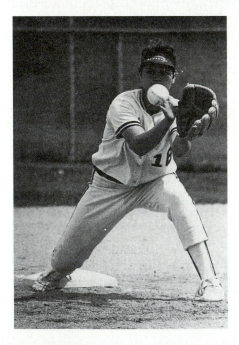

Figure 19-32

Sports such as baseball can produce finger injuries.

ward. Any dislocation of the third joint of the finger can lead to complications and require the immediate care of an orthopedist. All hand dislocations must be x-rayed to rule out fracture.

Fractures of the hand The mechanism that produces strains, sprains, and dislocations can cause fractures of the metacarpal bones and phalanges. Other mechanisms include crushing injuries.

Fractures of the metacarpal bones Fractures of the metacarpal bones (Figure 19-33) are common in contact sports. They arise from striking an object with the fist or from having the hand stepped on. There is often pain, deformity, swelling, and abnormal mobility. In some cases no deformity occurs, and palpation fails to distinguish between a severe contusion and a fracture. In this situation digital pressure should be placed on the knuckles and the long axes of the metacarpal bones. Pressure often will reveal pain at the fracture site. After the fracture is located, the hand should be splinted over a gauze roll splint, cold and pressure applied, and the athlete referred to a physician.

Fractures of the phalanges Fractures of the phalanges are among the most common fractures in sports and can occur as the result of a variety of mechanisms: the fingers being stepped on, hit by a ball, or twisted. The finger suspected of fracture should be splinted in flexion around a gauze roll or a curved splint to avoid full extension. Flexion splinting reduces the deformity by relaxing the flexor tendons. Fracture of the end phalanx is less complicated than fracture of the middle or third phalanx.[13] The major concerns are to control bleeding, apply a splint properly, and refer the athlete to a physician.

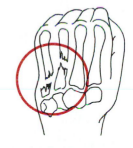

Figure 19-33

Fractures of the metacarpals.

Figure 19-34

The towel twist exercise.

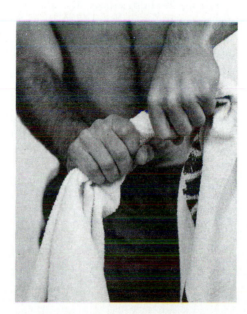

Reconditioning Exercises for the Forearm, Wrist, and Hand

Reconditioning of the hand, wrist, and forearm must commence as early as possible. Immobilization of the forearm or wrist requires that the muscles be exercised almost immediately after an injury occurs if atrophy and contractures are to be prevented. The athlete is not ready for competition until full strength and mobility of the injured joint have been regained. Grip strength is an excellent way to determine the state of reconditioning of the hand, wrist, and forearm. The hand dynamometer may be used to ascertain strength increments during the process of rehabilitation. Full range of movement and strength must be considered for all the major articulations and muscles.

Once ligamentous or tendinous injuries have healed to the point that movement will not disrupt them, active mobilization is performed. Exercise is graduated to increase grip and pinch strength. Some of the following exercises can be used with success. NOTE: All exercises should be performed in a pain-free range of motion. Such exercises should be performed in sets of 10, working toward an ultimate program of three sets of 10, two, or three times daily.

Suggested Forearm and Wrist Exercises

Proper forearm reconditioning is extremely important for injuries to the wrist and hand, as well as the forearm. An excellent beginning exercise is the towel twist, in which the athlete twists the towel in each direction as if wringing out water (Figure 19-34). A wrist roll exercise (Figure 19-35) against resistance is also an excellent forearm, wrist, and hand-strength developer. More specific strength development can be accomplished through the use of a resistance device such as a dumbbell. By stabilizing the bent elbow, the athlete can perform wrist flexion and extension and also forearm pronation and supination.

Wrist strength depends on forearm strength and freedom of movement in the wrist joint. Circumduction exercise helps to maintain joint integrity. Circling must be performed in each direction.

Suggested Hand and Wrist Exercises

Two exercises that are highly beneficial are gripping and spreading (Figure 19-36). Active opening and closing the hand can help reduce hand and/or wrist swelling.

A variety of resistance devices can be used to increase grip strength (Figure 19-37). Grip strength should be routinely monitored in a reconditioning program. A full return of strength is one indication of full recovery.

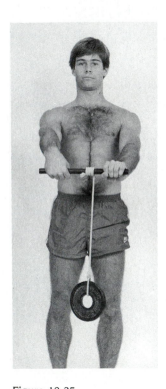

Figure 19-35

Wrist roll.

Figure 19-36

Finger spread and grip.

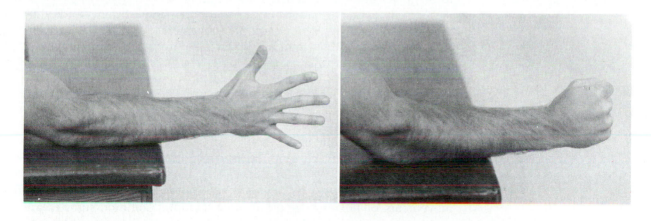

Figure 19-37

Devices for restoring grip
strength.

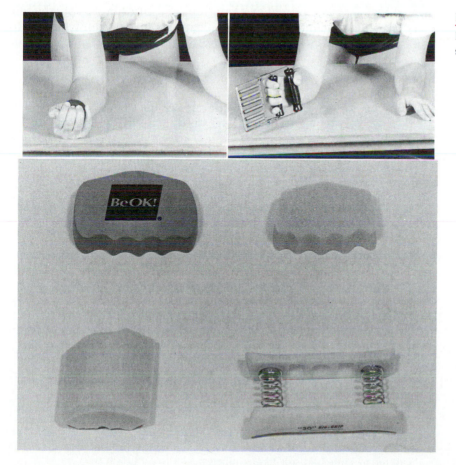

SUMMARY

The upper limb, including the elbow, forearm, wrist, and hand, is second to the lower limb in incidence of sports injuries.

The elbow is anatomically one of the more complex joints in the human body. The elbow joint allows the movements of flexion and extension and the radioulnar joint allows forearm pronation and supination. The major sports injuries of the elbow are contusions, strains, sprains, and dislocations. The chronic strain, which produces the pitcher's, tennis, javelin thrower's and golfer's elbows, is more formally known as epicondylitis.

The forearm is composed of two bones, the ulna and the radius, as well as associated soft tissue. Sports injuries to the region commonly consist of contusions, chronic forearm splints, acute strains, and fractures.

Injuries to the wrist usually occur as the result of a fall or repeated movements of flexion, extension, and rotation. Common injuries are sprains, lunate carpal dislocation, navicular carpal fracture, and hamate fracture.

Injuries to the hand occur frequently in sports activities. Common injuries include those caused by contusions and chronic pressure, by tendons receiving sustained irritation, which leads to tenosynovitis, and by tendon avulsions. Sprains, dislocations, and fractures of the fingers are also common.

REVIEW QUESTIONS AND CLASS ACTIVITIES

1. What are the bony and soft-tissue structures at the elbow? Why is a serious injury so devastating to the hand and wrist?
2. What are some common injuries of the elbow and how should they be managed?
3. How is a dislocation of the elbow managed?
4. What exercises can be used to recondition an injured elbow?
5. What muscles and associated structures are found in the forearm?
6. What are the common injuries of the forearm? What causes them, and how are they managed?
7. What bony and soft-tissue structures are in the wrist and hand?
8. What common injuries may occur in the wrist and hand? What causes them, and how are they managed? Which injuries can lead to serious complications?
9. How does the thumb differ from the other digits?
10. Why are finger and hand problems so often mismanaged?
11. Discuss the different finger injuries that can happen to an athlete. How are they managed? Discuss the pros and cons of reducing a dislocated finger.
12. How can a fracture be ruled out in the hand or fingers?
13. What specific exercises should be included in a total elbow, forearm, wrist, and hand rehabilitation program?
14. Each student should practice on-site injury evaluations at the elbow, forearm, wrist, and hand.
15. Invite a hand specialist to discuss injuries to the hand, serious complications that may arise if they are mishandled, and common surgical procedures that can repair bone and soft-tissue injuries.

REFERENCES

1. Allman FL, Carlson CA: Rehabilitation of elbow injuries. In Nicholas JA, Hershman EB, eds: *The upper extremity in sports medicine*, St Louis, 1990, Mosby-Year Book.
2. Andrews JR, Whiteside JA: Common elbow problems in the athlete, *J Orthop Sports Phys Ther* 17:289, 1993.
3. Bennett JB, Tullos HS: Acute injuries to the elbow. In Nicholas JA, Hershman EB, eds: *The upper extremity in sports medicine*, St Louis, 1990, Mosby-Year Book.
4. Curtis RJ, Corley FG, Jr: Fractures and dislocations of the forearm, *Clin Sports Med* 5, 1986.
5. Culver JE: Instabilities of the wrist, *Clin Sports Med* 5, 1986.
6. Gifeault JD: Mismanaging hand injuries can lead to long-term disability, *First Aider* 56:6, 1987.
7. Harding WG III: Use and misuse of the tennis elbow strap, *Phys Sports Med* 20:65, 1992.
8. Hoffman DF: Elbow dislocations, *Phys Sportsmed* 21:56, 1993.
9. Isani A, Melone CP, Jr: Ligamentous injuries of the hand in athletes, *Clin Sports Med* 5, 1986.
10. Jobe FW, Nuber G: Throwing injuries of the elbow, *Clin Sports Med* 5, 1986.
11. Kiefhaber TR et al: Upper extremity tendinitis and overuse syndrome in the athlete, *Clin Sports Med* 11, 1993.
12. Leach RE, Miller JK: Lateral and medial epicondylitis of the elbow, *Clin Sports Med* 6, 1987.
13. Leddy JP: Athletic injuries to the hand and wrist. *Post graduate advances in sports medicine*, I-IX, Pennington, NJ, 1986, Forum Medicos.
14. Mirabello ST et al: The wrist field evaluation and treatment, *Clin Sports Med* 11, 1992.
15. Nathan R: The jammed finger, *Sports Med Dig* 14:1, 1992.
16. Nirschl RP: Soft-tissue injuries about the elbow, *Clin Sports Med* 5, 1986.
17. Parks JC: Overuse injuries of the elbow. In Nicholas JA, Hershman EB, eds: *The upper extremity in sports medicine*, St Louis, 1990, Mosby-Year Book.
18. Regan WD: Lateral elbow pain in the athlete: a clinical review, *Clin Sports Med* 1:53, 1991.
19. Weinstein SM, Herring SA: Nerve problems and compartment syndromes in the hand, wrist, and forearm, *Clin Sports Med* 11, 1992.
20. Wright CS: Fractures and dislocations in the hand and wrist. In Welsh RP, Shephard RJ, eds: *Current therapy in sports medicine, 1985-1986*, Philadelphia, 1985, BC Decker.

ANNOTATED BIBLIOGRAPHY

Cailliet R: *Hand pain and impairment*, ed 3, Philadelphia, 1982, FA Davis.
  An excellent monograph on hand conditions. It offers a good review of key anatomy and causes of injury and pain.
Morray BF, ed: *The elbow and its disorders*, ed 2, Philadelphia, 1993, WB Saunders.
  A definitive text on biomechanics diagnosis, medical and surgical mechanics of the injured elbow.
Stanley BG, Tribuzi SM, eds: *Concepts in hand rehabilitation*, Philadelphia, 1992, FA Davis.
  A detailed text on all aspects of hand injury management.
Strickland JW, Rettig AC: *Hand injuries in athletics*, Philadelphia, 1992, WB Saunders.
  Covers the basic management of major hand injuries incurred in sports.

Other Health Concerns and the Athlete

When you finish this chapter, you will be able to:

- Explain the causes, preventions, and care of the most common skin infections in sports
- Describe respiratory tract illness common to athletes
- Describe gastrointestinal tract conditions seen in athletes
- Discuss how problems with the diabetic athlete should be avoided
- Discuss contagious viral diseases that may be seen in athletes
- Discuss what a coach should do with an athlete who is having a grandmal seizure
- Discuss the different anemias among athletes
- Contrast the different sexually transmitted diseases that athletes may have
- Discuss concerns of the female athlete in terms of menstruation, osteoporosis, and reproduction
- Explain the many concerns inherent in medical and nonmedical drug use among athletes

In addition to musculoskeletal injuries, the athlete is often exposed to many other common illnesses. Those that will be considered in this chapter include

SKIN INFECTIONS

The skin is the largest organ of the human body. It is composed of three layers—epidermis, dermis, and subcutis (Figure 20-1). The most common skin infections in sports are caused by viruses, bacteria, and fungi.

Viral Infections

Viruses are ultramicroscopic organisms that are parasitic to living cells. Common virus infections are the herpes simplex—labalis (cold sore), genital herpes (type 2 herpes simplex), and gladiatorum (side of the face, neck, or shoulders); the verruca virus (plantar and flat warts); and water warts (molluscum contagiosum).

Bacterial Infections

Bacteria are single-celled plantlike microorganisms that lack chlorophyll. There are three primary forms of bacteria: ovoid, rod-shaped, and spiral. The two types of ovoid forms associated with skin infections are

Common viruses that attack the skin of athletes:
  Herpes
  Verruca
  Molluscum contagiosum

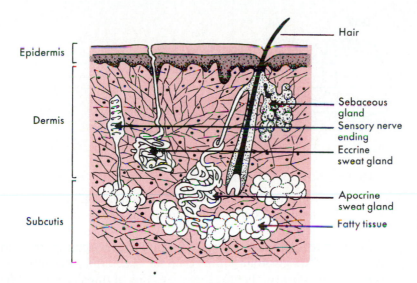

Epidermis
Dermis
Subcutis

Hair

Sebaceous
gland
Sensory nerve
ending
Eccrine
sweat gland

Apocrine
sweat gland
Fatty tissue

Figure 20-1

The skin is the largest organ
of the human body, weighing
6 to 7½ pounds in the adult.

Staphylococci aureus and streptococci (Figure 20-2), which cause impetigo contagiosa, boils, infected hair follicles, and infected sweat glands.

The bacillus bacterium causes a number of serious diseases. Among
them, tetanus is a major concern in athletics. Tetanus (lockjaw) is an
acute disease causing fever and convulsions. Tonic spasm of skeletal
muscles is always a possibility for any nonimmunized athlete. The tetanus bacillus enters an open wound as a spore and depending on individual susceptibility, acts on the motor end plate of the central nervous
system. After initial childhood immunization by tetanus toxoid, boosters
should be given every 10 years. An athlete not immunized should receive an injection of tetanus immune globulin (Hyper-Tet) immediately
after injury.[1]

The spiral bacterial form (spirilla and spirochete) is represented by
the spirochete of syphilis, a very serious venereal disease.

Fungal Infections

Fungi are plantlike organisms that can invade the skin's keratin; the most
common occurrence is ringworm. Ringworm (or tinea) is named for the
area of the infected skin such as tinea capitis (head), tinea corporis (body),
tinea unguium (toenails and fingernails), tinea cruris (jock rash), and
tinea pedis (athlete's foot).

Dermatophytes (Ringworm Fungi)

Dermatophytes, also known as *ringworm fungi,* are the cause of most skin,
nail, and hair fungal infections. Treatment usually consists of a topical
antifungal cream containing 1% clotrimazole.

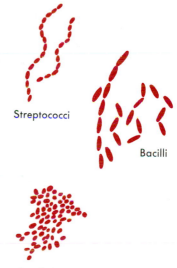

Streptococci

Bacilli

Staphylococci

Figure 20-2

Common disease organisms.

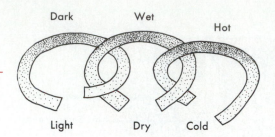

Figure 20-3

When managing a fungal infection, it is essential to break the chain of infection in one or more ways.

Tinea of the Groin (Tinea Cruris)

Tinea of the groin (tinea cruris), more commonly called "jock rash" or "dhobie itch," appears as a bilateral and often symmetrical brownish or reddish lesion resembling the outline of a butterfly in the groin area.

The athlete complains of mild to moderate itching, resulting in scratching and the possibility of a secondary bacterial infection.

Care One must be able to identify lesions of tinea cruris and handle them accordingly. Conditions of this type must be treated until cured (Figure 20-3). Infection not responding to normal management must be referred to the team physician. Most ringworm infections will respond to many of the nonprescription medications that contain such ingredients as undecylenic acid, triacetin, or propionate-caprylate compound, which are available as aerosol sprays, liquids, powders, or ointments. Powder, because of its absorbent qualities, should be the only medication vehicle used in the groin area. Medications that are irritating or tend to mask the symptoms of a groin infection must be avoided.

Athlete's Foot (Tinea Pedis)

The foot is the most common area of the body that is infected by dermatophytes, usually by tinea pedis, or athlete's foot. *Tricophyton mentagrophytes* infect the space between the third and fourth digits and enter the plantar surface of the arch. The same organism attacks toenails. *Trichophyton rubrum* causes scaling and thickening of the soles. The athlete wearing shoes that are enclosed will sweat, encouraging fungal growth. However, contagion is based mainly on the athlete's individual susceptibility. There are other conditions that may also be thought to be athlete's foot such as a dermatitis caused by allergy or an eczema-type skin infection.

Athlete's foot can reveal itself in many ways but appears most often as an extreme itching on the soles of the feet and between and on top of the toes. It appears as a rash, with small pimples or minute blisters that break and exude a yellowish serum (Figure 20-4). Scratching because of itchiness can cause the tissue to become inflamed and infected, manifesting a red, white, or gray scaling of the affected area.

Care Griseofulvin is the most effective management for tinea pedis. Of major importance is good foot hygiene. Topical medications used for tinea corporis can be beneficial (see box on facing page).[12]

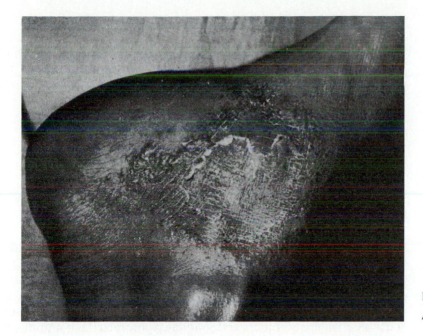

Figure 20-4

Athlete's foot (tinea pedis).

BASIC CARE OF ATHLETE'S FOOT

1. Keep the feet as dry as possible through frequent use of talcum powder.
2. Wear clean white socks to avoid reinfection, changing them daily.
3. Use a standard fungicide for specific medication. "Over-the-counter" medications such as Desenex and Tinactin are useful in the early stages of the infection. For stubborn cases see the team physician; a dermatologist may need to make a culture from foot scrapings to determine the best combatant to be used.

The best cure for the problem of athlete's foot is *prevention*. To keep the condition from spreading to other athletes, the following steps should be faithfully followed by individuals in the sports program:

1. All athletes should powder their feet daily.
2. One should dry the feet thoroughly, especially between and under the toes, after every shower.
3. One should keep sports shoes and street shoes dry by dusting them with powder daily.
4. All athletes should wear clean sports socks and street socks daily.
5. The shower and dressing rooms should be cleaned and disinfected daily.

ILLNESSES OF THE RESPIRATORY TRACT

The respiratory tract is an organ system through which various communicable diseases can be transmitted. It is commonly the port of entry for acute infectious diseases that are spread from person to person or by direct contact. Some of the more prevalent conditions affecting athletes are the common cold, sore throat, asthma, hay fever, and air pollution.

coryza
Profuse nasal discharge

malaise
Discomfort and uneasiness
caused by an illness

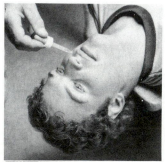

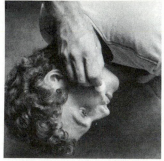

Figure 20-5

Proper applications of nose
drops. **A,** Head tilted back.
B, Head down.

The Common Cold (Coryza)

Upper respiratory tract infections, especially colds and associated conditions, are common in the sports program and can play havoc with entire teams. The common cold is attributed to a filterable virus, which produces an infection of the upper respiratory tract of a susceptible individual.[1]

The susceptible person is believed to be one who has, singly or in combination, any of the following characteristics:
1. Physical debilitation from overwork or lack of sleep
2. Chronic inflammation from a local infection
3. Inflammation of the nasal mucosa from an allergy
4. Inflammation of the nasal mucosa from breathing foreign substances such as dust
5. Sensitivity to stress

The onset of **coryza** is usually rapid; symptoms vary among individuals. The typical effects are a general feeling of **malaise** with an accompanying headache, sneezing, and nasal discharge. Some individuals may register a fever of 100° to 102° F (38° to 39° C) and have chills. Various aches and pains may also accompany the symptoms. The nasal discharge starts as a watery secretion and gradually becomes thick and discolored from the inflammation.[1]

Care Care of the cold is usually symptomatic, with emphasis on isolation, bed rest, and light eating. Palliative mediations include aspirin for relieving general discomfort, rhinitis tablets for drying the secreting mucosa, and nasal drops for an inhaler containing ephedrine to relieve nasal congestion (Figure 20-5). If a cough is present, various syrups may be given to afford relief.

Sore Throat (Pharyngitis)

The sore throat, or pharyngitis, is usually viral, streptococcal, pneumococcal, or staphylococcal. A sore throat usually is the result of postnasal drip associated with a common cold or sinusitis. It may also be an indication of a more serious condition. Frequently it starts as a dryness in the throat and progresses to soreness with pain and swelling. It is sometimes accompanied by a headache, a fever of 101° to 102° F (38° to 39° C), chills, coughing, and a general feeling of fatigue. On examination the throat may appear dark red and swollen, and mucous membranes may be coated.

Care In most cases bed rest is considered the best treatment, combined with symptomatic medications such as aspirin and a hot saltwater gargle. Antibiotics and a silver nitrate throat swab may be used by a physician if other measures are inadequate.

Influenza

Influenza, the "flu," is one of the most persistent and debilitating diseases. It usually occurs in various forms as an annual epidemic, causing severe illness among the populace.

Influenza is caused by myxoviruses classified A, B, and C. The virus enters the tissue's cell through its genetic material. Within the tissue, the virus multiplies and is released from the cell by a budding process, to be spread throughout the body. Not all athletes need influenza vaccines; however athletes engaging in winter sports, as well as basketball, wrestling, and swimming, may require them.

The athlete with the flu will have the following symptoms: fever, cough, headache, malaise, and inflamed respiratory mucous membranes with coryza. It should be noted that certain viruses can increase the body's core temperature. Flu generally has an incubation period of 48 hours and comes on suddenly, accompanied by chills and a fever of 39° to 39.5° C (102° to 103° F), which develops over a 24-hour period. The athlete complains of a headache and general aches and pains—mainly in the back and legs. The headache increases in intensity, along with photophobia and aching at the back of the skull. There is often sore throat, burning in the chest, and in the beginning, a nonproductive cough, which later may develop into bronchitis. The skin is flushed, and the eyes are inflamed and watery. The acute stage of the disease usually lasts up to 5 days. Weakness, sweating, and fatigue may persist for many days. Flu prevention includes staying away from infected persons maintaining good resistance through healthy living and annual vaccines.[27]

Care If the flu is uncomplicated, its management consists of bed rest. During the acute stage, the temperature often returns to normal. Symptomatic care such as aspirin, steam inhalation, cough medicines, and gargles may be given.

Allergic Rhinitis

Hay fever, or pollinosis, is an acute seasonal allergic condition that results from airborne pollens.

rhinitis
Inflammation of the nasal mucous lining

Hay fever can occur during the spring as a reaction to tree pollens such as oak, elm, maple, alder, birch, and cottonwood. During the summer grass and weed pollens can be the culprits. In the fall, ragweed pollen is the prevalent cause. Airborne fungal spores also have been known to cause hay fever.

In the early stages, the athlete's eyes, throat, mouth, and nose begin to itch, followed by watering of the eyes, sneezing, and a clear, watery, nasal discharge. The athlete may complain of a sinus-type headache, emotional irritability, difficulty in sleeping, red and swollen eyes and nasal mucous membranes, and a wheezing cough.[1] It should be noted that other common adverse allergic conditions are asthma, anaphylaxis, urticaria, angioedema, and rhinitis.[2,3,4]

Care Most athletes obtain relief from hay fever through oral antihistamines. To avoid the problem of sedation stemming from these drugs, the athlete may ingest a decongestant during the day and a long-reacting antihistamine before going to bed.

Bronchitis and Asthma

Bronchitis and asthma are two major respiratory problems that bother some athletes. Sports performance can be inhibited by both of these health problems.

Bronchitis (Acute)

An inflammation of the mucous membranes of the "bronchial tubes" is called bronchitis. It occurs in both acute and chronic forms. If occurring in an athlete, bronchitis is more likely to be in the acute form.

Acute bronchitis usually occurs as an infectious winter disease that follows a common cold or other viral infection of the upper respiratory region.[2] Secondary to this inflammation is a bacterial infection that may follow overexposure to air pollution. Fatigue, malnutrition, and/or becoming chilled could be predisposing factors.

The symptoms of an athlete with acute bronchitis usually start with an upper respiratory tract infection, nasal inflammation and profuse discharge, slight fever, sore throat, and back and muscle pains. A cough signals the beginning of bronchitis. In the beginning, the cough is dry, but in a few hours or days, a clear mucous secretion begins, becoming yellowish, indicating an infection. In most cases, the fever lasts 3 to 5 days, and the cough lasts 2 to 3 weeks or longer. The athlete may wheeze and rale when auscultation of the chest is performed. Pneumonia could complicate bronchitis.

To avoid bronchitis, it is advisable that an athlete not sleep in an area that is extremely cold or exercise in extremely cold air without wearing a face mask to warm inhaled air.

Care Management of acute bronchitis involves rest until fever subsides, drinking 3 to 4 L of water per day, and ingesting an antipyretic analgesic, a cough suppressor, and an antibiotic (when severe lung infection is present) daily.

Asthma

As one of the most common respiratory diseases, bronchial asthma can be produced from a number of stressors such as a viral respiratory tract infection, emotional upset, changes in barometric pressure or temperature, exercise, inhalation of a noxious odor, or exposure to a specific allergen.

Bronchial asthma is characterized by a spasm of the bronchial smooth muscles, edema, and inflammation of the mucous lining. In addition to asthma's narrowing of the airway, copious amounts of mucus are produced. Difficulty in breathing may cause the athlete to hyperventilate, resulting in dizziness. The attack may begin with coughing, wheezing, shortness of breath, and fatigue (see box).

Exercise-Induced Bronchial Obstruction (Asthma)

Etiology Exercise-induced bronchial obstruction is also known as *exercise-induced asthma (EIA)*. It is a disease that occurs almost exclusively

MANAGEMENT OF THE ACUTE ASTHMATIC ATTACK

Athletes who have a history of asthma usually know how to care for themselves when attack occurs. However, the athletic trainer must be aware of what to look for and what to do if called on.

Early Symptoms and Signs

Anxious appearance
Sweating and paleness
Flared nostrils
Breathing with pursed lips
Fast breathing
Vomiting
Hunched-over body posture
Physical fatigue unrelated to activity
Indentation in the notch below the Adam's apple
Sinking in of rib spaces as the athlete inhales
Coughing for no apparent reason
Excess throat clearing
Irregular, labored breathing or wheezing

Actions to Take

Attempt to relax and reassure the athlete.
If medication has been cleared by the team physician, have the athlete use it.
Encourage the athlete to drink water.
Have the athlete perform controlled breathing along with relaxation exercises.
If an environmental factor triggering the attack is known, remove it or the athlete from the area.
If these procedures do not help, immediate medical attention may be necessary.

in asthmatic persons.[28] An asthmatic attack can be stimulated by exercise in some individuals and can be provoked in others, only on rare occasions, during moderate exercise. The exact cause of EIA is not clear. Loss of heat and water causes the greatest loss of airway reactivity. Eating certain foods such as shrimp, celery, and peanuts can cause EIA. Sinusitis can also trigger an attack in an individual with chronic asthma.[20]

The athlete with EIA often displays an airway narrowing caused by bronchial-wall thickening and excess production of mucus. Athletes who have a chronic inflammatory asthmatic condition (bronchiectasis) characteristically have a constant dilation of the bronchi and/or bronchioles.

The athlete with EIA may show signs of swelling of the face (angioedema), swelling of the palms and soles of the feet, nausea, hypertension, diarrhea, fatigue, itching, respiratory stridor (high-pitched noise on respiration), headaches, and redness of the skin.[27]

Care Long continuous running causes the most severe bronchospasm. Swimming is the least bronchospasm producing, which may be a result of the moist, warm air environment. It is generally agreed that a

The athlete undergoing a sudden attack should
  Be relaxed and reassured
  Use a previously specified medication
  Drink water
  Perform controlled breathing
  Be removed from what might be triggering the attack

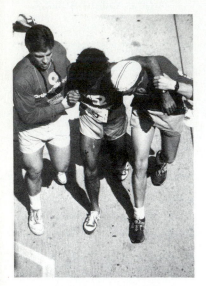

Figure 20-6

Long, continuous activity rather than intermittent activity causes most severe exercise-induced asthma.

A balanced diet is as important as brushing the teeth in preventing gum disease.

regular exercise program can benefit asthmatics and nonasthmatics. Fewer symptoms occur with short intense work followed by rest, as compared to sustained exercise. There should be gradual warm-up and cool down. The duration of exercise should build slowly to 30 to 40 minutes, four or five times a week. Exercise intensity and loading also should be graduated slowly. An example would be 10 to 30 seconds of work, followed by 30 to 90 seconds of rest.[22] Many athletes with chronic and/or EIA use the inhaled bronchodilator. Inhalation of B_2 agonists such as metaproterenol theophylline and its derivatives and cromolyn sodium relax bronchial smooth muscles and inhibit the chemical mediators of asthma. Metered-dose inhalers are preferred for administration.[22] It has also been found that prophylactic use of the bronchodilator 15 minutes before exercise delays the symptoms by 2 to 4 hours.[17] Asthmatic athletes who receive medication for their condition should make sure that what they take is legal for competition (Figure 20-6).

Exercise-Induced Bronchospasm

EIB (exercise-induced bronchospasm) is seen in individuals with chronic asthma and about half of those athletes having allergies. Bronchospasm is typical 5 to 15 minutes after cessation of physical activity with a spontaneous recovery in 20 to 60 minutes. The cause of EIB is a combination of airway cooling and drying of the airway. Prevention is a gradual pre-exercise warming and/or administration of a beta adrenergic agonist or other drug.

GASTROINTESTINAL TRACT CONDITIONS

Like any other individual, the athlete may develop various complaints of the digestive system as a result of poor eating habits or the stress engendered from competition. The responsibility of the coach in such cases is to be able to recognize the more severe conditions so that early referrals to a physician can be made. The following discussion of the digestive system disorders that are common in sports provides information on how to (1) give proper counsel to the athlete about the prevention of mouth and intestinal disorders, (2) recommend a proper diet, and (3) recognize deviations from the normal in these areas.

Mouth Disorders

Many different conditions involving the mouth appear during the course of a regular training program. Of them, the most commonly observed is dental caries (tooth decay), which is indicated by local decalcification of the tooth. Tooth decay is the result of an increase in mouth acids, usually from food fermentation. Proper oral hygiene is necessary and should include the following: (1) eating wholesome foods and (2) brushing the teeth properly immediately after meals.

The greatest single cause of tooth loss is gum disease. Infections associated with dental caries and gum disease can completely debilitate an athlete. Therefore an immediate referral to a dentist is important.

Indigestion (Dyspepsia)

Some athletes have certain food idiosyncrasies that cause them considerable distress after eating. Others develop reactions when eating before competition. The term given to digestive upset is *indigestion (dyspepsia)*.

Indigestion can be caused by any number of conditions. The most common in sports are emotional stress, esophageal and stomach spasms, and/or inflammation of the mucous lining of the esophagus and stomach.

These conditions cause an increased secretion of hydrochloric acid (sour stomach), nausea, and flatulence (gas).

Care   Care of acute dyspepsia involves the elimination of irritating foods from the diet, development of regular eating habits, and avoidance of anxieties that may lead to gastric distress.

Constant irritation of the stomach may lead to chronic and more serious disorders such as gastritis, an inflammation of the stomach wall, or ulcerations of the gastrointestinal mucosa. Athletes who appear nervous and high-strung and suffer from dyspepsia should be examined by the sports physician.

Diarrhea

Diarrhea is abnormal stool looseness or passage of a fluid, unformed stool and is categorized as acute or chronic, according to the type present.

Diarrhea can be caused by problems in diet, inflammation of the intestinal lining, gastrointestinal infection, ingestion of certain drugs, or even stress.

Diarrhea is characterized by abdominal cramps, nausea, and possibly vomiting, coupled with frequent elimination of stools, ranging from 3 to 20 a day. The infected person often has a loss of appetite and a light brown or gray, foul-smelling stool. Extreme weakness caused by fluid dehydration is usually present.

Diarrhea could lead to fluid dehydration.

Care   The cause of diarrhea is often difficult to establish. It is conceivable that any irritant may cause the loose stool. This can include an infestation of parasitic organisms or an emotional upset. Management of diarrhea requires a knowledge of its cause. Less severe cases can be cared for by (1) omitting foods that cause irritation, (2) drinking boiled milk, (3) eating bland food until symptoms have ceased, and (4) using pectins (such as apples) two or three times daily for the absorption of excess fluid.

Constipation

Some athletes are subject to constipation, the failure of the bowels to evacuate feces.

There are numerous causes of constipation, the most common of which are (1) lack of abdominal muscle tone, (2) insufficient moisture in the feces, causing it to be hard and dry, (3) lack of a sufficient proportion of roughage and bulk in the diet to stimulate peristalsis, (4) poor bowel habits, (5) nervousness and anxiety, and (6) overuse of laxatives and enemas.

Laxatives and enemas should not be used to relieve constipation.

The best means of overcoming constipation is to regulate eating patterns to include foods that will encourage normal defecation. Cereals, fruits, vegetables, and fats stimulate bowel movement, whereas sugars and carbohydrates tend to inhibit it. Some persons become constipated as the result of psychological factors. In such cases it may be helpful to try to determine the causes of stress and, if need be, to refer the athlete to a physician or school psychologist for counseling. Above all, laxatives or enemas should be avoided unless their use has been prescribed by a physician.

Hemorrhoids (Piles)

Hemorrhoids are varicosities of hemorrhoidal veins related to the anus. There are both internal and external anal veins.

Chronic constipation or straining at the stool may tend to stretch the anal veins, resulting in either a protrusion (prolapse) and bleeding of the internal or external veins or a **thrombus** in the external veins.

Often hemorrhoids are painful nodular swellings near the sphincter of the anus. There may be slight bleeding and itching. The majority of hemorrhoids are self-limiting and spontaneously heal within 2 to 3 weeks.

thrombus

blood clot that blocks small blood vessels or a cavity of the heart

DIABETES MELLITUS

Diabetes mellitus is a complex hereditary or developmental disease of carbohydrate metabolism. Decreased effectiveness of insulin or an insufficient amount is responsible for most cases. Until recently diabetics were usually discouraged from or forbidden competitive sports participation. Today an ever-increasing number of diabetics are active sports participants, functioning effectively in almost all sports. Since the key to the control of diabetes is the control of blood sugar, the insulin-dependent athlete must constantly juggle food intake, insulin, and exercise to maintain the blood sugar in its proper range if he or she is to perform to maximum. Diet, exercise, and insulin are the major factors in the everyday life-style of the diabetic athlete, who out of necessity must develop an ordered and specific living pattern to cope with the demands of daily existence and strenuous physical activity.

Diabetic athletes engaging in vigorous physical activity should eat before exercising and if the exercise is protracted, should have hourly glucose supplementation. As a rule the insulin dosage is not changed, but food intake is increased. The response of diabetics varies among individuals and depends on many variables. Although there are some hazards, with proper medical evaluation and planning by a consultant in metabolic diseases, diabetics can feel free to engage in most physical activities.

Management of the Diabetic Coma and Insulin Shock

It is important that those who work with athletes who have diabetes mellitus are aware of the major symptoms of diabetic coma and insulin shock and the proper actions to take when either one occurs.

Diabetic Coma

Without proper diet and intake of insulin, the diabetic athlete can develop acidosis. A loss of sodium, potassium, and ketone bodies through excessive urination produces ketoacidosis that can lead to coma. The signs of a diabetic coma include the following:

- Labored breathing or gasping for air
- Fruity-smelling breath caused by acetone
- Nausea and vomiting
- Thirst
- Dry mucous lining of the mouth and flushed skin
- Mental confusion or unconsciousness followed by coma

Care Because the diabetic coma threatens life, early detection of ketoacidosis is essential. The injection of insulin into the athlete will normally prevent coma.

Insulin Shock

Unlike diabetic coma, insulin shock occurs when too much insulin is taken into the body, resulting in hypoglycemia and shock. It is characterized by the following:

- Physical weakness
- Moist and pale skin
- Drooping eyelids
- Normal or shallow respirations

Care The diabetic athlete who engages in intense exercise and metabolizes large amounts of glycogen may inadvertently take too much insulin and thus have a severe reaction. To avoid this problem the athlete must adhere to a carefully planned diet that includes a snack before exercise. The snack should contain a combination of a complex carbohydrate and protein such as in cheese and crackers. Activities that last for more than 30 to 40 minutes should be accompanied by snacks and simple carbohydrates. Some diabetics carry with them a lump of sugar or have candy or orange juice readily available in the event an insulin reaction seems imminent.

Key questions to ask a diabetic athlete are the following:

1. Have you eaten today and when?
2. Have you taken your insulin today and when?

COMMON CONTAGIOUS VIRAL DISEASES

It is not within the scope of this text to describe in detail all the various infectious diseases to which athletes maybe prone. However, on occasion an athlete may exhibit recognizable symptoms of such a disease; one should know the symptoms and be able to identify them (Table 20-1). A player or other athlete with such symptoms should be referred to a physician without delay.

The virus is an extremely small organism that is visible only with an electron microscope. Viruses are a parasitic mode of **DNA** or **RNA** and reside in a cell. Along with the cell, viruses are provided with nutrition and their reproductive needs by the host systems.

TABLE 20-1 Some infectious viral diseases

Disease	Sites Involved	Mode of Transmission	Incubation Period	Chief Symptoms	Duration	Period of Contagion	Treatment	Prophylaxis
Measles (rubeola)	Skin, respiratory tract, and conjunctivae	Contact or droplet	7-14 days	Appearance—like common cold with fever, cough, conjunctivitis, photophobia, and spots in throat, followed by skin rash	4-7 days after symptoms appear	Just before coldlike symptoms through approximately 1 week after rash appears	Bed rest and use of smoked glasses; symptomatic	Vaccine available
German measles (rubella)	Skin, respiratory tract, and conjunctivae	Contact or droplet	14-21 days	Cold symptoms, skin rash, and swollen lymph nodes behind ear	1-2 days	2-4 days before rash through 5 days afterward	Symptomatic	Vaccine available; gamma globulin given in postexposure situations
Chicken pox (varicella)	Trunk; then face, neck and limbs	Contact or droplet	14-21 days	Mild cold symptoms followed by appearance of vesicles	1-2 weeks	1 day before onset through 6 days afterward	Symptomatic	Vaccine available, including zoster immune globulin (ZIG) or varicell-zoster immune globulin (VZIG)

Mumps (epidemic parotiditis)	Salivary glands	Prolonged contact or droplet	18-21 days	Headache, drowsiness, fever, abdominal pain, pain during chewing and swallowing, swelling of neck under jaw	10 days	1 week	Symptomatic	Temporary immunization by virus vaccine
Influenza (flu)	Respiratory tract	Droplet	1-2 days	Aching of low back, generalized aching, chills, headache, fever, and bronchitis	2-5 days	2-3 days	Symptomatic	Moderate temporary protection from polyvalent influenza virus
Cold (coryza)	Respiratory tract	Droplet	12 hours to 4 days	Mild fever, headache, chills, and nasal discharge	1-2 weeks	Not clearly identified	Symptomatic	Possible help from vitamins and/or cold vaccine; avoid exposure
Infectious mononucleosis	Trunk	Contact	4-7 weeks	Sore throat, fever, skin rash, general aching, and swelling of lymph glands	3-4 weeks	Low rate	Symptomatic	None; avoid extreme fatigue

More than 300 viruses have been isolated, some of which are harmless to humans. But others are related to infectious diseases such as the common cold, most childhood diseases, and a majority of the upper respiratory tract diseases. Infectious mononucleosis or "mono" is a common occurrence among athletes and is associated with Epstein-Barr virus.[10] Of special concern to the athletic population is the viral diseases of Hepatitis B and HIV producing AIDS (acquired immune deficiency syndrome). See p. 539.

Hepatitis B Infection

The B virus can produce a wide number of liver diseases. Virus B can be transmitted through intravenous, subcutaneous, intramuscular or mucosal routes. An athlete may be a chronic carrier. Incubation is about 4 to 25 weeks.

Hepatitis B infection varies from a minor flu-type illness to one that occurs rapidly a great strength to one that leads to fatal liver failure. Loss of appetite, physical discomfort, nausea and vomiting. A skin rash may occur. Later a dark-colored urine and yellowing of the skin and joint pain occur. Recovery, if uncomplicated, is 4 to 8 weeks.

Care   In most cases no special treatment is necessary. Appetite usually returns after a few days. The physician should clear the athlete for return to his or her sport. A vaccine consisting of immune globulin is available to prevent hepatitis B. It used to vaccinate individuals who may come in contact with persons who are carriers of the hepatitis B virus or with blood or bodily fluids.

It should be noted that hepatitis lasting for 6 months is considered to be chronic. Chronic hepatitis can be one that is persistent without major symptoms. An aggressive chronic hepatitis could, on the other hand, lead an eventual liver failure.

CONVULSIVE DISORDERS (EPILEPSY)

epilepsy
Recurrent paroxymal disorder characterized by sudden attacks of altered consciousness, motor activity, sensory phenomena, or inappropriate behavior

Epilepsy is not a disease but is a symptom that can be manifested by a large number of underlying disorders. **Epilepsy** is defined as "a recurrent paroxysmal disorder of cerebral function characterized by a sudden, brief attack of altered consciousness, motor activity, sensory phenomena, or inappropriate behavior."[1]

For some types of epilepsy there is a genetic predisposition and a low threshold to having seizures. In others, altered brain metabolism or a history of injury may be the cause. A seizure can range from extremely brief episodes (petit mal seizures) to major episodes (grand mal seizures), unconsciousness, and tonic-clonic muscle contractions.

Each person with epilepsy must be considered individually as to whether he or she should engage in competitive sports. It is generally agreed that if an individual has daily or even weekly major seizures, collision sports should be prohibited. This prohibition is not because hitting the head will necessarily trigger a seizure, but that unconsciousness during participation could result in a serious injury. If the seizures are properly controlled by medication or only occur during sleep, little, if any,

For individuals who have major daily or weekly seizures, collision-type sports may be prohibited.

sports restriction should be imposed except for scuba diving, swimming alone, or participation at a great height.[1]

Care   The athlete who commonly takes a anticonvulsant medication that is specific for the type and degree of seizures that occur. On occasions the athlete may experience some undesirable side effects from drug therapy such as drowsiness, restlessness, nystagmus, nausea, vomiting, problems with balance, skin rash, or other adverse reactions.

When an athlete with epilepsy becomes aware of an impending seizure measures should be taken to avoid injury such as immediately sitting or lying down. When a seizure occurs without warning, the following steps should be taken by the athletic trainer:

Be emotionally composed.

If possible, cushion the athlete's fall.

Keep the athlete away from injury-producing objects.

Loosen restricting clothing.

Prevent the athlete from biting the mouth by placing a soft cloth between the teeth.

Allow the athlete to awaken normally after the seizure.

ANEMIA IN ATHLETES

Athletes who engage in aerobic exercise generally experience a mild lowering of their **hemoglobin** concentration. It is not considered an adverse condition but one that is an adaptation to aerobic exercise. This occurrence may be noted in individuals immediately following exercise and is not true anemia. Another adaptation to exercise that is found in elite athletes is an increase in red cell mass.

hemoglobin
Coloring substance of red blood cells

Iron-Deficiency Anemia

Iron deficiency is the most common form of true anemia among athletes.

Three conditions occur during anemia: erythrocytes (red blood cells) are too small or too large, hemoglobin is decreased, and ferritin concentration is low. Ferritin is an iron-phosphorous-protein complex that normally contains 23% iron.

In the first stages of iron deficiency, the athlete's performance begins to decline. The athlete may complain of burning thighs and nausea from becoming anaerobic. Ice craving is also common. Athletes with mild iron-deficiency anemia may display some mild impairment in their maximum performance. Determining serum ferritin is the most accurate test of iron status. Two factors must be checked by the physician: (1) the athlete's mean corpuscular volume (MCV), which is the average volume of individual cells in a cubic micron, and (2) the relative sizes of the erythrocytes.

Care   For men, iron deficiency is usually caused by blood loss in the gastrointestinal tract. For women, the most common causes are menstruation and not enough iron in the diet. If the athlete is a vegetarian, he or she might lack iron. Aspirin or stress can irritate the gastrointestinal tract. The following are some ways to manage iron deficiency: (1) ensure proper diet, including more red meat or dark chicken; (2) avoid coffee or tea, which hampers iron absorption from grains; (3) ingest vitamin C sources, which enhance iron absorption; and (4) take an iron supplement, consisting of ferrous sulfate, 325 mg, three times per week.

Sickle Cell Anemia

Sickle cell anemia is a chronic hereditary hemolytic anemia. Approximately 35% of the black population in the United States has this condition; 8% to 13% are not anemic but carry this trait in their genes (sicklemia). The person with the sickle cell trait may participate in sports and never encounter problems until symptoms are brought on by some unusual circumstance.

In individuals with sickle cell anemia the red cells are sickle- or crescent-shaped. Within the red cells, an abnormal type of hemoglobin exists. It has been speculated that the sickling of the red blood cells results from an adaptation to malaria, which is prevalent in Africa. It is a recessive trait that is not sex-linked but is found in both parents.[18]

The sickle cell has less potential for transporting oxygen and is fragile when compared to normal cells. A sickle cell's life span is 15 to 25 days, compared to the 120 days of a normal red cell; this short life of the sickle cell can produce severe anemia in individuals with acute sickle cell anemia. The cell's distorted shape inhibits its passage through the small blood vessels and can cause clustering of the cells and, consequently, clogging of the blood vessels, producing **thrombi,** which block circulation. For individuals having this condition, death can occur (in the severest cases of sickle cell anemia) from a stroke, heart disease, or an **embolus** in the lungs. Conversely, persons with sickle cell anemia may never experience any problems.

An athlete may never experience any complications from having the sickle cell trait. However, a sickle cell crisis can be brought on by exposure to high altitudes or by overheating of the skin, as is the case with a high fever. Crisis symptoms include fever, severe fatigue, skin pallor, muscle weakness, and severe pain in the limbs and abdomen. Abdominal pain in the right upper quadrant may indicate a splenic syndrome in which there is an infarction. This is especially characteristic of a crisis triggered by a decrease in ambient oxygen while flying at high altitudes. The athlete may also experience headache and convulsions.

Care   Treatment of a sickle cell crisis is usually symptomatic. The physician may elect to give anticoagulants and analgesics for pain.

SEXUALLY TRANSMITTED DISEASES

Sexually transmitted diseases are of major concern in sports because many athletes are at an age during which they are more sexually active than they will be at any other time in their life. The venereal diseases with the highest incidence among the relatively young are nonspecific sexually transmitted infection (NSI), genital herpes, gonorrhea, genital candidiasis, condyloma acuminata (venereal warts), and acquired immune deficiency syndrome (AIDS).

thrombi
Plural of thrombus

emboli
Plural of embolus

Nonspecific Sexually Transmitted Infection

Nonspecific sexually transmitted infection (NSI), although not required to be reported to health officials, is considered by many the most common venereal disease in the United States. It is more common than gonorrhea.[1]

The two organisms associated with NSI are **Chlamydia trachomatis** and *Ureaplasma urealyticum*. NSI is most commonly called chlamydia.

In the male, inflammation occurs along with a purulent discharge, 7 to 28 days after intercourse.[1] On occasion, painful urination and traces of blood in the urine occur. Most females with this infection are asymptomatic, but some may experience a vaginal discharge, painful urination, pelvic pain, and pain and inflammation in other sites.

Care A bacteriological examination is given to determine the exact organism(s) present. Once identified, the infection must be treated promptly to prevent complications. Organism identification and treatment must take place immediately in women who are pregnant. Chlamydial opthalmia neonatorum can cause conjunctivitis and pneumonia in the newborn from an infected mother.[2] Uncomplicated cases are usually treated with antibiotics. Approximately 20% of the sufferers have one or more relapses.

Chlamydia trachomatis
A genus microorganism that can cause a wide variety of diseases in humans, one of which is venereal and causes nonspecific urethritis.

Genital Herpes

Genital herpes is a venereal infection that is currently widespread among the populace.

Type 2 herpes simplex virus is associated with genital herpes infection, which is now the most prevalent cause of genital ulcerations. Signs of the disease appear approximately 4 to 7 days after sexual contact.

The first signs in the male are itching and soreness, but women may be asymptomatic in the vagina and cervix. It is estimated that 50% to 60% of individuals who have had one attack of herpes genitalis will have no further episodes, or if they do, the lesions are few and insignificant. Like herpes labialis and gladiatorum, lesions develop that eventually become ulcerated with a red areola. Ulcerations crust and heal in approximately 10 days, leaving a scar.

Of major importance to a pregnant woman with a history of genital herpes is whether there is an active infection when she is nearing delivery. Herpes simplex can be fatal to a newborn child. There is also some relationship (although this is unclear) between a higher incidence of cervical cancer and the incidence of herpes genitalis.[1]

Care At this time there is no cure for genital herpes. Recently systemic medication, specifically antiviral medications such as acycloguanosine (Zovirax, Acyclovir) and vidarabine (Vira-A), are being used to lessen the early symptoms of the disease.[1]

Gonorrhea

Gonorrhea, commonly called "clap," is an acute venereal disease that can infect the urethra, cervix, and rectum.

The organism of infection is the gonococcal bacteria *Neisseria gonorrhoeae,* which is usually spread through sexual intercourse.

In men the incubation period is 2 to 10 days. The onset of the disease is marked by a tingling sensation in the urethra, followed in 2 or 3 hours by greenish-yellow discharge of pus and painful urination. Sixty percent of infected women are asymptomatic. For those who have symptoms, onset is between 7 and 21 days. In these cases symptoms are very mild with some vaginal discharge. Gonorrheal infection of the throat and rectum are also possible.

Because of embarrassment some individuals fail to secure proper medical help for treatment of gonorrhea, and, although the initial symptoms will disappear, such an individual is not cured and can still spread the infection. Untreated gonorrhea becomes latent and will manifest itself in later years, usually causing sterility and/or arthritis. Treatment consists of large amounts of penicillin or other antibiotics. Evidence of any of the symptoms should result in immediately remanding the individual to a physician for testing and treatment. *All sexual contact must be avoided* until it has been medically established that the disease is no longer active. Because of the latent residual effects that are the end result of several diseases in this group, including sterility and arthritis, immediate medical treatment is mandatory. Although outward signs may disappear, the disease is still insidiously present in the body. Additionally, such treatment will alleviate the discomfort that accompanies the initial stages of the disease.

Care Penicillin in high doses is usually the drug of choice. Other antibiotics may be used if the strain of bacteria is resistant to penicillin.

Trichomoniasis

Trichomoniasis is an infection that affects 20% of all females during their reproductive years, and 5% to 10% of males.

Trichomoniasis is caused by the flagellate protozoan *Trichomonas vaginalis.*

The female with trichomoniasis typically has a vaginal discharge that is greenish-yellow and frothy. The disease causes irritation of the vulva, perineum, and thighs. The female may also experience painful urination. Males are usually asymptomatic, although some may experience a frothy, purulent urethral discharge.

Care Metronidazole, taken for 7 days, is usually the drug of choice in the treatment of trichomoniasis. Complete cure is required before the individual can again engage in sexual intercourse.

Genital Candidiasis

Skin Disorders, Candida (a genus of yeastlike fungi) is commonly part of the normal flora of the mouth, skin, intestinal tract, and vagina.

The *Candida* organism is one of the most common causes of vaginitis in women of reproductive age. The infection is usually transmitted sexually but also can stem from the intestine.

As with other related conditions, the female complains of vulval ir-

> Trichomoniasis affects 20% of all females and 5% to 10% of all males.

ritation beginning with redness and severe pain, and a vaginal discharge (scanty). The male is usually asymptomatic but could develop some irritation and soreness of the glans penis, especially after intercourse. Rarely, a slight urethral discharge may occur.

Care Because of the highly infectious nature of this disease, all sexual contact should cease until completion of treatment. The drug nystatin (a fungicide) is usually inserted high into the vagina for 14 nights at bedtime. This treatment is immediately followed by application of nystatin cream to the labia, perineum, and perianal region.

Condyloma Acuminata (Veneral Warts)

Another sexually transmitted disease that should be recognized and referred to a physician is condyloma acuminata or venereal warts.

Etiology These warts are transmitted through sexual activity and commonly occur from poor hygiene. They appear on the glans penis, vulva, or anus.

Symptoms and signs This form of wart virus produces nodules that have a cauliflower-like lesion or can be singular. In their early stage they are soft, moist, pink or red swellings that rapidly develop a stem with a flowerlike head.

Care Moist condylomas are often carefully treated by the physician with a solution containing 20% to 25% podophyllin. Dry warts may be treated with a freezing process such as liquid nitrogen.

Acquired Immune Deficiency Syndrome (AIDS)

AIDS is a viral disease that attacks the T-helper lymphocytes of the immune system. This organism is known as *HIV*, or *human immunodeficiency virus*. It destroys the ability to defend against a variety of infections. Victims of AIDS are susceptible to infections caused by bacteria, protozoa, fungi, certain viruses, and cancers. A less severe condition is known as *AIDS-related complex*, or *ARC*.

At the beginning of infection a person with AIDS may feel healthy. It may take 10 years or longer for the disease to develop, or it may never develop at all. Infection, however, will last for a lifetime.

There are four main ways that AIDS can be contracted: sexual activity with an infected partner; sharing needles or syringes with an infected person; receiving infected blood during a transfusion; and from an infected mother, who may pass AIDS to her unborn child.

AIDS is not spread through casual contact. It cannot be contracted through hugging, shaking hands, using toilets, sinks, bathtubs, or swimming pools, sneezing, coughing, or spitting on someone, or by using objects used by a person infected with AIDS.[18]

AIDS can produce varying degrees of sickness that may consist of fever and night sweats, weight loss, swollen lymph glands in the neck, underarm, or groin, unusual fatigue, diarrhea, and/or white spots in the mouth. Anyone with one or more of these symptoms lasting longer than 2 weeks should see a physician.

Care The main means of managing AIDS is prevention (see box

AIDS is a fatal disease that attacks the body's immune system.

REDUCING THE RISK OF AIDS

1. Know your sex partner's name and address.
2. Limit the number of sex partners.
3. Consistently use condoms.
4. Avoid contact with others' body fluids, feces, and semen.
5. Curtail use of drugs that alter good judgment.
6. Never share hypodermic needles.
7. Avoid sex with drug abusers.
8. Avoid sex with AIDS victims, with those having symptoms and signs of AIDS, and with high-risk persons.
9. Get regular tests for STD infections.
10. Avoid inserting any foreign object into the rectum.
11. Practice good hygiene before and after sex.

above). Identifying AIDS-infected individuals through blood testing can help to prevent the spread of infection. There now is no cure or vaccine for AIDS. Some drugs such as azidothimidine (AZT), can help to alleviate symptoms or inhibit the multiplication of the virus.

It should be noted that every athletic training facility should have a infection control policy.[18] Latex surgical gloves are recommended at all times when the athletic trainer is exposed to mucous membrane secretions, noncontact skin, or any materials contaminated by blood or body fluids. Major caution should be taken to avoid needle or scalpel introjection to the body. All training room tables and other surfaces should be routinely cleansed with 10% bleach solution.[18]

It is extremely important that coaches and athletic trainers are fully aware of the general symptoms and signs, as well as the management, of venereal diseases. An athlete who is concerned about having contracted a venereal disease will often ask a coach or athletic trainer, "What does it look like when you have it?" or "What should one do if he or she thinks he or she has it?" As with recreational drugs, all sports programs should provide opportunities for education and counseling, as well as immediate medical referral, for an athlete with the possibility of a venereal disease.

MENSTRUAL IRREGULARITIES AND THE FEMALE REPRODUCTIVE SYSTEM

Because women in the United States participate more in sports and are training harder than ever before in history, the question arises as to what impact these factors have on menstruation and reproduction.

Prepubertal and Pubertal Factors

During the prepubertal period, girls are the equal of, and often superior to, boys of the same age in activities requiring speed, strength, and endurance. The difference between men and women is not too apparent

During the prepubertal period, girls are the equal of, and often superior to, boys of the same age in activities requiring speed, strength, and endurance.

until after puberty. With the advent of puberty the gulf begins to widen, with the males continuing in a slower, gradual increase in strength, speed, and endurance.

Menarche

Menarche, the onset of the menses, normally occurs between the tenth and the seventeenth year, with the majority of girls usually entering it between 13 and 15 years.[20]

There is some indication that strenuous training and competition may delay the onset of menarche. The greatest delay is related to the higher-caliber competition. The late-maturing girl commonly has longer legs, narrower hips, and less adiposity and body weight for her height, all of which are more conducive to sports.

The onset of menarche may be delayed by strenuous training and competition.

Menstruation

As interest and participation in girls' and women's sports grow, the various myths that have surrounded female participation and the effects of participation on menarche, menstruation, and childbirth are gradually being dispelled. Although the effects of sustained and strenuous training and competition on the menstrual cycle and the effects of menstruation on performance still cannot be fully explained.

Menstruation and Its Irregularities

Menarche may be delayed in highly physically active women. **Amenorrhea** (absence of menses) and oligomenorrhea (diminished flow) have been common in professional female ballet dancers, gymnasts, and long-distance runners.[6] Runners who decrease training, such as when they have an injury, often report a return of regular menses. Weight gain, together with less intense exercise, also are reported to reverse amenorrhea and oligomenorrhea. Because these irregularities may or may not be normal aspects of thinness and hard physical training, it is advisable that a physician be consulted. To date, there is no indication that these conditions will adversely affect reproduction. Almost any type of menstrual disorder can be caused by overly stressful and demanding sports activity—amenorrhea, dysmenorrhea, menorrhagia (excessive menstruation), oligomenorrhea, polymenorrhea (abnormal frequent menstruation), irregular periods, or any combination of these.

amenorrhea
Absence or suppression of menstruation

In general, childbirth is not adversely affected by a history of hard physical exercise.

Currently no experimental evidence indicates that sports training can delay menarche.[34] In general, menarche is not delayed but normally occurs later in some athletes.[34]

Dysmenorrhea

Dysmenorrhea (painful menstruation) apparently is prevalent among more active women; however, it is inconclusive whether specific sports participation can alleviate or produce dysmenorrhea. For women with moderate-to-severe dysmenorrhea gynecological consultation is warranted to rule out a pathological condition.[31]

Women who have moderate-to-severe dysmenorrhea require examination by a physician.

Dysmenorrhea is caused by ischemia (a lack of normal blood flow to the pelvic organs) or by a possible hormonal imbalance.[31] This syndrome, which is identified by cramps, nausea, lower abdominal pain, headache, and on occasion emotional lability, is the most common menstrual disorder. Mild-to-vigorous exercises that help ameliorate dysmenorrhea are usually prescribed by physicians. Physicians generally advise a continuance of the usual sports participation during the menstrual period, provided the performance level of the individual does not drop below her customary level of ability. Among athletes, swimmers have the highest incidence of dysmenorrhea; it, along with **menorrhagia,** occurs most often, quite probably as the result of strenuous sports participation during the menses. Generally, oligomenorrhea, amenorrhea, and irregular or scanty flow are more common in sports that require strenuous exertion over a long period of time. Because great variation exists among female athletes in respect to the menstrual pattern, its effect on physical performance, and the effect of physical activity on the menstrual pattern, each individual must learn to make adjustments to her cycle that will permit her to function effectively and efficiently with a minimum of discomfort or restriction.

Bone Density and Amenorrhea

There is some indication that women who have not menstruated for a long period of time may be losing bone density.[18] When there is a significant decrease in circulating estrogen, a decrease in bone mass may occur. Amenorrhea in athletes does respond to weight gain and reduction of work intensity. Another factor in amenorrhea is that women athletes may prematurely lose bone mass, a loss that may increase risks of fractures.[22,24] Three factors stand out in preventing bone weakness: proper amount of calcium, exercise, and estrogen. Girls require 1200 mg to 1500 mg of calcium per day; adult women require at least 1000 mg per day. Exercise should be regulated to prevent stopping menstruation and estrogen should be ingested to prevent further bone loss. There are also indications that women who have irregular menses have a higher incidence of musculoskeletal injury.[23] All women who stop menstruating should be examined by a physician.[23]

Contraceptives and Reproduction

Female athletes have been known to take extra oral contraceptive pills to delay menstruation during competition. This practice is not recommended because the pills should be taken no more than 21 days, followed by a 7-day break. Side effects range from nausea, vomiting, fluid retention, and amenorrhea to the extreme effects of hypertension, and double vision. It should be noted that some oral contraceptives make women hypersensitive to the sun. Any use of oral contraceptives related to physical performance should be under the express direction and control of a physician. However, oral contraceptive use is acceptable for females with no medical problems who have coitus at least twice a week.

AMERICAN COLLEGE OF OBSTETRICIANS AND GYNECOLOGISTS GUIDE-LINES FOR EXERCISE DURING PREGNANCY AND POSTPARTUM

1. Regular exercise (at least three times per week) is preferable to intermittent activity. Competitive activities should be discouraged.
2. Vigorous exercise should not be performed in hot, humid weather or during a period of febrile illness.
3. Ballistic movements (jerky, bouncy motions) should be avoided. Exercise should be done on a wooden floor or a tightly carpeted surface to reduce shock and provide a sure footing.
4. Deep flexion or extension of joints should be avoided because of connective tissue laxity. Activities that require jumping, jarring motions or rapid changes in direction should be avoided because of joint instability.
5. Vigorous exercise should be preceded by a 5-minute period of muscle warm-up. This can be accomplished by slow walking or stationary cycling with low resistance.
6. Vigorous exercise should be followed by a period of gradually declining activity that includes gentle stretching. Because connective tissue laxity increases the risk of joint injury, stretches should not be taken to the point of maximum resistance.
7. Heart rate should be measured at times of peak activity. Target heart rates and limits established in consultation with the physician should not be exceeded.
8. Care should be taken to gradually rise from the floor to avoid orthostatic hypotension. Some form of activity involving the legs should be continued for a brief period.
9. Liquids should be taken liberally before and after exercise to prevent dehydration. If necessary, activity should be interrupted to replenish fluids.
10. Women who have led sedentary life-styles should begin with physical activity of very low intensity and advance activity levels very gradually.
11. Activity should be stopped and the physician consulted if any unusual symptoms appear.

Pregnancy Only

1. Maternal heart rate should not exceed 140 beats per minute.
2. Strenuous activities should not exceed 15 minutes in duration.
3. No exercise should be performed in the supine position after the fourth month of gestation is completed.
4. Exercises that use the Valsalva maneuver should be avoided.
5. Caloric intake should be adequate to meet not only the extra energy needs of pregnancy but also of the exercise performed.
6. Maternal core temperature should not exceed 38° C.

The new low-dose preparations, containing less than 50 mg of estrogen, add negligible risks to the healthy woman.

During pregnancy women athletes exhibit high levels of muscle tonicity. It has been determined that women who suffer from a chronic disability after childbirth usually have a record of little or no physical exercise in the decade immediately preceding pregnancy. Generally, competition may be engaged in well into the third month of pregnancy unless bleeding or cramps are present and can frequently be continued until the seventh month if no handicapping or physiological complications arise. Such activity may make pregnancy, childbirth, and postparturition less stressful. Many women athletes do not continue beyond the third month because of a drop in their performance that can result from a number of reasons, some related to their pregnancy, others perhaps psychological. It is during the first 3 months of pregnancy that the dangers of disturbing the pregnancy are greatest. After that period there is less danger to the mother and fetus, since the pregnancy is stabilized. There is no indication that mild-to-moderate exercise during pregnancy is harmful to fetal growth and development or causes reduced fetal mass, increased perinatal or neonatal mortality, or physical or mental retardation.[6] It has been found, however, that extreme exercise may lower birth weight. (See the box on p. 543).

Many athletes compete during pregnancy with no ill effects. Most physicians, although advocating moderate activity during this period, believe that especially vigorous performance, particularly in activities in which there may be severe body contact or heavy jarring or falls, should be avoided.

NONMEDICAL SUBSTANCE USE

There is increasing concern about the number of athletes engaging in substance abuse. Some do so in an attempt to improve performance, whereas others engage in it as a recreational pursuit. Because of the inequities that result in competition and the health problems that can result, the use of these substances cannot be condoned.

Banned Substances and Methods

In sports medicine and athletic training, the administration of a drug that is designed to improve the competitor's performance is known as **"doping."**

The International Olympic Committee (IOC) defines doping as "the administration or use of substances in any form alien to the body or of physiological substances in abnormal amounts and with abnormal methods by healthy persons with the exclusive aim of attaining an artificial and unfair increase in performance in sports.[14]"

Stimulants

The intention of the athlete when he or she ingests a stimulant may be to increase alertness, to reduce fatigue, or, in some instances, to increase competitiveness and can produce hostility.[14] In general, some athletes respond to stimulants with a loss of judgment that may lead to personal injury or injury to others.

Amphetamines and cocaine are the psychomotor drugs most commonly used in sports. Cocaine is discussed in the section on *Recreational*

doping

The administration of a drug that is designed to improve the competitor's performance

Drug Abuse. These drugs present an extremely difficult problem in sports because they are commonly found in cold remedies, nasal and ophthalmic decongestants, and most asthma preparations.[14] The IOC has approved some substances to be used by asthmatics who develop exercise-induced bronchospasms. Before an athlete engages in Olympic competition, his or her team physician must notify the IOC Medical Subcommission in writing concerning their usage.[14]

Amphetamines Amphetamines are extremely powerful and dangerous drugs. They may be injected, inhaled, or taken as tablets. Amphetamines are among the most abused drugs used with the goal of enhancing sports performance. In ordinary doses, amphetamines can produce an increased sense of well-being and heightened mental activity—until fatigue sets in (from lack of sleep), accompanied by nervousness, insomnia, and anorexia. In high doses, amphetamines reduce mental activity and impair performance of complicated motor skills. The athlete's behavior may become irrational. The chronic user may be "hung up" or, in other words, get stuck in a repetitive behavioral sequence. This may last for hours, becoming increasingly more irrational. The long-term, or even short-term, use of amphetamines can lead to "amphetamine psychosis," manifested by auditory and visual hallucinations and paranoid delusions.

Physiologically, high doses of amphetamines can cause abnormal pupillary dilation, increased blood pressure, and hyperthermia.

In terms of their sports performance, athletes believe that amphetamines promote quickness and endurance, delay fatigue, and increase confidence, thereby causing increased aggressiveness. Studies indicate that there is no improvement in performance, but there is an increased risk of injury, exhaustion, and circulation collapse.

Caffeine Caffeine is found in coffee, tea, cocoa, and cola, and is readily absorbed into the body (see box).[7] It is a central nervous system stimulant and diuretic and also stimulates gastric secretion. One cup of coffee can contain from 100 to 150 mg of caffeine. In moderation, caffeine causes results in wakefulness and mental alertness. In larger amounts and in individuals who ingest caffeine daily, it raises blood pressure, decreases and then increases the heart rate. It affects coordination,

---

EXAMPLES OF CAFFEINE-CONTAINING PRODUCTS

Product	Dose
Coffee (1 cup)	100 mg
Diet Coke (12 oz)	45.6 mg
Diet Pepsi (12 oz)	36.0 mg
No-Doz (1)	100.0 mg
Anacin (1)	32.0 mg
Excedrin (1)	65.0 mg
Midol (1)	32.4 mg

sleep, mood, behavior, and thinking processes.[7] In terms of exercise and sports performance, caffeine is controversial. Like amphetamines, caffeine can affect some athletes by acting as an ergogenic aid during prolonged exercise. The IOC considers caffeine a stimulant if the concentration in the athlete's urine exceeds 12 mcg/ml. A habitual user of caffeine who suddenly stops may experience withdrawal, including headache, drowsiness, lethargy, rhinorrhea, irritability, nervousness, depression, and loss of interest in work. Caffeine also acts as a diuretic when hydration may be important.[7]

Narcotic Analgesic Drugs

Narcotic analgesic drugs are derived directly or indirectly from opium. Morphine and codeine (methylmorphine) are examples of substances made from opium. Narcotic analgesics are used for the management of moderate-to-severe pain. They have been banned by the IOC because of the high risk of physical and psychological dependency, as well as many other problems stemming from their use. It is believed that slight-to-moderate pain can be effectively dealt with by drugs other than narcotics.

Beta Blockers

The "beta" in beta blockers refers to the type of adrenergic drug that blocks sympathetic nerve endings. Medically, beta blockers are used for hypertension and heart disease. In sports, beta blockers have been used in sports that require steadiness, and signs of nervousness must be in control such as marksmanship, sailing, archery, fencing, ski jumping, and luge. Beta blockers produce relaxation of blood vessels. This relaxation, in turn, slows heart rate and decreases cardiac output. Therapeutically, beta blockers are used for a variety of cardiac diseases, as well as in the treatment of hypertension.

Diuretics

Diuretic drugs increase kidney excretion by decreasing the kidney's resorption of sodium. The excretion of potassium and bicarbonate may also be increased. Therapeutically, diuretics are used for a variety of cardiovascular and respiratory conditions (e.g., hypertension) in which elimination of fluids from tissues is necessary. Sports participants have misused diuretics mainly in two ways—to reduce body weight quickly or to decrease a drug's concentration in the urine (increasing its excretion to avoid the detection of drug misuse). In both cases, there are ethical and health grounds for banning certain classes of diuretics from use during Olympic competition.

Anabolic Steroids and Growth Hormone (GH)

Two substance classes related to the increase of muscle build, strength, power, and growth are the anabolic steroids and growth hormone (GH). Both are abused during sports participation.

Anabolic steroids Androgenic hormones are basically a product of the male testes. Of these hormones, testosterone is the principal one and possesses the ability to function androgenically (the ability to stimulate male characteristics) and anabolically (the ability to through an improved protein assimilation to increase muscle mass and weight, general growth, bone maturation, and virility). When prescribed by a physician to improve certain physiological conditions, these drugs have value. In 1984, the American College of Sports Medicine (ACSM) reported that anabolic androgenic steroids taken with an adequate diet could contribute to an increase in body weight, and with a heavy resistance program there can be a significant gain in strength.[33] However, in sports, they constitute a major threat to the health of the athlete (see box below). Anabolic steroids present an ethical dilemma for the sport world. It is estimated that over a million young male and female athletes are taking them, with most being purchased through the black market. Its been noted that over 700,000 high school students take or have taken anabolic steroids. This figure consists of 6.5 males and 1.4 females.[14] An estimated 2% to 20% of male intercollegiate athletes take anabolic steroids.[14]

If these drugs are given to the prepubertal boy, a decrease in his ultimate height, because of the cessation of long bone growth, is a most certain hazard. Acne, hirsutism, a deepening of the voice in the prepubescent boy, and in some cases, a swelling of the breasts called gynecomastia are among other androgen effects.[14] The ingestion of steroids by females can result in **hirsutism** and a deepening of the voice as a result of vocal cord alteration. When the dosage is halted, the hirsutism may cease, but the change of the vocal cords is irreversible. As the duration and dosage increase, the possibility of producing androgen effects also increases. Because self-administered overdosage seems to be the pattern of those who use steroids, the preceding statement is most significant. Abuse of these drugs may also lead to cancer of the liver and prostate glands, as well as heart disease.

Usage of anabolic steroids is a major problem in sports that involve strength. Powerlifting, the throwing events in track and field and Ameri-

hirsutism
Excessive hair growth and/or the presence of hair in unusual places

---

EXAMPLES OF DELETERIOUS EFFECTS OF ANABOLIC STEROIDS

Teens—premature closure of long bones, acne, hirsutism, voice deepening, enlarged mammary glands (gynecomastia) of the male
Males—male-pattern baldness, acne, voice deepening, mood swings, aggressive behavior, decreased high-density lipoprotein, increased cholesterol, reduction in size of testicle, reduced testosterone production, changes in libido[33]
Females—female-pattern baldness, acne, voice deepening (irreversible), increased facial hair, enlarged clitoris (irreversible), increased libido, menstrual irregularities, increased aggression, decreased body fat, increased appetite, decreased breast size
Abuse—may lead to liver tumors and cancer, heart disease, and hypertension

can football are some of the sports in which the use of anabolic steroids is a serious problem. Because female athletes are developing the attitude of "win at all costs," their abuse of anabolic steroids is also becoming a major health problem.

Human growth hormone (HGH)   Human growth hormone (HGH) is a polypeptide hormone produced by the somatrophic cells of the anterior region of the pituitary gland. It is released into circulation in a pulsating manner. This release can vary with age and the developmental periods of a person's life. A lack of HGH can result in dwarfism. In the past, HGH was in limited supply because it was extracted from cadavers. Now, however, it can be made synthetically and is more available.[14]

Experiments indicate that HGH can increase muscle mass, skin thickness, connective tissues in muscle, and organ weight and can produce lax muscles and ligaments during rapid growth phases. It also increases body length and weight and decreases body fat percentage.[14]

The use of HGH by athletes throughout the world is on the increase because it is more difficult to detect in urine than anabolic steroids.[14] There is currently a lack of concrete information about the effects of HGH on the athlete who does not have a growth problem. It is known that an overabundance of HGH in the body can lead to premature closure of long-bone growth sites or, conversely, can cause acromegaly, a condition that produces elongation and enlargement of bones of the extremities and thickening of bones and soft tissues of the face. Also associated with acromegaly is diabetes mellitus, cardiovascular disease, goiter, menstrual disorders, decreased sexual desire, and impotence. It decreases the life span by up to 20 years. As with anabolic steroids, HGH presents a serious problem for the sports world. At this time there is no proof that an increase of HGH combined with weight training contributes to strength and muscle hypertrophy.[14]

Other Drugs Subject to IOC Restriction

The IOC indicates that, although it does not expressly prohibit alcohol, breath or blood alcohol levels may be determined at the request of the committee. Local anesthetics that are injected (excluding cocaine) are permitted. Corticosteroids have been abused for their ability to produce euphoria and certain side effects. They are, therefore, banned except for topical use or for inhalation therapy and intra-articular injections during the Olympic Games.

Blood Reinjection (Blood Doping, Blood Packing, and Blood Boosting)

Endurance, acclimatization, and altitude make increased metabolic demands on the body, which responds by increasing blood volume and red blood cells to meet the increased aerobic demands.

Recently researchers have replicated these physiological responses by removing 900 ml of blood, storing it, and reinfusing it after 6 weeks. The reason for waiting at least 6 weeks before reinfusion is it takes that long for the athlete's body to reestablish a normal hemoglobin and red blood cell concentration. Using this method, endurance performance has been significantly improved. From the standpoint of scientific research such experimentation has merit and is of interest. However, not only is use of such methods in competition unethical, but use by nonmedical personnel could prove to be dangerous, especially when a matched donor is used.

There are serious risks with transfusing blood and related blood products. The risks include allergic reactions, kidney damage (if the wrong type of blood is used), fever, jaundice, the possibility of transmitting infectious diseases (viral hepatitis or acquired immune deficiency disease), or a blood overload, resulting in circulatory and metabolic shock.[13]

RECREATIONAL DRUG ABUSE

As is true with the general public, recreational drug use has become a part of the world of sports. Reasons for using these substances may include desire to experiment, temporarily to escape from problems, or just to be part of a group (peer pressure). For some, recreational drug use leads to abuse and dependence. There are two general aspects of dependence—psychological and physical. *Psychological dependence* is the drive to repeat the ingestion of a drug to produce pleasure or to avoid discomfort. *Physical dependence* is the state of drug adaptation that manifests as the development of *tolerance* and, when the drug is removed, causes a *withdrawal syndrome*. Tolerance of a drug is the need to increase the dosage to create the effect that was obtained previously by smaller amounts. The withdrawal syndrome consists of an unpleasant physiological reaction when the drug is abruptly stopped. Some drugs that are abused by the athlete overlap with those thought to enhance performance. Examples include amphetamines and cocaine. Tobacco (nicotine), alcohol, cocaine, and marijuana are the most abused recreational drugs. The coach might also come in contact with abuse by athletes of barbiturates, non-barbiturate sedatives, psychotomimetic drugs, or different inhalants.

Tobacco

There are a number of current problems related to tobacco and sports. They can be divided into two headings—cigarette smoking and the use of smokeless tobacco.

Cigarette Smoking

On the basis of various investigations into the relationship between smoking and performance, the following conclusions can be drawn:
1. There is individual sensitivity to tobacco that may seriously affect performance in instances of relatively high sensitivity. Because over one third of the men studied indicated tobacco sensitivity, it may be wise to prohibit smoking by athletes.
2. Tobacco smoke has been associated with as many as 4700 different chemicals, many of which are toxic.

3. As few as 10 inhalations of cigarette smoke cause an average maximum decrease in airway conductance of 50%. This occurs in nonsmokers who inhale smoke secondhand as well.

4. Smoking reduces the oxygen-carrying capacity of the blood. A smoker's blood carries from five to as much as 10 times more carbon monoxide than normal; thus the red blood cells are prevented from picking up sufficient oxygen to meet the demands of the body's tissues. The carbon monoxide also tends to make arterial walls more permeable to fatty substances, a factor in atherosclerosis.

5. Smoking aggravates and accelerates the heart muscle cells through overstimulation of the sympathetic nervous system.

6. Total lung capacity and maximum breathing capacity are significantly decreased in heavy smokers; this is important to the athlete, because both changes would impair the capacity to take in oxygen and make it readily available for body use.

7. Smoking decreases pulmonary diffusing capacity.

8. After smoking, an accelerated thrombolic tendency is evidenced.

9. Smoking is a carcinogenic factor in lung cancer and is a contributing factor to heart disease.

The addictive chemical of tobacco is nicotine, which is one of the most toxic drugs. When ingested, it causes blood pressure elevation, increased bowel activity, and an antidiuretic action. Moderate tolerance and physical dependence occur. It also has been noted that passive inhalation of cigarette smoke can reduce maximum aerobic power and endurance capacity.

Use of Smokeless Tobacco

It is estimated that 36% of athletes use smokeless tobacco, which comes in three forms—loose-leaf, moist or dry powder (snuff), and compressed.[28] The tobacco is placed between the cheek and the gum. Then it is sucked and chewed. Aesthetically, this is an unsavory habit during which an athlete is continually spitting into a container. Besides the unpleasant appearance, the use of smokeless tobacco proposes an extremely serious health risk. Smokeless tobacco causes bad breath, stained teeth, tooth sensitivity to heat and cold, cavities, gum recession, tooth bone loss, leukoplakia, and oral and throat cancer.[28] Aggressive oral and throat cancer and periodontal destruction (with tooth loss) have been associated with this habit. The major substance injested is nitrosonornicotine, which is the drug responsible for this habit's addictiveness. This chemical makes smokeless tobacco a more addictive habit than smoking. Smokeless tobacco increases heart rate but does not affect reaction time, movement time, or total response time among athletes or nonathletes.[13]

Coaches, athletic trainers, and professional athletes themselves must avoid the use of smokeless tobacco to present a positive role model.[13]

Alcohol

Alcohol is the number one abused drug in the United States.[14] Alcohol is absorbed directly into the bloodstream through the small intestine. It accumulates in the blood because alcohol absorption is faster than its oxidation. It acts as a central nervous system depressant, producing sedation and tranquility. Characteristically, alcohol consumption, at any time and in any amount, does not improve mental or physical abilities and should be completely avoided by athletes. Alcohol consumption on a large scale can lead to a moderate degree of tolerance. Alcohol has no place in sports participation.

Alcohol consumption, at any time or in any amount, does not improve mental or physical abilities and should be avoided by athletes.

Cocaine

Cocaine, sometimes called "coke," "snow," "toot," "happy dust," and "white girl," is a powerful central nervous system stimulant, as well as a local anesthetic and vasoconstrictor. Besides being a banned performance enhancer, it is one of the most abused recreational drugs. It can be inhaled, smoked, or injected (intravenously, subcutaneously, or intramuscularly).[14]

In high doses cocaine causes a sense of excitement and euphoria. On occasions it also produces hallucinations. Found in the leaves of the coca bush, when applied locally to the skin, it acts as an anesthetic; however, when taken into the body through inhalation, snorting, or injection, it acts on the central nervous system.

Crack

Crack, a highly purified form of cocaine, is smoked and known to produce a virtually instantaneous high.

Habitual use of cocaine will not lead to physical tolerance or dependence but will cause psychological dependence and addiction. When cocaine is used recreationally, the athlete feels alert, self-satisfied, and powerful. Heavy usage can produce paranoid delusions and violent behavior. Overuse can lead to overstimulation of the sympathetic nervous system and can cause tachycardia, hypertension, extra heartbeats, coronary vasoconstriction, strokes, pulmonary edema, aortic rupture, and sudden death.[4]

Marijuana

Marijuana is another one of the most abused drugs in Western society. It is more commonly called "grass," "weed," "pot," "dope," or "hemp." The marijuana cigarette is called a "joint," "j," "number," "reefer," or "root."

Marijuana is *not* a harmless drug. The components of marijuana smoke are similar to those of tobacco smoke and the same cellular changes are observed in the user.

Continued use leads to respiratory diseases such as asthma and bronchitis and a decrease in vital capacity of 15% to as much as 40% (certainly detrimental to physical performance). Among other deleterious effects are lowered sperm counts and testosterone levels. Evidence of interference with the functioning of the immune system and cellular metabolism has also been found. The most consistent sign is the increase in pulse rate, which averages close to 20% higher during exercise and is a definite factor in limiting performance. Some decrease in leg, hand, and finger strength has been found at higher dosages. Like tobacco, marijuana must be considered carcinogenic.

Psychological effects such as a diminution of self-awareness and judgment, a slowdown of thinking, and a shorter attention span appear early in the use of the drug. Postmortem examinations of habitual users reveal not only cerebral atrophy but alterations of anatomical structures, which suggest irreversible brain damage. Marijuana also contains unique substances (cannabinoids) that are stored, in very much the same manner as are fat cells, throughout the body and in the brain tissues for weeks and even months. These stored quantities result in a cumulative deleterious effect on the habitual user.

A drug such as marijuana has no place in sports. Claims for its use

IDENTIFYING THE SUBSTANCE ABUSER

The following are signs of drug abuse:
1. Sudden personality changes
2. Severe mood swings
3. Changing peer groups
4. Decreased interest in extracurricular and leisure activities
5. Worsening grades
6. Disregard for household chores and curfews
7. Feeling of depression most of the time
8. Breakdown in personal hygiene habits
9. Increased sleep and decreased eating
10. Clothes and skin smell of alcohol or marijuana
11. Sudden weight loss
12. Lying, cheating, stealing, etc.
13. Arrests for drunk driving or for possessing illegal substances
14. Truancies from school
15. Loses or changes jobs frequently
16. Becomes defensive at the mention of drugs or alcohol
17. Increased isolation (spends time in room)
18. Family relationship deteriorates
19. Drug paraphernalia (needles, empty bottles, etc.) found
20. Others make observations about negative behavior
21. Shows signs of intoxication
22. Constantly misses appointments
23. Falls asleep in class or at work
24. Has financial problems
25. Misses assignments or deadlines
26. Diminished productivity

are unsubstantiated, and the harmful effects, both immediate and long-term, are too significant to permit indulgence at any time.

SUMMARY

The most common skin infections in athletes are caused by viruses, bacteria, and fungi. Viral infections include herpes simplex (e.g., the cold sore), verruca (warts), and the molluscum contagiosum (water warts). Tetanus, which can cause lock jaw, is another major concern in athletics. Bacterial infections are represented by impetigo contagiosa, boils, and infected hair follicles and sweat glands. Ringworm, or tinea, is the fungus infection commonly attacking all areas of the body; tinea pedis (athlete's foot) is the most common.

The common cold, sore throat, hay fever, and asthma are respiratory tract illnesses that can adversely affect the athlete. Asthma can be chronic (e.g., bronchial) or induced by physical activity. Care of the athlete who is having an acute asthmatic attack requires understanding the early symptoms and signs and responding accordingly.

Gastrointestinal complaints such as indigestion, diarrhea, and constipation are as common among athletes as nonathletes. Minor problems should be distinguished from major complaints such as factors that may indicate appendicitis.

Diabetes mellitus is a complex hereditary or developmental disease of carbohydrate metabolism. Decreased effectiveness of insulin or an insufficient amount is responsible for most cases. The diabetic athlete must carefully monitor his or her energy output to ensure there is a balance of food intake and the burning of sugars via insulin. If this does not occur, diabetic coma or insulin shock may result.

Epilepsy is defined as "a recurrent paroxysmal disorder of cerebral function characterized by sudden, brief attacks of altered consciousness motor activity, sensory phenomena, or inappropriate behavior."[3] A coach or athletic trainer must recognize that an athlete is going into seizure and be able to provide proper immediate care.

Because communicable viral diseases such as German measles, mumps, and infectious mononucleosis can infect many athletes on a team, early recognition is necessary. When such a disease is suspected, the athlete should be isolated from other athletes and immediately referred to a physician for diagnosis. Hepatitis B, like HIV, can be spread by sexual contact.

The athlete with high blood pressure may have to be carefully monitored by the physician. Hypertension may require the avoidance of heavy resistive activities.

Anemia is a problem for some athletes. Most often, iron deficiency anemia is a condition found in women. In an athlete with iron deficiency anemia, the red blood cells are either too small or too large. Hemoglobin is decreased, and the ferritin concentration is low. The athlete with the sickle cells tract may have on adverse reaction at high altitudes where the sickle-shaped red blood cell is unable to transport oxygen adequately.

Sexually transmitted disease has its highest incidence among younger sexually active persons. Because the highest number of athletes are in this highest risk age group, there should be great concern about the spread of these diseases. Many of these diseases, such as genital herpes, condyloma acuminata, and acquired immune deficiency syndrome (AIDS), are caused by viral microorganisms. AIDS, a potentially fatal disease, presents a major challenge in prevention. Some are caused by bacteria (e.g., gonorrhea by Neisseria gonorrhoea and nonspecific sexually transmitted infection by Chlamydia trachomatis), whereas others may be caused by a yeast infection (candidiasis) or a protozoa (trichomoniasis). To avoid these infections, "safe sex" is suggested, which involves the use of a condom, the elimination of multiple partners, or even complete abstinence from sexual intercourse.

A major problem in sports participation is the extensive use of performance aids, consisting of drugs and blood doping. The International Olympic Committee (IOC) lists banned drugs under the headings of stimulants, narcotic analgesics, diuretics, and anabolic steroids. Blood doping has also been placed in the banned category.

A third area of concern is that of recreational drug abuse. This abuse is worldwide. It leads to serious psychological and physical health problems. The most prevalent substances that are abused are nicotine, cocaine, and marijuana.

REVIEW QUESTIONS AND CLASS ACTIVITIES

1. Describe the organism underlying the common skin infectious seen in athletes. Name a disease caused by each one.
2. Invite a dermatologist or other professional to speak to the class about skin conditions, skin disease, and their care. He or she may wish to discuss specific conditions that pose a serious threat to the athlete's health and to others.
3. What disorders or conditions of the gastrointestinal tract may cause discomfort or problems for the athlete? How do you manage each condition?
4. What is diabetes mellitus? What is the difference between diabetic coma and insulin shock? How is each managed?
5. What is epilepsy? At what point should an athlete trainer do for the athlete during a seizure? After it?
6. In a sports setting, what would be the indication that an athlete had a contagious disease?
7. Describe the anemias that most often affect the athlete. How should each be managed?
8. Discuss the etiology, symptoms, and signs of the most common sexually transmitted diseases. How can they be prevented?
9. Describe the AIDS virus, its transmission, and prevention.
10. Discuss menstrual irregularities that occur in highly active athletes. Why do they occur? How should they be managed? How do they relate to reproduction?
11. What are the implications of pregnancy to extensive physical activity?
12. Discuss the use of performance aids such as drugs.
13. How do stimulants enhance an athlete's performance? Do they, in fact, enhance it?

14. What are the deleterious effects of hormonal manipulation in sports?
15. Describe blood doping in sports. Why is it used? What are its dangers?
16. Have a member of the IOC explain the banned drug policy to the class.
17. List the dangers of smokeless tobacco. List the effects of nicotine on the body.
18. Select a recreational drug to research. What are the physiological responses to it, and what dangers does it pose to the athlete?
19. How can an athlete who is abusing drugs be identified? Describe behavioral identification, as well as drug testing.

REFERENCES

1. Berkow R, ed: *The Merck manual,* ed 10, Rahway, NJ, Merck.
2. Blumenthal MN: Sports-aggravated allergies, *Phys Sportmed* 18:12, 1990.
3. Briner WW, Jr: Introduction: Exercise and allergy, *Med Science Sports Exerc* 24:843, 1992.
4. Briner WW, Jr, Shiffer AL: Exercise-induced anaphylaxis *Med Science Sports Exerc* 24:849, 1992.
5. Burke AP: Sudden death in athletes, *Sports Med Dig* 15:2, 1993.
6. Clapp III JF et al: Exercise in pregnancy, *Med Sci Sports Exerc* 24:5294, 1992.
7. Coleman E: Diet and hypertension, *Sports Med Dig* 15:8, 1993.
8. Dalsky GP: Effect of exercise on bone: permissive influence of estrogen and calcium, *Med Sci Sports* 22:281; 1990.
9. Eichner ER: Infectious mononucleosis: recognition and management in athletes, *Phys Sportsmed* 15:61, 1987.
10. Eichner ER: Gastrointestinal bleeding in athletes, *Phys Sportsmed* 17:129, 1989.
11. Ekoe J-M: Overview of diabetes mellitus and exercise, *Med Sci Sports Exerc* 214, 1989.
12. Glover ED et al: Smokeless tobacco: questions and answers, *Ath Train* 25:10, 1990.
13. Gledhill N: Blood doping and performance. In Torg JS, Welsh RP, Shephard RJ, eds: *Current therapy in sports medicine,* vol 2, Philadelphia, 1990, BC Decker.
14. Guide to banned medications, United States Olympic Committee, Division of Sports Medicine, Drug Education, and Doping Control Program, Nov 1, 1990.
15. Health GW et al: Exercise and incidence of upper-respiratory infections, *Med Sci Sports Exerc* 23:152, 1991.
16. Jones NL: Exercise in chronic airway obstruction. In Torg JS et al, eds: *Current therapy in sports medicine,* Toronto, 1990, BC Decker.
17. Kark JA et al: Sickle-cell traits as a risk factor sudden death in physical training, *N Engl J Med* 317:781, 1987.
18. Landry GL: HIV infection and athletes—*Sports Med Dig* 15:1, 1993.
19. Loucks AB: Effects of exercise training on the menstrual cycle: existence and mechanisms, *Med Sci Sports Exerc* 22:275, 1990.
20. Loucks AB et al: The reproductive system and exercise in women, *Med Sci Sports Exerc* 24:5288, 1993.
21. Mahler DA: Exercise induced asthma, *Med Sci Sports Exerc* 25:554, 1993.
22. Marcus R et al: Osteoporosis and exercise in women, *Med Sci Sports Exerc* 24:5301, 1992.
23. Otis EL, Lynch L: How to keep your bones healthy, *Phys Sportsmed* 22:71, 1994.
24. Partin N: Exercise-induced asthma, *Ath Train* 24:250, 1989.
25. Partin N: Prevention and control of influenza, *NATA News,* Mar 1993 pg 23.
26. Partin N: Alternative for smokeless tobacco use in athletes, *NATA News,* June 1993, pg 24.

27. Robbins DC, Carleton S: Managing the diabetic athlete, *Phys Sportsmed* 17:45, 1989.

28. Shanghold MM: Special concerns of the female athlete. In Torg JS et al, ed: *Current therapy in sports medicine,* Toronto, 1990, BC Decker.

29. Shanghold MM: Dysmenorrhea and other pelvic pain, *Sports Med Dig* 15:5, 1992.

30. Shroyer JA: Getting tough on anabolic steroids: can we win the battle? *Phys Sportsmed* 18:106, 1990.

31. Shephard RJ, Shek PN: Athletic competition and susceptibility to infection, *Clin J Sports Med* 3:7, 1993.

32. Simons SM, Moriarity: Hypertrophic cardio-myopathy in a col-lege athlete, *Med Sci Sports Exerc* 24:1321, 1992.

33. Stager JM et al: Interpreting the relationship between age of menarche and prepubertal training, *Med Sci Sports Exerc* 22:54, 1990.

34. Stiene HA: Management of infections in athletes, *Sports Med Dig* 14:1, 1992.

35. Thomas RJ, Cantwell JD: Sudden death during basketball games, *Phys Sportsmed* 18:75, 1990.

36. Virant FS: Exercise-induced bronchospasm: epidemiology, pathology, and therapy, *Med Sci Sports Exerc* 24:851, 1992.

37. Webster DL, Kaiser DA: An infection control policy for the athletic training setting, *Ath Train* 26:70, 1991.

ANNOTATED BIBLIOGRAPHY

Berkow R, ed: The Merck Manual, ed 16, Rahway, NJ, Merck 1992.
   This text book is one of the classical medicine references available to health care professional. It covers most medical conditions.
Herbert DL: Legal aspects of sports medicine, Professional Report Corporation, Stephen Circle NW, Canton, OH 44718-3629.
   A major guide to sports medicine and the law including procedure, responsibilities of the sportsmedicine team.
Otis CL: *Campus health guide,* New York, 1989.
   Provides information on nutrition, exercise, medical and dental problems, sexual and emotional health, eating disorders, and drugs and alcohol.
Rosenberg JM et al, eds: *Athletic Drug Reference: 1992 Edition,* Durham NC: Clean Data Inc., 1992.
   A guide drug reference for athletes, coaches, trainers, drug and poison information centers, physician, pharmacists, nurses, and health care professionals.
US Olympic Committee Drug Education: *Handbook 1989-1992—Drug Free.*
   A handbook providing in a well-written and succinct manner the goals of the US Olympic Committee's Drug Education program.
Wright JE, Cowart VS: *Anabolic steroids: Altered states,* Carmel, Ind, 1990, Beuchmark Press.
   A straightforward to description of anabolic steroids their mechanism of action and health effects.

Appendix

A

Units of Measure

Temperature

To convert a Fahrenheit temperature to Celsius (centigrade):
$$°C = (°F - 32) \div 1.8$$
To convert a Celsius temperature to Fahrenheit:
$$°F = (1.8 \times °C) + 32$$

On the Fahrenheit scale, the freezing point of water is 32° G and the boiling point is 212° F. On the Celsius scale, the freezing point of water is 0°C and the boiling point is 100° C.

Distance

Equivalent Metric Unit	Equivalent English Unit
1 centimeter (cm)	0.3937 inch
2.54 centimeters	1 inch
1 meter (m)	3.28 feet; 1.09 yards
0.304 meters	1 foot
1 kilometer (km)	0.62 mile
1.61 kilometers	1 mile

Power and Energy

Power = Work divided by time; measured in horsepower (HP), watts, etc.

1 HP = 746 watts

Energy = Application of a force through a distance

1 kilocalorie (kcal) = Amount of energy required to heat 1 kilogram (kg) of water 1° Celsius

Vitamin Tables

Summary of fat-soluble vitamins

Vitamin	Physiological Functions	Results of Deficiency	Requirement	Food Sources
A				
Provitamin—β-carotene	Production of rhodopsin and other light-receptor pigments	Poor dark adaptation, night blindness, xerosis	Adult male—1000 μg RE* Adult female—800 μg RE	Liver, cream, butter, whole milk, egg yolk
Vitamin—retinol	Formation and maintenance of epithelial tissue Growth Reproduction Toxic in large amounts	Keratinization of epithelium Growth failure Reproductive failure	Pregnancy—800 μg RE Lactation—1300 μg RE Children—400-1000 μg RE	Green and yellow vegetables, yellow fruits Fortified margarine
D				
Provitamins—ergosterol (plants), 7-dehydrocholesterol (skin)	1,25-dihydroxy-cholecalciferol, a major hormone regulator of bone mineral (calcium and phosphorus) metabolism	Faulty bone growth—rickets, osteomalacia	Adult—5-10 μg cholecalciferol Pregnancy and lactation—10 μg, depending on age Children—10 μg	Fortified milk Fortified margarine Fish oils Sunlight on skin
Vitamins—D$_2$ (ergocalciferol) and D$_3$ (cholecalciferol)	Calcium and phosphorus absorption Toxic in large amounts			
E				
Tocopherols	Antioxidation Hemopoiesis Related to action of selenium	Anemia in premature infants	Adults—8-10 mg α TE* Pregnancy and lactation—10-12 mg α TE Children—3-10 mg α TE	Vegetable oils

*RE = retinol equivalent; TE = tocopherol equivalent

Continued.

Summary of fat-soluble vitamins (cont'd)

Vitamin	Physiological Functions	Results of Deficiency	Requirement	Food Sources
K K$_1$ (phylloquinone) K$_2$ (Menaquinone) Analog—K$_3$ (mena-dione)	Activation of blood-clotting factors (e.g., pro-thrombin) by car-boxylating glutamic acid res-idues Toxicity can be in-duced by water-soluble analogs	Hemorrhagic dis-ease of the new-born Defective blood clotting Deficiency symp-toms, which can be produced by coumarin antico-agulants and by antibiotic therapy	Adult—65-80 μg Children—15-65 μg Infants—5-10 μg	Cheese, egg yolk, liver Green leafy vegeta-bles Synthesized by in-testinal bacteria

Summary of B-complex vitamins

Vitamin	Coenzymes: Physiological Function	Requirement/Day	Food Source
Thiamine (B$_1$)	Carbohydrate metabolism, nervous system function	1.1-1.5 mg	Pork, beef, liver, whole or enriched grains, legumes
Riboflavin (B$_2$)	General metabolism, cellular en-ergy release, respiration	1.2-1.7 mg	Milk, liver, enriched cereals
Niacin (nicotinic acid, nicotinamide)	General metabolism—cellular en-ergy processes and respiration, carbohydrate metabolism, fat synthesis	15-19 mg NE*	Meat, peanuts, en-riched grains (pro-tein foods containing tryptophan)
Vitamin B$_6$ (pyridox-ine, pyridoxal, pyridoxamine)	General metabolism—amino acid and protein metabolism, RBC* formation	1.6-2.0 mg	Wheat, corn, meat, liver
Pantothenic acid	General metabolism—energy and tissue metabolism	4-7 mg	Liver, eggs, milk
Biotin	General metabolism—synthesis of glycogen and fat, amino acid me-tabolism	30-100 μg	Egg yolk, liver
Folic acid (folacin)	General metabolism—regulates tis-sue processes, RBC formation	Infants—25-35 μg Children—50-180 μg Adults—150-180 μg	Liver, green leafy veg-etables
Cobalamin (B$_{12}$)	General metabolism—maintenance of nerve tissue, RBC develop-ment	2.0 μg	Liver, meat, milk, eggs, cheese

*RBC = red blood cell; NE = niacin equivalent.

Glossary

abduction A movement of a body part away from the midline of the body

accident Occurring by chance or without intention

accommodating resistance Form of isokinetic exercises where speed is an element

acute injury An injury with sudden onset and short duration

ad libitum In the amount desired

adduction A movement of a body part toward the midline of the body

afferent nerve fibers Nerve fibers that carry messages toward the brain

agonist muscles Muscles directly engaged in contraction as related to muscles that relax at the same time

ambulation Move or walk from place to place

ameboid action A leukocyte moving through a capillary wall through the process of diapedisis

amenorrhea Absence or suppression of menstruation

amnesia Loss of memory

analgesia Pain inhibition

anesthesia Partial or complete loss of sensation

anomaly Deviation from the norm

anorexia Lack or loss of appetite; aversion to food

anorexia nervosa Eating disorder characterized by a distorted body image

anoxia Lack of oxygen

antagonist muscles Muscles that counteract the action of the agonist muscles

anterior Before or in front of

anterior cruciate ligament Stops external rotation

anteroposterior Refers to the position of front to back

anxiety A feeling of uncertainty or apprehension

apophysis A bone outgrowth to which muscles attach

arrhythmical movement Irregular movement

arthroscopic examination Viewing the inside of a joint via the arthroscope, which utilizes a small camera lens

articulation A joint

assumption of risk An individual, through expressed or implied agreement, assumes that some risk or danger will be involved in a particular undertaking

asymmetries (body) A lack of symmetry of sides of the body

atrophic necrosis Death of an area due to lack of circulation

atrophy Wasting away of tissue or of an organ; diminution of the size of a body part

automatism Automatic behavior before consciousness or full awareness has been achieved following a brain concussion

avascular necrosis Death of tissue resulting from a lack of blood supply

avulsion A tearing away

axial loading A blow to the top of the athlete's head while in 300 flexion

axilla Arm pit

bandage A strip of cloth or other material used to hold a dressing in place

bilateral Pertaining to both sides

biomechanics Branch of study that applies the laws of mechanics to living organisms and biological tissues

bipedal Having two feet or moving on two feet

bowlegged Bending outward of the lower joint

bradykinin Peptide chemical that causes pain in an injured area

bulimia Binge-purge eating disorder

bursa A fibrous sac between certain tendons and the bones beneath them that acts as a cushion and allows the tendon, as it contracts and relaxes, to move over the bone

bursitis Inflammation of a bursa, especially those bursae located between bony prominences and a muscle or tendon, such as those of the shoulder or knee

calcific tendinitis Deposition of calcium in a chronically inflamed tendon, especially the tendons of the shoulder

calisthenic Exercise involving free movement without the aid of equipment

calorie (large) Amount of heat required to raise 1 kg of water 1° C; term used to express the fuel or energy value of food or the heat output of the organism; the amount of heat required to heat 1 lb of water to 4° F

catastrophic injury A permanent injury to the spinal cord that leaves the athlete quadriplegic or paraplegic

cauterization A purposeful destruction of tissue

cerebrovascular accident Stroke

chondromalacia A degeneration of a joint's articular surface, leading to softening

chronic injury An injury with long onset and long duration

circumduct Act of moving a limb such as the arm or hip in a circular motion

clavus durum Hard corn

clavus molle Soft corn

clonic muscle contraction Alternating involuntary muscle contraction and relaxation in quick succession

clonic muscle cramp Involuntary muscle contraction marked by alternate contraction and relaxation in rapid succession

closed fracture Fracture that does not penetrate superficial tissue

collagenous tissue The white fibrous substance composing connective tissue

collision sport Athletes use their bodies to deter or punish opponents

commission (legal liability) Performing an act outside of an individual's legal jurisdiction

communicable disease A disease that may be transmitted directly or indirectly from one individual to another

concentric muscle contraction Refers to muscle shortening

conduction Heating by direct contact with a hot medium

conjunctivae Mucous membrane that lines the eyes

contact sport Athletes make physical contact, but not with the intent to produce bodily injury

contrecoup brain injury After head is struck, brain continues to move within the skull and becomes injured opposite the force

convection Heating indirectly through another medium, such as air or liquid

conversion Heating by other forms of energy (e.g., electricity)

convulsions Paroxysms of involuntary muscular contractions and relaxations

core temperature Internal, or deep body, temperature monitored by cells in the hypothalamus, as opposed to shell, or peripheral, temperature which is registered by the layer of insulation provided by the skin, subcutaneous tissues, and superficial portions of the muscle masses

corticosteroid A steroid produced by the adrenal cortex

coryza Profuse nasal discharge

counterirritant An agent that produces a mild inflammation and in turn acts as an analgesic when applied locally to the skin (e.g., liniment)

crepitation A crackling sound heard on the movement of ends of a broken bone

cryokinetics Cold application combined with exercise

cryotherapy Cold therapy

cubital fossa Triangular area on the anterior aspect of the forearm directly opposite the elbow joint (the bend of the elbow)

cyanosis Slightly bluish, grayish, slatelike, or dark purple discoloration of the skin due to a reduced amount of blood hemaglobin

cutaneous Of or pertaining to the skin

debride Removal of dirt and dead tissue from a wound

deconditioning A state in which the athlete's body loses its competitive fitness

degeneration Deterioration of tissue

dermatome A segmental skin area innervated by various spinal cord segments

diapedisis Passage of blood cells by ameboid action through the intact capillary wall

diaphragm A musculomembranous wall separating the abdomen from the thoracic cavity

diarthrodial joint Ball and socket joint

diastolic blood pressure The residual pressure when the heart is between beats

diplopia Seeing double

distal Farthest away from a point of reference

doping The administration of a drug that is designed to improve the competitor's performance

dorsiflexion Bending toward the dorsum or rear, opposite of plantar flexion

dorsum The back of a body part

dressing A material, such as gauze, applied to a wound

duration Length of time that an athlete works during a bout of exercise

dysmenorrhea Painful or difficult menstruation

dyspepsia Imperfect digestion

dyspnea Difficulty in breathing

eccentric muscle contraction Refers to muscle lengthening

ecchymosis Black and blue skin discoloration due to hemorrhage

ectopic Located in a place different from normal

ectopic bone formation Bone formation occurring in an abnormal place

edema Swelling as a result of the collection of fluid in connective tissue

electrolyte Solution that is a conductor of electricity

electrotherapy Treating disease by electrical devices

emboli Plural of embolus

encephalon The brain

endurance The ability of the body to undergo prolonged activity

entrapment Organ becomes compressed by nearby tissue

epidemiological approach The study of sports injuries involving the relationship of as many injury factors as possible

epilepsy Recurrent paroxysmal disorder characterized by sudden attacks of altered consciousness, motor activity, and sensory perception

epiphysis The cartilagenous growth region of a bone

epistaxis Nosebleed

etiology Pertaining to the cause of a condition

eversion of the foot To turn the foot outward

exostoses Benign bony outgrowths that protrude from the surface of a bone and are usually capped by cartilage

extraoral mouth guard A protective device that fits outside the mouth

extravasation Escape of a fluid from its vessels into the surrounding tissues

exudates Accumulation of a fluid in an area

fascia Fibrous membrane that covers, supports, and separates muscles

fasciitis Fascia inflammation

fibrinogen A protein present in blood plasma that is converted into a fibrin clot

fibroblast Any cell component from which fibers are developed

fibrocartilage A type of cartilage in which the matrix contains thick bundles of collagenous fibers (e.g., intervertebral disks)

fibrosis Development of excessive fibrous connective tissue; fibroid degeneration

foot pronation Combined foot movements of eversion and abduction

foot supination Combined foot movements of inversion and abduction

frequency Number of times per week that an athlete exercises

genitourinary Pertaining to the reproductive and urinary organs

genu recurvatus Hyperextension at the knee joint

genu valgum Knock knees

genu varum Bow legs

hemarthrosis Blood in a joint cavity

hematoma Blood tumor

hematuria Blood in the urine

hemoglobin Coloring substance of the red blood cells

hemoglobinuria Hemoglobin in the urine

hemophilia A hereditary blood disease in which coagulation is greatly prolonged

hemorrhage Discharge of blood

hemothorax Bloody fluid in the pleural cavity

hirsutism Excessive hair growth and/or hair in unusual places

homeostasis Maintenance of a steady state in the body's internal environment

hyperemia An unusual amount of blood in a body part

hyperextension Extreme stretching out of a body part

hyperflexibility Flexibility beyond a joint's normal range

hyperhidrosis Excessive sweating; excessive foot perspiration

hypermobility Mobility of a joint that is extreme

hypertension High blood pressure; abnormally high tension

hypertonic Having a higher osmotic pressure than a compared solution

hypertrophy Enlargement of a part caused by an increase in the size of its cells

hyperventilation Abnormally deep breathing that is prolonged, causing a depletion of carbon dioxide, a fall in blood pressure, and fainting

hypoallergenic Low allergy producing

hypoxia Lack of an adequate amount of oxygen

ICE-R *I*ce, *c*ompression, *e*levation, and *r*est

idiopathic Of unknown cause

injury An act that causes damage or hurt

innervation Nerve stimulation of a muscle

integument A covering or skin

intensity Increasing the work load

interosseous membrane Connective tissue membrane between bones

intervertebral Between two vertebrae

intramuscular bleeding Bleeding within a muscle

intraoral mouth guard A protective device that fits within the mouth and covers the teeth

intravenous Substances administered to a patient via a vein

inversion of the foot To turn the foot inward. Inner border of the foot lifts

ions Electrically charged atoms

ipsilateral Situated on the same side

ischemia Local anemia

isokinetic exercise Amount of resistance depends upon the extent of force applied by the athlete, and speed is constant

isokinetic muscle resistance Accommodating and variable resistance

isometric exercise Type of movement that contracts the muscle statically without changing its length

isometric muscle contraction Muscle contracts statically without a change in its length

isosceles triangle Triangle with two sides equal in length

isotonic exercise Form of exercise that shortens and lengthens the muscle through a complete range of motion

isotonic muscle contraction Muscle shortens and lengthens through a complete range of joint motion

joint Point where two bones join together

joint capsule Saclike structure that encloses the ends of bones in a diarthrodial joint

keloid An overgrowth of collagenous scar tissue at the site of a wound of the skin

keratolytic Pertaining to loosening the horny layer of skin

knock knee Bending inward of the lower joint

kyphosis Exaggeration of the normal thoracic spine

labile Unsteady; not fixed and easily changed

lateral Pertaining to point of reference away from the midline of the body

liability The legal responsibility to perform an act in a reasonable and prudent manner

lordosis Abnormal lumbar vertebral convexity

luxation Total dislocation

lysis Breakdown

macerated skin Skin softened by soaking

malaise Discomfort and uneasiness caused by an illness

margination Accumulation of leukocytes on blood vessel walls at the site of injury during early stages of inflammation

medial Pertaining to point of reference closest to the midline of the body

menarche Onset of menses

meninges Any one of the three membranes that enclose the brain and the spinal cord, comprising the dura mater, the pia mater, and the arachnoid

menorrhagia Abnormally heavy or long menstrual periods

metabolites Products left after metabolism has taken place

metatarsalgia Pain in the metatarsal

metatarsophalangeal joint Joint where the phalanges meet with the metatarsal bones

microtrauma Small musculoskeletal traumas that are accumulative

mononucleosis (infectious) A disease, usually of young adults, causing fever, sore throat, and lymph gland swelling

muscle Tissue that when stimulated contracts and produces motion

muscle contracture Abnormal shortening of muscle tissue in which there is a great deal of resistance to passive stretch

muscle cramps Clonic: involuntary muscle contraction with alternating relaxation; tonic: rigid muscle contraction with no relaxation

muscular endurance The ability to perform repetitive muscular contractions against some resistance

muscular strength The maximum force that can be applied by a muscle during a single maximal contraction

musculoskeletal Pertaining to muscles and the skeleton

myoglobin A respiratory pigment in muscle tissue that is an oxygen carrier

myositis Inflammation of muscle

myotatic reflex Stretch reflex

necrosis Death of tissue

negative resistance Slow eccentric muscle contraction against resistance with muscle lengthening

negligence The failure to use ordinary or reasonable care

nerve entrapment A nerve that is compressed between bone or soft tissue

neuritis Inflammation of a nerve

NOCSAE National Operating Committee on Standards for Athletic Equipment

noncontact sport Athletes are not involved in any physical contact

nystagmus A constant involuntary back and forth, up and down, or rotary movement of the eyeball

omission (legal) Person fails to perform a legal duty

open fracture Overlying skin has been lacerated by protruding bone fragments

orthosis Used in sports as an appliance or apparatus used to support, align, prevent, or correct deformities, or to improve function of a movable body part

osteoarthritis A chronic disease involving joints in which there is destruction of articular cartilage and bone overgrowth

osteoblasts Bone-forming cells

osteochondral Refers to relationship of bone and cartilage

osteochondritis Inflammation of bone and cartilage

osteochondritis dissecans Fragment of cartilage and underlying bone is detached from the articular surface

osteochondrosis A disease state of a bone and its articular cartilage

osteoclasts Cells that absorb and remove osseous tissue

osteoporosis Loss of the quantity of bone or atrophy of skeletal tissue

palpate To use the hands or fingers to examine

palpation Feeling an injury with the fingers

papule Pimple

paraplegia Paralysis of lower portion of the body and of both legs

paresthesia Abnormal sensation such as numbness, prickling, and tingling

pathology Study of the nature and cause of disease

pediatrician A specialist in the treatment of children's diseases

periosteum The fibrous covering of a bone

peristalis A progressive, wavelike movement that occurs in the alimentary canal

pes planus Flat feet

phagocytosis Process of ingesting microorganisms, other cells, or foreign particles, commonly by monocytes, or white blood cells

phalanges Bones of the fingers and toes

phalanx Any one of the bones of the fingers and toes

photophobia Unusual intolerance to light

plantarflexion The forepart of the foot is depressed relative to the ankle

plica A fold of tissue within the body

plyometric exercise An exercise that maximizes the stretch reflex

pneumothorax A collapse of a lung due to air in the pleural cavity

polymers Natural or synthetic substances formed by the combination of two or more molecules of the same substance

positive resistance Slow concentric muscle

contraction against resistance with muscle shortening

posterior Toward the rear or back

posterior cruciate ligament A ligament that stops internal rotation

post-traumatic amnesia A period of amnesia between a brain injury resulting in memory loss and the point at which memory functions are restored

power Ability to accelerate a load, depending on the level of strength and velocity of a muscle contraction

primary assessment Initial first aid evaluation

prophylactic Pertaining to prevention, preservation, or protection

prophylaxis Guarding against injury or disease

proprioceptive neuromuscular facilitation (PNF) Stretching techniques that involve alternating contractions and stretches

proprioceptors Organs within the body that provide the athlete with an awareness of where the body is in space (kinesthesis)

prostaglandin Acidic lipids widely distributed in the body; in musculoskeletal conditions it is concerned with vasodilation, histamine-like effect; it is inhibited by aspirin

prothrombin Interacts with calcium to produce thrombin

proximal Nearest to the point of reference

psychogenic Of psychic origin; that which originates in the mind

psychophysiological Involving the mind and the body

psychosomatic Showing effects of mind-body relationship; physical

disorder caused or influenced by the mind (i.e., by the emotions)

quadriplegia Paralysis affecting all four limbs

referred pain Pain that is felt at a point of the body other than at its actual origin

regeneration Repair, regrowth, or restoration of a part such as tissue

residual That which remains; often used to describe a permanent condition resulting from injury or disease (e.g., a limp or a paralysis)

resorption Act of removal by absorption

retrograde amnesia Memory loss for events occurring immediately before trauma

revascularize Restoration of blood circulation to an injured area

rhinitis Inflammation of the nasal mucus lining

rotation Turning around an axis in an angular motion

SAID principle *S*pecific *a*daptations to *i*mposed *d*emands

Scheuermann's disease (osteochondrosis) A degeneration of the vertebral epiphyseal endplates

sciatica Inflammatory condition of the sciatic nerve; commonly associated with peripheral nerve root compression

sclera White outer coating of the eye

scoliosis A lateral deviation curve of the spine

secondary assessment Follow up; a more detailed examination

seizure Sudden attack

sign Objective evidence of an abnormal situation within the body

sling psychrometer Instrument for establishing the wet-bulb, globe temperature index

spasm A sudden, involuntary muscle contraction

spica A figure-8, with one loop larger than the other

spondylolisthesis Forward slipping of a vertebral body, usually a lumbar vertebrae

spondylolysis A degeneration of the vertebrae and a defect in the pars intermedia of the articular processes of the vertebrae

staleness Deterioration in the usual standard of performance; chronic fatigue, apathy, loss of appetite, indigestion, weight loss, and inability to sleep or rest properly

staplylococcus A genus of micrococci, some of which are pathogenic, causing pus and tissue destruction

static stretching Passively stretching an antagonist muscle by placing it in a maximal stretch position and holding it in place

strength Ability of a muscular contraction to exert force to move an object (dynamic) or to perform work against a fixed object (static)

streptococcus Oval bacteria that appear in a chain

stress The positive and negative forces that can disrupt the body's equilibrium

stressor Anything that affects the body's physiological or psychological condition

stroke volume The heart's capacity to pump blood

subcutaneous Beneath the skin

subluxation Partial dislocation

subthreshold Below the point at which a physiological effect begins to be produced

symptom Subjective evidence of an abnormal situation within the body

syndrome Group of typical symptoms or conditions that characterize an injury, a deficiency, or a disease

synergy To work in cooperation with

synovia A transparent viscid lubricating fluid found in joints, bursae, and tendons

synovitis Inflammation of a synovial membrane

synthesis Buildup

systolic blood pressure The pressure caused by the heart's pumping

tendinitis Inflammation of the tendon

tendon Tough cord or band of white fibrous connective tissue that attaches muscle to bone

tenosynovitis Inflammation of the sheath covering a tendon

tetanus toxoid Tetanus toxin modified to produce active immunity against *Clostridium tetani*

thrombi Plural of thrombus

thromboplastin Substance within the body's tissues that accelerates blood clotting

thrombus Blood clots that blocks small blood vessels or a cavity of the heart

time-loss injuries Injuries that require the player to suspend activity within a day of an injury's onset

tinea Ringworm; skin fungus disease

tonic muscle cramp Continuous muscle contraction that is long in duration

tonic muscle spasm Rigid muscle contraction that lasts over a period of time

tonus (muscle) Residual state of muscle contraction

torque A twisting force produced by contraction of the medial femoral muscles that tends to rotate the thigh medially

torsional Rotating or twisting of a body part

tort Legal wrongs committed against the person or property of another

transitory paralysis Temporary inability to move

traumatic Pertaining to the course of an injury or wound

traumatic arthritis Arthritis stemming from repeated joint injury

traumatic asphyxia Result of a violent blow to, or compression of, the rib cage, causing cessation of breathing

trigger points Small

valgus Bent outward

variable resistance Resistance that fluctuates in intensity throughout the range of motion

varus Bent inward

vasoconstriction Decrease in the diameter of a blood vessel

vasodilation Increase in the diameter of a blood vessel

vasospasm Blood vessel spasm

venule Tiny vein fed by a capillary

verruca Virus causing a wart

viscera Internal organs

viscus (organs) Any internal organ enclosed within a cavity

volar Referring to the palm or the sole

water ad libitum Unlimited access to water

xerostomia Having a dry mouth

xiphoid process Smallest of three parts of the sternum

Photo Credits

Chapter 1

Fig 1-1 Anderson Hurt/Focus on Sports. **Fig 1-2** Courtesy Cramer Products, Gardner, KS. **Fig 1-5, Fig 1-6, and Fig 1-8** Adapted from American Academy of Pediatrics, Committee on Sports Medicine: Sports Medicine: health for young athletes, Nathan Smith (editor), 1983, Evanston, IL. **Fig 1-10** G. Robert Bishop. **Fig 1-11** L Childress. **Fig 1-12** top: Mike Powell/Allsport; middle: Allsport/Vandystadt; bottom left: Allsport; bottom right: Steve Powell/Allsport.

Chapter 2

Fig 2-2 Courtesy Al McDaniels from Mood, D., Musker F., Rink J.: Sports and recreational activities, ed 11, Mosby-Year Book, 1995. **Fig 2-3 and Fig 2-4** Courtesy Prentice W: Fitness for college and Life, ed 3, Mosby-Year Book, 1991. **Fig 2-5, Fig 2-7, Fig 2-8, and Fig 2-9** Courtesy of Robert Freligh, California State University, Long Beach. **Fig 2-12** Courtesy of Cybex, a division of Lumex, Inc. **Fig 2-16** Courtesy James Bryant from Coakley, J; Sport in society, ed 5, Mosby-Year Book, 1994.

Chapter 3

Fig 3-4 and Fig 3-5 Courtesy Cramer Products, Gardner, KS.

Chapter 4

Fig 4-4 Courtesy Cramer Products, Gardner, KS. **Fig 4-5** From Wardlaw, G and Insel, P.: Perspectives in nutrition, ed 2, Mosby-Year Book, 1990.

Chapter 5

Fig 5-1 and Fig 5-5 Courtesy Robert Freligh, California State University, Long Beach. **Fig 5-6** Robert Barclay/Renee Reavis Shingles, Central Michigan University. **Fig 5-8A** Courtesy Raili Mood from Mood, D., Musker F., and Rink J.: Sports and recreational activities, ed 10, Mosby-Year Book, 1991. **Fig 5-8B** Courtesy Raili Mood from Mood, D., Musker F., and Rink J.: Sports and recreational activities, ed 11, Mosby-Year Book, 1995. **Fig 5-10** Courtesy Donzis Protective Equipment, Houston, TX. **Fig 5-11 and Fig 5-12** From Nicholas J., and Hershman, E.: The upper extremity in sports medicine, Mosby-Year Book, 1990. **Fig 5-13** Courtesy G. Robert Bishop. **Fig 5-14 and Fig 5-15** Courtesy Denise Fandel, University of Nebraska at Omaha. **Fig 5-17, Fig 5-18, and Fig 5-19** from Nicholas, J., and Hershman, E.: The upper extremity in sports medicine, Mosby-Year Book, 1990. **Fig 5-20** Courtesy of Mueller Sports Medicine, Inc. **Fig 5-23, Fig 5-24, and Fig 5-25A** From Nicholas, J., and Hershman, E.: The upper extremity in sports medicine, Mosby-Year Book, 1990. **Fig 5-25 B** Courtesy of Cramer Products, Gardner, KS. **Fig 5-26, Fig 5-27, and Fig 5-28** From Nicholas, J., and Hershman, E.: The upper extremity in sports medicine, Mosby-Year Book, 1990. **Fig 5-29, Fig 5-30, and Fig 5-31,** (left and right) Courtesy Don Joy Orthopedic, Carlsbad, CA.

Chapter 6

Fig 6-1 bottom: Courtesy Cramer Products, Gardner, KS; top: Joe Patronite/Allsport. **Fig 6-2** From Booher, J., and Thibodeau, G.: Athletic injury assessment, Mosby-Year Book, 1989. **Fig 6-22** From Nicholas, J., and Hershman, E.: The upper extremity in sports medicine, Mosby-Year Book, 1990. **Fig 6-23** Courtesy Al McDaniels from Mood, D., Musker F., and Rink J.: Sports and recreational activities, ed 11, Mosby-Year Book, 1995.

Chapter 7

Fig 7-2, Fig 7-7, Fig 7-8, Fig 7-10, Fig 7-15A, Fig 7-18 B through G, Fig 7-20, Fig 7-21, and Fig 7-22: Robert Barclay and Renee Reavis Shingles, Central Michigan University.

Chapter 8

Fig 8-1 Courtesy Sherry Kimbro, University of Alabama. **Fig 8-3** Mark Dobson **Fig 8-4** A:© Nathan Billow; B: Focus on Sports; C: Allsport/Vandystadt; D and E: Tony Duffy/Allsport. **Fig 8-11** B From Prentice, W.: Therapeutic modalities in sports medicine, ed 2, Mosby-Year Book, 1990. **Fig 8-12** Courtesy Lossing Orthopaedic, Minneapolis, MN. **Fig 8-13** Courtesy Robert Freligh, California State University, Long Beach.

Chapter 9

Fig 9-1 From Booher, J., and Thibodeau, G.: Athletic injury assessment, Mosby-Year Book, 1989.

Chapter 11

Fig 11-11 From Nicholas, J., and Hershman, E.: The lower extremity and spine in sports medicine, vol 2, Mosby-Year Book, 1986.

Chapter 12

Fig 12-8 Cramer Products **Fig 12-10** (photo) From William, J.: Color atlas of injury in sport, ed 2, Mosby-Year Book, 1990. **Fig 12-17** Cramer Products. **Fig 12-18 and Fig 12-24** From Nicholas, J., and Hershman, E.: The lower extremity and spine in sports medicine, vol 2, Mosby-Year Book, 1986.

Chapter 13

Fig 13-1 Sherry Kimbro. **Fig 13-4** Courtesy McDavid Knee Guards, Clarendon Hills, IL. **Fig 13-7** From Nicholas, J., and Hershman, E.: The lower extremity and spine in sports medicine, vol 2, Mosby-Year Book, 1986. **Fig 13-10** G. Robert Bishop. **Fig 13-13** Robert Barclay and Renee Reavis Shingles, Central Michigan University. **Fig 13-14** From Booher, J., and Thibodeau, G.: Athletic injury asessment, Mosby-Year Book, 1985. **Fig 13-23** From Prentice, W.: Rehabilitation techniques in sports medicine, Mosby-Year Book, 1990. **Fig 13-24** (left) Courtesy BREG, Vista, CA. **Fig 13-25** Courtesy Don Joy Orthopedic, Carlsbad, CA.

Chapter 14

Fig 14-10 From Williams, J.: Color atlas of injury in sport, ed 2, Mosby-Year Book, 1990. **Fig 14-11** Courtesy Mueller Sports Medicine, Inc. **Fig 14-12** Courtesy Al McDaniels from Mood, D., Musker F., and Rink J.: Sports and recreational activities, ed 11, Mosby-Year Book, 1995. **Fig 14-15 and Fig 14-16** (photo) Robert Barclay and Renee Reavis Shingles, Central Michigan University. **Fig 14-17** Courtesy BRACE International, Phoenix, AZ. **Fig 14-20** Robert Barclay and Renee Reavis Shingles, Central Michigan University.

Chapter 15

Fig 15-1 G. Robert Bishop. **Fig 15-6** Michael Ponzini/Focus on Sports. **Fig 15-10** Robert Barclay and Renee Reavis Shingles, Central Michigan University.

Chapter 16

Fig 16-2 Donald O'Connor. **Fig 16-10** (bottom right) From Nicholas, J., and Hershman, E.: The lower extremity and spine in sports medicine, vol 2, Mosby-Year Book, 1986. **Fig 16-13** Courtesy Mueller Sports Medicine Inc. **Fig 16-19** C.H. Petit/Vandystadt/Allsport. **Fig 16-23** From Williams, J.: Color atlas of injury in sport, ed 2, Mosby-Year Book, 1990.

Chapter 17

Fig 17-2 Vandystadt/Allsport. Many head injuries incurred in sports have serious consequences. **Fig 17-13 and Fig 17-14** From Williams, J.: Color atlas of injury in sport, ed 2, Mosby-Year Book, 1990. **Fig 17-16** Focus on Sports. **Fig 17-21** Richard Mackson/Allsport.

Chapter 18

Fig 18-1 Diane Johnson/Allsport. **Fig 18-11** Cramer Products, Gardner, KS. **Fig 18-15** Courtesy BRACE International, Phoenix, AZ. **Fig 18-28** From Prentice, W: Rehabilitation techniques in sports medicine, ed 2, Mosby-Year Book, 1990. **Fig 18-30** Courtesy Healthsouth Rehabilitation Program, Birmingham, AL.

Chapter 19

Fig 19-8 From Nicholas, J., and Hershman, E.: The upper extremity in sports medicine, Mosby-Year Book, 1990. **Fig 19-19** From Booher, J. and Thibodeau, G.: Athletic injury assessment, Mosby-Year Book, 1989. **Fig 19-27 through 19-31** From Nicholas, J. and Hershman, E.: The upper extremity in sports medicine, Mosby-Year Book, 1990. **Fig 19-32** Robert Barclay/Renee Reavis Shingles. **Fig 19-37** From Nicholas, J. and Hershman, E.: The upper extremity in sports medicine, Mosby-Year Book, 1990.

Chapter 20

Fig 20-4 From Stewart, W., Danto, J., Madden, S.: Dermatology diagnosis and treatment of cutaneous disorders, ed 4, Mosby-Year Book, 1978. **Fig 20-6** Allsport.

Index

A

Abdomen, 390-398
  anatomy of, 390, *391-392*
  injuries to, 390, 392-398
  wall of, injuries to, 392-394
Abdominal curl, 53
Abrasion(s), 139, *140*, 245
  care of, 247*t*
  corneal, 460
Acceptance in response to loss, 81
Accident, 26
Accident insurance, 15
Accident-proneness, 77-78
Accommodating resistance, 55-56
Accommodating resistance machines, 61-62
Achilles tendon
  rupture of, 330-331
  strains of, 329-330
  taping of, 275-276
  tendinitis of, 330
Achilles tendon stretch, 44
Acquired immune deficiency syndrome (AIDS), 539-540
Acromioclavicular joint, *465*
  sprain of, 473-474
Acromioclavicular support, taping for, 285-286
Activity limitation for low back pain, 434
Acupressure, 233
Acupuncture, 233
Acute-onset muscle soreness, 143
Adhesive felt as pad material, 132
Adhesive tape; *see* Tape; Taping
Adolescent heel pain, 311-312
Agility in exercise reconditioning, 237
Air splints, 193
Airway
  in CPR, 177-178
  obstructed, management of, 180-182
Alarm stage in response to stress, 78
Alcohol use, 551
Allergic rhinitis, 525
Ambulatory aid for transporting injured athlete, *198*, 199
Ameboid action in acute inflammation, 215
Amenorrhea, 541
  bone density and, 542
Amnesia, 441
Amphetamines, 544-545
Anabolic steroids, 546-548
Analgesic drugs, narcotic, 546
Anaphylactic shock, *186*
Anemia, 535-536

Anger in response to loss, 81
Ankle, 316-332
  anatomy of, 316, *317-319*
  cloth wrap for, 249-250
  and foot, spica bandage for, 250-251
  fractures of, 328, *329*
  injured/painful, evaluation of, 322-325
  injuries to, 322-332
    acute, 322-331
    chronic, 331-332
    prevention of, 316-317, 320-322
      exercises in, 337-339
      wrapping, taping, and bracing in, 320-322
    reconditioning exercise for, 337-339
    sprains of, 322, *323, 324*
      eversion, 328
      inversion, grading of, 326-328
      management of, 325-326
    strains about, 329-331
    strength training for, 317, *320*
    supports for, commercial, 126-127
    taping of, 271-275
Annulus fibrosus, 407
Anorexia nervosa, 97
Anoxia from blow to solar plexus, 395
Anterior cruciate ligament, 342-343, *344*
Anxiety, staleness and, 76
Apophysis, 152
Apophysitis, 151
  calcaneal, 311
Appendicitis, 394-395
Arch of foot
  fallen, 305-306
  high, 306-307
  strain of, 303-304
  taping for, 267-270
Arm
  lower, 501-504; *see also* Forearm
  upper, injuries to, 479-481
Arterial pulses in shoulder complex evaluation, 467
Arteries of elbow joint, *492*
Arthritis, traumatic, 152
Articular cartilage, 147
Articular disks, 147
Articulation, 147
Articulations; *see also* Joint(s)
  of shoulder complex, *465*
Asphyxia, traumatic, 403
Assumption of risk, 11
Asthma, 526
  exercise-induced, 526-528

Electrical muscle stimulation, 231
Electrolytes in training diet, 90
Electrotherapy, 231-233
Elevation
    for external bleeding, 183
    in musculoskeletal injury, 191
Embolus in sickle cell anemia, 536
Emergency
    assessment principles in, 173-176
    environmental stress and, 200-210
    plan for, 172-173
    primary survey in, 176-186
    procedures for, 172-241
    secondary survey in, 186-196
Emotional reaction to injury, emergency care for, 80*t*
Endomorph, 95
Endosteum, 154
Endurance
    cardiorespiratory, 64-65
    in conditioning, 38
    muscle, 64
    stamina and, 63-65
Energy, units for measurement of, A0
Environmental stress, 200-210
    cold-related, 206, 208-210
    heat-related, 201-206, 207-208*t*
Epicondylitis, 497-498
Epidemic parotiditis, 533*t*
Epidemiological approach to sports injury data, 28-29
Epidural hemorrhage, 442
Epilepsy, 534-535
Epiphyseal fracture, 481
Epiphyseal growth plate in long bone, 154, *155*
Epiphyseal injuries in young athlete, 69-70
Epiphysis, 154
    capital femoral, slipped, 383
Equipment
    athletic training, 24
    protective, 104-134; *see also* Protective sports devices
Equipment personnel, 10
Examination, preparticipation, 16-21
Exercise(s)
    boot, 54
    free, 57
    for hip rehabilitation, *386-387, 388*
    isokinetic, 55-56
    isometric, definition of, 48
    isotonic, 49-54
    for low back pain, 434-435
    muscle contraction and, 48-57
    partner resistance, 57-58
    plyometric, 56-57
    progressive resistance, 55
    reciprocal resistance, 57-58
    reconditioning
        for foot, 312-314

Exercise—cont'd
    reconditioning—cont'd
        for knee, 361-364
    static, for flexibility, 43-46
Exercise physiologists, 10
Exercise reconditioning, 233-240
    advanced exercise phase in, 239
    agility in, 237
    coordination in, 237
    early exercise phase in, 238-239
    exercise overdosage in, 238
    flexibility in, 237
    initial sports reentry phase in, 239
    intermediate exercise phase in, 239
    muscle endurance in, 237
    muscular strength in, 235-237
    plan for, 239-240
    postsurgical/acute injury exercise phase in, 238
    presurgical exercise phase in, 238
    proprioception in, 237
    psychological aspects of, 237-238
    rehabilitative phases in, 238-239
    speed of movement in, 237
Exercise rehabilitation, 234
Exercise-induced bronchial obstruction, 526-528
Exercise-induced compartment syndrome, 336-337
Exhaustion stage in response to stress, 79
Exostoses of foot, 310, *311*
Extremity; *see* Arm; Leg; Limb(s)
Eye
    anatomy of, 456
    bandage for, 254-255
    black, 457-458
    foreign body in, 459-460
    injuries to, 456-460
    protection of, 457
        devices for, 112-114
Eye signs in cerebral trauma assessment, 444

F

Face, 447-460
    anatomy of, 447, *448*
    injuries to, 449-450
    protective sports devices for, 108-114
Face guards, 109-110
Fasciitis, 144
Fat(s)
    joint, 147
    lean body and, 38
    in training diet, 87
Fat pads, knee, 356
Felt as pad material, 132
Female reproductive system, 540-544
Femoral groove, kneecap and, pain related to, 358
Femoral hernias, 393